CW01597625

Australian Nurses' Dictionary
3rd edition

Medical knowledge is constantly changing. As new information and technologies become available, changes in management, procedures, equipment, and the use of drugs become necessary. The editors, contributors, and publishers have taken care to ensure information given in this text is accurate and that the information is current. However, readers are strongly advised to confirm that information, especially with regard to drug usage, complies with the latest legislation and standards of practice.

Australian Nurses' Dictionary
3rd edition

Rhonda Hawley
PhD (Syd.), RN, RMN, Cardio-Thoracic Cert., Dip Nurs Ed.
(Arm. CAE), BA (UNE), MEd (Syd.)
Senior Lecturer, Department of Clinical Nursing,
University of Sydney

Jennie King
RN, BA (Hons)
Research Fellow, Department of Clinical Nursing,
University of Sydney

Barbara F Weller
MSC, RGN, RSCN, RNT
Independent Nurse Consultant,
Honorary Consultant Lecturer,
Thames Valley University, London

Baillière
Tindall

Sydney Edinburgh London New York
Philadelphia St Louis Toronto

ELSEVIER

BAILLIÈRE TINDALL
is an imprint of Elsevier

Elsevier Australia
30–52 Smidmore Street, Marrickville, NSW 2204

This edition © 2004, reprinted 2004
by Elsevier Australia
A division of Reed International Books Australia Pty Ltd ABN 70 001 002 357
1st UK edition 1912; 23rd UK edition 2000
1st Australian edition 1991; 2nd Australian edition 1998

This publication is copyright. Except as expressly provided in the Copyright Act 1968 and the Copyright Amendment (Digital Agenda) Act 2000, no part of this publication may be reproduced, stored in any retrieval system or transmitted by any means (including electronic, mechanical, microcopying, photocopying, recording or otherwise) without prior written permission from the publisher.

National Library of Australia Cataloguing-in-Publication Data

---

Australian nurses' dictionary.
3rd ed.
ISBN 0 7295 3721 8.

1. Nursing–Australia–Dictionaries. 2. Nursing–Dictionaries. 3. Medicine–Australia–Dictionaries. 4. Medicine – Dictionaries. I. King, Jennifer. II. Title: Australian nurses' and allied health dictionary. 2nd ed. 1998.

610.7303

Publisher: Vaughn Curtis
Publishing Editor: Meg O'Hanlon
Developmental Editor: Rhiain Hull
Publishing Services Manager: Helena Klijn
Edited by Ross Gilham
Cover design by Avril Makula
Text design and typesetting by Egan-Reid Limited
Revised artwork by Joe Lucia
Printed in Hong Kong by China Translation & Printing Services Ltd

Contents

Preface

The revision of *Baillière's Nurses' Dictionary* for Australian nurses has been a challenging exercise. Editions of the dictionary have been an integral part of the repertoire of Australian nurses for more than fifty years, and this revision reflects the changes that have been occurring in Australian nursing over the past decade.

The guiding principles in the revision have been to establish direct relevance to Australian conditions, and to provide a quick reference source for students and nurses in the clinical setting. For more extensive background to specific entries, the reader is referred to encyclopaedic nursing dictionaries.

One aspect of Australian nursing has been the incorporation of certain terminology and spelling from our American colleagues, and the revision has attempted to include this in a balanced way.

This edition has relied upon the support of nurses and allied health personnel in many areas. In particular the following have acted as consultants in the revisions of the entries and appendices: Rosemary Brooker, Wendy Grey, Andrea Marshall, Terry Maunsell, and Tracey Thornley.

Rhonda Hawley, Jennie King, Barbara F Weller.

Publisher's Acknowledgments

The publisher would like to thank the following for their kind permission to reproduce material in this dictionary: Saunders Company for figures in airway, cell, fluid, leukocytes, and Trousseau's sign; American College of Surgeons, figure in Lund and Browder chart; McGraw-Hill, figure in injection.

We are grateful to the following Baillière Tindall authors for their kind permission to use material from their texts: Ann Faulkner, for Maslow's hierarchy of needs (from Faulkner, A., *Nursing: A Creative Approach*, 1985); Sheila Jackson and Penelope Bennett, for figures in ear, endometrium, hair, and heart (from Jackson, S. and Bennett, P., *Physiology with Anatomy for Nurses*, 1988).

References

Dorland's Illustrated Medical Dictionary, 30th edn, 2003, Philadelphia, Saunders.

Forrester, K. & Griffiths, D. (2001), *Essentials of Law for Health Professionals*, Sydney, Mosby.

Gatford, J. D. & Phillips, N. (2002) *Nursing Calculations,* 6th edn, Edinburgh, Churchill Livingstone.

Mosby's Medical, Nursing and Allied Health Dictionary, 6th edn, St Louis, Mosby.

Schneider, Z., Elliott, D., LoBiondo-Wood, G. & Haber, J. (2003), *Nursing Research Methods, critical appraisal and utilization*, 2nd edn, Sydney, Mosby.

Publisher's Acknowledgements

References

Pronunciation Guide

Introduction

The pronunciations are transcribed using ordinary English-spelling letters. So that the guide is consistent and unambiguous, these characters have been combined together in precise ways (see below). The avoidance of the use of phonetic symbols (with the exeption of the upside-down 'e' or 'schwa' (ə)) ensures that the guide is more-or-less immediately, and to some extent intuitively, understandable.

Style of transcription

All pronunciations are found in parentheses immediately following the bold main entry word (or variant, if one exists). The pronunciations reflect general Australian English. Furthermore, transcriptions given reflect *current, spoken usage* of the terms rather than how the term 'should' be pronounced, i.e. the guide does not attempt to be didactic or prescriptive.

Variant pronunciations and spellings. Where alternative pronunciations for a word are given, or where alternative spellings or synonyms are given, these are separated by commas. For example:

> **medicine** (ˈmedəsən, ˌmedsən)
> **neurone (neuron)** (ˌnyoo·rohn, ˌnyoo·ron)

Alternative pronunciations are often given in a truncated form with the use of hyphens: For example:

> **encephalic** (ˈenkəˌfalik, -ˌensə-)

Entries with repeated words. Note that once a transcription for a particular word has been given, subsequent entries that use the same word do not have a repeated transcription of that word.

Characters and combinations used to represent sound. In the pronunciation guide, single letters represent single sounds and where two or more characters are combined, as in the accompanying tables, these also represent precise sounds.

Pronunciation style guide

	Vowel sounds	*Nearest International Phonetic Alphabet Character*
a	as in **bad** (bad)	æ
ah	as in **father** ('fahthə)	a:
air	as in **hair** (hair)	ɛa or eə
aw	as in **water** ('wawtə)	ɔ:
ay	as in **fatal** ('fayt'l)	eɪ
e	as in **bed** (bed)	ɛ or e
ee	as in **fetus** ('feetəs)	i:
i	as in **film** (film)	ɪ
ie	as in **bite** (biet)	aɪ
i·ə	as in **chloropsia** (klaw'ropsi·ə)	i:ə (unstressed)
iə	as in **fear** (fiə)	ɪə
ieə	as in **diet** ('dieət)	aɪə
o	as in **body** (ˌbodee)	ɒ
oh	as in **choke** (chohk)	əʊ
oo	as in **boot** (boot)	u:
ooə	as in **cure** (kyooə)	u:ə
ow	as in **now** (now)	aʊ
owə	as in **hour** (owə)	aʊə
oy	as in **goitre** ('goytə)	ɔɪ
oyə	as in **soya** ('soyə)	ɔɪə
u	as in **tongue** (tung)	ʌ
uh	as in **foot** (fuht)	ʊ
ə	as in **mother** ('muthə)	ə
ər	as in **bird** (bərd)	ɜ:
y	as in **yet** (yet)	j (semi-vowel)

	Consonant sounds	
b	as in **baby** ('baybee)	b
ch	as in **chat** (chaht)	tʃ

	Vowel sounds	*Nearest International Phonetic Alphabet Character*
d	as in **digit** ('dijət)	d
f	as in **fever** ('feevə)	f
g	as in **gag** (gag)	g
h	as in **heal** (heel)	h
j	as in **jump** (jump)	dʒ
k	as in **king** (king)	k
l	as in **light** (liet)	l
m	as in **man** (man)	m
n	as in **need** (need)	n
ng	as in **sung** (sung)	ŋ
nh	as in **en passant** (onh 'pasonh)	õ (from French)
ny	as in **nutrition** (nyoo'trishən)	nj
p	as in **pelvis** ('pelvəs)	p
r	as in **rod** (rod)	r
s	as in **sac** (sak)	s
sh	as in **fish** (fish)	ʃ
t	as in **test** (test)	t
th	as in **thirst** (thərst)	θ
v	as in **vein** (vayn)	v
w	as in **weight** (wayt)	w
z	as in **zero** ('ziə·roh)	z
zh	as in **pleasure** ('plezhə)	ʒ

Stress marks. These are used where the word or term has more than one syllable, with the stress mark placed *before* the syllable to be stressed. The primary stressed syllable is indicated by a superior stress mark (') and secondary stress by a subscript stress mark (ˌ). For example:

respiration (ˌrespə'rayshan)
respirator ('respəˌraytə)
respiratory (rəs'pirətree)

Syllabic apostrophe. Where a consonant is preceded by an apostrophe, this indicates that the consonant should be pronounced as a separate syllable. For example:

hospital ('hospət'l)

The use of the centred dot. Where two letters occur together that may be mistaken for a different sound from that intended, a centred full point is added to separate the characters. For example:

myopia (miə'ohpi·ə)

Sub-entries

The term being sought may be a main entry or a sub-entry under the main entry. Sub-entries are listed alphabetically under the main entry, with the initial letter(s) of the main entry repeated. For example:

abdomen . . .

Acute a. . . .

Pendulous a. . . .

Scaphoid (navicular) a. . . .

Aa

A abbreviation for accommodation; adenine; anode (anodal); anterior; axial; symbol for ampere and mass number.

abacterial (ˌaybak'tiə·ri·əl) indicating a condition not caused by bacteria.

abarticulation (ˌabahˌtikyə'layshən) dislocation of a joint.

abasia (ə'bayzi·ə) the inability to walk.

abatement (ə'baytmənt) a decrease in the severity of a pain or a symptom.

abdomen ('abdəmən, 'ab'doh-) the belly. The cavity between the diaphragm and the pelvis, lined by a serous membrane, the peritoneum, and containing the stomach, intestines, liver, gallbladder, spleen, pancreas, kidneys, suprarenal glands, ureters, and bladder. For descriptive purposes, its area can be divided into nine regions (*see* figure). *Acute a.* any abdominal condition urgently requiring treatment, usually surgical. *Pendulous a.* a condition in which the anterior part of the abdominal wall hangs down over the PUBIS. *Scaphoid* (navicular) *a.* a hollowing of the anterior wall commonly seen in grossly emaciated people.

abdominal (ab'domin'l) pertaining to the abdomen. *A. aneurysm* a dilation of the abdominal aorta. *A. aorta* that part of the aorta below the diaphragm. *A. breathing* deep breathing; HYPERPNOEA. *A. reflex* reflex contraction of abdominal wall muscles observed when skin is lightly stroked. *A. section* incision through the abdominal wall. *A. thrust, see* HEIMLICH MANOEUVRE.

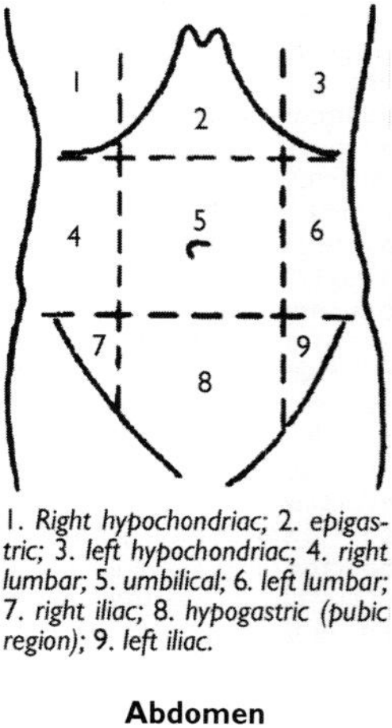

1. Right hypochondriac; 2. epigastric; 3. left hypochondriac; 4. right lumbar; 5. umbilical; 6. left lumbar; 7. right iliac; 8. hypogastric (pubic region); 9. left iliac.

Abdomen

abdominocyesis (abˌdominoh-ˈsieˈeesəs) an abdominal pregnancy.

abdominopelvic (abˌdomənoh-ˈpelvik) concerning the abdomen and the pelvic cavity.

abdominoperineal (abˌdomənoh-ˌperiˈneeəl) pertaining to the abdomen and the perineum. *A. excision* an operation performed through the abdomen and the perineum for the excision of the rectum or bladder; often done as a synchronised operation by two surgeons, one working at each approach.

abdominoposterior (abˌdomənoh-poˈstiə·ri·ə) indicating a position of the fetus with its abdomen turned towards the maternal back.

abduce (abˈdyoos) to abduct (or draw away).

abducent (abˈdyoosənt) leading away from the midline. *A. muscle* the external rectus muscle of the eye, which rotates it outwards. *A. nerve* the cranial nerve that supplies this muscle.

abduction (abˈdukshən, əb-) movement of a limb away from the body.

abductor (abˈduktə) a muscle that draws a limb away from the midline of the body. The opposite of ADDUCTOR.

aberrant (aˈberənt) taking an unusual course. Used of blood vessels and nerves.

aberration (ˌabəˈrayshən) deviation from the normal. In optics, failure to focus rays of light. *Mental a.* mental disorder of an unspecified kind.

ability (əˈbilətee) the power to perform an act, either mental or physical, with or without training. *Innate a.* the ability with which a person is born.

ablation (abˈlayshən) removal or destruction, by surgical or radiological means, of neoplasms or other body tissue. *Catheter a.* a technique to interrupt conduction through accessory atrioventricular pathways and ablate arrythmogenic foci responsible for TACHYCARDIA.

abnormal (ˌabˈnawmˈl) varying from what is regular or usual.

abort (əˈbawt) 1. to terminate a process or disease before it has run its normal course. 2. to give birth to a fetus earlier than the 20th week of pregnancy. Other criteria can include no breathing or heartbeat, and a fetal weight of less than 400 g.

abortifacient (əˌbawtiˈfayshənt) an agent or drug that can induce abortion.

abortion (əˈbawshən) 1. premature cessation of a normal process. 2. emptying of the pregnant uterus before the end of the 20th week. 3. the product of such an abortion. *Complete a.* one in which the contents of the uterus are expelled intact. *Criminal a.* the termination of a pregnancy for reasons other than those permitted by law (i.e. danger to mental or physical health of mother or child or family) and without medical approval. *Incomplete a.* that in which some part of the fetus or placenta is retained in the uterus. *Induced a.* the intentional emptying of the uterus. *Inevitable a.* condition in which profuse bleeding is accompanied by pains, dilated cervix, and the contents of the uterus able to be felt. *Missed a.* condition in which all signs of pregnancy disappear and the uterus later discharges a blood clot surrounding a shrivelled fetus, i.e. a CARNEOUS MOLE. *Septic a.* abortion associated with infection. *Therapeutic* (legal) *a.* abortion induced on medical advice because continuation of the pregnancy would involve risk to the life of the pregnant woman, or of injury to the physical or mental health of the pregnant woman or any existing children of her family, greater than if the pregnancy were terminated; or because there is a substantial risk that if the child were born it would suffer from such physical or mental abnormalities as to be seriously handicapped. *Threatened a.* the appearance of signs of premature expulsion of the fetus; bleeding is slight, the cervix is closed. *Tubal a.* the termination of a tubal pregnancy caused by rupture of the uterine tube.

abrasion (ə'brayzhən) a superficial injury in which the skin or mucous membrane is rubbed or torn. *Corneal a.* condition in which the surface of the cornea has been removed, e.g. by a scratch or other injury.

abreaction (ˌabri'akshən) the reliving of a past painful experience, with the release of repressed emotion.

abruptio placentae (əˌbrupshioh plə'sentee, -tioh) premature detachment of the placenta, causing maternal shock.

abscess ('absəs) a collection of pus in a cavity. Caused by the disintegration and replacement of tissue damaged by mechanical, chemical, or bacterial injury. *Alveolar a.* an abscess in a tooth socket. *Brodie's a.* a bone abscess, usually in the head of the tibia. *Cold a.* the result of chronic tubercular infection; so called because there are few, if any, signs of inflammation. *Psoas a.* a cold abscess that has tracked down the psoas muscle from caries of the lumbar vertebrae. *Subphrenic a.* an abscess situated under the diaphragm.

absolute zero (ab'səˌlut 'zi ə·roh) the temperature at which all molecular activity ceases: –273°C (–460°F).

absorbent (əb'sawbənt, -'zaw-) 1. able to take in, or suck up and incorporate. 2. a tissue structure involved in absorption. 3. a substance that absorbs or promotes absorption.

absorption (əb'sawpshən,-'zaw-) 1. in physiology, the taking up by suction of fluids or other substances by the tissues of the body. 2. in psychology, great mental concentration on a single object or activity. 3. in radiology, uptake of radiation by body tissues.

abstinence ('abstənəns) a refraining from the use of (or indulgence in) food, stimulants, or coitus. *A. syndrome* withdrawal symptoms.

abstract ('abstrakt) a brief, comprehensive summary of a research study or other academic report.

abuse (ə'byoos) misuse, maltreatment, or excessive use. *Child a.* the non-accidental use of physical force or the non-accidental act of omission by a parent or other custodian responsible for the care of a child. *Drug a.* use of illegal drugs or misuse of prescribed drugs. *Solvent a.* the deliberate inhalation of volatile chemicals with the aim of inducing intoxication.

acanthoma (ˌakən'thohma) a tumour originating in the prickle cell layer of the epidermis, usually benign epithelial tumours.

acanthosis (ˌakən'thohsis) hyperplasia of the prickle cell layer of the epidermis, as seen in PSORIASIS.

acaricide (a'karisied) an agent that destroys mites.

Acarus ('akə·rəs) a genus of small mites. *A. scabiei* (Sarcoptes scabiei) the cause of scabies.

acatalepsy (ˌay'katəˌlepsee) lack of understanding.

acataphasia (ˌaykatə'fayzi·ə) loss of the ability to express connected thought, resulting from a cerebral lesion.

accessory (ak'sesə·ri, 'ək-) supplementary. *A. nerve* the 11th cranial nerve; it is made up of two portions: the cranial and the spinal.

accommodation (əˌkomə'dayshən) adjustment. In ophthalmology, the term refers specifically to adjustment of the ciliary muscle, which controls the shape of the lens. In *negative a.* the ciliary muscle relaxes and the lens becomes less convex, providing long-distance vision; in *positive a.* the ciliary muscle contracts and the lens becomes more convex, providing near vision.

accouchement (ə'kooshmonh) childbirth.

accountable (ə'kowntəb'l) liable to be held responsible for a course of action. A qualified nurse has a duty of care according to law; in nursing, being *accountable* refers to the responsibility taken by a qualified nurse for prescribing and initiating nursing care. Nurses are *accountable* to their patients, their peers, and their employing authority, according to professional codes of conduct.

accreditation ('əkredəˌtayshən) a process of evaluation whereby an institution or an individual undergoes regular appraisal against agreed criteria, which, if met, result in the individual or institution being given official recognition by the accrediting organisation.

accretion (ə'kreeshən) growth. The accumulation of deposits (e.g. of salts) to form a calculus in the bladder. In dentistry, the growth of tartar on the teeth.

ACE inhibitors (ays in'hibətəz) a group of drugs used in the treatment of hypertension. The name angiotensin converting enzyme (ACE) inhibitors, explains part of their mode of action, although it is thought that some of their other actions might also be important in reducing blood pressure.

acephalic (ˌaykə'falik, -sə-) without a head.

acetabuloplasty (ˌasə'tabyəloh-ˌplastee) an operation performed to improve the depth and shape of the hip socket in correcting congenital dislocation of the hip or in treating osteoarthritis of the hip.

acetabulum (ˌasə'tabyələm) the cup-like socket in the innominate bone, in which the head of the femur moves.

acetate ('asəˌtayt) a salt of ACETIC ACID.

acetazolamide (əˌsetə'zoləmied) a sulphonamide compound which is an oral diuretic and is used in the treatment of congestive heart failure and GLAUCOMA.

acetic acid (ə'seetik) the acid of vinegar. It can be used as an antidote to alkaline poisons.

acetoacetic acid (ˌasətoh·ə'seetik, əˌsee-) diacetic acid. A product of fat metabolism. It occurs in excessive amounts in diabetes and starvation, giving rise to acetone bodies in the urine.

acetonaemia (ˌasətə'neemi·ə, əˌsee-) the presence of acetone bodies in the blood.

acetone ('asəˌtohn) a colourless inflammable liquid with a characteristic odour. Traces are found in the blood and in normal urine. *A. bodies* are ketones found in the blood and urine of patients with uncontrolled diabetes and also in those with acute starvation as a result of the incomplete breakdown of fatty and amino acids.

acetonuria (ˌasətə'nyoo·ri·ə, əˌsee-) the presence of an excess quantity of acetone bodies in the urine.

acetylcholine (ˌasətiel'kohleen, ˌasitil-) a chemical transmitter that is released by some nerve endings at the synapse between one neurone and the next or between a nerve ending and the effector organ it supplies. These nerves are said to be cholinergic, e.g. the parasympathetic nerves and the lower motor neurones to skeletal muscles. It is rapidly destroyed in the body by cholinesterase (an enzyme).

acetylcholinesterase (ˌasətielˌ-kohlən'estə·rayz) an enzyme that reduces or prevents excessive firing of neurons at neuromuscular junctions (also known as cholinesterase).

acetylcoenzyme A (ˌasətiel-koh'enziem, ˌasətəl-) active form of acetic acid, to which carbohydrates, fats, and amino acids that are not needed for protein synthesis are converted.

acetylsalicylic acid ('asətielˌsaləsilik, 'asətəl-) aspirin. An analgesic, antipyretic, and antirheumatic drug. It is available in its pure form or in combination with other drugs.

achalasia (akə'layzi·ə) failure of relaxation of a muscle sphincter causing dilatation of the part above, e.g. of the oesophagus above the cardiac sphincter.

ache (ayk) a dull continuous pain.

Achilles (ə'kileez) Greek mythological hero who could be wounded only in the heel. *A. tendon* tendocalcaneus, connecting the soleus and gastrocnemius muscles of the calf to the heel bone (os calcis). Tapping the *A. tendon* normally produces the *A. reflex* (or ankle jerk).

achlorhydria (ˌayklor'hiedri·ə) the absence of free hydrochloric acid in the stomach. Can be found in pernicious anaemia, pellagra, and gastric cancer.

acholia (ay·kohli·ə) a lack of secretion of bile.

acholuria (ˌaykə'lyoo·ri·ə) absence of bile in the urine.

acholuric (ˌaykə'lyoo·rik) pertaining to ACHOLURIA. *A. jaundice* jaundice without bile in the urine.

achondroplasia (ayˌkondroh-'playzi·ə) an inherited condition in which there is early union of the epiphysis and diaphysis of long bones. Growth is arrested, resulting in short stature.

achromasia (ˌaykroh'mayzi·ə) 1. lack of colour in the skin. 2. absence of normal reaction to staining in a tissue or cell.

achromatopsia (ˌaykrohmə'topsi·ə) complete colour blindness caused by disease or trauma. It can be congenital.

achylia (ay'kieli·ə) absence of hydrochloric acid and enzymes in the gastric secretions. *A. gastrica* a condition in which gastric secretion is reduced or absent.

acid ('asəd) 1. sour or sharp in

taste. 2. a substance which, when combined with an alkali, will form a salt. Any acid substance will turn blue litmus red. Individual acids are given under their specific names. *A.-alcohol-fast* descriptive of stained bacteria that are resistant to decolourisation by both acid and alcohol. *A.-base balance* the normal ratio between the acid ions and the basic (or alkaline) ions required to maintain the pH of the blood and body fluids.

acidaemia (ˌasə'deemi·ə) abnormal acidity of the blood, which contains an excess of hydrogen ions.

acidity (ə'sidətee) 1. sourness or sharpness of taste. 2. the state of being acid.

acidosis (ˌasə'dohsəs) a condition in which the relation of alkalinity to acidity of the blood is disturbed, with an increase in the hydrogen ion concentration. It is characterised by vomiting, drowsiness, hyperpnoea, acetone odour (of new-mown hay) of breath, and acetone bodies in the urine. It is indicated by a blood pH below the lower limit of the normal range. It can occur in DIACETES mellitus owing to incomplete metabolism of fat. *See also* KETOSIS.

acidotic (ˌasə'dotik) 1. pertaining to acidosis. 2. one suffering from acidosis.

aciduria (ˌasə'dyoo·ri·ə) a condition in which acid urine is excreted.

acinus ('asənəs) a minute saccule or alveolus of a compound gland, lined by secreting cells. The secreting portion of the mammary gland consists of acini.

acme ('akmee) 1. the highest point. 2. the crisis of a fever when the symptoms are fully developed.

acne ('aknee) an inflammatory condition of the sebaceous glands in which blackheads (comedones) are usually present together with papules and pustules. *A. keratitis* inflammation of the cornea associated with acne rosacea. *A. rosacea* a redness of the forehead, nose, and cheeks due to chronic dilatation of the subcutaneous capillaries, which becomes permanent with the formation of pustules in the affected areas. *A. vulgaris* a form of acne that occurs commonly in adolescents and young adults, affecting the face, chest, and back.

acneiform (ak'nee·əˌfawm) resembling acne.

acousma (ə'koosmə) the hearing of illusory sounds.

acoustic (ə'koostik) relating to sound or the sense of hearing.

acquired (ə'kwieəd) pertaining to disease, habits, or immunity developed after birth; not inherited.

acquired immune deficiency syndrome (abbreviated AIDS). *See* AIDS.

acrid ('akrəd) bitter; pungent; irritating.

acrocephalia (ˌakrohke'fayli·ə, -se-) malformation of the head, in which the top is pointed. Oxycephaly.

acrocyanosis (ˌakrohˌsieə'nohsəs) persistent cyanosis, coldness of the hands and feet, and profuse sweating of the digits; often associated with a vasomotor defect.

acrodynia (ˌakroh'dini·ə) an allergic reaction to mercury in children, causing pain and erythema in the fingers and toes. Pink disease.

acromegaly (ˌakrho'megəlee) a chronic condition producing gradual enlargement of the hands, feet, and bones of the head and chest.

Associated with overactivity of the anterior lobe of the pituitary gland in adults.

acromioclavicular (əˌkrohmiohˌklə'vikyələ) pertaining to the joint between the acromion process of the scapula and the lateral aspect of the clavicle.

acromion (ə'krohmi·ən) the outwards projection of the spine of the scapula, forming the point of the shoulder.

acroosteolysis (ˌakroostəohləsəs) an occupational disease that affects people working with polyvinylchloride (PVC) plastics.

acroparaesthesia (ˌakrohˌparəs'theezi·ə) condition in which pressure on the nerves of the brachial plexus causes numbness, pain, and tingling of the hand and forearm.

acrophobia (ˌakroh'fohbi·ə) morbid terror of being at a height.

acrosclerosis (ˌakrohsklə'rohsəs) a type of SCLERODERMA that affects the hands, feet, face, or chest.

acrosome ('akrəˌsohm) part of the head of a spermatozoon.

acrylics (ə'kriliks) synthetic plastic materials derived from acrylic acid, from which dental and medical prostheses are made. Used in ophthalmology for making artificial eyes, implants, and lenses.

ACTH adrenocorticotrophic hormone; corticotrophin.

actigraph ('aktəˌgraf) an instrument that records changes in the activity of an organism and produces a graphic record of the process.

actin ('aktən) the protein of myofibrils responsible for contraction and relaxation of muscles.

actinism ('aktəˌnizəm) the ability of rays of light to produce chemical changes.

actinodermatitis (ˌaktənohˌdərmə'tietəs) inflammation of the skin due to the action of ultraviolet or X-rays.

Actinomyces (ˌaktənə'mieseez) a genus of branching, spore-forming, vegetable parasites which can give rise to actinomycosis and from which many antibiotic drugs are produced, e.g. streptomycin.

actinomycin (ˌaktənoh'miesən) a group of cytotoxic drugs used in the treatment of malignant disease.

actinomycosis (ˌaktənohmie'kohsəs) a chronic infective disease of cattle that is also found in humans. Granulated tumours occur, chiefly on the tongue and jaws.

actinotherapy (ˌaktənoh'therəpee) treatment of disease by rays of light, e.g. artificial sunlight.

action ('akshən) the accomplishment of an effect, whether mechanical or chemical, or the effect so produced. *Cumulative a.* the sudden and markedly increased action of a drug after administration of several doses. *Reflex a.* an involuntary response to a stimulus conveyed to the nervous system and reflected to the periphery, passing below the level of consciousness (*see also* reflex).

activator (ˌaktə'vaytə) a substance, hormone, or enzyme that stimulates a chemical change, although it might not take part in the change. In chemistry, a catalyst. For example, yeast is the activator in the process by which sugar is converted into alcohol; the digestive secretions are activated by hormones to carry out normal digestion.

active ('aktiv) causing change; energetic. *A. immunity* an immunity in which the individual has been stimulated to produce his or her own antibodies. *A. movements* movements made by the patient, as distinct from passive movements. *A. principle* the ingredient in a drug that is primarily responsible for its therapeutic action.

activities of daily living (ak'tivəteez əv 'daylee 'living) abbreviated ADL. The activities usually performed in the course of a person's normal daily routine, such as eating, cleaning teeth, washing, and dressing.

actomyosin (ˌaktoh'mieəsən) muscle protein complex; the myosin component acts as an enzyme which causes the release of energy.

acuity (ə'kyooətee) sharpness. *A. of hearing* an acute perception of sound. *A. of vision* clear focusing ability.

acupressure (akyuh'preshə) the application of digital pressure on designated points on the body to produce anaesthesia, relieve pain, or regulate a body function.

acupuncture ('akyəˌpungchə) a system which originated in China whereby the insertion of special needles into specific points along the 'meridians' of the body is used for the production of anaesthesia, the relief of pain, and the treatment of certain conditions.

acute (ə'kyoot) a term applied to a disease in which the attack is sudden and of short duration.

acyclic (ay'sieklik) occurring independently of a natural cycle of events.

acyclovir (ay'sieklohviə) an antiviral agent used to treat HERPES viruses. Uses include the treatment of varicella (herpes zoster) and herpes simplex. It is effective only if started at the onset of the infection. Can also be used as prophylaxis in immunocompromised persons and for prevention of recurrence. It is available as a cream, ophthalmic ointment, suspension, tablets, and intravenous infusion.

adactylia (ˌaydak'tili·ə) congenital absence of fingers or toes.

Adam's apple ('adəmz) the laryngeal prominence, a protrusion of the front of the neck formed by the thyroid cartilage.

adamantine (ˌadə'manteen, -tien) pertaining to the enamel of the teeth.

adaptation (ˌadəp'tayshən) 1. the process of modification that a living organism undergoes when adjusting itself to new surroundings or circumstances. 2. adaptation was understood by the nurse theorist Roy (1976) as being a function of the stimulus to which the individual is exposed and of the individual's adaptation to the situation. Roy maintained that there are four modes of adaptation: physiological needs, role functions, 'self' concept, and interdependence relations. 3. the process of overcoming difficulties and adjusting to changing circumstances. Neuroses and psychoses are often associated with failure of adaptation. 4. used in ophthalmology to mean the adjustment of visual function according to the ambient illumination. *Colour a.* 1. changes in visual perception of colour with prolonged stimulation. 2. adjustment of vision to degree of brightness or colour tone of illumination. *Dark a.* adaptation of the eye to vision in reduced illumination. *Light a.* adaptation of the eye to vision in bright illumination (photopia), with reduction in the concentration of the photosensitive pigments of the eye.

addict ('adikt) a person exhibiting ADDICTION.

addiction (ə'dikshən) the taking of drugs or alcohol leading to physiological and psychological dependence with a tendency to increase use of the drug. *See* DEPENDENCE and DRUG (addiction).

Addisonian crisis *see* ADRENAL CRISIS

Addison's anaemia ('adəsənz) *T. Addison, British physician, 1793–1860.* Pernicious anaemia.

Addison's disease ('adəsənz) deficiency disease caused by partial or complete failure of adrenocortical function; There is wasting, brown pigmentation of the skin, and extreme debility.

adducent (ə'dyoosənt) leading towards the midline. *A. muscle* the medial rectus muscle of the eye, which turns it inwards.

adduction (ə'dukshən) movement of a limb towards the body.

adductor (ə'duktə) a muscle that draws a limb towards the midline of the body. The opposite of abductor.

adenectomy (ˌadə'nektəmee) excision of a gland.

adenine ('adəˌneen) one of the purine bases found in DNA.

adenitis (ˌadə'nietəs) inflammation of a gland or lymph node.

adenocarcinoma (ˌadənohˌkahsə'nohmə) a malignant new growth of glandular epithelial tissue.

adenofibroma (ˌadənohfie'brohmə) a benign tumour of connective tissue which contains glandular structures.

adenohypophysis (ˌadənoh·hie'pofəsəs) the anterior lobe of the pituitary gland.

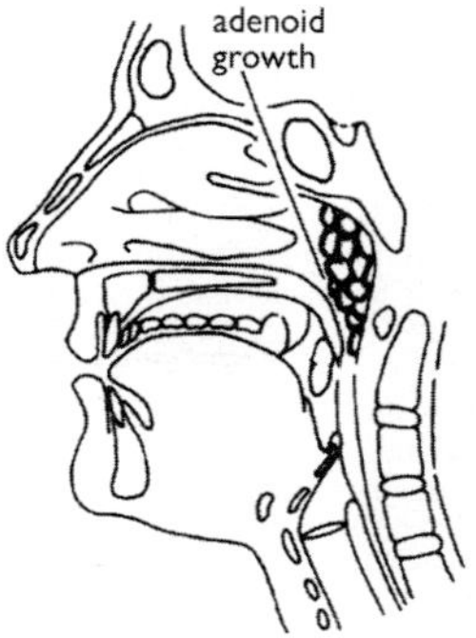

Adenoid Growth

adenoid ('adəˌnoyd) resembling a gland. Generally applied to abnormal lymphoid growth in the nasopharynx (*see* figure).

adenoidectomy (ˌadənoy'dektəmee) the surgical removal of adenoid tissue from the nasopharynx.

adenoma (ˌadə'nohmə) a non-malignant tumour of glandular tissue.

adenomatome (ˌadə'nohməˌtohm) an instrument for the removal of adenoids.

adenomyoma (ˌadənohmie'ohmə) an innocent new growth involving both endometrium and muscle tissue; found in the uterus or uterine ligaments.

adenopathy (ˌadə'nopəthee) enlargement of any gland, especially those of the lymphatic system.

adenosarcoma (ˌadənohsah'kohmə) a malignant tumour of connective and glandular tissue. *Embryonal a.* NEPHROBLASTOMA.

adenosclerosis (ˌadənohsklə'rohsəs)

hardening of a gland. Usually the result of calcification.

adenosine (a'denə,seen) a nucleoside consisting of adenine and D-ribose (a pentose sugar). *A. triphosphate* (abbreviated ATP) a compound containing three phosphoric acids that is present in all cells and serves as a store for energy.

adenosis (,adə'nohsəs) a disease in a gland.

adenovirus (,adənoh'vierəs) a virus of the Adenoviridae family. Many types have been isolated, some of which cause respiratory tract infections whereas others are associated with conjunctivitis, epidemic keratoconjunctivitis, and gastrointestinal infections.

adeps ('adeps) [L.] lard, a foundation fat for ointments. *A. lanae hydrosus* lanolin.

ADH antidiuretic hormone. Vasopressin.

adhesion (əd'heezhən) union between two surfaces normally separated. Usually the result of inflammation when fibrous tissue forms, e.g. peritonitis can cause adhesions between organs. A possible cause of intestinal obstruction.

adiaphoresis (ay,dieəfə'reesəs) deficiency in secretion of sweat.

adiaphoretic (ay,dieəfər'retik) an antihidrotic agent. A drug that prevents the secretion of sweat.

adipocele ('adəpoh,seel) a hernia, with the sac containing fatty tissue.

adipose ('adə,pohs, -z) of the nature of fat. Fatty.

adiposity (,adə'posətee) the state of being too fat. Obesity.

adiposuria (,adəpoh'syoori·ə) the presence of fat in the urine. Lipuria.

aditus ('adətəs) an opening or passageway; often applied to that between the middle ear and the mastoid antrum.

adjustment (ə'justmənt) in psychology, the ability of a person to adapt to changing circumstances or environment.

adjuvant ('ajəvənt) 1. any treatment used in conjunction with another to enhance its efficacy. 2. a substance administered with a drug to enhance its effect.

ADL activities of daily living.

Adler's theory ('adləz) *A. Adler, Austrian psychiatrist, 1870–1937.* The theory that neuroses develop as a compensation for feelings of inferiority, either social or physical.

adnexa (ad'neksə) appendages. *Uterine adnexae* the ovaries and tubes.

adolescence (,adə'lesəns) The stage in human growth from the onset of puberty to the attainment of full physical development.

adrenal (ə'dreen'l) 1. near the kidneys. 2. a triangular endocrine gland situated above each kidney. *A. cortex* the outer and greater portion of the adrenal gland. *A. crisis* an acute life-threatening state of profound adrenocortical insufficiency requiring immediate therapy. Also called Addisonian crisis.

adrenalectomy (ə'dreenə'lektəmee) surgical excision of adrenal gland.

adrenaline (ə'drenələn) a hormone secreted by the medulla of the adrenal gland. Has an action similar to normal stimulation of the sympathetic nervous system causing: (a) dilatation of the bronchioles; (b) raised blood pressure by constriction of surface vessels and stimulation of the cardiac output; and (c) release of glycogen from the liver. It is therefore used to treat such conditions as asthma, collapse, and hypoglycaemia. It acts as a haemostatic agent in local anaesthetics.

adrenergic (ˌadrə'nərjik) pertaining to nerves that release the chemical transmitter noradrenaline to stimulate the muscles and glands they supply.

adrenocortical (əˌdreenoh'kawtikəl) pertaining to the adrenal cortex·.

adrenocorticotrophin (əˌdreenohˌkawtikoh'trohfən) adrenocorticotrophic hormone (ACTH) secreted by the anterior lobe of the pituitary body. Stimulates the adrenal cortex to produce cortisol. Corticotrophin.

adrenogenital (əˌdreenoh'jenət'l) relating to both the adrenal glands and the gonads. *A. syndrome* a condition of masculinisation caused by overactivity of the adrenal cortex resulting in precocious puberty in the male infant and masculinisation in the female. Both sexes are liable to Addisonian crises.

adrenolytic (ə'dreenoh'litik) a drug that inhibits the stimulation of the sympathetic nerves and the activity of adrenaline.

adsorbent (əd'sawbənt, -'zawb-) a substance that has the power of attracting gas or fluid to itself.

adsorption (əd'sawpshən, -'zawp-) the power of certain substances to attach gases or other substances in solution to their surface and so concentrate them on that surface. Used in chromatography.

adult (ə'dult, 'adult) mature. A mature person.

adulteration (ə'dultə'rayshən) addition of an impure, cheap, or unnecessary ingredient to cheat, cheapen, or falsify a preparation.

advancement (əd'vahnsmənt, əd'vans-) in surgery, an operation to detach a tendon or muscle and reattach it in a forward position. Used in the treatment of STRACISMUS and uterine retroversion.

adventitia (ˌadvən'tish·ə, -'tishə) the outer coat of an artery or vein.

adventitious (ˌadvən'tishəs) 1. accidental or acquired. 2. arising sporadically.

advocacy ('advəkəsee) the process whereby a nurse provides a patient and/or the patient's family with information to enable them to make an informed decision relating to care. The nurse is then able to provide support (in accordance with the patient's decision) to other professionals and to incorporate the informed decision into care planning.

aeration (air'rayshən) supplying with air. Used to describe the oxygenation of blood which takes place in the lungs.

aerobe ('air·rohb) an organism that can live and thrive only in the presence of oxygen.

aeropathy (air'ropəthee) commonly called the bends (decompression sickness).

aerophagy (air'rofajee) the excessive swallowing of air.

aerosol ('air·rəˌsol) finely divided particles or droplets. *A. sprays* used in medicine to humidify air or oxygen, or for the administration of drugs by inhalation.

Æsculapius ('eeskyə'laypi·əs, 'es-) the god of healing in Roman mythology.

aetiology (ˌeeti'oləjee) the science of the cause of disease.

afebrile (ay'feebriel, -'feb-) without fever.

affect (ə'fekt) in psychiatry, the feeling experienced in connection with an emotion or mood.

affection (ə'fekshən) 1. a morbid condition or disease state. 2. a positive feeling for someone or something.

affective (ə'fektiv) pertaining to the emotions or moods. *A. psychoses* major mental disorders in which there is grave disturbance of the emotions.

afferent ('afə·rənt) conveying towards the centre. *A. nerves* the sensory nerve fibres that convey impulses from the periphery towards the brain. *A. paths* or *tracts* the course of the sensory nerves up the spinal cord and through the brain. *A. vessels* arterioles entering the GLOMERULUS of the kidney, or lymphatics entering a lymph gland. *See* EFFERENT.

affinity (ə'finətee) in chemistry, the attraction of two substances to each other, e.g. haemoglobin and oxygen.

afibrinogenaemia (ˌayfiebrinəjə'neemi·ə) absence of fibrinogen in the blood, causing the clotting mechanism of the blood to be impaired.

aflatoxins ('afləˌtoksənz) a group of toxic and carcinogenic factors produced by certain food moulds.

African tick fever ('afrikən) disease caused by a spirochaete *Borrelia duttonii*. Transmitted by ticks. *See* RELAPSING FEVER.

afterbirth ('ahftəˌbərth) a lay expression used to describe the placenta, cord, and membranes expelled after childbirth.

aftercare ('ahftəˌkair) social, medical, or nursing care provided after a period of hospital treatment.

afterimage ('ahftəˌimij) a visual impression that remains briefly after the cessation of sensory stimulation.

afterload ('ahftəˌlohd) the resistance against which the left ventricle ejects its blood during a contraction.

afterpain ('ahftəˌpayn) pain due to uterine contraction after childbirth.

afunctional (ay'fungkshənəl) lacking function.

agammaglobulinaemia (ayˌgaməˌglobyuhlə'neemi·ə) a condition in which there is no gamma-globulin in the blood. The patients are therefore susceptible to infections because of an inability to form antibodies.

agar ('aygah) a gelatinous substance prepared from seaweed. Used as a culture medium for bacteria and as a laxative because it absorbs liquid from the digestive tract and swells, so stimulating peristalsis.

age ('ayj) 1. the duration of or the measure of time of the existence of a person or object. 2. to undergo change as a result of the passage of time. *achi*evement a. 1. *see* DEVELOPMENTAL (milestones). 2. proficiency in study expressed in terms of the chronological age of a normal child showing the same degree of attainment. 3. acquirement of a new skill or interest in old age or a praiseworthy accomplishment by an aged person. Chronological a. the actual measure of time elapsed since a person's birth. Gestational a. an expression of age of a developing fetus, usually given in weeks. It is measured from the date of the mother's last menstrual period and so is approximately 2 weeks longer than time from conception. Mental a. the age level of mental ability of a person as gauged by standard intelligence tests.

ageing ('ayjing) the structural changes that take place with time and that are not caused by accident or disease.

ageism ('ayjizəm) the systematic discrimination against people on the grounds of age, based on stereotyping of the elderly as helpless, infirm, confused, and requiring health care and supportive social services.

agenesis (ay'jenəsəs) failure of a structure to develop properly.

agent ('ayjənt) any substance or force capable of producing a physical, chemical, or biological effect. *Alkylating a.* a cytotoxic preparation. *Chelating a.* a chemical compound that binds metal ions. *Wetting a.* a substance that lowers the surface tension of water and promotes wetting.

Agent Orange a mixture of two herbicides: 2,4-D and 2, 4, 5-T used during the Vietnam War. Believed to cause cancer and birth defects.

agglutination (əˌglootə'nayshən) the collecting into clumps, particularly of cells suspended in a fluid and of bacteria affected by specific immune serum. *Cross a.* a simple test to decide the group to which a blood belongs (*see* BLOOD GROUP). *A. test* a means of aiding diagnosis and identification of bacteria. If serum containing known agglutinins comes into contact with the specific bacteria, clumping will take place (*see* WIDAL REACTION).

agglutinin (ə'glootənən) any substance causing agglutination (clumping together) of cells, particularly a specific antibody formed in the blood in response to the presence of an invading agent. Agglutinins are proteins (*see* IMMUNOGLOCULINS) and function as part of the immune mechanism of the body. When the invading agents that bring about the production of agglutinins are bacteria, the agglutinins produced bring about agglutination of the bacterial cells.

agglutinogen (ˌagluh'tənəjən) any substance that, when present in the bloodstream, can cause the production of specific antibodies or agglutinins.

aggregation (ˌagrə'gayshən) the massing together of materials, as in clumping. *Familial a.* the increased incidence of cases of a disease in a family compared with that in control families. *Platelet a.* the clumping together of platelets; can be induced by a number of agents, such as thrombin and collagen.

aggression (ə'greshən) animosity or hostility shown towards another person or object in response to opposition or frustration.

agitation (ˌajə'tayshən) 1. shaking. 2. mental distress causing extreme restlessness.

aglossia (ay'glosi·ə) absence of the tongue.

aglutition (ˌaygloo'tishən) difficulty in the act of swallowing. Dysphagia.

agnathia (ag'naythi·ə) absence or defective development of the jaw.

agnosia (ag'nohzi·ə) an inability to recognise objects because the sensory stimulus cannot be interpreted, in spite of the presence of a normal sense organ.

agonad (ay'gonad) having no sex glands.

agonal ('agənəl) related to dying.

agonist ('agənəst) the prime mover.

A muscle opposed in action by another (the antagonist).

agony ('agənee) extreme suffering, either mental or physical.

agoraphobia (ˌagə·rə'fohbi·ə) a fear of open spaces, especially of leaving the closed environment of home.

agranulocyte (ay'granyələˌsiet) a white blood cell without granules in its cytoplasm. Includes monocytes and lymphocytes.

agranulocytosis (ayˌgranyəloh-sie'tohsəs) a condition in which there is a marked decrease or complete absence of granular leucocytes in the blood, leaving the body defenceless against bacterial invasion. Can result from: (a) the use of drugs, e.g. gold salts, sulphonamides, thiouracil, and benzol preparations; (b) irradiation. Characterised by a sore throat, ulceration of the mouth and pyrexia. It can result in severe prostration and death.

agraphia (ay'grafi·ə) loss of the power of expressing thought in writing. It arises from a lack of muscular coordination or as a result of a cerebral lesion.

ague (ˌaygyoo) a fever, especially that due to malaria.

AHF antihaemophilic factor (clotting factor VIII).

AHG antihaemophilic globulin (clotting factor VIII).

AID artificial insemination of a woman with donor semen.

AIDS (aydz) acquired immune deficiency syndrome. It is the extreme end of the spectrum of disease caused by human immunodeficiency virus (HIV) infection, and impairs the body's cellular immune system. This can allow infection by organisms of otherwise low pathogenicity (opportunistic infections), principally Pneumocystis carinii pneumonia (PCP) or the development of unusual tumours, namely Kaposi's sarcoma (KS). A. related complex (ARC) recurrent symptoms such as lymphadenopathy, night sweats, diarrhoea, weight loss, malaise, and chest infections. Examination of the blood might show abnormally low platelet and neutrophil counts, as well as low lymphocyte counts.

AIH artificial insemination of a woman by her husband's semen.

ailment ('ailmənt) any minor disorder of the body.

air (air) a mixture of gases that make up the earth's atmosphere. It consists of: non-active nitrogen 79%; oxygen 21%, which supports life and combustion; traces of neon, argon, hydrogen, etc.; and carbon dioxide 0.03%, except in expired air, in which 6% is exhaled as a result of diffusion that has taken place in the lungs. Air has weight and exerts pressure, which aids in syphonage from body cavities. *A.bed* a rubber mattress inflated with air. *Complemental a.* additional air that can be inhaled with inspiratory effort. *A. embolism* an embolism caused by air entering the circulatory system. *A. encephalography* radiological examination of the brain after the injection of air into the subarachnoid space. *A. hunger* a form of dyspnoea in which there are deep sighing respirations, characteristic of severe haemorrhage or acidosis. *Residual a.* air remaining in the lungs after deep expiration. *Stationary a.* retained in the lungs after normal expiration. *Supplemental a.* the extra air forced out of the lungs with expiratory effort. *Tidal a.* that which passes in and out of the lungs in normal respiratory action.

airway ('air,way) 1. the passage by which the air enters and leaves the lungs. 2. a mechanical device (tube) used for securing unobstructed respiration during general anaesthesia or on other occasions when the patient is not ventilating or exchanging gases properly. It can be passed through the mouth or nose. The tube prevents a flaccid tongue from resting against the posterior pharyngeal wall thus causing obstruction of the airway (*see* figure).

akinesia (,aykə'neezi·ə) loss of muscle power. This can be the result of a brain or spinal cord lesion or, temporarily, due to anaesthesia.

akinetic (,aykə'netik) relating to states or conditions in which there is lack of movement.

alacrima (ay'lakrəmə) a deficiency or absence of secretion of tears.

alalia (ə'layli·ə) loss or impairment of the power of speech due to muscle paralysis or a cerebral lesion.

alanine ('alə,neen, -nien) an amino acid formed by the ingestion of dietary protein.

alarm reaction (ə'lahm) the mobilisation of the defence mechanisms of the body to cope with stress.

albinism ('albə,nizəm) a condition in which there is congenital absence of pigment in the skin, hair, and eyes. It can be partial or complete.

albino (al'beenoh) a person affected with albinism.

Albright's syndrome ('awlbriets) *F. Albright, American physician, 1900–69.* Condition in which there is abnormal development of bone, excessive pigmentation of the skin and, in females, precocious sexual development.

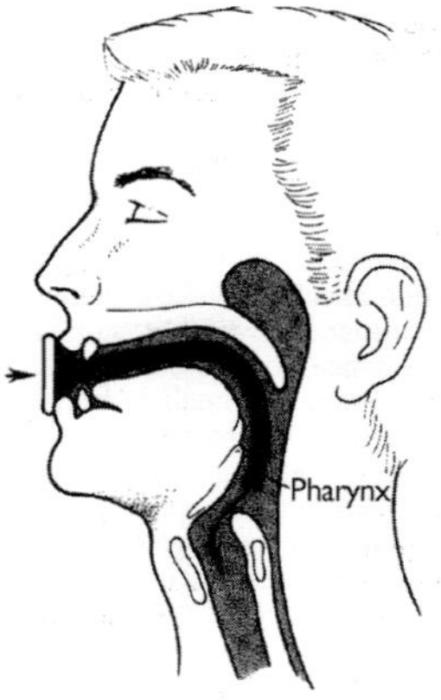

Oropharyngeal Airway

albumin ('albyəmən) 1. any protein that is soluble in water and moderately concentrated salt solutions and is coagulable by heat, e.g. egg white. 2. serum albumin; a plasma protein, formed principally in the liver and constituting about four-sevenths of the 6–8% protein concentration in the plasma. Albumin is a very important factor in regulating the exchange of water between the plasma and the interstitial compartment (space between the cells). A drop in the amount of albumin in the plasma results in an increase in tissue fluid, which, if severe, becomes apparent as oedema. Albumin serves also as a transport protein.

albuminuria (alˌbyoomə'nyoo·ri·ə) the presence of albumin in the urine, occurring e.g. in renal disease, in most feverish conditions and, sometimes, in pregnancy. *Orthostatic* or *postural a.* a non-pathological form that affects some individuals after prolonged standing but disappears after bed rest for a few hours.

albumose ('albyəˌmohs, -ˌmohz) a substance, formed during gastric digestion, intermediate between albumin and peptone.

alcohol ('alkəˌhol) a volatile liquid distilled from fermented saccharine liquids and forming the basis of wines and spirits. The official British Pharmacopoeia (BP) preparation of ethyl alcohol (ethanol) contains 95% alcohol and 5% water. Used: (a) as an antiseptic; (b) in the preparation of tinctures; (c) as a preservative for anatomical specimens. Taken internally, it acts as a temporary heart stimulant and, in large quantities, as a depressant poison. It has some value as a food, 33 mL brandy producing about 400 J. *Absolute a.* that which contains not more than 1% by weight of water. *A.-fast* pertaining to bacteria that, once having been stained, are resistant to decolourisation by alcohol.

alcoholic (ˌalkə'holik) 1. pertaining to alcohol. 2. a person addicted to excessive, uncontrolled alcohol consumption. This results in loss of appetite and vitamin B deficiency, leading to peripheral neuritis with eye changes and cirrhosis of the liver and to progressive deterioration in personality.

alcoholism ('alkəˌholizəm) the state of poisoning resulting from alcoholic addiction.

aldosterone (ˌaldoh'stiə·rohn, al'dostəˌrohn) a compound, isolated from the adrenal cortex, that aids the retention of sodium and the excretion of potassium in the body, and by so doing aids the maintenance of electrolyte balance.

aldosteronism (al'dostə·rəˌnizəm) an excess secretion of aldosterone caused by an adrenal neoplasm. The serum potassium is low, and the patient has hypertension and severe muscular weakness.

aleukaemia (ˌayloo'keemi·ə) an acute condition in which there is an absence or deficiency of white cells in the blood.

Alexander technique (ə'ləks·andə) a mental health therapy that focuses mainly on posture and breathing.

alexia (ə'leksi·ə, ay-) a form of aphasia in which there is inability to recognise written or printed words. Word blindness.

algae ('aljee, -gee) simple forms of plant life.

algesia (al'jeezi·ə) excessive sensitiveness to pain.

algodystrophy (ˌalgoh'distrəfee) a painful wasting of the muscles, especially in the hands.

algor ('algor) chill or rigor; coldness.

alienation (ˌayli·ə'nayshən) a feeling of estrangement or separation from others or from self. A symptom of schizophrenia in which the sufferer feels that his or her thoughts are under the control of someone else. Depersonalisation.

alignment (ə'lienmənt) the state of being arranged in a line, i.e. in correct anatomical position.

aliment ('aləmənt) food or nourishment.

alimentary (ˌalə'mentə·ree, -tree)

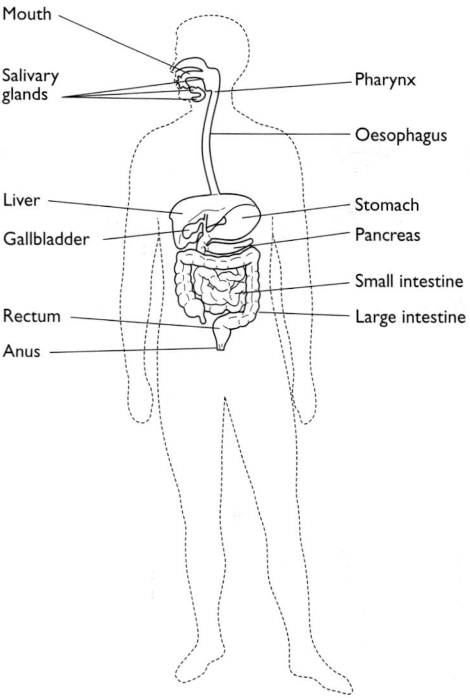

Alimentary Canal

relating to the system of nutrition. *A. canal* or *tract* the passage through which the food passes, from mouth to anus. *A. system* the alimentary tract together with the liver and other organs concerned in digestion and absorption (*see* figure).

alimentation (ˌaləmən'tayshən) giving or receiving of nourishment. The process of supplying the patient's need for nutrition.

aliquot ('aləˌkwot) one of a number of equal parts forming a compound or solution.

alkalaemia (ˌalkə'leemi·ə) an increase in the alkali content of the blood. The pH is above 7. 4. Alkalosis.

alkali ('alkəˌlie) a substance capable of uniting with acids to form salts, and with fats and fatty acids to form soaps. Alkaline solutions turn red litmus paper blue. *A. reserve* the ability of the combined buffer systems of the blood to neutralise acid. The pH of the blood is normally slightly on the alkaline side, between 7.35 and 7.45. The principal buffer in the blood is bicarbonate; the alkali reserve is essentially represented by the plasma bicarbonate concentration.

alkaline ('alkəˌlien) having the reactions of an alkali. *A. phosphatase* an enzyme localised on cell membranes that hydrolyses phosphate esters, liberating inorganic phosphate, and has an optimal pH of about 10.0. Serum alkaline phosphatase activity is elevated in obstructive jaundice and bone disease.

alkalinity (ˌalkə'linətee) 1. the quality of being alkaline. 2. the combining power of a base, expressed as the maximum number of equivalents of acid with which it reacts to form a salt.

alkaloid ('alkəˌloyd) one of a group of active nitrogenous compounds that are alkaline in solution. They usually have a bitter taste and are characterised by powerful physiological activity. Examples are morphine, cocaine, atropine, quinine, nicotine, and caffeine. The term is also applied to synthetic substances that have structures similar to plant alkaloids, such as procaine.

alkalosis (ˌalkə'lohsəs) an increase in the alkali reserve in the blood. It can be confirmed by estimation of the blood carbon dioxide content and treated by giving normal saline or ammonium chloride intravenously to encourage the excretion of bicarbonate by the kidneys.

alkapton (al'kapton) an abnormal product of protein metabolism, from the amino acid, tyrosine.

alkaptonuria (alˌkaptə'nyoo·ri·ə) the excretion of alkapton, an abnormal product of protein metabolism, in the urine. On exposure to air, oxidation takes place, giving a dark-brown colour to the urine.

alkylating agent ('alkəˌlayting) a drug that damages the deoxyribonucleic acid (DNA) molecule of the nucleus of the cell. Many are nitrogen mustard preparations and can be termed 'chromosome poisons'; they are used in cancer chemotherapy.

allantois (ə'lantoh·s) a membranous sac projecting from the ventral surface of the fetus in its early stages. It eventually helps to form the placenta.

allele ('aleel, ə'leel) allelomorph. One of a pair of genes that occupy the same relative positions on homologous chromosomes and produce different effects on the same process of development.

allelomorph (ə'leeləˌmawf) ALLELE.

Allen test ('alən) a test for the patency of the radial artery after the insertion of an arterial cannula.

allergen ('aləˌjən) a substance that can produce an allergy or manifestation of an immune response.

allergy ('aləjee) a hypersensitivity to some foreign substances that are normally harmless but which produce a violent reaction in the patient. Asthma, hayfever, angioneurotic oedema, migraine, and some types of urticaria and eczema are allergic states. *See* ANAPHYLAXIS.

alloaesthesia (ˌaloh·əs'theezi·ə) allocheiria. A response or sensation felt on (referred to) the opposite side from that to which a stimulus is applied.

allocate ('aləˌkayt) to assign for a particular purpose.

allocation (ˌalə'kayshən) the act of allocating. *Clinical a.* a period of time spent in a ward/department/unit in which there are patients/clients. *Patient a.* a patient or group of patients designated to be in the care of a particular nurse for a spell of duty. *Task a.* a set of patient care responsibilities in a ward/unit designated to be the responsibility of each nurse in a group of nurses. Each nurse is allocated a specific nursing activity (task), e.g. one nurse in the clinical area might be responsible for bed baths whereas another is responsible for taking and recording vital signs for the same group of patients.

allograft ('alləˌgrahft) tissue transplanted from one person to another. *Non-viable a.* skin, taken from a cadaver, that cannot regenerate. *Viable a.* living tissue transplanted.

allopurinol (ˌaloh'pyroorəˌnol) a drug that reduces the serum and urinary levels of uric acid. Used in the long-term treatment of gout to lessen the frequency and severity of attacks.

all-or-none law (ˌawlaw'nun) principle that states that in individual cardiac and skeletal muscle fibres there are only two possible reactions to a stimulus: either there is no reaction at all or there is a full reaction, with no gradation of response according to the strength of the stimulus. Whole muscles can grade their response by increasing or decreasing the *number* of fibres involved.

alloy ('aloy) a mixture of two or more metals.

aloes ('alohz) a drug made from the leaves of the aloe. An irritant purgative likely to cause griping. It is contraindicated in pregnancy.

alopecia (ˌalə'peeshi·ə) baldness. Loss of hair. The cause of simple baldness is not yet fully understood, although it is known that the tendency to become bald is limited almost entirely to males, runs in certain families, and is more common in certain racial groups than in others. Baldness is often associated with ageing. *A. areata* hair loss in sharply defined areas, usually the scalp or beard. *Cicatricial a., a. cicatrisata* irreversible loss of hair associated with scarring, usually on the scalp. *Male-pattern a.* loss of scalp hair, genetically determined and androgen-dependent, beginning with frontal recession and progressing symmetrically to leave, ultimately, only a sparse peripheral rim of hair.

alpha ('alfə) the first letter of the Greek alphabet, α. *A. cells* cells found in THE ISLET OF LANGERHANS in the pancreas. They produce the hormone glucagon. *A. fetoprotein* abbreviated AFP. A plasma protein originating in the fetal liver and gastrointestinal tract. The serum AFP level is used to monitor the effectiveness of cancer treatment; the amniotic fluid AFP level is used in the prenatal diagnosis of neural tube defects. *A. receptors* tissue receptors associated with the stimulation (contraction) of smooth muscle. A. wave one of the four types of brain waves.

Alport's syndrome ('awlpawts) *A. C. Alport, South African physician, 1880–1959.* An hereditary disorder marked by progressive nerve deafness, progressive PYELONEPHRITIS or GLOMERULONEPHRITIS, and occasionally ocular defects.

alternating current ('awltə,nayting) an electrical current that runs alternately from the negative and positive poles.

altitude sickness (,altə,tyood) condition caused by hypoxia that occurs as a result of lower oxygen pressure at high altitudes.

altruism ('altroo,izəm) a sense of unconditional concern for the welfare of others.

alum ('aləm) a powerful astringent and styptic, composed of aluminium and potassium or ammonium sulphate. Used as a styptic or haemostatic and, for its astringent properties, as a mouthwash. *A. precipitated toxoid* abbreviated APT. A preparation used for diphtheria immunisation.

aluminium (,alyə'mini·əm, ,alə-) *symbol* Al. A silver-white metal with a low specific gravity, compounds of which are astringent and antiseptic. *A. hydroxide* compound used as an antacid in the treatment of gastric conditions. *A. silicate* kaolin; used as a dusting powder or as a poultice. Refined kaolin can be given orally as an antidiarrhoeal.

alveolar (,alvi'ohlə) concerning an alveolous. *A. air* air found in the alveoli or air sacs of the lungs.

alveolitis (,alvioh'lietəs) inflammation of the alveoli. *Extrinsic allergic a.* inflammation of the alveoli lung caused by inhalation of an antigen, such as pollen.

Alzheimer's cells ('alts·hieməz) *A. Alzheimer, German neurologist, 1864–1915.* 1. giant astrocytes with large prominent nuclei found in the brain in hepatolenticular degeneration and hepatic comas. 2. degenerated astrocytes.

Alzheimer's disease a progressive form of neuronal degeneration in the brain and the most common cause of dementia in people of all ages. It is more common in older than younger people and is not just a form of presenile dementia, as was originally thought. The degeneration of neurons is accompanied by changes in the brain's biochemistry. At present this condition is irreversible and there is no effective treatment.

amalgam (ə'malgəm) a compound of mercury and other metals. *Dental a.* used for filling teeth.

amantadine (ə'mantə,deen) an antiviral agent used against the influenza A virus; also used as an antidyskinetic in the treatment of PARKINSON'S DISEASE.

amaurosis (,amaw'rohsəs) loss of vision, sometimes following excessive blood loss, especially after prolonged bleeding, e.g. haematuria. The visual loss can be partial or complete, temporary or permanent.

amaurotic (,amaw'rotik) pertaining to amaurosis. *A. family idiocy* Tay-Sachs disease. A familial metabolic disorder starting in infancy or childhood. Characterised by progressive mental deterioration, blindness, and spastic paralysis.

ambidextrous (ˌambi'dekstrəs) equally skilful with either hand.
ambivalence (am'bivələns) the existence of contradictory emotional feelings towards an object, commonly of love and hate for another person. If these feelings occur to a marked degree, they lead to psychological disturbance.
amblyopia (ˌambli'ohpi·ə) dimness of vision without any apparent lesion of the eye. Uncorrectable by optical means.
ambulant ('ambyələnt) able to walk.
ambulatory (ˌambyə'laytə·ree) having the capacity to walk. *A. treatment* or *care* health services provided on an outpatient basis.
ameba (ə'meebə) *see* AMOEBA.
amelia (ay'meeli·ə) congenital absence of the limbs.
amelioration (əˌmeelyə'rayshən) improvement of symptoms; a lessening of the severity of a disease.
amenorrhoea (aˌmenə'reeə, ayˌ-men-) absence of menstruation. *Primary a.* the non-occurrence of the menses. *Secondary a.* the cessation of the menses after they have been established, owing to disease or pregnancy.
amentia (ay'menshi·ə) mental subnormality. Can be due to hereditary factors, failure of development of the embryo, or birth trauma.
Ames test (ay'mz) a test to indicate the carcinogenic potential of substances.
amethocaine ('amethəˌkayn) a local anaesthetic for mucous membranes. *A. pastille* a lozenge that, after being dissolved slowly in the mouth, aids the passage of a bronchoscope or gastroscope.
ametropia (ˌaymə'trohpi·ə) defective vision. A general word applied to incorrect refraction.

Essential Amino Acids

1. Threonine
2. Lysine
3. Methionine
4. Value
5. Phenylalanine
6. Leucine
7. Tryptophan
8. Isoleucine
9. Histidine
10. Arginine

amikacin (ˌamə'kaysin) a semi-synthetic aminoglycoside antibiotic derived from kanamycin, used in the treatment of a wide range of infections due to susceptible organisms.
amiloride (ə'miləried) a weak but potassium-retaining diuretic drug.
amino acid (ə'meenoh) a chemical compound containing both NH_2 and COOH groups. The end-product of protein digestion. *Essential a. a.* one required for replacement and growth but which cannot be synthesised in the body in sufficient amounts and which must therefore be obtained in the diet (*see* table). *Non-essential a. a.* one necessary for proper growth but which can be synthesised in the body and is therefore not specifically required in the diet.
aminoacidopathy (ə'meenohˌasə-'dopəthee, əˌmienoh-, əˌminoh-) any

inborn error of amino acid metabolism producing a metabolic block that results in accumulation of one or more amino acids in the blood (aminoacidaemia) or excess excretion in the urine (aminoaciduria) or both.

aminoglutethimide (ˌameenoh-gloo'tethəˌmied) drug which inhibits adrenal hormone synthesis. Its use is sometimes referred to as 'medical adrenalectomy'. The effects are reversible when the drug is discontinued. Used to treat metastatic breast and prostate cancers.

aminoglycoside (əˌmeenoh'glieka-ˌsied) any of a group of bacterial antibiotics, derived from various species of *Streptomyces*, that interfere with the function of bacterial ribosomes. The aminoglycosides include gentamicin, netilmicin, streptomycin, tobramycin, amikacin, kanamycin, and neomycin. They are used to treat infections caused by Gram-negative organisms and are classified as bactericidal agents because of their interference with bacterial replication. All the aminoglycoside antibiotics are highly toxic, requiring monitoring of blood serum levels and careful observation of the patient for early signs of toxicity, particularly OTOTOXICITY and NEPHROTOXICITY.

aminophylline (ˌamə'noflən) an alkaloid from camellia, it relaxes plain muscle spasm of the bronchioles and coronary arteries. It can be given by mouth, intravenously, or as a suppository, and is useful in treating asthma and heart failure.

aminosalicylic acid (ˌamənohˌsalə-'silik) *see* PARA-AMINOSALICYCLIC ACID.

amitosis (ˌamə'tohsəs) multiplication of cells by simple division or fission.

amitriptyline (ˌamə'triptəˌleen) an antidepressant drug that is chemically related to imipramine. It is useful in relieving tension and anxiety, but can cause dizziness and hypotension.

ammonia (ə'mohni·ə) NH_3. A colourless pungent gas. In solution, used as a cardiac stimulant.

ammonium (ə'mohni·əm) NH_4^+.A chemical group that combines to form salts similar to those of the alkaline metals. *A. chloride* used as a mild diuretic and to render the urine acid. Widely used in mixtures as an expectorant.

amnesia (am'neezi·ə, am'neezha) partial or complete loss of memory. *Anterograde a.* loss of memory of events that have taken place since an injury or illness. *Retrograde a.* loss of memory for events prior to an injury. It often applies to the time immediately preceding an accident.

amniocentesis (ˌamneeohsən'teesəs) the withdrawal of fluid from the uterus through the abdominal wall by means of a syringe and needle. It is primarily used in the diagnosis of chromosome disorders in the fetus and in cases of HYDRAMNIOS.

amniography (ˌamnee'ogrəfee) radiography of the gravid uterus.

amnion ('amni·ən) the innermost membrane enveloping the fetus and enclosing the liquor amnii, or amniotic fluid.

amnioscope ('amni·əˌskohp) instrument for examining the fetus and the amniotic fluid by means of a tube passing through the abdominal wall.

amnioscopy (ˌamnee'oskəpee)

inspection of the amniotic sac using an amnioscope.

amniotic (ˌamnee'otik) pertaining to the amnion. *A. fluid* the albuminous fluid contained in the amniotic sac. LIQUOR amnii.

amoeba (ə'meebə) a minute unicellular protozoon. It is able to move by pushing out parts of itself (called pseudopodia). Capable of reproduction by amitotic fission. Infection of the intestines by *Entamoeba histolytica* causes 'amoebic dysentery'.

amoebiasis (ˌami'bieəsəs) infection with amoeba, particularly *Entamoeba histolytica.*

amoebic (əˌmeebik) pertaining to, caused by, or of the nature of an amoeba. *A. abscess* an abscess cavity of the liver resulting from liquefaction necrosis due to entrance of *Entamoeba histolytica* into the portal circulation in amoebiasis; amoebic abscesses can affect the lung, brain, and spleen. *A. dysentery* a form of dysentery caused by *Entamoeba histolytica* and spread by contaminated food, water, and flies; called also amoebiasis. Amoebic dysentery is mainly a tropical disease but many cases occur in temperate countries. Symptoms are diarrhoea, fatigue, and intestinal bleeding. Complications include involvement of the liver, liver abscess, and pulmonary abscess. Several drugs are available for treatment, for example, emetine hydrochloride and chloroquine, which can be used singly or in combination.

amoeboid (ə'meeboyd) resembling an amoeba in structure or movement.

amorphous (ə'mawfəs) without definite shape. The term can be applied to fine powdery particles, as opposed to crystals.

amoxycillin (əˌmoksee'silən) a penicillin analogue similar in action to ampicillin but more efficiently absorbed from the gastrointestinal tract and therefore requiring less frequent dosage and not as likely to cause diarrhoea. It also penetrates sputum more readily than ampicillin.

ampere ('ampair) *symbol* A. The unit of intensity of an electrical current.

amphetamine (amˌfetəˌmeen, -min) a synthetic drug that stimulates the central nervous system. It is addictive and is now seldom used except in the treatment of NARCOLEPSY; ATTENTION DEFICIT/HYPERACTIVE DISORDER (ADHD).

amphiarthrosis (ˌamfeeah'throhsəs) a form of joint in which the bones are joined together by fibrocartilage, e.g. the junctions of the vertebrae.

amphoric (am'for·rik) pertaining to a bottle. Used to describe the sound sometimes heard on auscultation over cavities in the lungs, which resembles that produced by blowing across the mouth of a bottle.

amphotericin (ˌamfə'terəsən) an antifungal drug which is not absorbed by the gut. The only polyene antibiotic that can be given parenterally. Active against most yeasts and other fungi. Side-effects of fever, nausea, and vomiting are common when the drug is given parenterally.

ampicillin (ˌampə'silən) a broad-spectrum penicillin of synthetic origin, used in the treatment of a number of infections, and available in oral preparations as well as for intramuscular injection. It is active against many of the Gram-negative pathogens, in addition to the usual Gram-positive organisms that are sensitive to penicillin.

ampoule ('ampyool) a small glass or plastic phial in which sterile drugs of specified dose for injection are sealed.

ampulla (am'puhlə) the flask-like dilatation of a canal, e.g. of a uterine tube.

amputation (ˌampyə'tayshən) surgical removal of a limb or other part of the body, e.g. the breast.

amputee (ˌampyə'tee) a person who has had one or more limbs amputated.

amyl ('aməl) the radical C_5H_{11}. *A. nitrite* vasodilator and heart stimulant, prescribed for inhalation in cases of ANGINA PECTORIS. Capsules can be broken into a handkerchief and the fumes inhaled.

amylase ('aməˌlayz) an enzyme that reduces starch to maltose. Found in saliva (ptyalin) and pancreatic juice (amylopsin).

amylobarbitone (əˌmieloh'bah-bətohn) one of the barbiturates, used as a short-acting hypnotic and sedative. Effects develop rapidly and the drug is eliminated more quickly than other barbiturates. Regular use can lead to habituation, and overdosage can produce narcosis and death.

amyloid ('aməˌloyd) 1. pertaining to starch. 2. a waxy starch that forms in certain tissues. *A. degeneration* amyloidosis.

amylopsin (ˌamə'lopsən) an enzyme found in the pancreas. Amylase.

amylum ('amələm) [L.] *starch.*

amyotonia (ayˌmieoh'tohni·ə) atonic condition of the muscles. *A. congenita* any of several rare congenital diseases marked by general hypotonia of the muscles; called also Oppenheim's disease or 'floppy baby syndrome'.

anabolic (ˌanə'bolik) relating to anabolism. *A. compound* a substance that aids in the repair of body tissue, particularly protein. Androgens can be used in this way.

anabolism (ə'nabəˌlizəm) the building up or synthesis of cell structure from digested food materials. *See* METABOLISM.

anacidity (ˌanə'sidətee) decrease in normal acidity.

anaclisis (ˌanə'klisəs) generally reclining or leaning; typically an emotional dependence on others.

anaclitic (ˌanə'klitik) denoting the dependence of the infant on the mother or mother-substitute for its sense of wellbeing. *A. choice* a psychoanalytical term for the adult selection of a loved one who closely resembles one's mother (or another adult on whom one depended as a child). *A. depression* severe and progressive depression found in children who have lost their mothers and have not found a suitable substitute.

anacrotism (ə'nakrəˌtizəm) an abnormal pulse evidenced by the presence of a prominent notch on the ascending limb of the pulse wave tracing. *adj.*, anacrotic.

anaemia (ə'neemi·ə) deficiency in either quality or quantity of red cells in the blood, giving rise especially to symptoms of anoxaemia. There is pallor, breathlessness on exertion with palpitations, slight oedema of the ankles, lassitude, headache, giddiness, albuminuria, indigestion, constipation, and amenorrhoea. Anaemia can be due to many causes.

Aplastic a. the bone marrow is unable to produce red blood cells. A rare condition of unknown cause in most cases, but it can arise from the administration of certain drugs. *Deficiency a.* any type that is due to the lack of the necessary factors for red cell formation, e.g. hormones or vitamins. Haemolytic a. a variety in which there is excessive destruction of red blood cells caused by antibody formation in the blood (*see* RHESUS FACTOR) by drugs or by severe toxaemia, as in extensive burns. Iron-deficiency a. the most common type of anaemia; due to a lack of absorbable iron in the diet, excessive or chronic blood loss, or to poor absorption of dietary iron. *Macrocytic a.* a type in which the cells are larger than normal; present in pernicious anaemia. *Microcytic a.* a variety in which the cells are smaller than normal, as in iron deficiency. Pernicious a. a variety caused by the inability of the stomach to secrete the intrinsic factor necessary for the absorption of vitamin B_{12} from the diet. *Sickle-cell a.* an hereditary haemolytic anaemia seen most commonly in black people living in or originating from the Caribbean islands, Africa, Asia, the Middle East, and the Mediterranean. The red blood cells are sickle shaped. *Splenic a.* a congenital, familial disease in which the red blood cells are fragile and easily broken down. Increasingly, with the advent of electronic cell counters, anaemia is now classified according to the morphological characteristics of the ERYTHROCYTES.

anaerobe (an'air·rohb, 'anə͵rohb) a microorganism that can live and thrive in the absence of free oxygen. These organisms are found in body cavities or wounds in which the oxygen tension is very low. Examples are the bacilli of tetanus and gas gangrene. *Facultative a.* a microorganism that can live and grow with or without molecular oxygen. *Obligate a.* an organism that can grow only in the complete absence of molecular oxygen.

anaesthesia (͵anəs'theezi·ə) loss of feeling or sensation in a part or in the whole of the body, usually induced by drugs. *Basal a.* basal narcosis. Loss of consciousness, although supplemental drugs have to be given to ensure complete anaesthesia. *Epidural a.* injection into the extradural space between the vertebral spines and beneath the ligamentum flavum. *General a.* unconsciousness produced by inhalation or injection of a drug. *Hysterical a.* a common symptom in hysteria, in which the insensibility to touch or pain has local distribution unrelated to the nerve supply. *Inhalation a.* a form of general anaesthesia in which drugs or gas used are administered by a face mask or endotracheal tube. *Intravenous a.* unconsciousness produced by the introduction of a drug. e.g. hexobarbitone, into a vein. *Local a.* local analgesia. Nerve conduction is blocked by injection of a local anaesthetic, or by freezing with ethyl chloride or by topical application. *Spinal a.* injection of anaesthetic agent into the spinal subarachnoid space.

anaesthetic (͵anəs'thetik) a drug causing anaesthesia.

anaesthetist (ə'neesthətəst) a person who is medically qualified to administer an anaesthetic.

anal ('ayn'l) pertaining to the anus. *A. eroticism* sexual pleasure derived from anal functions. *A. fissure see* FISSURE. *A. fistula see* FISTULA.

analeptic (ˌanə'leptik) a drug that stimulates the central nervous system.

analgesia (ˌan'l'jeezi·ə) insensibility to pain, especially the relief of pain without causing unconsciousness. *Patient-controlled a.* a preset dose of analgesic, which the patient controls according to need. In-built safety measures prevent accidental overdose.

analgesic (ˌan'l'jeezik, -sik) 1. relating to analgesia. 2. a remedy that relieves pain. *A. cocktail* an individualised mixture of drugs used to control pain.

analogue ('anəˌlog) 1. an organ with different structure and origin but the same function as another organ. 2. a compound with similar structure to another but differing in respect of a particular element.

analysis (ə'naləsəs) 1. the act of determining the component parts of a substance. 2. in psychiatry, the method of trying to determine the reasons for an individual's behaviour by understanding his or her complex mental processes, experiences, and relationships with other individuals or groups of individuals. *A of covariance* (ANCOVA) a statistic that measures differences among group means and uses a statistical technique to equate the groups under study in relation to another given variable. A *of variance* (ANOVA) a statistic that tests whether groups differ from each other, rather than testing each pair of means separately, ANOVA considers the variation among all groups.

anaphase ('anəˌfayz) part of the process of MITOSIS or MEIOSIS.

anaphylaxis (ˌanəfə'laksəs) anaphylactic shock. A severe reaction, often fatal, occurring when a second injection of a particular foreign protein is given, e.g. horse serum. The symptoms are severe dyspnoea, rapid pulse, profuse sweating, and collapse. The condition can be avoided by giving a test dose before all serum injections. If the patient has any reaction, he or she can be desensitised by giving repeated small doses.

anaplasia (ˌanə'playzi·ə) a change in the character of cells, seen in tumour tissue.

anarthia (an'ahthri·ə) inability to articulate speech sounds owing to a brain lesion or damage to peripheral nerves innervating articulatory muscles.

anastomosis (əˌnastə'mohsəs) in surgery, any artificial connection of two hollow structures, e.g. GASTROENTEROSTOMY. In anatomy, the joining of the branches of two blood vessels.

anatomy (ə'natəmee) the science of the structure of the body.

ANCOVA abbreviation for analysis of covariance. *See* ANALYSIS OF COVARIANCE.

Ancylostoma (ˌansi'lostəmə) a genus of nematode roundworms which can inhabit the duodenum and cause extreme anaemia. *A. duodenale* a hookworm, very widespread in tropical and subtropical areas.

androgen ('andrəˌjən) one of a group of hormones secreted by the testes and adrenal cortex. They are steroids which can be synthesised and produce the secondary male characteristics and the building up of protein tissue.

android ('androyd) resembling a man. *A. pelvis* a female pelvis shaped like a male pelvis with a wedge-shaped entrance and narrow anterior segment.

anemia *see* ANAEMIA.

anencephaly (ˌanən'kefəlee, -'sef-) congenital absence of the cranial vault, with the cerebral hemispheres completely missing r reduced to small masses.

anergic (a'nərjik) sluggish, inactive.

anesthesia *see* ANAESTHESIA.

aneurine ('anyəˌreen) thiamine. An essential vitamin involved in carbohydrate metabolism. The main sources are unrefined cereals and pork. Vitamin B_1.

aneurysm ('anyəˌrizəm) a local dilatation of a blood vessel, usually an artery (*see* figure). Atherosclerosis is responsible for most arterial aneurysms; any injury to the arterial wall can predispose to the formation of a sac. Other diseases that can lead to an aneurysm include syphilis, certain non-specific inflammations, and congenital defect in the artery. The pressure of blood causes it to increase in size and rupture is likely. Sometimes excision of the aneurysm or ligation of the artery is possible. Dissecting a. a condition in which a tear occurs in the aortic lining when the middle coat is necrosed and blood gets between the layers, stripping them apart. *Fusiform a.* a spindle-shaped arterial aneurysm. *Saccular a.* a dilatation of only a part of the circumference of an artery.

angiitis (ˌanjee'ietəs) inflammation of a blood or lymph vessel.

angina (an'jienə, 'anjienə) 1. a tight

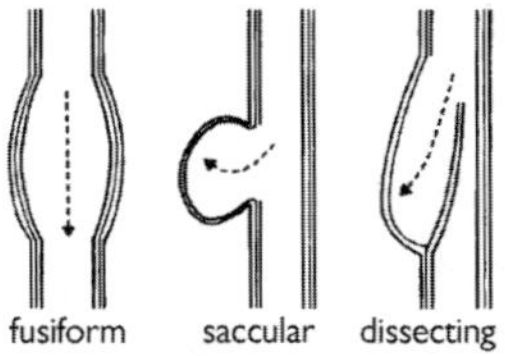

Types of Aneurysm

strangling sensation or pain. 2. an inflammation of the throat causing pain on swallowing. *A. cruris* intermittent claudication. Severe pain in the leg after walking. *A. pectoris* cardiac pain that occurs on exertion owing to insufficient blood supply to the heart muscles. *Ludwig's a.* acute pharyngitis with swelling and abcess formation. *Prinzmetal a.* spasm of blood vessel/s supplying heart muscle resulting in transient reduction in coronary blood flow. *Vincent's a.* infection and ulceration of the tonsils by a spirochaete, *Borrelia vincentii*, and a bacillus, *Fusiformis fusiformis*.

angiocardiography (ˌanjeeohˌkahdee'ogrəfee) radiological examination of the heart and large blood vessels by means of cardiac catheterisation and an opaque contrast medium.

angioectasis (ˌanjeeoh'ektəsəs) abnormal enlargement of capillaries.

angiography (ˌanjee'ogrəfee) radiological examination of the blood vessels using an opaque contrast medium.

angioma (ˌanjee'ohmə) a benign tumour composed of dilated blood vessels.

angioneurosis (ˌanjeeohnyə'rohsəs) a neurosis affecting the blood vessels, which can produce paralysis.

angioneurotic (ˌanjeeohnyə'rotik) pertaining to angioneurosis. *A. oedema see* OEDEMA.

angioplasty (ˌanjeeohˌplastee) plastic surgery of blood vessels.

angiosarcoma (ˌanjeeohsah'kohmə) a malignant vascular growth.

angiospasm ('anjeeohˌspazəm) a spasmodic contraction of an artery, causing cramping of the muscles.

angiotensin (ˌanjeeoh'tensən) a substance that raises the blood pressure. It is a polypeptide produced by the action of renin on plasma globulins. Hypertensin.

angiotensinogen (ˌanjeeohten-'sinəjən) the precursor to angiotensin, produced in the liver.

Ångström unit ('angstrom) *A. J. Ångström, Swedish physicist, 1814–74. Symbol* Å. A non-SI unit of wavelength of light equal to 10^{-10} metre or 0.1 nanometre.

anhidrosis (ˌanhə'drohsəs) marked deficiency in the secretion of sweat.

anhidrotic (ˌanhə'drotik) an agent that decreases perspiration. An adiaphoretic.

anhydraemia (ˌanhie'dreemi·ə) deficiency of water in the blood.

anhydrous (an'hiedrəs) containing no water.

aniline ('anəˌleen, -lən) a chemical compound derived from coal tar, used for making antiseptic dyes. It is an important cause of serious industrial poisoning associated with bone marrow depression as well as METHAEMOGLOBINAEMIA.

anima ('animə) 1. the soul. 2. Jung's term for the unconscious or inner being of the individual, as opposed to the personality presented to the world (persona). In Jungian psychoanalysis, the more feminine soul or feminine component of a man's personality.

anion ('anˌieən) a negatively charged ion which travels against the current towards the anode, e.g. chloride (Cl^-), carbonate (CO_3^{2-}). *See* CATION.

anisocoria (anˌiesoh'koh·ri·ə) inequality of diameter of the pupils of the two eyes.

anisocytosis (anˌiesohsie'tohsəs) inequality in the size of the red blood cells.

anisometropia (anˌiesohmə'trohpi·ə) a marked difference in the refractive power of the two eyes.

ankle ('angkəl) the joint between the leg and foot, formed by the tibia and fibula articulating with the talus.

ankyloblepharon (ˌangkəloh-'blefə·ron) adhesions and scar tissue on the ciliary borders of the eyelids, giving the eye a distorted appearance.

ankylosing spondylitis ('angkə-ˌlohzing ˌspondə'lietəs) a chronic inflammatory disease, primarily affecting the sacroiliac and intervertebral joints, causing back pain and progressive stiffness. Often results in fusion of the joints.

ankylosis (ˌangkə'lohsəs) consolidation, immobility and stiffness of a joint as a result of disease.

Annelida (ə'nelidə) a phylum of metazoa, the segmented worms, including the leeches.

annular ('anyələ) ring-shaped.

anoci-association (aˌnohsee əˌsohsee-'ayshən, -ˌsohshi-) the exclusion of pain, fear, and shock in surgical operations, brought about by means of local anaesthesia and basal narcosis.

anode ('anohd) the positive pole of an electric battery. *See* CATHODE.

anodyne ('anə͵dien) a drug that relieves pain.

anomaly (ə'noməlee) considerable variation from the normal.

anomie ('anəmee) a feeling of hopelessness and lack of purpose.

anonychia (͵anə'niki·ə) congenital absence of nails.

anoopsia (a'nopsee·ə) the tendency of one or both eyes to turn upwards.

Anopheles (ə'nofə͵leez) a genus of mosquito. Many are carriers of the malarial parasite and by their bite infect humans. Other species transmit FILARIASIS.

anophthalmia (͵anof'thalmee·ə) congenital absence of a seeing eye. Some portion of the eye, e.g. the conjunctiva, is always present.

anorchism (an'awkizəm) a condition in which the testicles have failed to develop or to descend.

anorexia (͵anə'reksi·ə) loss of appetite for food. *A. nervosa* a condition in which there is complete lack of appetite, with extreme emaciation. It is due to psychological causes and usually occurs in young women, leading them to perceive themselves as fat and to take extreme forms of dietary control in order to lose weight.

anosmia (an'ozmi·ə) loss of the sense of smell.

ANOVA abbreviation for analysis of variance. *See* ANALYSIS OF VARIANCE.

anovular (an'ohvyələ) applied to the absence of ovulation. Usually refers to uterine bleeding when there has been no ovulation, the result of taking contraceptive pills.

anoxaemia (͵anok'seemi·ə) complete lack of oxygen in the blood.

anoxia (an'oksi·ə) lack of oxygen to an organ or tissue.

antacid (ant'asəd) a substance neutralising acidity, particularly of the gastric juices.

antagonist (an'tagənəst) 1. a muscle that has an opposite action to another, e.g. the biceps to the triceps. 2. in pharmacology, a drug that inhibits the action of another drug or enzyme, e.g. methotrexate is a folic acid antagonist. 3. in dentistry, a tooth in one jaw opposing one in the other jaw.

antecubital (͵antee'kyoobətəl) at the bend of the elbow.

anteflexion (͵antee'flekshən) a bending forwards, as of the body of the uterus. *See* RETROFLEXION.

antenatal (͵antee'nayt'l) before birth.

antepartum (͵antee'pahtəm) shortly before birth, i.e. in the last three months of pregnancy. *A. haemorrhage* bleeding occurring before parturition. *See* PLACENTA PRAEVIA.

anterior (an'tiə·ri·ə) situated at or facing towards the front. The opposite of 'posterior'. *A. capsule* the anterior covering of the lens of the eye. *A. chamber of the eye* the space between the cornea in front and the iris and lens behind.

anterograde ('antə·roh͵grayd) extending or moving forwards.

anteversion (͵antee'vərzhən) the forwards tilting of an organ, e.g. the normal position of the uterus. *See* RETROVERSION.

anthelmintic (anthelminthic) (͵ant·hel'mintik, ͵anthel-) 1. destructive to worms. 2. an agent destructive to worms.

anthracosis (͵anthrə'kohsəs) a disease of the lungs, caused by inhalation of coal dust. A form of PNEUMOCONIOSIS. 'Miner's lung'.

anthrax ('anthraks) an acute, notifiable, infectious disease due to

Bacillus anthracis, acquired through contact with infected animals or their byproducts, such as carcases, bones or skin, usually by occupational exposure. The incubation period is 2–5 days.

anthropoid ('anthrə,poyd) resembling man. *A. pelvis* female pelvis in which the anteroposterior diameter exceeds the transverse diameter.

anthropology (,anthrə'poləjee) the study of human beings that focuses on origins, historical, and cultural development, and races. *Cultural a.* that branch of anthropology that is concerned with the individuals and their relationship to others and to their environment. *Medical a.* biocultural discipline concerned with both the biological and sociocultural aspects of human behaviour, and the ways in which the two interact to influence health and disease. *Physical a.* that branch of anthropology that concerns the physical and evolutionary characteristics of human beings.

anthropometry (,anthrə'pomətree) the science that deals with the comparative measurement of parts of the human body, such as height, weight, body fat, etc.

antiarrhythmic (,anteeay'ridhmik) an agent used to treat cardiac ARRYTHMIAS.

antibacterial (,anteebak'tiə·ri·əl) a substance that destroys or suppresses the growth of bacteria.

antibiotic (,anteebie'otik) substances (e.g. penicillin), produced by certain bacteria and fungi, that prevent the growth of, or destroy, other bacteria.

antibody ('antee,bodee) a specific form of blood protein produced in the lymphoid tissue and able to counteract the effects of bacterial antigens or toxins.

anticholinergic (,antee,kohlin'ərjik) a drug that inhibits the action of acetylcholine.

anticholinesterase (,antee,kohlə'n-estə,rayz) an enzyme that inhibits the action of acetylcholinesterase, thereby potentiating the action of acetylcholine at postsynaptic receptors in the parasympathetic nervous system, thus allowing return of normal muscle contraction.

anticoagulant (,anteekoh'agyələnt) a substance that prevents or delays blood from clotting, e.g. heparin.

anticonvulsant (,anteekən'vulsənt) a substance that arrests or prevents convulsions. Anticonvulsant drugs such as phenytoin are used in the treatment of epilepsy and other conditions in which convulsions occur.

anti-D gamma-globulin (,antee'dee) anti-rhesus antibody which is given to a rhesus-negative woman within 72 hours of delivery of her infant or following termination of her pregnancy, miscarriage, or invasive investigations, such as AMNIOCENTESIS, to prevent haemolytic disease of the newborn in the next pregnancy. *See* RHESUS FACTOR.

antidepressant (,anteedə'presənt) one of a group of drugs which elevate mood, often diminish anxiety, and increase coping behaviour. Selective serotonin reuptake inhibitors (SSRIs) are now considered the first-line drugs in the treatment of major depression. Examples are fluoxetine (Prozac 20), sertraline (Zoloft), paroxetine (Aropax 20), fluvoxamine (Luvox), and citalopram (Cipramil). SSRIs have camparable efficacy to tricyclic antidepressants (TCAs). However, the TCAs have been found to be more effective in the treatment of conditions such as melancholic or severe depression. Monoamine oxidase inhibitors (MAOIs) are less commonly used because of the dietary restriction necessary and the toxic side-effects.

antidiuretic (ˌanteeˌdieyə'retik) a substance that reduces the volume of urine exreted. *A. hormone* abbreviated ADH. A hormone which is secreted by the posterior pituitary gland. VASOPRESSIN.

antidote ('antəˌdoht) an agent that counteracts the effect of a poison.

antiembolic (ˌantee·em'bolik) against embolism. Antiembolic hose/stockings are worn to prevent the formation or decrease the risk of deep vein thrombosis, especially in patients after surgery or those confined to bed.

antiemetic (ˌantee·ə'metik) a drug that prevents or overcomes nausea and vomiting.

antigen ('antəˌjen, -jən) any substance, bacterial or otherwise, which in suitable conditions can stimulate the production of antibodies.

antigen-antibody reaction ('antəˌjen, -jən 'anteeˌbodee) the combination of an antibody with its specific antigen; it forms the basis of the immune system.

antiglobulin (ˌantee'globyələn) an antibody against human globulin.

antihaemophilic (ˌanteeˌheemoh'filik) 1. effective against the bleeding tendency in hameophilia. 2. an agent that counteracts the bleeding tendency in HAEMOPHILIA. *A. factor* abbreviated AHF. One of the clotting factors, deficiency of which causes classic, sex-linked haemophilia; called also factor VIII and antihaemophilic globulin. It is available in a preparation for preventive and therapeutic use.

antihistamine (ˌantee'histəˌmeen, -min) any one of a group of drugs which block the tissue receptors for histamine. They are used to treat allergic conditions, e.g. drug rashes, hayfever and serum sickness. They include promethazine and mepyramine.

antihypertensive (ˌanteeˌhiepə'tensiv) 1. effective against hypertension. 2. an agent that reduces high blood pressure.

anti-inflammatory (ˌantee·in'flamətə·ree, -tree) an agent that counters inflammation.

antimetabolite (ˌanteeme'tabəliet) one of a group of chemical compounds which prevent the effective utilisation of the corresponding metabolite, and interfere with normal growth or cell mitosis if the process requires that metabolite.

antimycotic (ˌanteemie'kotik) a preparation effective in treating fungal infections.

antineoplastic (ˌanteeˌneeoh'plastik) effective against the multiplication of malignant cells.

antiperistalsis (ˌanteeˌperi'stalsəs) contrary contractions which propel the contents of the intestines backwards and upwards.

antipruritic (ˌanteeˌproo'ritik) an external application or drug that relieves itching.

antipyretic (ˌanteepie'retik) an agent that reduces fever.

anti-rhesus serum (ˌantee'reesəs) a substance containing rhesus agglutinins produced in the blood of those who are rhesus-negative if the rhesus-positive antigen obtains access to it, e.g. by blood transfusion. Haemolysis and jaundice are the result. *See* RHESUS FACTOR.

antisepsis (ˌantee'sepsəs) the prevention of infection by destroying or arresting the growth of harmful microorganisms.

antiseptic (ˌantə'septik) 1. preventing sepsis. 2. any substance that inhibits the growth of bacteria, in contrast to a germicide, which kills bacteria outright.

antiserum (ˌantee'siə·rəm) a serum prepared against a specific disease by immunising an animal so that antibodies are formed. These can then be used to create a passive immunity or to treat the infection in humans.

antisocial (ˌantee'soshəl) against society. *A. behaviour* in psychiatry, the refusal of an individual to accept the normal obligations and restraints imposed by the community upon its members.

antispasmodic (ˌanteespaz'modik) any measure used to prevent or relieve the occurrence of muscle spasm.

antistatic (ˌantee'statik) relating to measures taken to prevent the build-up of static electricity.

antitoxin (ˌantee'toksən) a substance produced by the body cells as a reaction to invasion by bacteria, which neutralises their toxins. Serum from immunised animals contains these antitoxins and is used in the treatment of specific diseases such as diphtheria, tetanus, etc. *See* IMMUNITY.

antitussive (ˌantee'tusiv) 1. effective against cough. 2. an agent that suppresses coughing.

antivenin (ˌanteevə'neen) an antitoxic serum to neutralise the poison injected by the bite of a snake or insect.

antrectomy (an'trektəmee) excision of an antrum.

antrostomy (an'trostəmee) surgical opening of an antrum, particularly the maxillary antrum, for drainage purposes.

antrum ('antrəm) a cavity in bone. *Mastoid a.* the tympanic antrum, which is an air-conditioning cavity in the mastoid portion of the temporal bone. *Maxillary a.* antrum of Highmore. The air sinus in the upper jaw bone.

anuria (ə'nyoo·ri·ə) cessation of the secretion of urine.

anus ('aynəs) the extremity of the alimentary canal, through which the faeces are discharged. *Imperforate a.* one where there is no opening because of a congenital defect.

anxiety (ang'zieətee) a chronic state of tension, which affects both mind and body. *A. neurosis see* NEUROSIS.

anxiolytic (ˌanzieoh'litik) a substance, such as diazepam, used for relief of anxiety. Anxiolytics can quickly cause dependence and are not suitable for long-term administration. Called also anti-anxiety agent and minor tranquilliser.

aorta (ay'awtə) the large artery rising out of the left ventricle of the heart and supplying blood to all the body. *Abdominal a.* that part of the artery lying in the abdomen. *Arch of the a.* the curve of the artery over the heart. *Thoracic a.* that part which passes through the chest.

aortic (ay'awtik) pertaining to the aorta. *A. incompetence* owing to previous inflammation the aortic valve has become fibrosed and is unable to close completely, thus allowing backwards flow of blood (a. regurgitation) into the left ventricle during diastole. A. stenosis a narrowing of the aortic valve. *A. valve* the valve between the left ventricle of the heart and the ascending aorta, which prevents the backwards flow of blood through the artery.

aortic body small structure on the aortic arch containing neural tissue sensitive to changes in blood oxygen content and triggering an increase in respiratory rate.

aortitis (ˌay·aw'tietəs) inflammation of the aorta.

aortography (ay·aw'togrəfee) radiographic examination of the aorta. A radio-opaque contrast medium is injected into the blood to render visible lesions of the aorta or its main branches.

APACHE abbreviation for Acute Physiology and Chronic Health Assessment. A classification system for indicating severity of illness in intensive-care patients.

apathy ('apəthee) an appearance of indifference, with no response to stimuli or display of emotion.

aperient (ə'piəri·ənt) a drug that produces an action of the bowels. A laxative.

aperistalsis (ˌayperi'stalsəs) lack of peristaltic movement of the intestines.

Apert's syndrome (a'pairz) *E. Apert, French paediatrician, 1868–1940.* A congenital abnormality in which there is fusion at birth of all the cranial sutures, in addition to syndactyly (webbed fingers).

apex ('aypeks) the top or pointed end of a cone-shaped structure. *A. beat* the beat of the heart against the chest wall which can be felt during systole. *A. of the heart* the end closing the left ventricle. *A. of the lung* the extreme upper part of the organ.

Apgar score ('apgah) *V. Apgar, American anaesthetist, 1909–74.* A system used in the assessment of the newborn: reflex irritability and colour. The Apgar score is assessed 1 minute after birth and again at 5 minutes. Most healthy infants score 9 at birth. A score below 7 indicates cause for concern (*see* table p. 34).

aph antepartum haemorrhage.

aphagia (ə'fayji·ə, ay-) loss of the power to swallow.

aphakia (ay-, ə'fayki·ə, -'fak-) absence of the lens of the eye. Aphacia.

aphasia (ə'fayzi·ə, ay-) a communication disorder due to brain damage; characterised by complete or partial disturbance of language comprehension, formulation or expression. Partial disturbance is also called dysphasia. *Broca's a.* disorder in which verbal output is impaired, and in which verbal communication can also be affected. Speech is slow and laboured and writing is often impaired. *Developmental a.* a childhood failure to acquire normal language when deafness, learning difficulties, motor disability, or severe emotional disturbance are not causes.

aphonia (ə'fohni·ə, ay-) inability to produce sound. The cause can be organic disease of the larynx or the problem can be purely functional.

aphrodisiac (ˌafrə'diziak) a drug which excites sexual desire.

aphthae ('apthee) small ulcers surrounded by erythema on the

APGAR SCORE

Sign	Score		
	0	*1*	*2*
Colour	Blue, pale	Body pink, limbs blue	Completely pink
Respiratory effort	Absent	Slow, irregular, weak cry	Strong cry
Heart rate	Absent	Slow, less than 100 bpm	Over 100 bpm
Muscle tone	Limp	Some flexion of limbs	Active movement
Reflex response to flicking foot	Absent	Facial grimace	Cry

inside of the mouth (aphthous ulcers).

apical ('aypikəl) pertaining to the apex of a structure.

apicectomy ('aypee'sektəmee) excision of the root of a tooth. Root resection.

aplasia (ə'playzi·ə, ay-) incomplete development of an organ or tissue or absence of growth.

aplastic (ay'plastik) without power of development. *A. anaemia see* ANAEMIA.

apnea ('apni·ə) *see* APNOEA.

apneustic centre (ap'nyoostik) nerve tissue in the pons that controls the inspiratory rate of respiration.

apnoea ('apni·ə) cessation of respiration. *Cardiac a.* the temporary cessation of breathing caused by a reduction of the carbon dioxide tension in the blood, as seen in Cheyne-Stokes respiration. *A. of the newborn* apnoeic periods occurring in the respiration of newborn infants in whom the respiratory centre is immature or depressed; *A. mattress* designed to sound an alarm if the infant lying on it ceases breathing. *A. monitors* are designed to give an audible signal when a certain period of apnoea has occurred. *Sleep a.* transient attacks of failure of autonomic control of respiration, becoming more pronounced during sleep.

apocrine ('apəkrien, -krin) pertaining to modified sweat glands that develop in hair follicles, such as are mainly found in the axillary, pubic, and perineal areas.

apomorphine (ˌapoh'mawfeen) a derivative of morphine which produces vomiting.

aponeurosis (aˌpohnyə'rohsəs) a sheet of tendon-like tissue which connects some muscles to the parts that they move.

apophysis (ə'pofəsəs) a prominence or excrescence, usually of a bone.

apoplexy (ˈapəˌpleksee) a sudden fit of insensibility, usually caused by rupture of a cerebral blood vessel or its occlusion by a blood clot. The symptoms are coma, accompanied by stertorous breathing, and a varying degree of paralysis of the opposite side of the body to the lesion.

apparition (ˌapəˈrishən) a hallucinatory vision, usually the phantom appearance of a person. A spectre.

appendectomy (ˌapənˈdektəmee) appendicectomy.

appendicectomy (əˌpendəˈsektəmee) removal of the vermiform appendix.

appendicitis (əˌpendəˈsietəs) inflammation of the vermiform appendix.

appendix (əˈpendiks) a supplementary or dependent part. *A. epiploicae* small tag-like structures of peritoneum containing fat, which are scattered over the surface of the large intestine, especially the transverse colon. *Vermiform a.* a worm-like tube with a blind end, projecting from the caecum in the right iliac region. It can be from 2.5 cm to 15 cm in length.

apperception (ˌapəˈsepshən) conscious reception and recognition of a sensory stimulus.

appetite (ˈapəˌtiet) the desire for food. It is stimulated by the sight, smell, or thought of food, and is accompanied by the flow of saliva in the mouth and gastric juice in the stomach. The stomach wall receives extra blood supply in preparation for its digestive activity. Appetite is psychological, and is dependent on memory and associations, in contrast to hunger, which is physiologically aroused by the body's need for food. Appetite can be discouraged by unattractive food, surroundings or company, and by emotional states such as anxiety, irritation, anger, and fear.

appliance (əˈplieəns) a device used for performing a particular medical function.

applicator (ˈapliˌkaytə) any device used to apply medication or treatment to a particular part of the body.

apposition (ˌapəˈzishən) the bringing into contact of two structures, e.g. fragments of bone in setting a fracture.

apprehension (ˌaprəˈhenshən) a feeling of dread or fear.

apraxia (əˈpraksi·ə) the inability to perform correct movements because of a brain lesion and not because of sensory impairment or loss of muscle power in the limbs. *Oral a.* inability to perform volitional movements of the tongue and lips in the absence of paralysis or paresis. Involuntary movements can, however, be observed, e.g. the patient might purse lips in order to blow out a match.

APT alum precipitated toxoid.

aptitude (ˈaptəˌtyood) the natural ability or capacity to acquire mental and physical skills. *a. test* the evaluation of a person's ability for learning certain skills or carrying out specific tasks.

apyrexia (ˌaypieˈreksi·ə) the absence of fever.

aqua (ˈakwə) [L.] *water. A. destillata* distilled water. *A. fortis* nitric acid.

aqueduct (ˈakwəˌdukt) a canal for the passage of fluid. *A. of Sylvius* the canal connecting the third and fourth ventricles of the brain.

aqueous (ˈakwi·əs, ˈay-) watery. *A. humour* the fluid filling the anterior and posterior chambers of the eye.

Arachis ('arəkis) a genus of leguminous plants. *A. oil* peanut oil; used as a substitute for olive oil.

arachnodactyly (əˌraknə'daktəlee) abnormally long and thin fingers and toes. A congenital condition (Marfan's Syndrome).

arachnoid (ə'raknoyd) 1. resembling a spider's web. 2. a weblike membrane covering the central nervous system between the DURA and PIA MATER.

arborisation (ˌahbə·rie'zayshən) the branching terminations of many nerve fibres and processes.

arbovirus (ˌahboh'vierəs) one of a large group of viruses transmitted by insect vectors (arthropod borne), e.g. mosquitoes, sandflies or ticks. The diseases caused include many types of encephalitis, and yellow, dengue, sandfly, and Rift Valley fevers.

arcus ('ahkəs) [L.] *bow, arch. A. senilis* an opaque circle appearing round the edge of the cornea in old age.

ards adult respiratory distress syndrome. Also known as non-cardiogenic pulmonary oedema.

areola (ə'reeələ) 1. a space in connective tissue. 2. a ring of pigmentation, e.g. that surrounding the nipple.

argentum (ah'jentəm) [L.] *silver.*

arginase ('ahjəˌnayz) an enzyme of the liver that splits arginine into urea and ornithine.

arginine ('ahjəˌneen, -ˌnin) an essential amino acid produced by the digestion of protein. It forms a link in the excretion of nitrogen, being hydrolysed by the enzyme arginase

argon ('ahgon) *symbol* Ar. An inert gaseous element; less than 0.1% in the atmosphere.

Argyll Robertson pupil (ah'giel 'robətsən) *D. Argyll Robertson, British ophthalmologist, 1837–1909. See* PUPIL.

Arnold–Chiari deformity (ˌahnəld-ˌkee'ahree) *J. Arnold, German pathologist, 1835–1915; H. Chiari, German pathologist, 1851–1916.* Herniation of the cerebellum and elongation of the MEDULLA oblongata; occurs in HYDROCEPHALUS associated with spina bifida.

aromatherapy (ərohmə'therəpee) the therapeutic use of specially prepared essential or aromatic oils obtained from the different parts of plants, including the flowers, leaves, seeds, wood, roots, and bark. The oils can be diluted for use in massage, baths, or infusions.

arousal (ə'rowzəl) a state of alertness and increased response to stimuli.

arrachment (ˌarash'monh) the extraction of a membranous cataract via a corneal incision.

arrector pili (ə'rektə) small muscle attached to the hair follicle of the skin. When contracted, causes the hair to become erect, producing the appearance known as goose flesh.

arrest (ə'rest) a cessation or stopping. *Cardiac a.* cessation of ventricular contractions. *Developmental a.* discontinuation of a child's mental or physical development at a certain stage. *Respiratory a.* cessation of breathing.

arrhenoblastoma (ə'reenohbla-'stohmə) a rare ovarian tumour that causes masculinisation in women, with male distribution of hair and coarsening of the skin.

arrhythmia (ə'ridhmi·ə, ay-) variation from the normal rhythm, e.g. in the heart's action. *Sinus a.* an abnormal pulse rhythm due to disturbance of the sinoatrial node, causing quickening of the heart on inspiration and slowing on expiration.

arsenic ('ahsnik) *symbol* As. A metallic element, organic preparations of which have been widely used in medicine. These have been replaced for the most part by antibiotics, which are less toxic.

art therapy ('aht 'therəpee) the use of art as a medium to encourage patients to express their feelings when unable to do so verbally.

artefact ('ahtə,fakt) something that is man made or introduced artificially.

arterial blood gas (ah'tiə·ri·əl) the oxygen and carbon dioxide in the arterial blood, measured to assess acid–base balance and adequacy of ventilation.

arteriectomy (ah,tiə·ri'ektəmee) the removal of a portion of artery wall, usually followed by anastomosis or a replacement graft. *See* ARTERIOPLASTY.

arteriography (ah'tiə·ree'ografee) radiography of arteries after the injection of a radio-opaque contrast medium.

arteriole (ah'tiə·ree,ohl) a small artery.

arterioplasty (ah'tiə·reeoh,plastee) the reconstruction of an artery by means of replacement surgery.

arteriorrhaphy (ah'tiə·ree'o·rəfee) ligature of an artery.

arteriosclerosis (ah,tiə·reeoh-sklə'rohsəs) a gradual loss of elasticity in the walls of arteries due to thickening and calcification. It is accompanied by high blood pressure, and precedes the degeneration of internal organs associated with old age or chronic disease.

arteriotomy (ah,tiə·ree'otəmee) an incision into an artery.

arteriovenous (ah,tiə·reeoh'vennəs) both arterial and venous; pertaining to both artery and vein, e.g. an arteriovenous aneurysm, fistula or shunt for HAEMODIALYSIS.

arteritis (,ahtə'rietəs) inflammation of an artery. *Giant cell a.* a variety of polyarteritis resulting in partial or complete occlusion of a number of arteries. The carotid arteries are often involved. *Temporal a.* occlusion of the extracranial arteries, particularly the carotid arteries.

artery (ahtə·ree) a tube of muscle and elastic fibres, lined with endothelium, which distributes blood from the heart to the capillaries throughout the body.

arthralgia (ah'thralji·ə) neuralgic pains in a joint.

arthrectomy (ah'threktəmee) excision of a joint.

arthritis (ah'thrietəs) inflammation of one or more joints. Movement in the joint is restricted, with pain and swelling. *Acute rheumatic a.* rheumatic fever. *Osteo-a.* a degenerative condition attacking the articular cartilage and aggravated by an impaired blood supply, previous injury or overweight, mainly affecting weight-bearing joints and causing pain. *Rheumatoid a.* a chronic inflammation, usually of unknown origin. The disease is progressive and incapacitating, owing to the resulting ankylosis and deformity of the bones. Usually affects the elderly. A juvenile form is known as STILL'S DISEASE.

arthroclasia (,ahthrə'klayzi·ə) the breaking down of adhesions in a joint to produce freer movement.

arthrodesis (,ahthrə'deesəs) the

fixation of a movable joint by surgical operation.

arthrodynia (ˌahthrə'dini·ə) painful joints. Arthralgia.

arthrography (ah'throgrəfee) the examination of a joint by means of X-rays. An opaque contrast medium can be used.

arthrogryposis (ˌahthrohgrie'pohsəs) 1. a congenital abnormality in which fibrous ankylosis of some or all of the joints in the limbs occurs. 2. a tetanus spasm.

arthrology (ah'throləjee) scientific study or description of the joints.

arthroplasty ('ahthrəˌplastee) plastic surgery for the reorganisation of a joint. *Cup a.* reconstruction of the articular surface, which is then covered by a vitallium cup. *Excision a.* excision of the joint surfaces affected, so that the gap thus formed then fills with fibrous tissue or muscle. *Girdlestone a.* an excision arthroplasty of the hip. *McKee Farrar a.* replacement of both the head and the socket of the femur; *Charnley's a.* is similar. *Replacement a.* partial removal of the head of the femur and its replacement by a metal prosthesis.

arthroscope ('ahthrəˌskohp) an endoscope for examining the interior of a joint.

arthrotomy (ah'throtəmee) an incision into a joint.

articular (ah'tikyələ) pertaining to a joint.

articulation (ah'tikyə'layshən) 1. a junction of two or more bones. 2. the enunciation of words.

artifact ('artəˌfakt) anything that is unwanted or irrelevant.

artificial (ˌahtə'fishəl) not natural. *A. feeding* 1. the giving of food other than by placing it directly in the mouth. It may be provided via the mouth, using an oesophageal (Ryle's) tube; the food can be introduced into the stomach through a fine tube via the nostril (the nasal route). An opening through the abdominal wall into the stomach (i.e. a gastrostomy) can allow direct introduction; or food can be injected intravenously (*see* PARENTERAL). 2. in reference to the feeding of infants, giving food other than human milk. A. insemination the insertion of sperm into the uterus by means of syringe and cannula instead of coitus. Husbands (AIH) or donor (AID) semen can be used. *A. respiration* a means of resuscitation from asphyxia.

arytenoid (ˌarə'teenoyd) resembling the mouth of a pitcher. *A. cartilages* two cartilages of the larynx; their function is to regulate the tension of the vocal cords attached to them.

asbestos (as'bestos, -təs) a fibrous non-combustible silicate of magnesium and calcium that is a good non-conductor of heat. If inhaled can lead to pulmonary fibrosis. Continuous exposure to asbestosis fibres can cause mesothelioma

asbestosis (ˌasbes'tohsəs) a form of pneumoconiosis caused by the inhalation of asbestos dust.

ascariasis (ˌaskə'rieəsəs) the condition in which roundworms are found in the gastrointestinal tract.

Ascaris ('askə·ris) a genus of roundworm. Some types can infest the human intestine.

Aschoff's nodules or **bodies** ('ashofs) *K. A. L. Aschoff, German pathologist, 1866–1942.* The nodules present in heart muscle in rheumatic MYOCARDITIS.

ascites (ə'sieteez) free fluid in the

peritoneal cavity. It can be the result of local inflammation or venous obstruction, or be part of a generalised oedema.

ascorbic acid (əs'kawbik) vitamin C. This acid is found in many vegetables and fruits and is an essential dietary constituent for humans. Vitamin C is destroyed by heat and deteriorates during storage. It is necessary for connective tissue and collagen fibre synthesis and promotes the healing of wounds. Deficiency causes scurvy.

asemia (ay'seemi·ə) inability to understand or to use speech or signs as a result of a cerebral lesion. Aphasia.

asepsis (ay'sepsəs) freedom from pathogenic microorganisms.

aseptic (ay'septik) free from sepsis. *A. technique* a method of carrying out sterile procedures so that there is the minimum risk of introducing infection. Achieved by the sterility of equipment and a non-touch technique.

asexual (ay'seksyooəl, a'sek-) without sex. *A. reproduction* the production of new individuals without sexual union, e.g. by cell division or budding.

asiderosis (ˌaysidə'rohsəs) iron deficiency, relating to anaemia.

asparaginase (ə'sparəjəˌnayz) an enzyme that catalyses the deamination of asparaginase; used as an antineoplastic agent against cancers, e.g. acute lymphocytic leukaemia, in which the malignant cells require exogenous asparagine for protein synthesis.

aspartame (ə'spahtaym) a synthetic compound of two amino acids (L-aspartyl-L-phenylalanine methyl ester) used as a low-calorie sweetener. It is 180 times as sweet as sucrose (table sugar); the amount equal in sweetness to a teaspoon of sugar contains 0.1 calorie (4.2 J). Aspartame does not promote the formation of dental caries. The amount of phenylalanine in aspartame must be taken into account in the low-phenylalanine diet for patients with PHENYLKETONURIA.

aspartate transaminase (AST) (ə'spahtayt) an enzyme, formerly SGOT, found particularly in heart and skeletal muscle, brain, liver, and kidney. Following myocardial infarction AST rises over 12 hours, peaks at 24–36 hours, and returns to normal from the third to the fifth day.

aspect ('aspekt) that part of a surface facing in a particular direction. *Dorsal a.* that facing and seen from the back. *Ventral a.* that facing and seen from the front.

aspergillosis (ˌaspəjə'lohsəs) a bronchopulmonary disease in which the mucous membrane is attacked by the fungus, *Aspergillus*.

Aspergillus (ˌaspə'jiləs) a genus of fungi. *A. fumigatus* a common cause of aspergillosis, found in soil and manure.

aspermia (ay'spərmi·ə) absence of sperm.

asphyxia (as'fiksi·ə) a deficiency of oxygen in the blood and an increase in carbon dioxide in the blood and tissues. Symptoms include irregular and disturbed respirations, or a complete absence of breathing, and pallor or cyanosis. Asphyxia can occur whenever there is an interruption in the normal exchange of oxygen and carbon dioxide between the lungs and the outside air. Common causes are drowning, electric shock, lodging of a foreign body in the air passages, inhalation of smoke and poisonous gases, and trauma to, or disease of, the lungs or air passages. Treatment includes immediate remedy of the situation (*see* RESPIRATION ARTIFICIAL) and removal of the underlying cause whenever possible.

aspiration (ˌaspəˈrayshən) 1. the act of inhaling. 2. the drawing off of fluid from a cavity by means of suction.

aspirator (ˈaspəˌraytə) any apparatus for withdrawing fluid or gases from a cavity of the body by means of suction.

aspirin (ˈasprən) acetylsalicylic acid. It reduces temperature and relieves pain. *Soluble a.* a combination of aspirin with citric acid and calcium carbonate, which is less irritating to the gastric mucosa.

assay (ˈasay, əˈsay) a quantitative examination to determine the amount of a particular constituent of a mixture, or of the biological or pharmacological potency of a drug.

assertiveness (əˈsərtivnəs) a form of behaviour characterised by a confident declaration or affirmation of a statement without need of proof. To assert oneself is to compel recognition of one's rights or position without either aggressively transgressing the rights of another, and assuming a position of dominance, or submissively permitting another to deny one's rights or rightful position. *A. training* instruction and practice in techniques for dealing with interpersonal conflicts and threatening situations in an assertive manner, avoiding the extremes of aggressive and submissive behaviour.

assessment (əˈsesmənt) 1. the critical analysis and valuation or judgment of the status or quality of a particular condition, situation, or other subject of appraisal. In the nursing process, assessment involves the gathering of information about the health status of the patient/client, analysis and synthesis of these data, and the making of a clinical nursing judgment (*see* NURSING PROCESS). The outcome of the nursing assessment is the establishment of a nursing DIAGNOSIS, the identification of the nursing problems. 2. an examination set by an examining authority to test a candidate's nursing skills and knowledge.

assimilation (əˌsiməˈlayshən) the process of transforming food so that it can be absorbed and utilised as nourishment by the tissues of the body.

association (əˌsohsiˈayshən, -ˌsohshi-) coordination of function of similar parts. *A. fibres* nerve fibres linking different areas of the brain. *Free a.* a method employed in psychoanalysis in which the patient is encouraged to express freely whatever comes to mind. By this method material that is in the unconscious can be recalled. *A. of ideas* a mental impression in which a thought or any sensory impulse calls to mind another object or idea connected in some way with the former.

associative play (əˌsohsee·ətiv) a form of play in which a group of children participates in similar activities without formal organisation or direction.

asterixis (ˌaystə'riksəs) involuntary jerking movements, especially in the hands; frequently associated with hepatic coma.

asthenia (as'theni·ə) want of strength. Debility. Loss of tone.

asthenic (as'thenik) description of a type of body build: pale, lean, narrowly built person with poor muscle development.

asthenopia (ˌasthe'nohpi·ə) eye strain giving rise to an aching, burning sensation, and headache. Likely to arise in long-sighted people when continual effort of accommodation is required for close work.

asthma ('asmə) paroxysmal dyspnoea characterised by wheezing, coughing, tighness in the chest, and difficulty in expiration. *Bronchial a.* attacks of dyspnoea in which there is wheezing and difficulty in expiration due to muscular spasm of the bronchi, inflammation, and increased mucus production. The attacks can be precipitated by hypersensitivity to foreign substances, chest infections, cold air, vigorous exercise, or cigarette smoke. There is often a family history of asthma or other allergic condition such as eczema or hayfever. Attacks can accompany chronic bronchitis. *Cardiac a.* attacks of dyspnoea and palpitation, arising most often at night, associated with left-sided heart failure and pulmonary congestion. *Renal a.* dyspnoea occurring in kidney disease, which can be a sign of developing URAEMIA. It is unrelated to true asthma.

astigmatism (ə'stigməˌtizəm) inequality of the refractive power of an eye, due to curvature of its corneal meridians. The curve across the front of the eye from side to side is not quite the same as the curve from above downwards. The focus on the retina is then not a point but a diffuse and indistinct area. Can be congenital or acquired.

astringent (ə'strinjənt) an agent causing contraction of organic tissues, thereby checking secretions, e.g. silver nitrate, tannic acid.

astrocytoma (ˌastrohsie'tohmə) a malignant tumour of the brain or spinal cord. It is slow growing. A GLIOMA.

asymmetry (ay'simətree, a-) inequality in size or shape of two normally similar structures or of two halves of a structure normally the same.

asymptomatic (ˌaysimptə'matik, a-) without symptoms.

asynchronous (ay'sinkrəˌnəs) uncoordinated; events not occurring in time with each other.

asynergy (ay'sinəˌjee) lack of coordination of structures which normally act in harmony.

asystole (ay'sistəlee) absence of heartbeat. Cardiac arrest.

at risk (ət 'risk) a situation whereby an individual or population is vulnerable to a particular disease, hazard, or injury. At risk situations include those involving problems that might be preventable with appropriate intervention, or, if they should occur, might be amenable to treatment.

ataractic (atə'raktik) 1. pertaining to or characterised by ataraxia. 2. an agent that induces ataraxia; a tranquilliser.

ataraxia (ˌatə'raksi·ə) a state of detached serenity with depression of mental faculties or impairment of consciousness.

atavism ('atə,vizəm) the reappearance of some hereditary peculiarity which has missed a few generations.

ataxia, ataxy (ə'taksi·ə) failure of muscle coordination resulting in irregular and jerky movements. *Hereditary a.* Friedrich's ataxia. *Locomotor a.* or *tabes dorsalis* a degenerative disease of the spinal cord; a manifestation of tertiary syphilis. Among signs and symptoms are uncoordinated movements of the legs in walking, absence of reflexes, and loss of sphincter control. The disease is chronic and progressive but can be controlled by antisyphilitic treatment.

atelectasis (,atə'lektəsəs) a collapsed or airless state of the lung, which can be acute or chronic and can involve all or part of the lung: (a) from imperfect expansion of pulmonary alveoli at birth (congenital a.); (b) as the result of disease or injury.

atheroma (,athə'rohmə) an abnormal mass of fatty or lipid material with a fibrous covering, existing as a discrete, raised plaque within the intima of an artery.

atherosclerosis (,athə·rohsklə'rohsəs) a condition in which the fatty degenerative plaques of atheroma are accompanied by arteriosclerosis, a narrowing and hardening of the vessels.

athetosis (,athee'tohsəs) a recurring series of slow, writhing movements of the hands, usually due to a cerebral lesion.

athlete's foot ('athleets) a fungal infection between the toes, easily transmitted to other people. Tinea pedis.

atlas ('atləs) the first cervical vertebra, articulating with the occipital bone of the skull.

atmosphere ('atməs,fiə) 1. the gases that surround the earth, extending to an altitude of 16 km. 2. the air or climate of a particular place, e.g. a smoky atmosphere. 3. mental or moral environment, tone or mood.

atmospheric pressure (,atməs'ferik) pressure exerted by the air in all directions. At sea level it is about 100 kPa.

atom ('atəm) the smallest particle of an element that retains all the properties of that element. It is made up of a central positively charged nucleus and, moving around it in a orbit, negatively charged electrons.

atomiser ('atə,miezə) an instrument by which a liquid is divided to form a fine spray or vapour (nebuliser).

atony ('atənee) lack of tone, e.g. in a muscle.

atopy ('atəpee) a state of hypersensivity to certain antigens. There is an inherited tendency that includes asthma, eczema, and hayfever.

atp adenosine triphosphate.

atracurium (,atrə'kyoo·ri·əm) a neuromuscular blocking agent of the non-depolarising type spontaneously broken down in the blood by the HOFFMAN REACTION. It has a relatively short duration of action and is particularly useful for providing muscle relaxation in patients with kidney or liver disease undergoing surgery.

atresia (ə'treezi·ə) absence of a natural opening or tubular structure, e.g. of the anus or vagina; usually a congenital malformation.

atrial ('aytri·əl) relating to the atrium. *A. fibrillation* overstimulation of the atrial walls so that many areas of excitation arise and the atrioventricular node is bombarded with impulses, many of which it cannot transmit, resulting in a highly irregular pulse. *A. flutter* rapid regular action of the atria. The atrioventricular node transmits alternative impulses or one in three or four. The atrial rate is usually about 300 beats per minute. *A. septal defect* the non-closure of the foramen ovale at the time of birth, giving rise to a congenital heart defect.

atrioventricular (aytreeohven'trikyələ) pertaining to the atrium and ventricle. *A. bundle see* BUNDLE OF HIS. *A. node* a node of neurogenic tissue situated between the two and transmitting impulses. *A. valves* the bicuspid and tricuspid valve on the left and right sides of the heart respectively.

atrium ('aytree·əm) *pl.* atria. 1. a cavity, entrance or passage. 2. one of the two upper chambers of the heart. Formerly called auricle.

atrophy ('atrəfee) wasting of any part of the body, due to degeneration of the cells, from disuse, lack of nourishment, or of nerve supply. *Acute yellow a.* massive necrosis of liver cells. A rare condition that can follow acute hepatitis or ECLAMPSIA or be precipitated by certain drugs. *Progressive muscular a.* (motor neurone disease) degeneration of the motor neurones with wasting of muscle tissue.

atropine ('atrə,peen, -pin) the active principle of belladonna. An alkaloid which inhibits respiratory and gastric secretions, relaxes muscle spasm and dilates the pupil.

ats antitetanus serum. *See* TETANUS.

attack (ə'tak) an episode or onset of illness. *A. rate* number of cases of a disease in a particular group, e.g. a school, over a given period, related to the population of that group. Transient ischaemic a's brief attacks (less than a few hours) of cerebral dysfunction of vascular origin, without lasting neurological deficit.

attention deficit syndrome (ə'tenshən) a disorder of childhood characterised by marked failure of attention, impulsiveness, and increased motor activity.

attenuation (ə'tenyoo'ayshən) a bacteriological process by which organisms are rendered less virulent by culture in artificial media through many generations, exposure to light, air, etc. used for vaccine preparations.

attitude ('atə,tyood) 1. a posture or position of the body; in obstetrics, the relation of the various parts of the fetal body to one another. 2. a pattern of mental views established by cumulative prior experience.

atypical (ay'tipikəl) irregular; not conforming to type.

audiogram ('awdeeoh,gram) a graph produced by an audiometer.

audiologist (,awdee'oləjist) an allied health professional specialising in audiology, who provides services that include: (a) evaluation of hearing function to detect hearing impairment and, if there is a hearing disorder, to determine the anatomical site involved and the cause of the disorder; (b) selection of appropriate hearing aids; and (c) training in lip reading, hearing aid use, and maintenance of normal speech.

audiology (,awdee'oləjee) the science concerned with the sense of hearing, especially the evaluation and measurement of impaired hearing and the rehabilitation of those with impaired hearing.

audiometer (ˌawdee'omətə) an instrument for testing hearing, whereby the threshold of a patient's hearing can be measured.

audit ('awdət) systematic review and evaluation of records and other data to determine the quality of the services or products provided in a given situation. *Medical a.* the systematic critical analysis of the quality of medical treatment and care, including the procedures for diagnosis and treatment, the use of resources, outcomes, and the resultant quality of life for the patient. *Nursing a.* an evaluation of structure, process, and outcome as a measurement of the quality of nursing care. *Concurrent a's* are conducted at the time the care is being provided to clients/patients. They can be conducted by means of observation and interview of clients/patients, review of open charts, or conferences with groups of consumers and providers of nursing care. *Retrospective a's* are conducted after the patient's discharge. Methods include the study of closed patients' charts and nursing care plans, questionnaires, interviews, and surveys of patients and families.

aura ('awrə) the premonition, peculiar to an individual, which often precedes an epileptic fit or attacks of migraine.

aural ('awrəl) referring to the ear.

auricle ('awrikəl, 'or-) 1. the external portion of the ear. 2. obsolete term for the atrium.

auriscope ('awrəˌskohp, 'or-) an instrument for examining the drum of the ear. An otoscope.

aurum ('awrəm) [L.] *gold.*

auscultation (ˌawskəl'tayshən) examining the internal organs by listening to the sounds that they give out. In *direct* or *immediate a.* the ear is placed directly against the body. In *mediate a.* a stethoscope is used.

Australia antigen (o'strayli·ə) hepatitis B surface antigen found in the blood of a patient with serum hepatitis or who is a carrier of the virus. Dilute concentrations of the antigen can cause the disease, and healthcare personnel must take adequate precautions to avoid inoculation accidents. Blood banks routinely screen for the antigen to exclude infected blood donations.

autism ('awtizəm) self-absorption. Abnormal dislike of the society of others. *Infantile a.* failure of a child to relate to people and situations, leading to complete withdrawal into a world of private fantasies.

autistic (aw'tistik) pertaining to autism.

autoagglutination ('awtoh·əˌglootiˌnayshən) 1. clumping or agglutination of cells by an individual's own serum, as in autohaemagglutination. Autoagglutination occurring at low temperatures is called cold agglutination. 2. agglutination of particulate antigens, e.g. bacteria, in the absence of specific antigens.

autoantibody ('awtoh'anteeˌbodee) an antibody formed in response to, and reacting against, an antigenic constituent of the individual's own tissues.

autoantigen (ˌawtoh'antəjən) a tissue constituent that stimulates production of autoantibodies in the organism in which it occurs.

autoclave (ˈawtəˌklayv) a steam-heated sterilising apparatus in which the temperature is raised by reducing the air pressure inside it; steam is injected under pressure, bringing about efficient sterilisation.

autodigestion (ˌawtohdieˈjeschən, -di-) dissolution of tissue by its own secretions.

autoeroticism (ˌawtoh·əˈrotəˌsizəm) sexual pleasure derived from self-stimulation of erogenous zones (the mouth, the anus, the genitals, and the skin).

autogenous (awˈtojənəs) generated within the body and not acquired from external sources.

autograft (ˈawtəˌgrahft) the transfer of skin or other tissue from one part of the body to another to repair some deficiency.

autoimmune disease (ˌawtoh·əˈmyoon) condition in which the body develops antibodies to its own tissues, e.g. in autoimmune thyroiditis (HASHIMOTO'S DISEASE).

autoimmunisation (ˌawtohˈ-imyənieˈzayshən) the formation of antibodies against the individual's own tissue.

autoinfection (ˌawtoh·inˈfekshən) self-infection, transferred from one part of the body to another by fingers, towels, etc.

autoinoculation (ˌawtoh·əˌnokyəˈlayshən) inoculation with a micro-organism from the body itself.

autointoxication (ˌawtoh·inˌtoksəˈkayshən) poisoning by toxins generated within the body itself.

autologous (awˈtoləgəs) related to self; belonging to the same organism. *A. blood transfusion* abbreviated ACT. The patient donates blood before elective surgery for transfusion postoperatively. ACT can also be obtained as a blood salvage procedure during operation or postoperatively. Avoids cross-matching, compatibility, and transfusion infection problems.

autolysis (awˈtoləsəs) a breaking up of living tissues, e.g. as can occur if pancreatic ferments escape into surrounding tissues. It also occurs after death.

automatic (ˌawtəˈmatik) performed without the influence of the will.

automatism (awˈtoməˌtizəm) performance of non-reflex acts without apparent volition, and of which the patient might have no memory afterwards, as in somnambulism. *Post-epileptic a.* automatic acts following an epileptic fit.

autonomic (ˌawtəˈnomik) self-governing. *A. nervous system* the sympathetic and parasympathetic nerves that control involuntary muscles and glandular secretion, over which there is no conscious control.

autoplasty (ˈawtohˌplastee) 1. replacement of missing tissue by grafting a healthy section from another part of the body. 2. in psychoanalysis, instinctive modification within the psychic systems in adaptation to reality.

autopsy (awˈtopsee, ˈawtəp-) post-mortem examination of a body to determine the cause of death.

autosome (ˈawtohˌsohm) any chromosome other than the sex chromosomes. In humans there are 22 pairs of autosomes and 1 pair of sex chromosomes.

autosuggestion (ˌawtohsəˈjeschən) suggestion arising in one's self. Uncritical acceptance of ideas arising in the individual's own mind.

autotransfusion (ˌawtohtrans'fyoozhən, -trahns-) reinfusion of a patient's own blood.

autotransplantation (ˌawtohˌtransplahn'tayshən) transfer of tissue from one part of the body to another part.

avascular (ay'vaskyuhlə) not vascular. Bloodless. *A. necrosis* death of bone owing to deficient blood supply, usually following an injury.

aversion (ə'vərzhən) intense dislike. *A. therapy* a method of treating addictions by associating the craving for what is addictive with painful or unpleasant stimuli.

avitaminosis (ayˌvitəmə'nohsəs) a condition resulting from an insufficiency of vitamins in the diet. A deficiency disease.

avoidance (ə'voydəns) a conscious or unconscious defence mechanism whereby an individual seeks to escape or avoid certain situations, feelings or conflicts.

avulsion (ə'vulshən) the tearing away of one part from another. *Phrenic a.* a tearing away of the phrenic nerve. It paralyses the diaphragm on the affected side.

axilla (ak'silə) an armpit.

axis ('aksəs) 1. a line through the centre of a structure. 2. the second cervical vertebra.

axon ('akson) the process of a nerve cell along which electrical impulses travel. The nerve fibre.

axonotmesis (ˌaksonət'meesəs) nerve injury characterised by disruption f the axon and myelin sheath but with preservation of the connective tissue fragments, resulting in degeneration of the axon distal to the injury site; regeneration of the axon is spontaneous.

azathioprine (ˌazə'thieəˌpreen) an immunosuppressive drug widely used for transplant recipients and also as treatment for autoimmune conditions.

azoospermia (ˌayzoh·oh'spərmi·ə) absence of spermatozoa in the semen.

azygos ('azəˌgos, ə'ziegəs) something that is unpaired. *A. vein* an unpaired vein that ascends the posterior MEDIASTINUM and enters the superior VENA CAVA.

Bb

Ba symbol for *barium.*

Babinski's reflex or **sign** (bə'binskee) *J.F.F. Babinski, French neurologist, 1857–1932.* On stroking the sole of the foot, the great toe bends upwards instead of downwards (dorsal instead of plantar flexion). Present in disease or injury to the upper motor neurone. Babies who have not walked react in the same way, but normal flexion develops later.

baby ('baybee) an infant as yet unable to walk. *Battered b.* one suffering from the result of continued violence; extensive bruising, fractures of limbs, rib and skull, an internal trauma may be found. *Blue b.* one suffering from cyanosis at birth as a result of ATELECTASIS or congenital heart malformation.

bacillaemia (ˌbasəl'leemi·ə) the presence of bacilli in the blood.

bacilluria (ˌbasə'lyoo·ri·ə) the presence of bacilli in the urine.

Bacillus (bə 'siləs) a genus of aerobic, spore-bearing Gram-positive bacteria. *B. anthracis* the causative agent of ANTHRAX.

bacillus (bə'siləs) loosely, the cause of any bacterial infection by a rod-shaped microorganism, e.g. *Escherichia coli*, the colon bacillus.

back (bak) dorsum. Posterior trunk from neck to pelvis. *B. bone* the vertebral column. *Hunch b.* KYPHOSIS. *B. slab* plaster or plastic splint in which a limb is supported.

backache ('bakˌayk) any pain in the back, usually the lower part. The pain is often dull and continuous, but sometimes sharp and throbbing. Backache, or lumbago, is one of the most common ailments and can be caused by a variety of disorders. Nurses are at particular risk and one in six are thought to experience back pain.

backward failure (bakˌwəd'faylyə) cardiac failure characterised by raised venous pressure and low-ered arterial pressure.

bacteraemia (ˌbaktə'reemi·ə) the presence of bacteria in the bloodstream.

bacterial (bak'tiə·ri·əl) pertaining to bacteria.

bactericidal (bakˌtiə·ri'sied'l) capable of killing bacteria; e.g. disinfectants, great heat, intense cold, or sunlight.

bactericide (bak'tiə·rə'sied) an agent that kills bacteria.

bacteriologist (bakˌtiə·ree'oləjəst) one who is qualified in the science of bacteriology.

bacteriology (bakˌtiə·ree'oləjee) the scientific study of bacteria.

bacteriolysin (bakˌtiə·ree'oləsən, -rioh'liesin) an antibody produced in the blood to assist in the destruction of bacteria. The action is specific.

bacteriolysis (bak,tiə·ree'oləsəs) the dissolution of bacteria by a bacteriolytic agent.

bacteriolytic (bak,tiə'reeə'litik) capable of destroying or dissolving bacteria.

bacteriophage (bak'tiə·ree·ə,fayj, -fahzh) a virus that infects only bacteria. Many strains exist, some of which are used for identifying types of STAPHYLOCOCCI and SALMONELLAE.

bacteriostat (bak,tiə·reeoh'stat) an agent that inhibits the growth of bacteria.

bacteriostatic (bak,tiə·reeoh'static) inhibiting the growth of bacteria.

bacterium (bak'tiə·ree·əm) a general name given to a minute vegetable organism which might live on organic matter. There are many varieties, only some of which are pathogenic to man, animals, and plants. Each bacterium consists of a single cell and, given favourable conditions, multiplies by subdivision. Bacteria (*see* figure) are classified according to their (A) shape (i) rod-shaped (bacillus, plu. Bacilli — example: Staphyloccus epidermidis); (ii) spherical (coccus, plu. cocci — example: Escherichia coli); and (iii) spiral (spirillum, plu. spirilla — example: Treponema pallidum); (B) whether they form (i) chains (streptococci); (ii) groups (staphylococci); or (iii) pairs (diplococci); and (C) their Gram staining properties that is: (i) Gram-negative — examples: *Bacteroides fragilis*, *Brucella abortus*, *Escherichia coli*, *Haemophilus influenzae*, *Neisseria gonorrhoeae*; or (ii) Gram-positive —examples: *Bacillus anthracis*, *Clostridium* species, *Mycobacterium tuberculosis*, *Staphylococcus aureus*. *Pathogenic b.* one whose growth in the body gives rise to disease, either by destruction of tissue or by formation of toxins, which circulate in the blood. Pathogenic bacteria thrive on organic matter in the presence of warmth and moisture.

bacteriuria (bak,tiə·ree'yoo·ri·ə) the presence of bacteria in the urine.

bag (bag) a sac or pouch. *Colostomy b.* a receptacle worn over the stoma by the patient, to receive the faecal discharge. *Douglas b.* a receptacle for the collection of expired air, permitting measurement of respiratory gases. *Ice b.* a rubber or plastic bag half-filled with pieces of ice and applied near or to a part of the body. *Ileostomy b.* any of various plastic or latex pouches attached to the stoma for the collection of faecal material after ILEOSTOMY. *Politzer b.* a soft bag of rubber for inflating the pharyngotympanic tube. *Urine b.* a receptable used for urine by ambulatory patients with urinary incontinence. *B. of waters* the membranes enclosing the AMNIOTIC (fluid) and the developing fetus in utero.

Bainbridge reflex ('baynbrij) *F.A. Bainbridge, British physiologist, 1874–1921.* An increase in the heart rate caused by an increase in right atrial pressure.

balanitis (,balə'nietəs) inflammation of the glans penis and of the prepuce, usually associated with PHIMOSIS. Balanoposthitis.

balantidiasis (,baləntə'diezəsəs) a rare form of colitis or dysentery

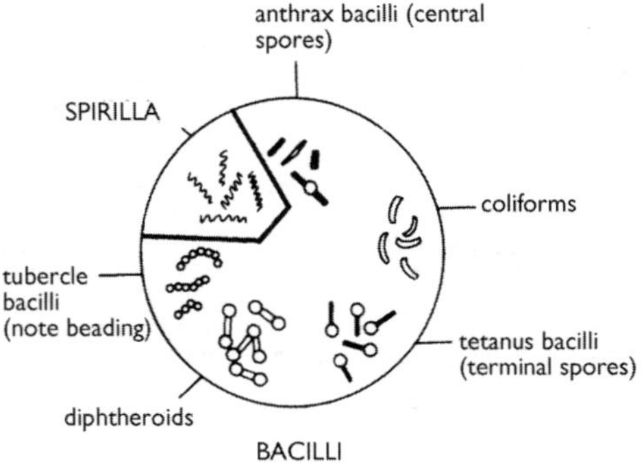

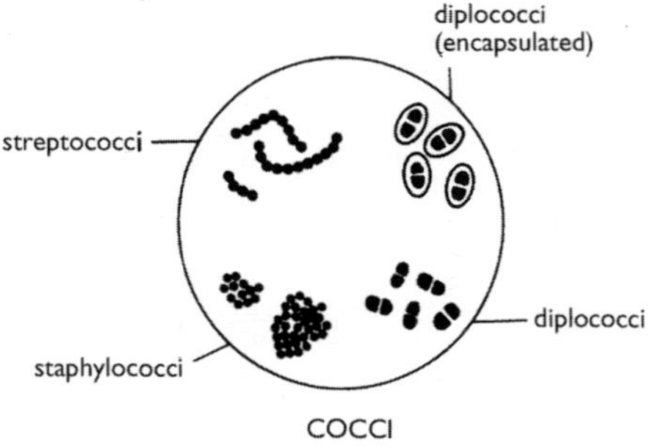

Bacteria

caused by intestinal infestation by *Balantidium coli*, a protozoon.

baldness ('bawldnəs) absence of hair, especially from the scalp. ALOPECIA.

Balkan frame ('bawlkən) a framework fitted over a bed to carry pulleys and slings or splints for the support of a limb undergoing surgical treatment. Used chiefly in the treatment of fractures.

balloon angioplasty (bə'loon 'anjeeoh,plastee) method of reopening or dilating an obstructed blood vessel.

ballottement (bə'lotmənt) [Fr.] a method of testing for a floating object, e.g. abdominal palpation of the uterus when testing for pregnancy. The uterus is pushed upwards by a finger in the vagina and, if a fetus is present, it will fall back again like a heavy body in water.

balsam ('bawlsəm) an aromatic vegetable juice. *Friar's b.* a compound containing tincture of benzoin. Used for steam inhalations. *Peru b.* used externally as an antiseptic ointment and in *tulle gras*. *Tolu b.* used as an expectorant. A constituent of friar's balsam.

bandage ('bandij) 1. a strip or roll of gauze or other material for wrapping or binding any part of the body. 2. to cover by wrapping with such material. Bandages can be used to stop the flow of blood, to provide a safeguard against contamination, or to hold a dressing in place. They can also be used to hold a splint in position or otherwise immobilise an injured part of the body to prevent further injury and to facilitate healing.

banding ('banding) placing a band around a vessel to restrict flow from it. *Pulmonary arterial b.* a palliative operation used in treating infants with ventricular septal defects.

Bandl's ring ('band'lz) a pathological contraction ring at the junction of the upper and lower segments of the uterus occurring at any stage of dysfunctional labour.

bank (bank) an institution offering services, or a store of donated human tissues for use in the future by other individuals, e.g., *blood b.*, *human milk b.*, *sperm b.* *Nurse b.* a group of nurses who are known to the employing authority and available for employment on an on-call basis.

Bankart's operation ('bangkhahts) *A.S.B. Bankart, British orthopaedic surgeon, 1879–1951*. An operation to repair a defect in the glenoid cavity that causes repeated dislocation of the shoulder joint.

Banti's disease ('banteez) *G. Banti, Italian pathologist, 1852–1925*. A clinical syndrome characterised by SPLENOMEGALY, cirrhosis of the liver, anaemia, leukopaenia, and gastrointestinal bleeding.

Barbados leg (bah'baydəs, -dos, -dohs) swelling and enlargement of the leg. A form of ELEPHANTIASIS.

barbiturates (bah'bityə·rəts, -'rayts) a large group of sedative and hypnotic drugs derived from barbituric acid, e.g. phenobarbitone, amylobarbitone. Prolonged use can lead to addiction.

barbotage (ˌbahbə'tahzh) [Fr.] a method of spinal anaesthesia by which some of the anaesthetic is injected, followed by partial withdrawal and then reinjection with more of the drug. This process is repeated until the full amount has been given, allowing dilution and mixing with the cerebrospinal fluid.

barium ('bair·ree·əm) *symbol* Ba. A soft silvery metallic element. *B. sulphate* a heavy mineral salt that is comparatively impermeable to X-rays and can therefore be used as a contrast medium, given as a meal or as an enema. Used to demonstrate abnormality in the stomach or intestines, and to show peristaltic movement. *B. sulphide* the chief constitutent of depilatory preparations, i.e. those that remove hair.

baroreceptors (ˌbarohree'septəz) the sensory branches of the glossopharyngeal and vagus nerves that influence the blood pressure. The receptors are situated in the walls of the carotid sinus and aortic arch.

barotrauma (ˌbaroh'trawmə) injury due to pressure, such as to structures of the ear, owing to differences between atmospheric and intratympanic pressures.

Barr body (bah) *M.L. Barr, Canadian anatomist, 1908–95.* Small, dark-staining area underneath the nuclear membrane of female cells. Represents an inactive X chromosome.

Barré–Guillain syndrome (ˌbaray-'giyanh) *J.A. Barré, French neurologist, 1880–1967; G. Guillain, French neurologist, 1876–1961.* Acute febrile polyneuritis. Called also Guillain–Barré syndrome.

barrier ('baree·ə) an obstruction. *Blood–brain b.* the selective barrier which separates the circulating blood from the cerebrospinal fluid. *B. contraceptive* mechanical barrier preventing the sperm entering the cervical canal, e.g. diaphragm, sheath. *B. nursing* precautions taken by nurses to prevent infection from a patient spreading to other patients and/or staff. This normally involves nursing the patient in a separate room or cubicle. *Placental b.* semipermeable membrane between maternal and fetal blood. *Protective b.* radiation-absorbing shield, e.g. lead, concrete, to protect the body against ionising radiations. *Reverse b. nursing* a technique used by nurses to prevent the transmission of infection to the patient who might be especially vulnerable, e.g. the immunosuppressed patient.

Bartholin's glands ('bahtəlinz) *C.T. Bartholin, Danish anatomist, 1655–1738.* Two glands situated in the LABIA MAJORA, with ducts opening inside the vulva.

basal ('baysəl) 1. fundamental. 2. referring to a base. *B. ganglia* the collections of nerve cells or grey matter in the base of the cerebrum. They consist of the caudate nucleus and putamen, forming the corpus striatum, and the GLOBUS PALLIDUS. Such cells are concerned with modifying and coordinating voluntary muscle movements. *B. metabolic rate* abbreviated CMR. An indirect method of estimating the rate of metabolism in the body by measuring the oxygen intake and carbon dioxide output on breathing. The age, sex, weight, and size of the patient have to be taken into account.

base (bays) 1.the lowest part or foundation. 2. the main constituent of a compound. 3. an alkali or other substance that can unite with an acid to form a salt.

basement membrane ('baysmənt) a thin layer of modified connective tissue supporting layers of cells, found at the base of the epidermis and underlying mucous membranes.

basilar ('basələ) situated at the base. *B. artery* midline artery at the base of the skull, formed by the junction of the vertebral arteries.

basilic (bə'silik) prominent. *B. vein* a large vein on the inner side of the arm.

basophil ('baysəˌfil) adj. *basophilic*. 1. any structure, cell, or histological element staining readily with basic dyes. 2. a granular leukocyte with an irregularly shaped, relatively pale-staining nucleus that is partially constricted into two lobes, and with cytoplasm containing coarse bluish-black granules of variable size. 3. a beta cell of the ADENOHYPOPHYSIS.

basophilia (ˌbaysəˈfili·ə) 1. an affinity of cells or tissues for basic dyes. 2. the reaction of relatively immature erythrocytes to basic dyes whereby the stained cells appear blue, grey, or greyish-blue, or bluish granules appear. 3. abnormal increase of basophilic leukocytes in the blood. 4. basophilic leukocytosis.

Batchelor plaster (ˈbachələ) *J.S. Batchelor, British surgeon*. A double abduction plaster of Paris splint used in the correction of congenital dislocation of the hip.

bath (bahth) 1. a medium, e.g. water, vapour, sand, or mud, with which the body is washed or in which the body is wholly or partially immersed for therapeutic or cleansing purposes; application of such a medium to the body. 2. the equipment or apparatus in which a body or object may be immersed. *Bed b***.** washing a patient in bed. *Emollient b.* a bath in a soothing and softening liquid, used in various skin disorders. It is prepared by adding soothing agents such as gelatin, starch, bran or similar substances to the bath water, for the purpose of relieving skin irritation and pruritis. The patient is dried by patting rather than rubbing the skin. Care must be taken to avoid chilling. *Hot b.* one in water at 36–44°C. Care must be taken to avoid faintness. *Sponge b.* one in which the patient's body is not immersed but is wiped with a wet cloth or sponge. Sponge baths are most often employed for reduction of body temperature in the presence of a fever, in which case the water used is tepid and might contain alcohol to increase evaporation of moisture from the skin. *Tepid b.* one in water at 30–33°C. *Warm b.* one in water at 32–40°C. *Whirlpool b.* (Jacuzzi) one in which the water is kept in constant motion by mechanical means. It has a gentle massaging action that promotes relaxation.

BCG vaccine (ˌbeeceeˈgee) bacille Calmette–Guérin vaccine, a tuberculosis vaccine containing live, attenuated bovine tubercle bacilli (*Mycobacterium bovis*).

'bearing down' (ˌbair·ringˈdown) 1. the expulsive pains in the second stage of labour. 2. a feeling of heaviness and downwards strain in the pelvis, present with some uterine growths or displacements.

beat (beet) pulsation of the heart or an artery. *Apex b.* pulsation of the heart felt over its apex. The beat of the heart is felt against the chest wall. *Dropped b.* the occasional loss of a ventricular beat. *Ectopic b.* one that originates somewhere other than the SINOATRIAL NODE.

Beck inventory of depression (bek) abbreviated BID. A self-scoring system used to determine the presence of depression.

beclomethasone dipropionate (ˌbeklohˈmethəzohn) a glucocorticoid administered by aerosol inhalation or spinhaler to patients who require corticosteroids for control of bronchial asthma symptoms.

becquerel (ˈbekərəl) abbreviated Bq. The SI unit of radioactivity equal to the quantity of material undergoing one disintegration per second; 3.7×10^{10} becquerels is equal to 1 curie.

bed (bed) 1. a supporting structure

or tissue. 2. a couch or support for the body during sleep. *Capillary b.* the capillaries of a tissue, area or organ considered collectively, and their volume capacity. *B. cradle* a frame placed over the body of a bed patient. *See* CRADLE. *Fracture b.* a bed for the use of patients with broken bones. *Nail b.* the area of modified epidermis beneath the nail over which the nail plate slides as it grows.

bedbug ('bed,bug) a bug of the genus *Cimex*, a flattened, oval, reddish insect that inhabits houses, furniture and neglected beds, and feeds on humans, usually at night.

bedpan ('bed,pan) a shallow vessel used for defaecation or urination by patients confined to bed.

bed rest ('bed,rest) limiting the patient to staying in bed for a prescribed period for therapeutic reasons.

bedsore ('bed,saw) an ulcer-like sore caused by prolonged pressure of the patient's body. Pressure sore is now the preferred term because these sores are primarily due to pressure and can also occur in patients who are not confined to bed. A decubitus ulcer.

bed-wetting ('bed,weting) enuresis; involuntary voiding of urine. *See also* ENURESIS.

bee sting (bee sting) injury caused by the venom of a bee. Symptoms of a severe allergic reaction, such as collapse or swelling of the body, indicate ANAPHYLAXIS and require that medical help be sought.

behaviour (bee'hayvyə, bə-) the way in which an organism reacts to an internal or external stimulus. *B. disorders* can take many forms, such as truancy, stealing, temper tantrums. *Incongruous b.* behaviour that is out of keeping with the person's normal reaction or has the opposite to that consciously desired. *B. modification* an approach to correction of undesirable behaviour that focuses on changing observable actions. Modification of the behaviour is accomplished through systematic manipulation of the environmental and behavioural variables related to the specific behaviour to be changed. *B. therapy* a therapeutic approach in which the focus is on the patient's observable behaviour rather than on conflict and unconscious processes presumed to underlie the maladaptive behaviour. This is accomplished through systematic manipulation of the environmental and behavioural variables related to the specific behaviour to be modified; operant conditioning, systematic desensitisation, token economy, aversive control, flooding, and implosion are examples of techniques that can be used in behaviour therapy.

behaviourism (bee'hayvyə,rizəm, bə-) the purely objective study and observation of the behaviour of individuals.

bejel ('bayjəl) a non-venereal infectious form of syphilis caused by a TREPONEMA indistinguishable from that causing syphilis. Occurs mainly in children of Africa and the Middle East. The primary lesion is on the mouth, spreading to the trunk, arms and legs. Treated with penicillin.

belching ('belching) the noisy expulsion of gas from the stomach through the mouth. Eructation.

beliefs (,bə'leefs) thoughts, ideas, and concepts developed by an individual over a period of time from cultural influences, education, religion, parents, and family. *Health b.* those beliefs held by an individual regarding the maintenance of his or her state of physical wellbeing, which can be at variance with those beliefs held by the healthcare practitioner, possibly leading to conflict and non-compliance with prescribed treatment.

belladonna (ˌbelə'donə) a drug from the deadly nightshade plant. Used as an antispasmodic in colic, to check secretions, and to dilate the pupil of the eye.

Bell's palsy (belz) *Sir C. Bell, British physiologist, 1774–1842*. Facial paralysis due to oedema of the facial nerve.

belle indifference (ˌbel in'difə·ronhs) [Fr.] an indication of conversion hysteria, in which the patient describes symptoms, appearing not to be distressed by them.

Bendrofluazide (ˌbendroh'flooəˌzied) an oral diuretic of the thiazide group. Used primarily to treat mild hypertension and cardiac failure.

bends (bendz) a colloquial term for caisson disease. Decompression sickness.

benign (bə'nien) 1. the opposite to malignant. 2. describes a non-invasive condition or illness that is not serious even though treatment might be required for health or cosmetic reasons.

benorylate (bə'nawrəlayt) an ester of paracetamol and aspirin used as an anti-inflammatory and analgesic.

benzalkonium chloride (ˌbenzal'kohnee·əm) a quaternary ammonium compound used as a surface disinfectant and detergent and as a topical antiseptic and antibiotic preservative. Incompatible with soap.

benzathine penicillin (ˌbenzətheen pene'silən) a long-acting antibiotic. Used in treatment of Gram-positive infections. Can be given orally or intramuscularly.

benzene ('benzeen) benzol. A coal-tar derivative widely used as a solvent.

benzhexol (benz'heksol) an antispasmodic drug that helps to overcome the tremors and ridigity of PARKINSON'S DISEASE.

benzocaine ('benzəˌkayn) a surface anaesthetic used for the relief of pain or to anaesthetise the oropharynx or anus. Available as lozenges or ointment.

benzyl benzoate (ˌbenzəl'benzoh·ayt, -ziel) an emulsion used in the treatment of scabies.

benzylpenicillin (ˌbenzəlˌpenə'silən, ˌbenziel-) a widely used soluble penicillin that is quickly absorbed. High blood levels can therefore be obtained.

bereavement (bə'reev·mənt) the experience of suffering loss, usually of a loved one by death or separation, but can also include the loss of previous good health, position, or wealth. Produces a psychological reaction that has recognised 'stages' that can overlap, including anger, denial, disbelief and, finally, acceptance. Collectively recognised as mourning.

beriberi (ˌberee'beree) a deficiency disease due to insufficiency of vitamin B_1 (thiamine) in the diet. The disease is more common in areas where refined rice is the main staple in the diet. It is a form of neuritis, with pain, paralysis, and oedema of the extremities.

berry aneurysm (bəree 'anyə,rizəm) small, saccular dilation of the wall of a cerebral artery.

beryliiosis (bə,rilee'ohsəs) an industrial lung disease due to inhalation of the metallic element beryllium. Interstitial fibrosis arises, impairing lung function.

beta ('beetə) the second letter in the Greek alphabet, β. *B. blockers* drugs used to block the action of adrenaline on beta-adrenergic receptors in cardiac muscle, thus decreasing the workload of the heart. *B. cells* insulin-producing cells found in the ISLETS OF LANGERHANS in the pancreas. *B. rays* electrons used therapeutically for treatment of lesions of the cornea and iris. *B. receptors* associated with the inhibition (relaxation) of smooth muscle. They also bring an increase in the force of contraction and rate of the heart.

Betadine ('betə,deen, -din) trade name for preparations of povidone-iodine, which have a longer antiseptic action than most iodine solutions.

betamethasone (beetə'methə,zohn) a synthetic glucocorticoid which is the most active of the anti-inflammatory steroids.

bethanechol (bə'thanə,kol) a derivative of a choline-like substance, used in the treatment of abdominal distension and urinary retention. Hypotension and DYSPNOEA can occur as side-effects.

bethanidine (bə'thanə,deen) an adrenergic blocking agent used in the treatment of hypertension.

Betnovate ('betnəvayt) trade name for preparations containing betamethasone. Used in the treatment of severe inflammatory skin disorders unresponsive to less potent corticosteroids.

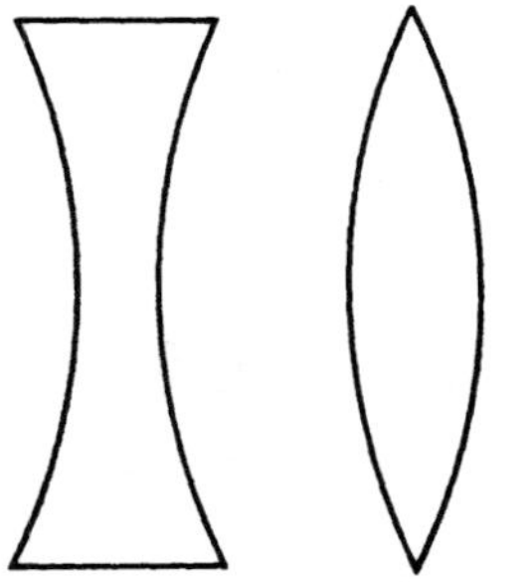

Betz cells (bets) *V.A. Betz, Russian anatomist, 1834–1894.* The pyramidal cells in the precentral area of the cerebrum.

bezoar ('beezaw) a mass of hair, fruit, or vegetable fibres sometimes found in the stomach or intestines.

bias ('bieəs) a distortion in the results of data analysis.

bicarbonate (bie'kahbə,nayt, -nət) any salt containing the HCO_3^- anion. *Blood b., plasma b.* the bicarbonate of the blood plasma, an important parameter of ACID–CASE CALANCE measured in blood gas analysis.

bicellular (bie'selyələ) composed of two cells.

biceps ('bieseps) a muscle with two heads; a flexor of the arm; one of the hamstring muscles of the thigh.

biconcave (bie'konkayv) pertaining to a lens or other structure with a hollow or depression on each surface (*see* figure).

biconvex (bie'konveks) pertaining to a lens or other structure that protrudes on both surfaces (*see* figure on p. 55).

bicornuate (bie'kawnyooət) having two horns. *B. uterus* a congenital malformation in which there is a partial or complete vertical division into two parts of the body of the uterus.

bicuspid (bie'kuspəd) having two cusps or projections. *B. teeth* the premolars. *B. valve* the mitral valve of the heart between the left atrium and left ventricle.

bidet ('beeday) a low narrow basin on a stand for washing the perineum and genitalia.

bifid ('biefəd) divided or cleft into two parts.

bifocal (bie'fohkəl) having two foci, as with spectacles in which the lenses have two different foci.

bifurcate (bie'fərkayt) to divide into two branches; arteries bifurcate frequently, thereby getting smaller.

bifurcation (ˌbie'jemən') the junction where a vessel divides into two branches, e.g. where the aorta divides into the right and left iliac vessels.

bigeminal (ˌbie'jemən'l) double. *B. pulse* two pulse beats which occur together, regular in time and force. A regular irregularity.

biguanides (bie'gwahniedz) oral hypoglycaemic agents for treating diabetes. They exert their effect by decreasing GLUCONEOGENESIS in muscle tissue. Effective only in those diabetics with functioning ISLET OF LANGERHANS cells. Most commonly used in non-insulin dependent diabetics, especially those who are overweight.

bilateral (bie'latə·rəl) pertaining to both sides.

bile (biel) a secretion of the liver, greenish-yellow to brown in colour. It is concentrated in the gall bladder and passes into the small intestine, where it assists digestion by emulsifying fats and stimulates peristalsis. *B. ducts* the canals or passageways that conduct bile. The hepatic and cystic ducts join to form the common bile duct. *B. pigments* bilirubin and biliverdin, produced by haemolysis in the spleen. Normally these colour the faeces only, but in jaundice the skin and urine can also become coloured. *B. salts* sodium taurocholate and sodium glycocholate, which cause the emulsification of fats.

Bilharzia (bil'hahtsi·ə) *T.M. Bilharz, German physician, 1825–62.* A genus of blood fluke now known as *Schistosoma*.

bilharziasis (ˌbilhaht'sieəsəs) SCHISTOSOMIASIS.

biliary ('bilyə·ree) pertaining to bile. *B. colic* spasm of muscle walls of the bile duct causing excruciating pain when gallstones are blocking the tube. Pain is in the right upper quadrant of the abdomen and referred to the shoulder. *B. fistula* an abnormal opening between the gall bladder and the surface of the body.

biliousness ('bileeəsˌnəs) a symptom complex comprised of nausea, abdominal discomfort, headache, and constipation.

bilirubin (ˌbilee'roobən) an orange bile pigment produced by the breakdown of haem and reduction of biliverdin; it normally circulates in plasma and is taken up by liver cells and conjugated to form bilirubin diglucuronide, the water-soluble pigment excreted in the bile. Bilirubin can be classified as indirect ('free' or unconjugated) while en route to the liver from its site of formation by reticuloendothelial cells, and direct (bilirubin diglucuronide) after its conjugation in the liver with glucuronic acid. Normally the body produces a total of about 260 mg of bilirubin per day. Almost 99% of this is excreted in the faeces; the remaining 1% is excreted in the urine as UROBILINOGEN. The typical yellowness of jaundice is caused by the accumulation of bilirubin in the blood and body tissues.

bilirubinaemia (ˌbileeˌroobə'nee-mi·ə) the presence of bilirubin in the blood.

biliuria (ˌbilee'yoo·ri·ə) bile or bile salts in the urine.

biliverdin (ˌbilee'vərdən) a green bile pigment, the oxidised form of bilirubin.

Billings method ('bilingz) a method of contraception. Ovulation time is estimated by observing changes in the cervical mucus that occur during the menstrual cycle.

bimanual (bie'manyooəl) using both hands. *B. examination* examination with both hands. Used chiefly in gynaecology, when the internal genital organs are examined between one hand on the abdomen, and the other hand or a finger within the vagina.

binary ('bienə·ree) made up of two parts. *B. fission* the multiplication of cells by division into two equal parts. *B. scale* one used in calculating, in which only two digits, 0 and 1, are used. Digital computers use this scale.

binaural (bie'nawrəl) pertaining to both ears. *B. stethoscope. See* STETHOSCOPE.

Binet's test ('beenayz) *A. Binet, French physiologist, 1857–1911.* A method of ascertaining the mental age of children or young persons by using a series of questions standardised on the capacity of normal children at various ages.

Bing test (bing) *A. Bing, German otologist, 1844–1922.* A vibrating tuning fork is held to the mastoid process and the auditory meatus is alternately occluded and left open; an increase and decrease in loudness (positive Bing) is perceived by the normal ear and in sensorineural hearing impairment, but in conductive hearing impairment no difference in loudness is perceived (negative Bing).

binocular (bə'nokyələ, bie-) relating to both eyes.

binovular (bə'novyələ) derived from two ova. *B. twins* twins, who might or might not be of different sexes.

bioassay (ˌbieoh'asay) biological assay. The use of animals or an isolated organ preparation to determine the effect of the active power of a sample of a drug. Comparison is made with the effect of a standard preparation.

biochemistry (ˌbieoh'keməstree) the chemistry of living matter.

biofeedback (ˌbieoh'feedˌbak) visual or auditory evidence provided to an individual of the satisfactory performance of an autonomic body function, e.g. sounding a tone when blood pressure is at a satisfactory level, so that, through conditioning, the patient might assert control over that function.

biogenesis (ˌbieoh'jenəsəs) 1. the origin of life. 2. the theory that living organisms can originate only from those already living and cannot be artificially produced.

biohazard ('bieoh,hazəd) any hazard arising from inadvertent human biological processes, e.g. accidental inoculation, needle-stick injury.

biology (bie'oləjee) the science of living organisms, dealing with their structure, function and relations with one another.

biometrics, biometry (,bieə'metriks; bie'omətree) 1. anthropometry. 2. the use of statistics in biological science.

biomicroscopy (,bieohmie'kroskəpee) a microscopic examination of living tissues, e.g. of the structures of the anterior of the eye during life. *See* SLIT LAMP.

bionics (bie'oniks) the application of electronic devices to medical problems, e.g. artificial pacemakers.

bioplasm ('bieoh,plazəm) protoplasm. The active principle in matter which produces living organisms.

biopsy ('bieopsee) the removal of some tissue or organ from the living body, e.g. a lymph gland, for examination to establish a diagnosis. *Aspiration b.* biopsy in which the tissue is obtained by suction through a needle and syringe. *Cone b.* biopsy in which an inverted cone of tissue is excised, as from the uterine cervix. *Excisional b.* removal of an entire lesion and significant portion of normal-looking tissue for examination. *Needle b.* tissue obtained by the puncture of a lesion with a needle. Rotation of the needle removes tissue within the lumen of the needle. *Punch b.* tissue obtained by a punch.

biorhythm ('bieoh,ridhəm) any cyclic, biological event, e.g. sleep cycle and menstrual cycle, affecting daily life.

biosensors ('bieoh,sensəz) non-invasive instruments that measure the result of biological processes, e.g. body temperature.

biostatistics (,bieohstə'tistiks) that branch of biometry that deals with the data and laws of human mortality, morbidity, natality, and demography; called also vital statistics.

biosynthesis (,bieoh'sinthəsəs) the creation of a compound within a living organism.

biotin ('bieətən) formerly termed vitamin H, now part of the vitamin B complex and present in all normal diets.

biparietal (biepə'rieət'l) pertaining to both parietal eminences or bones.

biparous (bie'parəs) giving birth to two infants at a time.

biphasic (bie'fazik) having two parts or aspects.

bipolar (bie'pohlə) with two poles. *B. nerve cells* cells having two nerve fibres, e.g. ganglionic cells.

birth (bərth) the act of being born. *B. control* limiting the size of the family by abstention from sexual intercourse or the use of contraceptives. *B. mark* a naevus present from birth.

birthing chair ('bərthing) a specially designed chair for use in labour and delivery to promote greater mobility for the mother.

birthing pool ('bərthing) a specially designed pool allowing mothers to give birth under water.

bisacodyl (,bisə'kohdəl) a laxative that acts directly on the rectum. Given as tablets or in the form of suppositories.

bisexual (,bie'sekshyooəl) 1. having gonads of both sexes. 2. hermaphrodite. 3. having both active and passive sexual interests or characteristics. 4. capable of the function of both sexes. 5. both heterosexual and homosexual. 6. an individual who is both heterosexual and homosexual. 7. of, relating to or involving both sexes, as in bisexual reproduction.

bismuth ('bizməth) symbol Bi. A greyish metallic element. Certain of its salts are used as gastric sedatives.

bistoury ('bistə·ree) a slender surgical knife, sometimes curved.

bite (biet) 1. to seize with the teeth. 2. a wound made by biting. 3. an impression made by the teeth on a thin sheet of malleable material such as wax.

Bitot's spots ('beetohz) *P.A. Bitot, French physician, 1822–88.* Collections of dried epithelium, microorganisms, etc., forming shiny, greyish spots on the cornea. A sign of vitamin A deficiency.

bivalve (bie,valv) 1. having two valves, as the shells of molluscs such as oysters. 2. to cut a plaster cast into an anterior and a posterior section. *B. speculum* a vaginal speculum with two blades that can be adjusted for easy insertion.

blackhead ('blak,hed) a COMEDO.

blackout ('blakowt) momentary failure of vision and unconsciousness due to cerebral circulatory insufficiency.

blackwater fever ('blak,wawtə) a form of malignant malaria in which severe haemolysis causes a dark discolouration of the urine.

bladder ('bladə) a membranous sac for holding fluid or gas. *Atonic b.* a condition in which there is lack of tone in the bladder wall, which might be the result of incomplete emptying over a long period. *Gall b.* the reservoir for bile. *Irritable b.* a condition in which there is frequent desire to micturate. *Urinary b.* the reservoir for urine. *B. worm* a cysticercus.

Blalock–Taussig operation (,blaylok'tawsig) *A. Blalock, American surgeon, 1899–1964; H.B. Taussig, American paediatrician, 1898–1986.* Operation in which the subclavian artery is anastomosed to the pulmonary artery. Performed in Fallot's tetralogy.

bland (bland) non-stimulating. *B. fluids* mild and non-irritating fluids such as barley water and milk.

blast (blahst) 1. an immature cell. 2. a wave of high air pressure caused by an explosion.

blastocyst ('blastə,sist) BLASTULA.

blastocyte ('blastə,siet) an embryonic cell that has not yet become differentiated into its specific type.

blastoderm ('blastə,derm) the germinal cells of the embryo consisting of three layers: the ectoderm, mesoderm, and entoderm.

blastolysis (bla'stoləsəs, ,blastə'liesəs) the destruction of germ substance.

blastomycosis (,blastohmie'kohsəs) a fungal infection which, after invasion of the skin, can cause granulomatous lesions in the mouth, pharynx, and lungs.

blastula ('blastyələ) BLASTOCYST. An early stage in the development of the fertilised ovum. This stage precedes the gastrula.

bleb (bleb) a blister.

bleeder ('bleedə) 1. a popular name for one who suffers from HAEMOPHILIA. 2. a vessel that is difficult to seal at operation.

bleeding ('bleeding) 1. escape of blood from an injured vessel. 2. venesection. *Functional b.* bleeding from the uterus when no organic lesion is present. *B. time* the time taken for oozing to cease from a sharp prick of the finger or ear lobe. The normal value is 1–3 min.

blennorhagia (ˌblenə'rayji·ə) 1. an excessive discharge of mucus, e.g. LEUCORRHOEA. 2. GONORRHOEA.

blennorrhoea (ˌblenə'reeə) blenorrhagia.

bleomycin (ˌblio'miesən) an anti-tumour antibiotic drug especially effective against squamous cell carcinoma.

blepharitis (ˌblefə'rietəs) inflammation of the eyelids. *Allergic b.* that associated with response to drugs or cosmetics applied to the eye or eyelids. *Squamous b.* that associated with dandruff of the scalp.

blepharon ('blefə·ron) the eyelid.

blepharophimosis (ˌblefə·rohfie-'mohsəs) abnormal narrowing of the aperture between the eyelids. Usually congenital but can arise from chronic inflammation.

blepharoptosis (ˌblefə·rop'tohsəs) drooping of the upper eyelid.

blepharospasm (ˌblefə·roh'spazəm) prolonged spasm of the orbicular muscles of the eyelids.

blind (bliend) without sight. *B. spot* the point where the optic nerve leaves the retina, which is insensitive to light. PUNCTUM caecum.

blind loop syndrome (bliend 'loop) a condition of stasis in the small intestine, which aids bacterial multiplication, leading to diarrhoea and salt deficiencies. The cause might be intestinal obstruction or surgical ANASTOMOSIS.

blindness ('bliendnəs) lack or loss of ability to see; lack of perception of visual stimuli. Legally, blindness is defined as less than 6/60 vision with glasses (vision of 6/60 is the ability to see only at 6 metres what the normal eye can see at 60 metres).

blister ('blis'tə) a bleb or vesicle. A collection of serum between the epidermis and the skin. *Blood b.* a blister containing blood, usually caused by a pinch or bruise.

bloat (bloht) filling with gas.

block (blok) a stoppage or obstruction. The term is used to describe (1) various forms of regional anaesthesia, e.g. epidural block; (2) obstruction to the passage of a nervous impulse due to disease, e.g. heart block (*see* HEART); (3) an interruption of mental function.

blood (blud) the fluid that circulates through the heart and blood vessels, supplying nutritive material to all parts of the body and carrying away waste products. Blood is a red viscid fluid and consists of plasma in which are suspended erythrocytes (red blood cells), leucocytes (white blood cells) and lymphocytes, and platelets or thrombocytes. (a) The red corpuscles or ERYTHROCYTES contain haemoglobin, which combines with oxygen in passing through the lungs. This oxygen is released into the tissues from the capillaries and oxidation takes place. (b) The white corpuscles or LEUKOCYTES defend against invading mircoorganisms, which they have power to destroy. (c) Blood platelets or THROMCOCYTES are concerned with the clotting of blood. Plasma also contains many other specialised substances that have important roles

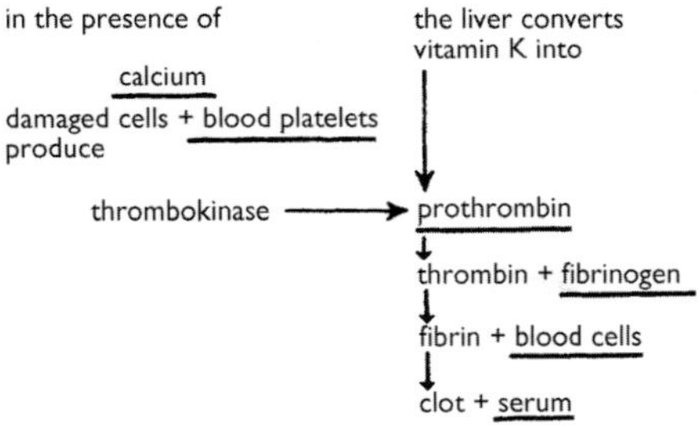

Clotting of Blood
Underlined substances are normally present in blood

to play in immunity and clotting of blood.

blood bank 1. a place of storage for blood. 2. an organisation that collects, processes, stores, and transfuses blood. In most hospitals the blood bank is located in the pathology laboratory.

blood–brain barrier abbreviated BBB. The membranous barrier separating the blood from the brain. It is permeable to water, oxygen, carbon dioxide, glucose, alcohol, general anaesthetics, and some drugs.

blood casts casts of coagulated red blood cells formed in the renal tubules and found in the urine.

blood clotting, coagulation the formation of a jelly-like substance over the ends or within the walls of a blood vessel, with resultant stoppage of the blood flow. Clotting is one of the natural defence mechanisms of the body when injury occurs. A clot will usually form within 5 minutes of a blood vessel being damaged. The exact process of clotting is not known but it is believed that the mechanism is triggered by the platelets, which disintegrate as they pass over rough places in the injured surface. If normal amounts of calcium, platelets, and tissue factors are present (*see* figure), prothrombin is converted to thrombin. Thrombin then acts as a catalyst for the change of fibrinogen into a mesh of insoluble fibrin, in which are embedded erythrocytes and leukocytes and small amounts of fluid (serum). Plasma coagulation factors are:

I Fibrinogen
II Prothrombin
III Tissue thromboplastin
IV Calcium ions
VII Factor VII
VIII Antihaemophilic factor (afh)
IX Christmas factor
X Stuart factor (Power factor)
XI Plasma thromboplastin antecedent (PTA)
XII Hageman factor
XIII Fibrin-stabilising factor

ABO system

Group	*Antigen present in red cell*	*Antibody present in plasma*
AB	A and B	—
A	A	Anti-B (β)
B	B	Anti-A (α)
O	—	Anti-A and Anti-B (α and β)

blood count the number of blood cells in a given sample of blood, usually expressed as the number of cells per litre of blood (as the red blood cell, white blood cell, or platelet count). A differential white cell count determines the number of various types of leukocyte in a sample of blood, *see* appendix 4.

blood gas gas dissolved in the liquid part of the blood, including oxygen, carbon dioxide, and nitrogen.

blood glucose the amount of glucose present in the blood. The normal range is 3.0–5.8 mmol/litre. When the amount exceeds 10 mmol/litre, glucose is excreted in the urine, as in DIABETES mellitus. *B. g. meter* instrument used to monitor blood glucose levels. *See* GLUCOMETER.

blood group ABO system (*see* table). In clinical practice there are four main blood types: A, B, O, and AB. In addition to this major grouping there is a rhesus (Rh) system that is important in the prevention of haemolytic disease of the newborn resulting from incompatibility of blood groups in mother and fetus. In determining blood group, a sample of blood is taken and mixed with specially prepared sera. One serum, anti-A agglutinin, causes blood of group A to agglutinate; another serum, anti-B agglutinin, causes blood of group B to agglutinate. Thus, if anti-A serum alone causes clumping, the blood is group A; if anti-B serum alone causes clumping, the blood group is B. If both cause clumping, the blood group is AB, and if it is not clumped by either, it is identified as group O. Transfusion with an incompatible ABO group causes severe haemolytic reaction and death can occur.

blood pressure abbreviated BP. The pressure exerted on the artery walls by the blood as it flows through them. It can be measured in milligrams of mercury using a sphygmomanometer. Two readings are made. Arterial pressure fluctuates with each heartbeat. One measure records the pressure while the heart is in SYSTOLE (when the heart is ejecting blood into the arteries); this is the higher, or systolic, pressure. The other measure records the pressure while the heart is in DIASTOLE (when the aortic and pulmonary valves are closed and the heart is relaxed); this is the lower, or diastolic, pressure. The range of normal blood pressure recording varies according to age and body size, but in the normal young adult is approximately: 100–120/70–80 mm Hg.

blood sugar *See* BLOOD GLUCOSE.

blood transfusion introduction of blood from the vein of one person (donor) or from a blood bank into the vein of another (recipient) in cases of severe loss of blood, trauma, septicaemia, etc. It is used to supplement the volume of blood and also to introduce constituents, such as clotting factors or antibodies, that are deficient in the patient. Clotting must be prevented in the transition stage. This is usually done by admixture with sodium citrate (1 g to 459 mL of blood). Too much sodium citrate tends to produce a reaction: rigor and shock can occur.

blood urea excretory product of protein present in the blood. The normal range is 3–7 mmol/litre; this increases in renal failure when the kidneys cease to function normally.

'blue baby' (bloo) a child born with a very blue colour. The colour can be due to ATELECTASIS or to a defect in the heart, in consequence of which arterial and venous blood become mixed. *See* FALLOT'S TETRALOGY.

blush (blush) growing redness of the face, usually a reaction to emotion or heat.

BMR basal metabolic rate.

body ('bodee) 1. the trunk, or animal frame, with its organs. 2. the largest and most important part of any organ. 3. any mass or collection of material.

body image the total concept, including conscious and unconscious feelings, thoughts, and perceptions, that a person has of his or her own body as an object in space, which is independent and apart from other objects.

body language the expression of thoughts or emotions by means of posture or gestures. Body language can include unintended 'signs' as well as intended communication. Detailed studies of human nonverbal communication have been documented by several observers.

body mass index abbreviated BMI. The weight (kg) divided by the square of the height (m).

Boeck's disease (beks) *C.P.M. Boeck, Norwegian dermatologist, 1845–1917.* SARCOIDOSIS.

boil (boyl) an acute staphylococcal inflammation of the skin and subcutaneous tissues around a hair follicle. It causes a painful swelling with a central core of dead tissue (slough), which is eventually discharged. A FURUNCLE.

bolus ('bohləs) 1. a large pill. 2. a rounded mass of masticated food immediately before being swallowed or one passing through the intestines. 3. a quantity of a drug injected directly to raise its concentration in the blood to a therapeutic level.

bonding ('bonding) the attachment process that occurs between an infant and its parents, especially the mother, during the first hours and days following birth. Bonding is a reciprocal process and is a biological need for the future of both the physical and the emotional development of the infant.

bone (bohn) the dense connective tissue forming the skeleton. It is composed of cartilage or membrane impregnated with mineral salts, chiefly calcium phosphate and calcium carbonate. This is arranged as an outer hard compact tissue and an inner network of cells (cancellous tissue), in the spaces of which is red bone marrow. In the shaft of long bones is a medullary cavity containing yellow marrow. Microscopically, the bone tissue is perforated with minute HAVERSIAN CANALS containing blood vessels and lymphatics for the maintenance and repair of the cells (*see* figure). Bone is covered by a fibrous membrane, the PERIOSTEUM, containing blood vessels and by which the bone grows in girth. *B. graft* transplantation of a healthy piece of bone to replace missing or repair defective bone. *B. marrow* substance which fills the marrow cavities of bones. Basically there are two types: yellow and red marrow. The red marrow is responsible for producing the blood cells. *B. marrow transplantation* a procedure used to treat aplastic anaemia, acute leukaemia, and some rare congenital disorders, with varying success. Healthy bone marrow is taken from the donor and infused into the bloodstream of the recipient, where it 'homes' into the bone marrow, where it will grow. Histocompatibility between the donor (usually a sibling) and recipient is essential.

borax ('baw·raks) a compound of soda and boric acid. Used as a mild antiseptic and as a mouthwash.

borborygmus (ˌbawbə'rigməs) a rumbling sound caused by gas in the intestines.

Bordetella (ˌbawdə'telə) a genus of bacteria. *B. pertussis* the causal agent of whooping cough.

boric acid ('baw·rik) a mild antiseptic.

Bornholm disease ('bawnˌholm) an epidemic myalgia with pleural pain due to Coxsackie virus infection. It is named after the Danish island of Bornholm where there was an outbreak in 1930.

botulism ('botyəˌlizəm, 'bochə-) an extremely severe form of food poisoning due to a neurotoxin (botulin) produced by *Clostridium botulinum*, sometimes found in improperly canned or preserved foods. The symptoms include vomiting, abdominal pain, headache, weakness, constipation, and nerve paralysis, which causes difficulty in seeing, breathing, and swallowing. Death is usually due to paralysis of the respiratory organs.

bougie ('boozhee, boo'zhee) a flexible cylindrical instrument use to dilate a stricture, as in the oesophagus or urethra. *Medicated b.* a soluble form impregnated with a medicinal substance. Used for urethral treatment.

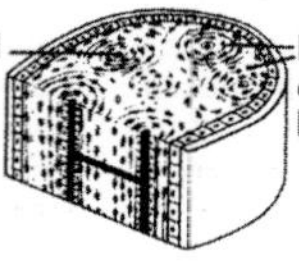

Structure of Compact Bone

bovine ('bohvien) relating to the cow or ox. *B. tuberculosis* that caused by infection from infected cows' milk, usually affecting glands and bones.

bowel ('bowəl) the intestine. *B. sounds* relatively high-pitched abdominal sounds caused by the propulsion of the intestinal contents through the lower alimentary canal.

bowleg ('boh͵leg) deformity in which there is an outwards curvature of one or both legs near the knee. This results in a gap between the knees on standing. *Genu varum*.

Bowman's capsule ('bohmənz) *Sir W.P. Bowman, British physician, 1816–92.* The expanded end of the kidney tubule, which surrounds the GLOMERULUS.

Boyle's anaesthetic machine (boylz) *H.E.G. Boyle, British surgeon, 1875–1941.* Apparatus by which gases, including chloroform, ether, nitrous oxide, and cyclopropane, can be administered.

Boyle's law *R. Boyle, British physicist, 1627–91.* Law stating that at any determined temperature a known mass of gas varies in volume inversely with the pressure.

brace (brays) 1. a support used in orthopaedics to hold parts of the body in their correct positions. 2. an orthodontic appliance to correct the alignment of teeth.

brachial ('brayki·əl, 'brak-) relating to the arm. *B. artery* the continuation of the axillary artery along the inner side of the upper arm. *B. plexus* a network of nerves at the root of the neck supplying the upper limb.

brachytherapy (͵braki'therəpee) radiotherapy delivered into or adjacent to a tumour by means of an intracavitary or interstitial radioactive source.

bradycardia (͵bradə'kahdi·ə) abnormally low rate of heart contractions and consequent slow pulse (fewer than 60 beats per minute).

bradykinin (͵bradə'kienən) peptide formed from the degradation of protein by enzymes. It is a powerful vasodilator that also causes contraction of smooth muscle.

braille (brayl) a method of printing developed by *Louis Braille* (1809–52) for the blind. Letters of the alphabet are represented by patterns of raised dots. These dots are read by passing the fingertips over them.

brain (brayn) that part of the central nervous system contained in the skull. It consists of the cerebrum, midbrain, cerebellum, MEDULLA OBLONGATA and PONS VAROLII.

brain stem the part of the central nervous system that connects the cerebral hemispheres with the spinal cord.

bran (bran) the husk of grain. The coarse outer coat of cereals. High in roughage and vitamins of the B complex. Frequently recommended as a dietary component both for those with alimentary disorders and for those in normal health.

branchial ('brangki·əl) relating to the clefts (branchia) that are present in the neck and pharynx in the developing embryo. Normally they disappear. *B. cyst* a cystic swelling arising from a branchial remnant in the neck. *B. sinus* (lateral cervical sinus) a track leading from the posterior cervical region to open in the lower neck in front of the sternomastoid muscle.

Braun's frame ('brawnz fraym) *H.F.W. Braun, German surgeon, 1862–1934.* A metal frame which incorporates one or more pulleys and is used to elevate the lower limb and to apply skeletal traction for a compound fracture of tibia and fibula.

Braxton Hicks contractions ('braks-tən hiks) *Braxton Hicks, British gynaecologist, 1823–97.* Painless uterine contractions occurring during pregnancy, becoming increasingly rhythmic and intense during the third trimester. Sometimes called 'false labour'.

breast (brest) 1. the anterior or front region of the chest. 2. the mammary gland. *B. access* formation of pus in the mammary gland. *B. bone* the sternum. *B. cancer* the breast is the most common site of malignant tumours in women. *B. feeding* the method of feeding a baby with milk directly from the mother's breasts. Midwives and paediatricians agree that breastfeeding is usually better for the baby and the mother, both physically and emotionally. *B. self-examination* a procedure in which a woman examines her breasts and accessory structures for evidence of change that could indicate a malignant process (*see* figure) *Pigeon b.* prominent sternum, a deformity resulting from rickets. *B. pump* an apparatus for removal of milk from the breast.

breath (breth) the air taken in and expelled by the expansion and contraction of the thorax.

breathing ('breedhing) the alternate inspiration and expiration of air into and out of the lungs (*see also* RESPIRATION).

breech (breech) the buttocks. *B. presentation* a position of the fetus in the uterus such that the buttocks present.

bregma ('bregmə) the anterior fontanelle. The membranous junction between the coronal and sagittal sutures.

bridge (brij) in dentistry, an irremovable prosthesis carrying false teeth that bridges gaps left when natural teeth are extracted.

Bright's disease (briets) *B. Bright, British physician, 1789–1858.* A broad description, once used for inflammation of the kidneys. Nephritis.

British Pharmacopoeia ('british ˌfahməkə'peeə) abbreviated BP. List of 'official' drugs, published by HM Stationery Office (UK).

broad ligaments (brawd) folds of peritoneum extending from the uterus to the sides of the pelvis, and supporting the blood vessels to the uterus and uterine tubes.

Broca's area of speech ('brohkəz) *P.P. Broca, French surgeon, 1824–80.* The motor centre for speech, situated in the left cerebral hemisphere. Damage to the nerve cells contained in it can impair speech.

Brodie's abscess (ˌbrohdeez) *Sir B.C. Brodie, British surgeon, 1783–1862.* A chronic abscess of bone.

bromhidrosis (ˌbromhə'drohsəs) offensive and fetid sweat.

bromide ('brohmied) a compound of bromide. Bromides are sedatives that are strongly depressant, cumulative in action, and can cause mental disturbances.

bromocriptine (ˌbrohmohˌkripteen) a dopamine agonist used in the treatment of Parkinsonism in cases in which LEVODOPA is not well tolerated.

Brompton cocktail ('bromptən 'koktayl) name given to mixtures containing various combinations of

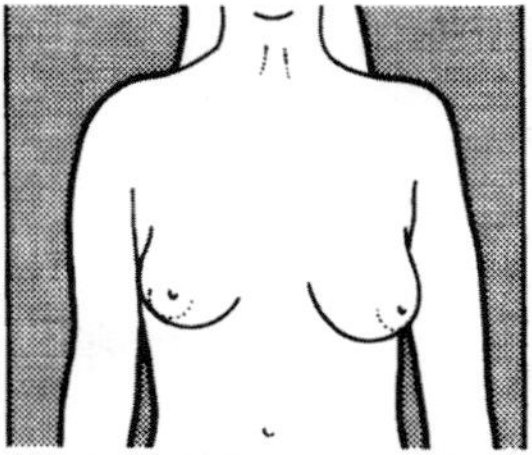

Any change in the shape and size of either breast or nipple should first be noted by looking in the mirror

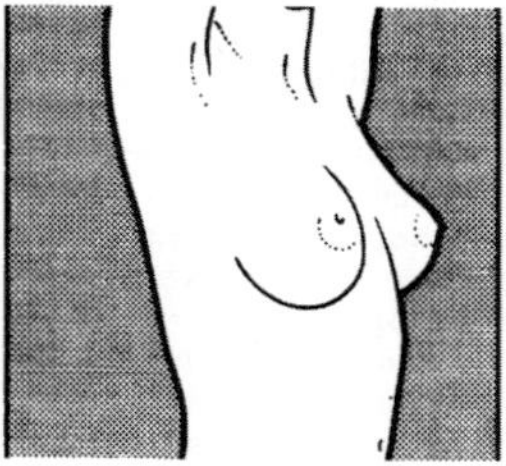

In front of the mirror, and with arms raised, view the breasts from different angles

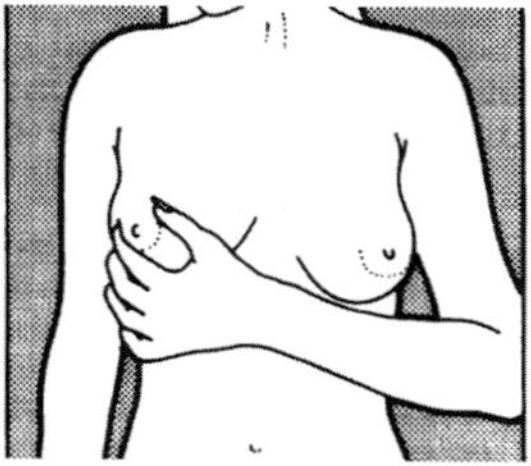

Squeeze each nipple gently, noting any discharge or bleeding

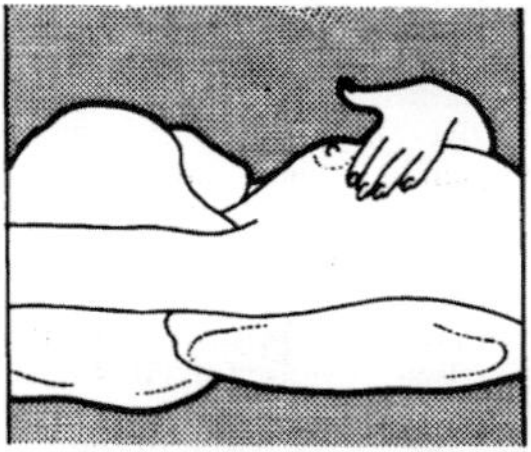

Lying down with a pillow or towel placed under the shoulder helps to spread the breast tissue for easier self-examination

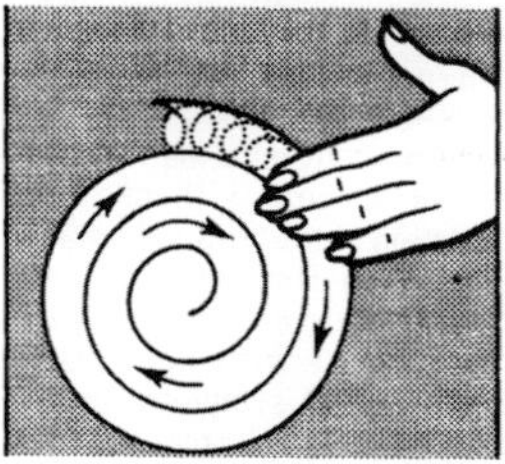

Rotate fingers in small circles and trace a spiral route around the breast to check for any lumps or unusual thickening

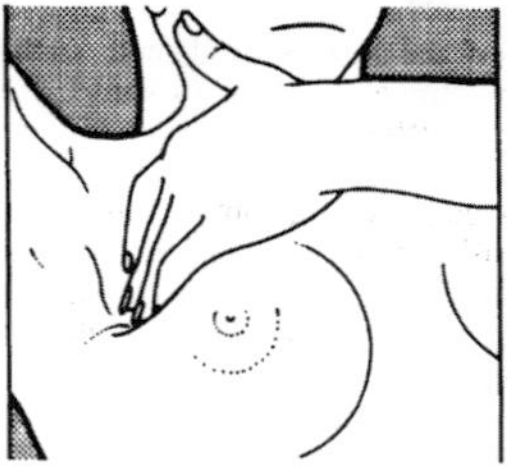

Finally, examine the armpits using the spiral technique and note any unusual findings

Breast Self-Examination

morphine, diamorphine, and cocaine. These mixtures often contained gin and/or chlorpromazine. They were used in the relief of pain in terminal care, but have now been replaced by a simple solution of morphine in chloroform water.

bromsulphthalein (ˌbromsulf'thayleen) a dye used in certain tests for liver function.

bronchi ('brongkee) plural of bronchus.

bronchiectasis (ˌbrongkee'ektəsəs) chronic dilatation of the bronchi and bronchioles with secondary infection, usually involving the lower lobes of the lung. The condition can occur as a congenital malformation of the alveoli with resultant dilatation of the terminal bronchi. Most often it is an acquired disease secondary to partial obstruction of the bronchi with necrotising infection. The symptoms include a chronic cough and purulent sputum.

bronchiole ('brongkee'ohl) one of the smallest of the subdivisions of the bronchi.

bronchiolitis (ˌbrongkeeoh'lietəs) inflammation of the bronchioles.

bronchitis (ˌbrong'kietəs) inflammation of the bronchi. *Acute b.* a short-lived infection, common in young children and the elderly. It is a descending infection from the common cold, influenza, measles, and other upper respiratory conditions. *Chronic b.* a chronic infection, usually associated with infection of the upper respiratory tract. It can, in time, lead to emphysema.

bronchoadenitis (ˌbrongkohˌadə'nietəs) inflammation of the bronchial glands.

bronchodilator (ˌbrongkohdie'laytə) any agent that causes dilatation of the bronchi.

bronchography (brong'kogrəfee) radiography of the bronchial tree after introduction of a radio-opaque medium.

bronchomycosis (ˌbrongkohmie'kohsəs) an industrial disease chiefly affecting agricultural workers, stablemen, etc., due to inhalation of microfungi which infect the air passages. Causes can be *Actinomyces* or *Aspergillus* species. Symptoms are similar to those of pulmonary tuberculosis.

bronchophony (brong'kofənee) resonance of the voice as heard in the chest over the bronchi on auscultation.

bronchopneumonia (ˌbrongkohnyoo'mohni·ə) *see* PNEUMONIA.

bronchopulmonary (ˌbrongkoh'pulmənə·ree, -'puhl) relating to the lungs, bronchi, and bronchioles.

bronchorrhoea (ˌbrongkə'reeə) an excessive discharge of mucus from the bronchi.

bronchoscope ('brongkohˌskohp) an endoscope that enables the operator to see inside the bronchi. It can also be used to wash out the bronchi, to remove foreign bodies, or to take a biopsy.

bronchoscopy (brong'koskəˌpee) examination of the bronchi by means of a bronchoscope.

bronchospasm (ˌbrongkohˌspazəm) difficulty in breathing caused by the sudden constriction of smooth muscle in the walls of the bronchi. This can occur in asthma or chronic bronchitis.

bronchospirometer (ˌbrongkohspie'romətə) an instrument used to measure the capacity of one lung or of one lobe of the lung, or of each lung separately.

bronchotracheal (ˌbrongkoh-'trakeeəl, ˌbrongkohtrə'keeəl) relating to both the trachea and the bronchi. *B. suction* the removal of mucus with the aid of suction.

bronchus (ˌbrongkəs) any of the larger passages conveying air to (right or left principal bronchus) and within (lobar and segmental bronchi) the lungs.

brow (brow) the forehead. *B. presentation* a position of the fetus such that the forehead appears at the cervix first.

brown fat (brown) special type of adipose tissue found in the newborn infant, and which is widely distributed throughout the body. The tissue is highly vascular and owes its colour to the large number of mitochondria found in the cytoplasm of its cells. It allows the infant to increase its metabolic rate and thus its heat production when subjected to cold. At the same time the fat itself is used up.

Brown-Séquard's syndrome (brown 'saykahdz) *C.E. Brown-Séquard, French physiologist, 1818–94*. Paralysis and loss of discriminatory and joint sensation on one side of the body and of pain and temperature sensation on the other, due to a lesion involving one side of the spinal cord.

Brucella (broo'selə) a genus of bacteria primarily pathogenic in animals but which can affect humans.

brucellosis (ˌbroosə'lohsəs) a generalised infection involving primarily the reticuloendothelial system, marked by remittent undulant fever, malaise, headache, and anaemia. It is caused by various species of *Brucella* and is transmitted to humans from domestic animals such as pigs, goats, and cattle, especially through infected milk or contact with the carcass of an infected animal. The disease is also called undulant fever because one of the major symptoms in humans is a fever that fluctuates widely at regular intervals. Prevention is best accomplished by the pasteurisation of milk and a program of testing, vaccination, and elimination of infected animals. Called also Malta fever, abortus fever, and Mediterranean fever.

Brudzinski's sign (broo'jinskeez) *J. Brudzinski, Polish physician, 1874–1917*. 1. passive flexion of one thigh causing spontaneous flexion of the opposite thigh. 2. flexion of the neck causing bilateral flexion of the hips and knees. These signs are indicative of meningeal irritation.

bruise (brooz) a superficial injury to tissues produced by sudden impact in which the skin is unbroken. A contusion.

bruit ('brooee) [Fr.] an abnormal sound or murmur heard on auscultation of the heart and large vessels.

Brunner's glands ('bruhnəz) *J.C. Brunner, Swiss anatomist, 1653–1727*. Small compound tubular glands in the mucous membrane of the duodenum.

bruxism ('brooksizəm) teeth clenching, particularly during sleep. This occurs in persons under tension and can cause headaches as a result of muscle fatigue.

bubo ('byooboh) inflammation of the lymphatic glands of the axilla or groin. Typical of bubonic plague (see plague) and venereal infections.

buccal ('bukəl) pertaining to the cheek or to the mouth.

buccinator ('buksə,naytə) a muscle of the cheek, between the mandible and the maxilla.

Budd–Chiari syndrome (,budkee-'ah·ree) *G. Budd, British physician, 1808–82; H. Chiari, Austrian pathologist, 1851–1916*. A condition in which thrombosis of the hepatic vein causes vomiting, jaundice, enlargement of the liver, and ascites.

Buerger's disease ('bərgəz) *L. Buerger, American physician, 1879–1943*. Thromboangiitis obliterans.

buffalo hump ('bufəloh hump) excess fat in the upper thoracic area of the back; associated with excessive adrenocortical hormone production or therapy.

buffer ('bufə) 1. a physical or physiological system that tends to oppose change within that system, e.g. the reflexes involved in blood pressure homeostasis. 2. a chemical system that acts to prevent change in the concentration of another chemical substance. Sodium bicarbonate is the chief buffer of the blood and tissue fluids. 3. anything that is used to reduce shock or jarring upon contact.

buggery ('bugə·ree) anal intercourse, either heterosexual or homosexual. In law the term also includes sexual contact with an animal.

bulbar ('bulbə) pertaining to the MEDULLA OBLONGATA. *B. paralysis see* PARALYSIS.

bulbourethral (,bulbohyə'reethrəl) relating to the bulb of the urethra (bulb of the penis). B. glands small glands opening into the male urethra. Cowper's glands.

bulimia (byoo'limi·ə) abnormal increase in the sensation of hunger. *B. nervosa* a pattern of 'binge eating', or episodes of uncontrolled and compulsive overeating occurring in response to stress. Bulimic 'binges' often occur in ANOREXIA NERVOSA.

bulla ('buhlə) a large, fluid-containing blister.

bumetanide (byoo'metə,nied) a diuretic drug which prevents the resorption of urine from HENLE'S LOOP in the renal tubule.

bundle ('bund'l) a collection of nerve fibres all running in the same direction. *B. branch block* the delay in conduction along either branch of the atrioventricular bundle of the heart. The abnormality is detected by an ECG recording.

bundle of His ('bund'l əv 'his) *L. His Jr, German physiologist, 1863–1934.* The band of neuromuscular fibres which, passing through the spectrum of the heart, divides at the apex into two parts, these being distributed into the walls of the ventricles. The impulse of contraction is conducted through the structure. Atrioventricular bundle.

bunion ('bunyən) a prominence of the head of the metatarsal bone at its junction with the great toe, caused by inflammation and swelling of the bursa at that joint. Usually due to shoes that distort the natural shape of the foot.

buphthalmos (buf'thalməs) abnormal enlargement of the eyes in congenital GLAUCOMA.

Burkitt's tumour (bərkits) *D.P. Burkitt, Irish surgeon, 1911–93.* African lymphoma. A lymphosarcoma, frequently of the jaw, occurring almost exclusively in children living in low-lying moist areas. Occurs in New Guinea and Central Africa. The Epstein–Barr virus (EB virus), a herpesvirus, has been isolated from Burkitt's lymphoma cells in culture, and has been implicated as a causative agent.

burn (bərn) an injury to tissues caused by: (a) physical agents, the sun, excess heat or cold, friction, nuclear radiation; (b) chemical agents, acids, or caustic alkalis; (c) electrical current. Burns are described as being partial thickness (involving only the epidermis) or full thickness (involving the dermis and underlying structures). Clinically, emphasis is placed on the percentage of the body affected by the burn. The treatment of shock and prevention of infection and malnutrition need special attention.

burn out a term used to describe the result of chronic stress among workers and, commonly, in members of the helping professions. Burn out is characterised by chronic low energy, defensiveness, and emergence of manoeuvres designed to create distance between helper and patient/client. Dissatisfaction and tension can be carried over from the work situation into the personal life, and self-esteem and confidence can suffer.

burr (bər) a bit for a surgical drill, used for cutting bone or teeth. *B. hole* a circular hole drilled in the cranium to permit access to the brain or to release raised intracranial pressure.

bursa ('bərsə) a small sac of fibrous tissue, lined with synovial membrane and containing synovial fluid. It is situated between parts that move upon one another at a joint to reduce friction.

bursitis (bər'sietəs) inflammation of the bursa. It produces pain and can impede movement of the joint. *Prepatellar b.* housemaid's knee.

busulphan (byoo'sulfən) a cytotoxic drug that depresses the bone marrow and can be used to treat myeloid leukaemia.

butobarbitone (ˌbyootoh'bahbəˌtohn) an intermediate-acting barbiturate, formerly much used as a sedative. Now used only in severe insomnia.

buttock ('butək) either of the two prominences formed by the flesh-covered gluteal muscles at either side of the lower spine.

butyrophenone (ˌbyootəroh'feenohn) a chemical class of major tranquillisers, especially useful in the treatment of manic and moderate to severe agitated states and in the control of the vocal utterances and tics of GILLES DE LA TOURETTE'S SYNDROME.

bypass ('bieˌpahs) diversion of flow. Formation of a shunt. *Aortocoronary b.* diversion of flow from the aorta to the coronary arteries via a saphenous vein or artificial graft. *Femoropopliteal b.* diversion of flow from the femoral to the popliteal artery to overcome an occlusion.

byssinosis (ˌbisə'nohsəs) an industrial disease caused by inhalation of cotton or linen dust in factories. A type of PNEUMOCONIOSIS.

Cc

C symbol for carbon, Centigrade or Celsius, and cytosine.

Ca symbol for *calcium.*

cachexia (kə'keksi·ə) a condition of extreme debility. The patient is emaciated, and has skin that is loose and wrinkled from rapid wasting, but shiny and tense over bone. The eyes are sunken, the skin yellowish, and there is a grey 'muddy' complexion. The mucous membranes are pale and anaemia is extreme. The condition is typical of the late stages of chronic diseases.

cadaver (kə'davə, -'dah-) a corpse. A dead body used for dissection.

caecostomy (see'kostəmee) the making of a surgical fistula into the caecum by incision through the abdominal wall.

caecum ('seekəm) the blind pouch forming the beginning of the large intestine. The vermiform appendix is attached to it.

caesarean section (sə'zairi·ən) delivery of a fetus by an incision through the abdominal wall and uterus. Performed for the safety of either the mother or the infant. Tradition has it that Julius Caesar was born in this way.

caesium ('seezi·əm) *symbol* Cs. A metallic element. *Caesium-137* radioactive caesium; a fission product from uranium. Sealed in a suitable container it can be used instead of cobalt for beam therapy; sealed in needles, tubes or applicators it can be used for local application.

café-au-lait spot ('kafay oh lay) pigmented macules of a distinctive light-brown colour, like coffee with milk, as in NEUROFIBROMATOSIS and ALBRIGHT'S SYNDROME.

caffeine ('kafeen) an alkaloid of tea and coffee which acts as a nerve stimulant and diuretic. Mixed with aspirin and codeine, it is used as an analgesic.

caffeinism (kafˌee·ənizəm) an agitated state due to excessive ingestion of caffeine.

caisson disease ('kaysən) decompression sickness.

CAL chronic airways limitation; formerly chronic obstructive airways disease (COAD); now known as chronic obstructive pulmonary disease (COPD).

calamine ('kaləˌmien) preparation of zinc carbonate or zinc oxide coloured pink with ferric oxide. It is an astringent and antipruritic used in lotion or ointment form for skin diseases.

calcaneum (kal'kayni·əm) the heel bone. Calcaneus.

calcareous (kal'kair·ri·əs) chalky. Containing lime.

calciferol (kal'sifə·rol) the chemical name for vitamin D.

calcification (ˌkalsifə'kayshən) 1. the deposit of lime in any tissue, e.g. in the formation of callus. 2. the deposit of lime salts in cartilage as part of the normal process of bone formation. *Dystrophic c.* the deposition of calcium in abnormal tissue, such as scar tissue or atherosclerotic plaques, without abnormalities of blood calcium.

calcitonin (ˌkalsə'tohnən) a polypeptide hormone, produced by the parafollicular or C cells of the thyroid gland, which regulates blood calcium levels.

calcium ('kalsi·əm) *symbol* Ca. A metallic element necessary for the normal development and functioning of the body. Calcium is the most abundant mineral in the body, and is a constituent of bones and teeth. Deficiency or excess of serum calcium causes nerve and muscle dysfunction and abnormalities in blood clotting. The concentration is regulated by hormones. *C. carbonate* chalk. *C. channel blocker* a drug that reduces the flow of calcium in smooth muscle, diminishing the risk of spasms. *C. gluconate* used as an antacid. A compound that is easily absorbed and can be given by intramuscular or intravenous route to raise the blood calcium. *C. lactate* a compound that increases the coagulability of blood; used orally as a calcium supplement. *C. pump* an energy-requiring mechanism that facilitates the movement of calcium across a cell membrane.

calculus ('kalkyələs) a stony concretion which may be formed in any of the secreting organs of the body or their ducts. *Arthritic c.* gouty deposits in or near joints. *Biliary c.* gallstone. *Coral c.* a large stone in the kidney, with branches resembling coral. *Mulberry c.* a gallstone made of calcium oxalate and shaped like a mulberry. *Renal c.* one formed in the kidney. *Salivary c.* stone in a salivary duct. *Staghorn c.* a many-branched stone sometimes found in the renal pelvis. *Urinary c.* one found anywhere in the urinary tract. *Vesical c.* stone formed in the urinary bladder.

calibrator (ˌkalə'braytə) 1. an instrument for measuring the size of openings. 2. an instrument used to dilate a tube, e.g. in urethral stricture.

caliper ('kaləpə) a two-pronged instrument used to exert traction on a part. *Walking c.* an appliance fitted to a boot or shoe to give support to the lower limb. It can be used when the muscles are paralysed or in the repair stage of fractures.

calipers ('kaləpəz) compasses for measuring diameters and curved surface. *Skinfold c.* an instrument used in nutritional assessment for determining the amount of body fat. A fold of skin and subcutaneous tissue, usually over the triceps muscle, is pinched away from the underlying muscle using the thumb and forefinger (*see* figure on p. 74).

callisthenics (ˌkaləs'theniks) mild gymnastics for developing the muscles and producing a graceful carriage.

callosity (kə'losətee) the plaques of thickened skin often seen on the soles of the feet or the palms of the hand, areas subject to friction.

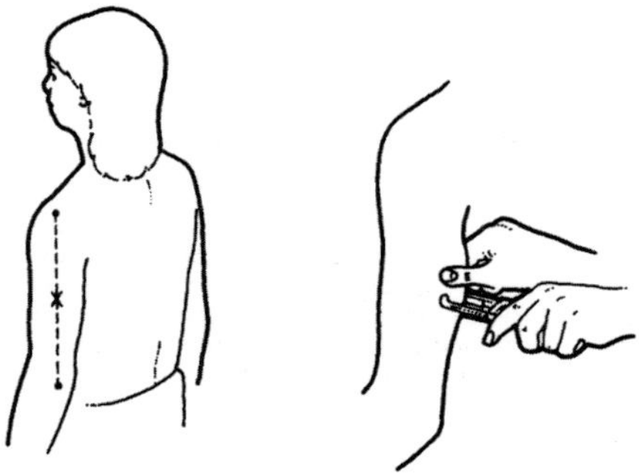

Triceps skinfold is measured at midpoint between acromion and olecranon

Skin is pinched and calipers are placed over skinfold

Skinfold Calipers

callous ('kaləs) hard and thickened.

callus ('kaləs) 1. a callosity. 2. the tissue that grows round fractured ends of bone and develops into new bone to repair the injury.

Calmette–Guérin bacillus (ˌkalmet geˌranh bə'siləs) *A.L.C. Calmette, French bacteriologist, 1863–1933; C. Guérin, French bacteriologist, 1872–1961.* A deactivated tuberculosis bacillus from which the antituberculosis vaccine, BCG vaccine, is made.

calor ('kalə) [L.] *heat*; one of the signs of inflammation.

caloric (kə'lor·rik, 'kalə·rik) pertaining to heat or calories.

calorie ('kalə·ree) *symbol* cal. A unit of heat. Used to denote physiological values of various food substances, estimated according to the amount of heat they produce on being oxidised in the body. *See* OXIDISATION. A Calorie with an initial capital letter (a Cal or kilocalorie) represents the heat required to raise the temperature of 1 kg (1000 g) of water by 1°C. A calorie (with a lower-case initial letter) represents the heat required to raise the temperature of 1 g of water by 1°C. In the SI system the calorie is replaced by the joule (1 Cal = 4.18 kJ).

calorific (ˌkalə'rifik) heat-producing.

calorimeter (ˌkalə'rimətə) an apparatus for measuring the heat that is produced or lost during a chemical or physical change.

calvaria (kal'vair·ri·ə) the upper, dome-like part of the skull.

calvities (kal'visheeˌeez) baldness.

calx (kalks) calcium oxide or lime. The basis of slaked lime, bleaching powder, and quicklime.

calyx ('kayliks, 'kal-) any cup-shaped vessel or part. *C. of kidney* the cup-like terminations of the ureter in the renal pelvis surrounding the pyramids of the kidney.

camphor ('kamfə) a crystalline substance prepared from the camphor laurel. It is used internally as a carminative. *Camphorated oil* is 1 part camphor to 4 parts of oil, prepared for external application as a rubefacient.

Campylobacter ('kampəloh,baktə) a genus of bacteria, family Spirillaceae, made up of Gram-negative, non-spore-forming, motile, spirally curved rods. Causes an intestinal illness lasting several days. Usually associated with unpasteurised milk, partially cooked meat and poultry.

canal (kə'nal) a tubular passage. *Alimentary c.* the passage along which the food passes on its way through the body. *Cervical c.* that through the cervix of the uterus. *Haversian c.* one of the minute channels that are present in bone. *C. of Ponti* carries chemical messages through the body. *C. of Schlemm* that which drains the aqueous humour. *Semicircular c.* one of the three canals in the middle ear responsible for maintenance of balance.

canaliculus (,kanə'likyələs) a small channel or canal.

cancellous ('kansələs) being porous or spongy. Applied to the honeycomb type of bone tissue in the ends of long bones and in flat and irregular bones.

cancer ('kansə) a general term to describe malignant growths in tissue, of which CARCINOMA is of epithelial and SARCOMA of connective tissue origin, as in bone and muscle. A cancerous growth is one that is not encapsulated, but infiltrates into surrounding tissues, the cells of which it replaces with its own. It is spread by the lymph and blood vessels and causes metastases in other parts of the body. Death is caused by destruction of organs to a degree incompatible with life, to extreme debility and anaemia, or to haemorrhage. *See* MALIGNANT.

cancroid ('kangkroid) 1. resembling cancer. 2. a skin tumour of moderate degree of malignancy.

cancrum oris (,kangkrəm'orəs) gangrenous STOMATITIS. An ulceration of the mouth that is a rare complication of measles in debilitated children. NOMA.

Candida ('kandədə) a genus of small fungi, formerly called *Monilia*. *C. albicans* the variety which causes CANDIDIASIS.

candidiasis (,kandə'dieəsəs) infection by the *Candida* fungus. Occurs particularly in moist areas, such as mouth, vagina, and skin folds. Popularly known as 'thrush'. Candidiasis can occur as a result of a debilitating illness or immunosuppressive therapy and/or cytotoxic drugs. The infection can also occur as a result of disturbed intestinal flora, and in pregnancy. Oral infection can be due to poor hygiene, carious teeth, or badly fitting dentures.

canine ('kaynien) 1. pertaining to a dog. 2. an 'eye tooth'. There is one on each side of both the upper jaw and the lower jaw between the incisors and the molars.

cannabis ('kanəbəs) an illegal drug which can be swallowed or smoked and produces hallucinations and a temporary sense of wellbeing, followed by extreme lethargy. Alternative terms for cannabis include marijuana, hashish, blow, draw, hash, grass, pot, the weed, ganga, kaya, kif, and bhang.

cannula ('kanyələ) a hollow tube for insertion into the body by which fluids are introduced or removed. Usually a trocar is fitted into it to facilitate its introduction.

canthus ('kanthəs) the angle formed by the junction of the upper and lower eyelids.

capacitance vessels (kə'pasətəns) the vessels that hold the major portion of the intravascular blood volume.

CAPD CONTINUOUS AMBULATORY PERITONEAL DIALYSIS.

capeline bandage ('kayplien) a caplike covering of two interwoven bandages used for protecting the head or a limb stump.

capillarity (ˌkapə'larətee) the action by which a liquid rises upwards in a fibrous substance or in a fine tube. Capillary attraction.

capillary (kə'pilə·ree) 1. hair-like. 2. a minute vessel connecting an arteriole and a venule. 3. a minute vessel of the lymphatic system.

capitellum (ˌkapə'teləm) capitulum. 1. the small rounded head at the elbow end of the humerus. 2. the bulb of a hair.

capreomycin (ˌkaprioh'miesən) a polypeptide antibiotic produced by *Streptomyces capreolus*, which is active against human strains of *Myobacterium tuberculosis* and has four microbiologically active components.

capsular ('kapsyələ) relating to a capsule. *C. ligaments* those that completely surround a movable joint, forming a capsule that loosely encloses the bones and is lined with synovial membrane which secretes a fluid for lubrication of the articular surfaces. Also called articular capsule.

capsule ('kapsyool) 1. a fibrous or membranous sac enclosing an organ. 2. a small soluble case of gelatin in which a nauseous medicine can be enclosed. 3. the gelatinous envelope that surrounds and protects some bacteria.

capsulectomy (ˌkapsyə'lektəmee) surgical excision of a capsule.

capsulitis (ˌkapsyə'lietəs) inflammation of the capsule of a joint.

capsulotomy (ˌkapsyə'lotəmee) the incision of a capsule, particularly that of a joint or of the lens of the eye.

caput ('kapuht) head. *C. succedaneum* a transient soft swelling on an infant's head, due to pressure during labour, which disappears within the first few days of life.

carbachol ('kahbəˌkol) a drug related to and acting like acetylcholine, but more stable. It causes contraction of plain muscle and relaxation of the voluntary sphincter, so relieving post-operative retention of urine. Also used in the treatment of glaucoma.

carbamazepine (ˌkahbə'mazəˌpeen) a drug used to control epilepsy and to relieve pain; used in the treatment of trigeminal neuralgia.

carbaminohaemoglobin (kahˌbamənohˌheemə'glohbən) a compound of carbon dioxide and haemoglobin, present in the blood.

carbenicillin ('kahbənə'silən) a

synthetic penicillin which is principally used in the treatment of serious infections caused by *Pseudomonas aeruginosa* and other Gram-negative organisms. Large doses, which need to be given intravenously, are required to obtain sufficiently high concentrations in the blood and tissues to be effective.

carbenoxolone (ˌkahbəˈnoksəˌlohn) an anti-inflammatory drug used in the treatment of gastric ulcers.

carbidopa (ˌkahbəˈdohpə) an inhibitor of the decarboxylation of LEVODOPA (L-dopa) in peri-pheral tissues, which does not cross the blood–brain barrier. It is used in combination with levodopa to control the symptoms of PARKINSON'S DISEASE. In the presence of carbidopa, levodopa enters the brain in larger quantities, thus avoiding the need for excessively high doses.

carbimazole (kahˈbiməˌzohl) an antithyroid drug that is used to stabilise a patient with THYROTOXICOSIS.

carbohydrate (ˌkahbohˈhiedrayt) a compound of carbon, hydrogen, and oxygen. Carbohydrates are classified into mono-, di-, tri-, poly- and heterosaccharides. In food they are an important and immediate source of energy for the body: 1 g of carbohydrate yields 17 kJ (4 kcal). They are synthesised by all green plants. In the body they are absorbed immediately or stored in the form of glycogen.

carbolic acid (kahˈbolik) phenol.

carbon (ˈkahbən) *symbol* C. A non-metallic element. *C. dioxide* a gas which, dissolved in water, forms weak carbonic acid. As a product of metabolism by the oxidation of carbon, it leaves the body by the lungs. It can be compressed until it freezes, and then forms a solid (carbon dioxide snow) used as an escharotic in various skin conditions. Also known as dry ice. Inhalations of the gas in a 5–7% mixture with oxygen are useful for stimulating the depth of respiration. *C. monoxide* a colourless gas that is very poisonous. It is a major constituent of coal gas and is usually present in the exhaust gases from petrol and diesel engines. In poisoning, there is vertigo, flushed face with very red lips, loss of consciousness, and convulsions. The blood is bright red because of the formation of carboxyhaemoglobin. *C. tetrachloride* a powerful anthelmintic used in treating hookworm and whipworm. Used also in cleaning fluids; the inhalation of its vapours in solvent abuse can depress central nervous system activity and cause degeneration of the liver and kidneys.

carbonic anhydrase (kahˈbonik anˈhiedrayz) an enzyme that catalyses the decomposition of carbonic acid into carbon dioxide and water, facilitating transfer of carbon dioxide from tissues to blood and from blood to alveolar air.

carboxyhaemoglobin (kahˈbokseeˌheeməˈglohbən) the combination of carbon monoxide with haemoglobin in the blood in carbon monoxide poisoning.

carbuncle (ˈkahbungkəl) an acute staphylococcal inflammation of subcutaneous tissues, which causes local thrombosis in the veins and death of tissue with several discharging sinuses. In appearance it resembles a collection of boils.

carcinogen (ˈkahsənəˌjən, kahˈsi-nəjən) any substance or agent that can produce a cancer.

carcinogenic (ˌkahsinohˈjenik) pertaining to substances or agents that produce or predispose to cancer. Crude oils are said to contain a *c. factor*.

carcinoid (ˈkahsəˌnoyd) *C. syndrome* a rare condition associated with certain bowel tumours, which spread to other parts of the body. Marked by attacks of severe cyanotic flushing of the skin and by diarrhoea, bronchoconstrictive attacks, pain, serious heart damage, sudden drops in blood pressure, oedema, and ascites. Symptoms are caused by serotonin, prostaglandins, and other biologically active substances secreted by the tumour.

carcinoma (ˌkahsəˈnohmə) a malignant growth of epithelial tissue. Microscopically the cells resemble those of the tissue in which the growth has arisen. Adenoic c. ADENOCARCINOMA. Basal cell c. a rodent ulcer (*see* ULCER). *Epithelial c.* EPITHELIOMA. *Squamous cell c.* one arising from the squamous epithelium of the skin.

carcinomatosis (ˌkahsəˌnohməˈtohsəs) the condition in which a carcinoma has given rise to widespread metastases.

cardia (ˈkahdi·ə) the cardiac orifice of the stomach.

cardiac (ˈkahdeeˌak) 1. pertaining to the heart. 2. pertaining to the cardia. *C. arrest* the cessation of the heart beat. *C. arrhythmia* an abnormal rate or rhythm of myocardial conduction. *C. asthma see* ASTHMA. *C. atrophy* fatty degeneration of the heart muscle. *C. bed* one that can be manipulated to form a chair shape for those who are comfortable only when sitting up. *C. catheterisation* a procedure whereby a radio-opaque catheter is passed from an arm vein to the heart. Its passage through the heart can be watched on a screen. Also blood pressure readings and specimens can be taken, thus aiding diagnosis of heart abnormalities. *C. cycle* the sequence of events, lasting about 0.8 seconds, during which the heart completes one contraction. *C. failure see* HEART FAILURE. *C. massage* rhythmic compression of the heart performed in order to re-establish circulation of the blood in cardiac arrest. *C. monitor* equipment used to monitor and visually record the cardiac cycle. *C. pacemaker* an electrical device that stimulates the heart muscle to maintain myocardial contractions. *See* PACEMAKER. *C. stimulant* a pharmacological agent that increases the action of the heart. Cardiac glycosides, e.g. digoxin and digitalis, increase myocardial contractions and decrease the heart rate and conduction velocity, thus allowing more time for the ventricles to relax and fill with blood. *C. tamponade* compression of the heart by a collection of fluid or blood in the pericardial sac.

cardialgia (ˌkahdeeˈalji·ə) pain in the region of the heart. Cardiodynia.

cardinal (ˈkahdənˈl) of first importance. Fundamental. *C. ligaments* deep transverse cervical ligaments. Mackenrodt's ligaments.

cardiogenic (ˌkahdeeohˈjenik) originating in the heart. *C. shock* shock caused by disease or failure of heart action.

cardiography (ˌkahdeeˈogrəfee) the

recording of the force and movements of the heart.

cardiologist (ˌkahdee'oləjəst) a medically qualified person skilled in the diagnosis of heart disease.

cardiology (ˌkahdee'oləjee) the study of the heart: how it works and its diseases.

cardiolysis (ˌkahdee'oləsəs) the breaking down of adhesions between the pericardium and chest wall by operation.

cardiomegaly (ˌkahdeeoh'megəlee) enlargement of the heart.

cardiomyopathy (ˌkahdeeohmie'opəthee) a chronic disorder of the heart muscle, especially one of unknown or non-specific origin.

cardiopathy (ˌkahdee'opəthee) any disease of the heart.

cardiopulmonary (ˌkahdeeoh'pulmənəree) relating to the heart and lungs. *C. bypass* the use of a heart–lung machine to oxygenate and pump the blood around the body while a surgeon operates on the heart.

cardioscope ('kahdeeohˌskohp) a flexible instrument with a lens and illumination attachment; used for examining the inside of the heart.

cardiospasm ('kahdeeoˌspazəm) spasm of the sphincter muscle at the cardiac end of the stomach. It can result in dilatation of the oesophagus, difficulty in swallowing solids and liquids, and regurgitation of undigested food. ACHALASIA.

cardiothoracic (ˌkahdeeohthə'rasik) pertaining to the heart and thoracic cavity. A specialised branch of surgery.

cardiotocography (ˌkahdeeohtə'kogrəfee) the simultaneous recording of the fetal heart rate, fetal movements, and uterine contractions in order to discover possible lack of oxygen (hypoxia) to the fetus. Fetal monitoring.

cardiotomy (ˌkahdee'otəmee) surgical incision into the heart or the cardia. *C. syndrome* an inflammatory reaction after heart surgery. There is PYREXIA, PERICARDITIS, and pleural effusion.

cardiotoxic (ˌkahdeeoh'toksik) anything that has a deleterious or poisonous effect on the heart.

cardiovascular (ˌkahdeeoh'vaskyələ) concerning the heart and blood vessels. *C. system* the heart together with the two chief networks of blood vessels: the systemic circulation and the pulmonary circulation.

cardioversion (ˌkahdeeoh'vərshən) a method of restoring an abnormal heart rhythm to normal (e.g., atrial fibrillation) by means of an electric shock.

carditis (kah'dietəs) inflammation of the heart.

caries ('kair·reez) suppuration and subsequent decay of bone, corresponding to ulceration in soft tissues. In caries, the bone dissolves; in necrosis, it separates in large pieces and is thrown off. *Dental c.* decay of the teeth due to penetration of bacteria through the enamel to the dentine. *Spinal c.* tuberculosis of the spine. Pott's disease.

carina (kə'rienə, -'reenə) a keel-like structure. Usually applied to the bifurcation of the trachea into the bronchi, because the terminal cartilage is keel-shaped.

carminative (kah'minətiv) an aromatic drug that relieves flatulence and associated colic. Cloves, ginger, cardamom, and peppermint are examples.

carneous ('kahnee·əs) fleshy. *C. mole*

a tumour of organised blood clot surrounding a dead fetus in the uterus. *See* ABORTION.

carotene ('karəˌteen) the colouring matter in carrots, tomatoes, and other yellow foods and in fats. It is a provitamin capable of conversion into vitamin A in the liver.

carotid (ka'rotəd) the principal artery on each side of the neck. *C. bodies* chemoreceptors in the bifurcation of both carotid arteries which monitor the oxygen content of the blood. *C. sinuses* dilated portions of the internal carotids containing the baroreceptors that monitor blood pressure.

carpal ('kahpəl) relating to the carpus or wrist. *C. tunnel syndrome* compression of the median nerve at the wrist causing numbing and tingling in the fingers.

carpopedal (ˌkahpə'ped'l) relating to the wrist and foot. *C. spasm* spasm of the hands and feet such as occurs in tetany.

carpus ('kahpəs) the eight bones forming the wrist and arranged in two rows: (a) scaphoid, lunate, triquetral, pisiform; (b) trapezium, trapezoid, capitate, hamate (*see* figure).

carrier ('kari·ə) 1. a person who harbours the microorganisms of an infectious disease but is not necessarily affected by it, although he or she can infect others. 2. one who carries and passes on an hereditary abnormality.

cartilage ('kahtəlij) a specialised, fibrous connective tissue present in adults and forming most of the temporary skeleton in the embryo. The three most important types are hyaline cartilage, elastic cartilage, and fibrocartilage. Also, a general term for a mass of such tissue in a particular site in the body. *Elastic c.* cartilage containing elastic fibres and forming the pinna of the ear, the epiglottis, and part of the nasal septum. *Fibro-c.* cartilage in which bundles of white fibres predominate, forming the intervertebral discs and costal cartilages. *Hyaline c.* flexible, somewhat elastic, semitransparent cartilage with an opalescent bluish tint, composed of a basophilic fibril-containing substance with cavities in which the CHONDROCYTES occur.

cartilaginous ('kahtə'lajənəs) of the nature of cartilage.

caruncle ('karəngkəl) a small fleshy swelling. *Lacrimal c.* a small reddish body situated at the medial junction of the eyelids. *Urethral c.* a small fleshy growth occurring at the urinary orifice in females and giving rise to great pain on micturition.

cascara (kas'kahrə) a laxative prepared from the bark of the Californian buckthorn. It can be prepared as an elixir or tablets.

case (kays) a particular instance of disease, as in 'a case of leukaemia'; sometimes used incorrectly to designate the patient with the disease. *C. conference* a meeting of professionals involved in the care of a particular person (sometimes including relatives or nominated carer of the patient), to agree patterns of action and to monitor progress. *C. control study* an epidemiological study in which the characteristics of cases of disease are compared with a matched control group of persons without the disease. Called also retrospective study, case referent study.

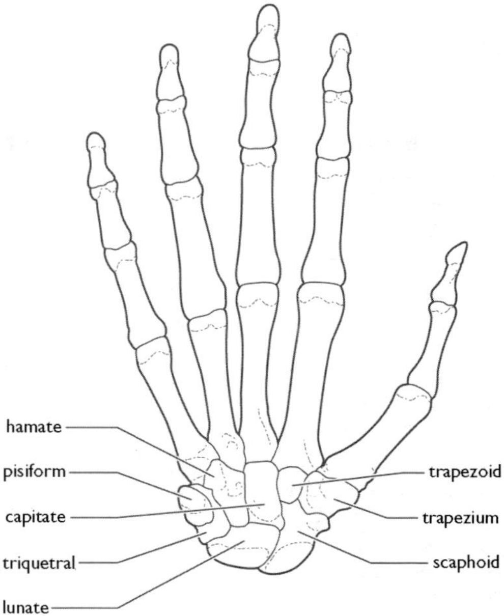

Carpus

C. fatality rate the number of persons dying of a particular disease expressed as a proportion of the total contracting the disease; usually expressed as a percentage. *C. history* the collected data concerning an individual, his or her family, and environment, including the medical history and any other information that might be useful in analysing and diagnosing the health issues or for instructional or research purposes. *C. mix* the groups of patients requiring similar procedures, tests and resources treated at a particular hospital. Used as a measure of hospital productivity. *C. studies* the study of a selected phenomenon that provides in-depth description of its dimensions and processes.

caseation (ˌkaysee'ayshən) degeneration of diseased tissue into a cheesy mass.

casein ('kayseeən, -seen) the chief protein of milk. It forms a curd from which cheese is made. *C. hydrolysate* a predigested concentrated protein; a useful supplement for a high protein diet.

cast (kahst) 1. a positive copy of an object, e.g. a mould of a hollow organ (a renal tubule, bronchiole, etc.), formed of effused plastic matter and extruded from the body, as a urinary cast; named, according to constituents, as epithelial, fatty, waxy, etc. 2. a positive copy of the tissues of the jaws, made in an impression, over which denture bases or other restorations can be fabricated. 3. to form an object in a mould. 4. a stiff dressing or casing, usually made of plaster of Paris, used to immobilise body parts. 5. STRABISMUS.

castor oil ('kahstə) a vegetable oil. Internally it is a purgative. Externally it is protective and soothing and can be used in ointments or in eye drops.

castration (ka'strayshən) removal or destruction of the testicles or the ovaries.

CAT computerised axial tomography. *See* COMPUTED TOMOGRAPHY.

cat-scratch disease (fever) (kat-skrach) a benign, subacute, regional LYMPHADENITIS resulting from a scratch or bite of a cat or a scratch from a surface contaminated by a cat. No specific causative agent has been isolated but a viral aetiology is suspected.

catabolism (kə'tabə,lizəm) the chemical breakdown of complex substances in the body to form simpler ones, with a release of energy. *See* METABOLISM.

catalase ('katə,layz) an enzyme found in body cells, including red blood cells and liver cells.

catalyst ('katələst) a substance that hastens or brings about a chemical change without itself undergoing alteration; for example, enzymes act as catalysts in the process of digestion.

cataplasm ('katə,plazəm) a poultice. It acts as a counter-irritant. Materials of which it can be made are: linseed, bread, and bran. Kaolin is more frequently used.

cataplexy ('katə,pleksee) sudden recurrent loss of muscle power without unconsciousness, often associated with narcolepsy. It can be produced by any strong emotion.

cataract ('katə,rakt) opacity of the crystalline lens of the eye causing partial or complete blindness. It can be congenital or can be due to degenerative changes, injury, or diabetes.

catarrh (kə'tah) chronic inflammation of a mucous membrane accompanied by an excessive discharge of mucus.

catatonia (,katə'tohni·ə) a syndrome of motor abnormalities occurring in schizophrenia, but less commonly in organic cerebral disease, characterised by stupor and the adoption of strange postures, or outbursts of excitement and hyperactivity. The patient might change suddenly from one of these states to another.

catecholamines (,katəkolə'meenz) a group of compounds that have the effect of sympathetic nerve stimulation. They have an aromatic and an amine portion and include dopamine, adrenaline, and noradrenaline.

catgut ('kat,gut) a substance prepared from the intestines of sheep and used in surgery for sutures and ligatures. It becomes gradually absorbed in the body at a variable rate, according to the preparation.

catharsis (kə'thahsəs) 1. a cleansing or purgation. 2. the bringing into consciousness and the emotional reliving of a forgotten (repressed) painful experience as a means of releasing anxiety and tension.

cathartic (kə'thahtik) a purgative drug.

catheter ('kathətə) a tubular, flexible instrument, passed through body channels for withdrawal of fluids from (or introduction of fluids into) a body cavity. Catheters are made of a variety of materials including plastic, metal, rubber, gum-elastic, and silicon. *Angiographic c.* one through which a contrast medium is injected for visualisation of the vascular system of an organ. *Arterial c.* one inserted into an artery and utilised as part of a catheter–transducer–monitor system for continuous observation of the BLOOD PRESSURE of critically ill patients. An arterial catheter can be inserted for radiological studies of the arterial system and for delivery of chemotherapeutic agents directly into the arterial supply of malignant tumours. *Cardiac c.* a long, fine catheter especially designed for passage, usually through a peripheral blood vessel, into the chambers of the heart under fluoroscopic control. *Central venous c.* a long, fine catheter inserted into a vein for the purpose of administering, through a large blood vessel, parenteral fluids (as in parenteral nutrition), antibiotics and other therapeutic agents. This type of catheter is also used in the measurement of central venous pressure (*see* CENTRAL venous pressure). *Eustachian c.* a silver catheter used to open up the PHARYNGOTYMPANIC TUBE. *Self-retaining c.* a catheter made in such a way that, after introduction, the blind end can be expanded such that it remains in the bladder. Useful for continuous or intermittent drainage or if frequent specimens are required. *Uretic c.* a fine gum-elastic catheter passed up the ureter to the renal pelvis and used to insert a contrast medium in retrograde urography.

catheterisation (ˌkathətə·rie-'zayshən) the insertion of a catheter into a body cavity.

cathode ('kathohd) 1. the negative electrode or pole of an electric current. 2. the negative pole of a battery. *See* ANODE.

cation ('katie·ən) a positively charged ion, which moves towards the cathode when an electric current is passed through an electrolytic solution, e.g. hydrogen (H^+), sodium (Na^+). *See* ANION.

cauda ('kawdah) a tail-like appendage. *C. equina* the bundle of coccygeal, sacral, and lumbar nerves with which the spinal cord terminates.

caudal ('kawd'l) referring to a cauda. *C. block* an anaesthetic agent injected into the sacral canal so that operations can be carried out in the peritoneal area without a general anaesthetic.

caul (kawl) the amnion, which occasionally does not rupture but envelops the infant's head at birth.

causalgia (kaw'zalji·ə) an intense burning pain which persists after peripheral nerve injuries.

caustic ('kostik, 'kaw-) a substance, usually a strong acid or alkali, capable of burning organic tissue. Silver nitrate (*lunar c.*), carbolic acid and carbon dioxide snow are those most commonly used.

cauterisation (ˌkawtə·rie'zayshən) the destruction of tissue with CAUTERY.

cautery ('kawtə·ree) 1. the application of searing heat by a hot instrument, an electric current, or other means such as a laser. 2. an agent so used. *Cold c.* cauterisation by carbon dioxide, called also cryocautery.

cavernous ('kavənəs, kə'vərnəs) having caverns or hollows. *C. breathing* sounds heard on auscultation over a pulmonary cavity. *C. sinus* a venous channel lying on either side of the body of the sphenoid bone through which pass the internal carotid artery and several nerves. *C. sinus thrombosis* a serious complication of any infection of the face, the veins from the orbit draining into the sinus and carrying the infection into the cranium.

cavitation (ˌkavə'tayshən) the formation of cavities, e.g. in the lung in tuberculosis.

cavity ('kavətee) a confined space or hollow or potential hollow within the body or one of its organs, e.g. the abdominal cavity or a decayed hollow in a tooth.

cefotaxime (ˌkefoh'takseem) a third-generation cephalosporin antibiotic having a broad spectrum of activity used to treat intra-abdominal infections, bone and joint infections, gonorrhoea, and other infections due to susceptible organisms, including penicillinase-producing strains.

cefoxitin (ke'foksətən) a semi-synthetic cephalosporin antibiotic, especially effective against Gram-negative organisms, with strong resistance to degradation by β-lactamase.

cell (sel) 1. the basic structural unit of living organisms (*see* figure). A microscopic mass of protoplasm consisting of a nucleus surrounded by cytoplasm and enclosed in a cell membrane from which all organic tissues are constructed. Each cell can reproduce itself by mitosis. 2. a small, more or less enclosed, space.

cellulitis (ˌselyə'lietəs) a diffuse inflammation of connective tissue, especially of subcutaneous tissue, which causes a typical brawny, oedematous appearance of the part; local abscess formation is not common.

cellulose ('selyəˌlohs, -ˌlohz) a carbohydrate forming the covering of vegetable cells, i.e. vegetable fibres. Not digestible in the alimentary tract of human beings but gives bulk and, as 'roughage', stimulates peristalsis.

Celsius scale ('selsi·əs) *A. Celsius, Swedish astronomer, 1701–44.* A temperature scale with the melting point of ice set at 0° and the boiling point of water at 100°. The normal temperature of the human body is 36.9°C. Formerly known as the Centigrade scale. *See* FAHRENHEIT SCALE.

cementum (sə'mentəm) cement. Connective tissue with a bone-like structure which covers the root of a tooth and supports it within the socket.

censor (ˌsensə) 1. a member of a committee on ethics or for critical

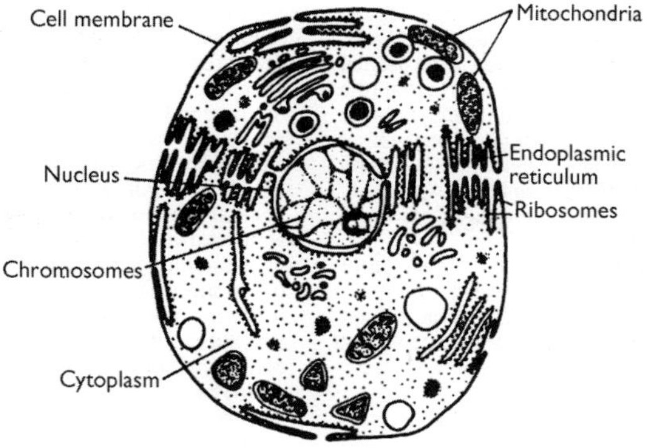

Major Parts of Cell

examination of a medical or other society. 2. the psychic influence that prevents unconscious thoughts and wishes coming into consciousness.

censorship ('sensə,ship) in psychiatry, the process of selecting, accepting or rejecting conscious ideas, memories, and impulses arising from the individual's subconscious.

Centigrade ('sentə,grayd) *see* CELSIUS SCALE.

central ('sentrəl) pertaining to the centre or midpoint. *C. nervous system* abbreviated CNS. The brain and spinal cord. *C. venous pressure* the pressure recorded by the introduction of a catheter into the right atrium to monitor the condition of a patient after a major operative procedure, such as heart surgery.

centrifugal (sentrə'fyoogəl) conveying away from a centre, such as from the brain to the periphery. Efferent.

centrifuge ('sentrə,fyooj) an apparatus that rotates at high speed. For example, if a test tubeis filled with a fluid, such as blood or urine, and rotated in a centrifuge, any bacteria, cells, or other solids in it are precipitated.

centripetal (sen'tripət'l, 'sentrə,-peet'l) the reverse of centrifugal. Conveying from the periphery to the centre. Afferent.

centromere ('sentrə,miə) the region(s) of the chromosomes which become(s) allied with the spindle fibres at MITOSIS and MEIOSIS.

centrosome ('sentrə,sohm) a body in the cytoplasm of most animal cells, close to the nucleus. It divides during mitosis, one half migrating to each daughter cell.

centrosphere ('sentrə,sfiə) the cell centre, in an area of clear cytoplasm near the nucleus.

cephalexin (,kefə'leksən, sef-)

cephalosporin antibiotic that can be administered orally.

cephalhaematoma (ˌkefəlˌheemə'tohmə, sef-) a swelling beneath the pericranium, containing blood, which might be found on the head of the newborn infant. Caused by pressure during labour. Gradually reabsorbed within the first few days of life.

cephalic (kə'falik, sə-) relating to or situated near the head.

cephalocaudal (ˌkefəloh'kawd'l) pertaining to the long axis of the body.

cephalocele ('kefəlohˌseel, 'sef-) cerebral hernia. *See* HERNIA.

cephalography (ˌkefə'logrəfee, ˌsef-) radiographic examination of the contours of the head.

cephalometry (ˌkefə'lomətree, ˌsef-) measurement of the dimensions of the head of a living person either directly or by radiography. *See* PELVIMETRY.

cephaloridine (ˌkefə'lo·rədeen, ˌsef-) an antibiotic; it is effective against a wide range of organisms.

cephalosporin (ˌkefəloh'spaw·rən, ˌsef-) any one of a group of broad-spectrum antibiotics derived from the mould *Cephalosporium*.

cephradine ('kefrədeen, 'sef-) a cephalosporin antibiotic similar in action to cephaloridine.

cerclage (sər'klahzh) [Fr.] encircling of a part with a ring or loop, as for correction of an incompetent cervix uteri or fixation of the adjacent ends of a fractured bone. *See* SHIRODKAR'S SUTURE.

cerebellum (ˌserə'beləm) the portion of the brain below the cerebrum and above the medulla oblongata. Its functions include the coordination of fine voluntary movements and posture.

cerebral ('serəbrəl) relating to the cerebrum. *C. cortex* the outer layer of the cerebrum, composed of neurones. *C. haemorrhage* rupture of a cerebral blood vessel. Likely causes are aneurysm and hypertension. *See* APOPLEXY. *C. hernia see* HERNIA. *C. irritation* a condition of general nervous irritability and abnormality, often with photophobia, which can be an early sign of meningitis, tumour of the brain, etc. It is also associated with trauma. *C. palsy* a condition caused by injury to the brain during or immediately after birth. Coordination of movement is affected, and can cause the child to be flaccid or athetoid, in which condition there is constant random and uncontrolled movement. *See* SPASTIC.

cerebration (ˌserə'brayshən) mental activity.

cerebrospinal (ˌserəbroh'spien'l) relating to the brain and spinal cord. *C. fluid* abbreviated CSF. The fluid made in the choroid plexus of the ventricles of the brain and circulating from them into the subarachnoid space around the brain and spinal cord.

cerebrovascular (ˌserəbroh'vaskylə) pertaining to the arteries and veins of the brain. *C. accident* a disorder arising from an embolus, thrombus, or haemorrhage in the cerebrum. *C. disease* any disorder of the blood vessels of the brain and its meninges.

cerebrum ('serəbrəm) the largest part of the brain, occupying the greater portion of the cranium and consisting of the right and left hemispheres divided by the longitudinal fissure (*see* figure). Each

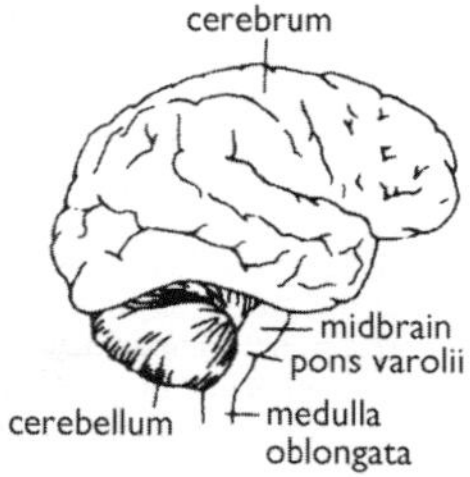

Cerebrum

hemisphere contains a lateral ventricle. The internal substance is white and the convoluted surface is grey. The centre of the higher functions of the brain.

cerumen (sə'roomən) a waxy substance secreted by the ceruminous glands of the auditory canal. Ear wax.

cervical ('sərvikəl, sə'vie-) pertaining to the neck or the constricted part of an organ, e.g. uterine cervix. *C. canal* the passage through the uterine cervix. *C. cancer* cancer of the uterine cervix. *C. collar* a rigid or semirigid immobilising support for the neck. *C. rib* a short extra rib, often bilateral, which sometimes occurs on the seventh cervical vertebra and may cause pressure on an artery or nerve. *C. smear* a test for disorders of the cervical cells; material is scraped from the uterine cervix and examined microscopically. *C. spondylosis* a degenerative disease of the intervertebral joints and discs of the neck. *C. vertebra* one of the seven bones forming the neck portion of the spinal column.

cervicitis (ˌservə'sietəs) inflammation of the neck of the uterus.

cervix ('sərviks) a constricted portion or neck. *C. uteri* the neck of the uterus; it is about 2 cm long and projects into the vagina. Capable of wide dilatation during childbirth.

cestode ('sestohd) tapeworm.

cetrimide ('setrəmied) cetyltrimethylammonium bromide (CTAB). A detergent and antiseptic widely used for preoperative skin preparation and the cleansing of wounds.

cevitamic acid (ˌsevə'tamik) ascorbic acid. Vitamin C.

chafe (chayf) irritation of the skin as caused by the friction between skinfolds. Occurs particularly in moist areas.

chalazion (kə'lazi·ən) a MEIBOMIAN or tarsal cyst. A swollen sebaceous gland in the eyelid. A small, hard tumour can develop.

chancre ('shangkə) 1. the initial lesion of syphilis developing at the site of inoculation. 2. a papular lesion occurring at the site of infection in tuberculosis or in sporotrichosis.

chancroid ('shangkroyd) soft chancre. A venereal ulceration, due to *Haemophilus ducreyi*, accompanied by inflammation and suppuration of the local glands.

character ('karəktə) the combination of traits and qualities distinguishing the unique nature of the individual. *C. change* indicates alteration in a person's recognised behaviour to one alien to the person's normal manner of conduct. *C. disorder* a chronic state in which the person exhibits maladaptive and unacceptable forms of behaviour and social response.

Charcot's disease or **joint** (shah'kohz) *J.M. Charcot, French* *neurologist, 1825–93*. A chronic progressive, degenerative disease of the stress-bearing portion of one or more joints. The disease is the result of an underlying neurological disorder, e.g. TABES DORSALIS from syphilis, diabetic neuropathy, or leprosy.

Charcot's triad nystagmus, intention tremor, and scanning speech. A triad of signs of disseminated sclerosis.

Charnley's arthroplasty ('chahnleez) *Sir J. Charnley, British orthopaedic surgeon, 1911–82*. The replacement of the hip joint using a plastic ACETABULUM and a steel femoral head. *See* ARTHROPLASTY.

chart ('chaht) a record in graphic or tabular form. *Reuss'c's* charts with coloured letters printed on coloured backgrounds, used in testing colour vision. *Snellen's c.* a chart printed with block letters in gradually decreasing sizes, used in testing visual acuity.

charting ('chahting) the keeping of a clinical record of the important facts about a patient and the progress of his or her illness. The patient's chart usually contains a medical history, a nursing history, results of physical examinations, laboratory reports, results of special diagnostic tests, and the observations of the nursing staff. Medical treatments, medications, and nursing approaches to problems are recorded on the chart, as is the patient's response to treatment. *See also* PROBLEM-ORIENTED RECORD.

cheiloschisis (kie'loskəsəs) cleft lip.

cheilosis (kie'lohsəs) maceration at the angles of the mouth; fissures can also occur. It can be associated with general debility or riboflavin deficiency.

cheiropompholyx (ˌkieroh'pomfohliks) a skin disease characterised by vesicles on the palms and soles.

chelate ('keelayt) a chemical compound in which an atom of a metal is held in a molecular ring.

chelating agent (kee'layting) a drug that has the power of combining with certain metals and so aiding excretion, to prevent or overcome poisoning. *See* DIMERCAPROL and PENICILLAMINE.

chemistry ('keməstree) the science of dealing with the elements and the atoms which compose them, and with the compounds they form.

chemoreceptor (ˌkeemohree'septə, ˌkem-) a sensory nerve ending or group of cells that are sensitive to chemical stimuli in the blood.

chemosis (kee'mohsəs) swelling of the conjunctiva due to the presence of fluid; an oedema of the conjuctiva.

chemosurgery (ˌkeemoh'sərjə·ree, ˌkem-) the destruction of tissue by chemical agents for therapeutic purposes, originally applied to chemical fixation of malignant, gangrenous or infected tissue with use of frozen sections to facilitate systematic microscopic control of its excision.

chemotaxis (ˌkeemoh'taksəs, ˌkem-) the reaction of living cells to chemical stimuli. These are either attracted (*positive c.*) or repelled (*negative c.*) by acids, alkalis, or other substances.

chemotherapy (ˌkeemoh'therəpee, ˌkem-) the specific treatment of disease by the administration of chemical compounds.

chest (chest) the thorax. *Barrel c.* one more rounded than usual, with raised ribs and, usually, KYPHOSIS.

It is often present in emphysema. *Flail c.* one in which part of the chest wall moves in opposition to respiration as a result of multiple fractures of the ribs. *C. leads* leads applied to the chest during the course of an electrocardiographic recording. *Pigeon c.* a chest with the sternum protruding forward.

Cheyne–Stokes respiration ('chayn'stohks) *J. Cheyne, British physician, 1776–1836; W. Stokes, British physician, 1804–1878.* Tidal respiration. A form of irregular but rhythmic breathing with temporary cessations (apnoea). It is likely to be present in cerebral tumour, in narcotic poisoning, and in advanced cases of ARTERIOSCLEROSIS and URAEMIA.

chiasma (kieˌazmə) a crossing point. *Optic c.* the crossing point of the optic nerves.

chickenpox ('chikənˌpoks) VARICELLA.

chilblain ('chilˌblayn) a condition resulting from defective circulation when exposure to cold causes localised swelling and inflammation of the hands or feet, with severe itching and burning sensations.

child (chield) the human young, from infancy to puberty. *C. abuse* the non-accidental use of physical force or the non-accidental act of omission by a parent or other custodian responsible for the care of a child. Child abuse encompasses malnutrition and other kinds of neglect through ignorance, as well as deliberate withholding from the child of necessary basic physical and emotional care, including medical and dental care necessary for the child to grow. Examples of physical abuse range from burns and exposure to extreme cold, to beating, poisoning, strangulation, and withholding food and water. *Deprived c.* a vague term usually implying that the child in question has been raised in a situation lacking in love, affection and consistent parenting responses from adults. Sometimes used to suggest that the child has experienced a generalised deficit of life opportunities, both interpersonal and social.

childbirth ('chield'bərth) the act or process of giving birth to a child. PARTURITION.

chiropody (ki'ropədee, shi-) the study and care of the feet and the treatment of foot diseases.

chiropractic (ˌkierə'praktik) a system of treatment employing manipulation of the spine and other bony structures.

Chlamydia (klə'midi·ə) a genus of bacteria comprised of two species: *C. trachomatis* which causes LYMPHOGRANULOMA venereum, trachoma, conjunctivitis, and non-gonococcal URETHRITIS; and *C. psittaci*, which causes psittacosis (parrot fever).

chi-square (kie skwair) (χ^2) a non-parametric statistic that is used to determine whether the frequency found in each category is different from the frequency that would be expected by chance.

chloasma (kloh'azmə) a condition in which there is brown, blotchy discolouration of the skin, appearing on the face, especially during pregnancy.

chloral ('klawrəl) an oily liquid formed by the reaction of chlorine and alcohol. Used in the production of *c. hydrate*, a drug used as a hypnotic; it is well tolerated by children and old people.

chlorambucil (klaw'rambyəsəl) an ankylating drug used in treating chronic leukaemia. A cytotoxic drug.

chloramphenicol (ˌklaw·ram-'fenəkol) an antibiotic. It gives rise to AGRANULOCYTOSIS and is used only for serious infectious diseases, such as typhoid fever. Used in drops and ointment for eye infections.

chlorcyclizine (klaw'sieklə,zeen) an antihistamine used for travel sickness.

chlorhexidine (klaw'heksə,deen) an antibacterial compound used for surgical scrub, preoperative skin preparation, and cleansing skin wounds.

chlorhydria (klaw'hiedri·ə) an excess of hydrochloric acid in the stomach.

chlorine ('klaw·reen) *symbol* Cl. A yellow, irritating poisonous gas. A powerful disinfectant, bleach, and deodorising agent. Used in hypochlorites for sterilisation purposes.

chlormethiazole (ˌklawmə'thieə-ˌzohl) a hypnotic and sedative drug used to treat insomnia, chiefly in elderly people.

chloroacetone (ˌklaw·roh'asə,tohn) chloracetone. Tear gas.

chlorocresol (ˌklaw·roh'kreesol) a coal tar product with a bacterial action more powerful than phenol and with a lower toxicity. Used as an antiseptic and as a preservative in injection fluids.

chloroform ('klo·rə,fawm) a colourless volatile liquid administered through inhalation as a general anaesthetic. Now rarely used.

chloroma (klaw'rohmə) a tumour having a greenish colour, usually found in skull bones. It is associated with MYELOID LEUKAEMIA.

chlorophyll ('klo·rə,fil) the green pigment of plants which absorbs solar energy for the synthesis of complex materials from the carbon dioxide and water taken in by the plant.

chloropsia (klaw'ropsi·ə) a form of colour blindness where all objects appear to have a greenish tinge.

chloroquine ('klaw·roh,kween) an antimalarial drug that has a strong suppressant action and is used in the treatment of amoebic hepatitis, rheumatoid arthritis, and LUPUS ERYTHEMATOSUS.

chlorothiazide ('klaw·roh'thieəzied) an oral diuretic used in the treatment of fluid retention and hypertension.

chlorotrianisene (ˌklaw·rohtrie-'anəseen) a long-acting oestrogen used in the treatment of menopausal symptoms and in cancer of the prostate.

chloroxylenol (ˌklaw·roh'zielənol) an antiseptic that is less irritating to the skin and mucous membranes than cresol and has a powerful disinfectant action.

chlorpheniramine (ˌklawfe'nirə-ˌmeen) an antihistamine drug used in the treatment of allergies such as hay fever and urticaria.

chlorpromazine (klaw'prohmə-ˌzeen) a sedative anti-emetic drug widely used to treat anxiety, agitation, and vomiting, particularly in the elderly, and in the management of psychiatric patients. It is also hypotensive and enhances the effect of analgesics and anaesthetics.

chlorpropamide (klaw'prohpə-ˌmied) an oral hypoglycaemic agent used in the treatment of type 2 diabetes.

chlorprothixene (ˌklawproh'thikseen) a tranquilliser used in the treatment of schizophrenia, psychoneuroses, and behaviour disorders.

chlortetracycline (ˌklawtetrə'siekleen) broad-spectrum antibiotic effective in treating many bacterial and protozoal infections.

chlorthalidone (klaw'thaləˌdohn) a diuretic used in the treatment of oedema and hypertension.

choana ('koh·anə, koh'ahnə) *pl* choanae [L.] 1. any funnel-shaped cavity or infundibulum. 2. *choanae* the paired openings between the nasal cavity and the nasopharynx.

cholaemia (ˌko'leemi·ə) the presence of bile in the blood.

cholangiography (kəˌlanji'ogrəfee) radiography of the hepatic, cystic, and bile ducts after the insertion of a radio-opaque contrast medium.

cholangitis (ˌkohlan'jietəs) inflammation of the bile ducts.

cholecystectomy (ˌkohləsi'stektəmee) excision of the gallbladder.

cholecystitis (ˌkohləsi'stietəs) inflammation of the gallbladder.

cholecystoduodenostomy (ˌkohləˌsistohˌdyooədə'nostəmee) an anastomosis between the gallbladder and the duodenum.

cholecystoenterostomy (ˌkohləˌsistohˌentə'rostəmee) the formation of an artificial opening from the gallbladder into the intestine. An operation performed in cases of irremovable obstruction of the bile duct.

cholecystography (ˌkohləsi'stogrəfee) radiography of the gallbladder after administration of a radio-opaque contrast medium.

cholecystokinin (ˌkohləˌsistoh'kienən) a hormone, released by the presence of fats in the duodenum, which causes contraction of the gallbladder.

cholecystolithiasis (ˌkohləˌsistohli'thiesəs) the presence of stones in the gallbladder.

cholecystotomy (ˌkohləsistotəmee) an incision into the gallbladder, usually to remove gallstones.

choledocholithiasis (ˌkohləˌdohkohlə'thieəsəs) the presence of stones in the bile duct.

choledocholithotomy (ˌkohləˌdohkohlə'thotəmee) incision into the bile ducts to remove stones.

choledochostomy (ˌkohlədoh'kostəmee) opening and draining of the common bile duct.

cholelithiasis (ˌkohləli'thieəsəs) presence of gallstones in the gallbladder or bile ducts.

cholera ('kolə·rə) an acute, notifiable, infectious enteritis which is endemic and epidemic in Asia and, more recently, in Africa. Caused by *Vibrio cholerae*, it is marked by profuse diarrhoea, muscle cramps, suppression of urine and severe prostration, and is often fatal. Travellers to areas where cholera is endemic should protect themselves by vaccination, although this provides only partial immunity. The local drinking water should be boiled and uncooked foods avoided.

cholestasis (ˌkohlə'staysəs) arrest of the flow of bile due to obstruction of the bile ducts.

cholesteatoma (ˌkohləˌsteeə'tohmə) a small tumour containing cholesterol; can occur in the middle ear. Also occurs in the meninges, central nervous system, and bones of the skull.

cholesterol (kə'lestəˌrol) a sterol found in nervous tissue, red blood-cells, animal fat, and bile. It is a precursor of bile acids and steroid hormones, and it occurs in the most common type of gallstone, in ATHEROMA of the arteries, in various cysts, and in carcinomatous tissue. Most of the body's cholesterol is synthesised, but some is obtained in the diet.

cholesterolosis (kəˌlestə·ro'lohsəs) a chronic form of cholecystitis in which the mucosa of the gallbladder is studded with deposits of cholesterol.

cholestyramine (ˌkohlə'stierəmeen) a drug that causes the excretion of bile salts by binding with them. Given to induce lower blood levels of cholesterol and other fats.

choline ('kohleen) an essential amine, found in the blood, cerebrospinal fluid, and urine, which aids fat metabolism. Formerly classified as a vitamin of the B complex. *C. theophyllinate* an antispasmodic drug used in respiratory conditions.

cholinergic (ˌkohlə'nərjik) pertaining to nerves that release acetylcholine, as the chemical stimulator, at their nerve endings. *C. drugs* drugs that inhibit CHOLINESTERASE and so prevent the destruction of acetylcholine.

cholinesterase (ˌkohlə'nestəˌrayz) an enzyme that rapidly destroys acetylcholine.

choluria (koh'lyoo·ri·ə) the presence of bile in the urine.

chondral ('kondrəl) pertaining to cartilage

chondritis (kon'drietəs) inflammation of cartilage.

chondroblast ('kondrəˌblast) an embryonic cell that forms cartilage.

chondrocyte ('kondrəˌsiet) a mature cartilage cell.

chondroma (kon'drohmə) an innocent new growth arising in cartilage.

chondromalacia (ˌkondrohmə'layshi·ə) a condition of abnormal softening of cartilage.

chondrosarcoma (ˌkondrohsah'kohmə) a malignant new growth arising from cartilaginous tissue.

chorda ('kawdə) a sinew or cord.

chordee (kaw'dee) downwards curvature of the penis caused by congenital anomaly (common in hypospadias) or urethral infection.

chorditis (kaw'dietəs) inflammation of the vocal or spermatic cords.

chordotomy (kaw'dotəmee) an operation on the spinal cord to divide the anterolateral nerve pathways for relief of intractable pain. Cordotomy.

chorea (ko'reeə) a symptom of disease of the basal ganglia whereby the individual suffers from spasmodic, involuntary, rapid movements of the face, shoulders, and hips. Huntington's c. (or Huntington's disease) a rare hereditary disorder which manifests itself in early middle age. The individual also suffers from progressive dementia, which often precedes a premature death. *Sydenham's c.* St Vitus's dance. Occurs in childhood and is associated with rheumatic fever.

choreiform (ko'ree·əfawm) resembling chorea.

choriocarcinoma (ˌko·riohˌkahsə'nohmə) formerly known as chorioepithelioma. A highly malignant NEOPLASM usually arising from the trophoblast of a hydatidiform mole (see hydatidiform mole). It can develop after an abortion or the evacuation of a hydatidiform mole or even in normal pregnancy. Metastases usually develop rapidly, but the disease usually has a good prognosis if early treatment is given.

chorioepithelioma (ˌko·riohˌepəˌtheeliˌohmə) CHORIOCARCINOMA.

chorion ('ko·reeon, 'kaw·ri·ən) the outer membrane enveloping the fetus; the placenta.

chorionic (ˌko·ree'onik) pertaining to the chorion. *C. gonadotrophin* human chorionic gonadotrophin (hcg). *C. villi* small protrusions on the chorion from which the placenta is formed. They are in close association with the maternal blood and, by diffusion, interchange of nutriment, oxygen, and waste matters is effected between the maternal and the fetal blood. *C. villus biopsy* tissue removed from the gestational sac early in pregnancy so that chromosomal and other inherited disorders can be identified. Can be carried out at an earlier stage than AMNIOCENTESIS.

chorioretinitis (ˌko·reeohˌretə'nietəs) choroidoretinitis.

choroid ('ko·royd) the pigmented and vascular coat of the eyeball, continuous with the iris and situated between the sclera and retina. It reduces the amount of light when it falls upon the retina. *C. plexus* specialised cells in the ventricles of the brain which produce cerebrospinal fluids. There is one choroid plexus in each ventricle.

choroiditis (ˌko·roy'dietəs) inflammation of the choroid.

choroidoretinitis (koˌroydohˌretən'nietəs) an inflammatory condition of both the choroid and retina of the eye.

Christmas disease ('krisməs) an hereditary bleeding disease similar to haemophilia. The name is derived from that of the first patient to be studied.

chromatography (ˌkrohmə'tografee) a method of chemical analysis by which substances in solution can be separated as they percolate down a column of powdered adsorbent or ascend an absorbent paper by capillary traction. A definite pattern is produced and substances can be recognised by the use of appropriate colour reagents. Amino acids can be identified in this way.

chromatometry (ˌkrohmə'tomətree) the measurement of colour perception.

chromatopsia (ˌkrohmə'topsi·ə) abnormal colour vision. Partial colour blindness.

chromic acid ('krohmik) a strong caustic sometimes used for the removal of warts.

chromicise ('krohməˌsiez) to impregnate with chromic acid; e.g. chromicised catgut, which is particularly strong and durable.

chromosome ('krohməˌsohm) in animal cells, a structure in the nucleus, containing a linear thread of DEOXYRIBONUCLEIC ACID, which transmits genetic information and is associated with RIBONUCLEIC ACID and histones. During cell division the material composing the chromosome is compactly coiled. Each organism of a species is normally characterised by the same number of chromosomes in its somatic cells, 46 being the number usually present in humans; 22 pairs of autosomes, and two sex chromosomes (XX or XY), which determine the sex of the organism. In the mature GAMETE (ovum or spermatozoa) the number of chromosomes is halved as a result of MEIOSIS.

chronic ('kronik) of long duration; the opposite of acute.

chrysarobin (ˌkrisə'rohbən) a derivative of Goa powder used in ointment form especially in the treatment of PSORIASIS It stains linen a yellow colour. *See* DITHRANOL.

Chvostek's sign (ˌvosteks) *F. Chvostek, Austrian surgeon, 1835–84*. A spasm of the facial muscles which occurs in tetany. It can be elicited by tapping the facial nerve.

chyle (kiel) digested fats which, as a milky fluid, are absorbed into the lymphatic capillaries (lacteals) in the villi of the small intestine.

chylothorax (ˌkieloh'thor·raks) the presence of effused chyle in the pleural cavity.

chyme (kiem) the semiliquid, acid mass of food that passes from the stomach to the intestines.

chymotrypsin (ˌkiemoh'tripsən) an enzyme secreted by the pancreas. It is activated by trypsin and assists in the breakdown of proteins.

Ci symbol for *curie*, a unit of radioactivity.

cicatrix ('sikətriks) the scar of a healed wound (see keloid).

cilia ('sili·ə) 1. the eyelashes. 2. microscopic filaments projecting from some epithelial cells, known as ciliated membranes, as in the bronchi, where cilia wave the secretion upwards.

ciliary ('sili·əˌree) hair-like. *C. body* a structure just behind the corneoscleral margin, composed of the ciliary muscle and processes. *C. muscle* the circular muscle surrounding the lens of the eye. *C. processes* the fringed part of the choroid coat arranged in a circle in front of the lens.

cimetidine (si'metəˌdeen) a histamine H_2-receptor antagonist which reduces gastric acid secretion; used in the treatment of peptic ulcers.

Cimex ('siemeks) a genus of blood-sucking bugs. *C. lectularius* the common bedbug.

CINAHL (Cumulative Index to Nursing and Allied Health Literature) a print or computerised database; computerised CINAHL is available on CD-Rom or on-line.

cinchocaine ('singkohkayn) a local anaesthetic agent.

cinchona (sing'kohnə) Peruvian bark, from which quinine is obtained.

cinchonism ('singkəˌnizəm) poisonous effect of cinchona. Quininism.

cineangiocardiography (ˌsinee-ˌanjiohˌkahdi'ogrəfee) angiography using a cine camera to show the movements of the heart and blood vessels.

cineradiography (ˌsineeˌraydee-'ogrəfee) the making of a motion picture record of successive images appearing on a fluoroscopic screen.

cinnamon ('sinəmən) an extract from the bark of an East Indian laurel, sometimes used as a digestive and carminative.

cinnarizine (si'narəˌzeen) an antihistamine drug which may also be used to treat nausea, vertigo, labyrinthine disorders, and motion sickness.

circadian (sər'kaydi·ən) denoting a period of 24 hours. *C. rhythm* the rhythm of certain biological activities that take place daily.

circinate (ˌsərsəˌnayt) having a circular outline. *Tinea circinata* is ringworm.

circle of Willis ('serkəl ə wiləs) *T. Willis, British physician and anatomist, 1621–75.* An anastomosis of arteries at the base of the brain, formed by the branches of the internal carotid and the basilar arteries.

circulation (ˌsərkyə'layshən) movement in a circular course, as of the blood. *Collateral c.* enlargement of small vessels establishing adequate blood supply when the main vessel to the part has been occluded. *Coronary c.* the system of vessels that supplies the heart muscle itself. *Extracorporeal c.* 1. removal of the blood by intravenous cannulae, passing it through a machine to oxygenate it, and then pumping it back into circulation. 2. the 'heart–lung' machine or pump respirator, used in cardiac surgery. *Lymph c.* the flow of lymph through lymph vessels and glands. *Portal c.* the passage of blood from the alimentary tract, pancreas, and spleen, via the portal vein and its branches through the liver and into the hepatic veins. *Pulmonary c.* passage of the blood from the right ventricle via the pulmonary artery through the lungs and back to the heart by the pulmonary veins. *Systemic c.* the flow of blood throughout the body. The direction of flow is from the left atrium to the left ventricle and through the aorta, with its branches and capillaries. Veins then carry it back to the right atrium, and so into the right ventricle.

circumcision (ˌsərkəmˌsizhən) excision of the prepuce or foreskin of the penis. An operation performed for religious reasons, or sometimes for phimosis or paraphimosis. *Female c.* excision of the labia minor and/or labia majora and sometimes the clitoris; still performed ritualistically in certain countries, the extent of the surgery varying from one culture to another.

circumduction (ˌsərkəm'dukshən) moving in a circle, e.g. the circular movement of the upper limb.

circumoral (ˌsərkəm'o·rəl) around the mouth. *C. pallor* a pale area around the mouth contrasting with the flushed cheeks, e.g. in scarlet fever.

circumvallate ('sərkəm'valayt) surrounded by a wall or raised ring. *C. papilla see* PAPILLA.

cirrhosis (sə'rohsəs) a degenerative change that can occur in any organ, but especially in the liver. Can be due to viruses, microorganisms, or toxic substances (*portal c.*). Fibrosis results and interferes with the working of the organ. In the liver it causes portal obstruction, with consequent ascites. *Alcoholic c.* the result of chronic alcoholism and nutritional deficiency which affects the liver. *Cardiac c.* cirrhosis of the liver following chronic heart failure. *Posthepatic c.* cirrhosis of the liver following hepatitis. *Pulmonary c.* cirrhosis of the lung tissue.

cisplatin ('sispləˌtin) an antineoplastic drug, containing platinum, used in the treatment of ovar-ian carcinomas and testicular TERATOMATA.

cisterna (si'stərnə) a space or cavity containing fluid. *C. chyli* the dilated portion of the thoracic duct containing chyle. *C. magna* the subarachnoid space between the cerebellum and MEDULLA oblongata.

cisternal (si'stərnəl) concerning the cisterna. *C. puncture* insertion of a hollow needle into the cisterna magna to withdraw cerebrospinal fluid.

citric acid ('sitrik) acid found in the juice of lemons, limes, etc. An antiscorbutic.

Cl symbol for *chlorine*.

clamp (klamp) a metal surgical instrument used to compress any part of the body.

clapping ('klaping) in physiotherapy, rhythmic beating with cupped hands. Frequently used over the chest to aid expectoration.

claudication (ˌklawdə'kayshən) lameness. *Intermittent c.* limping, accompanied by severe pain in the legs on walking, which disappears with rest. A sign of occlusive arterial disease.

claustrophobia (ˌklostrə'fohbi·ə, ˌklaw-) fear of confined spaces, such as small rooms.

clavicle ('klavikəl) the collar bone. A long bone, part of the shoulder girdle.

clavus ('klayvəs) a corn.

clawfoot (ˌklaw'fuht) a deformity of the foot in which the longitudinal arch is abnormally raised. PES CAVUS

clawhand (ˌklaw'hand) a deformity of the hand in which the fingers are bent and contracted, giving a claw-like appearance.

cleft (kleft) a fissure or longitudinal opening. *C. lip* a congenital fissure in the upper lip, often accompanied by cleft palate. *C. palate* a congenital defect in the roof of the mouth due to failure of the medial plates of the palate to meet. Often associated with cleft lip.

client ('klieənt) 1. recipient of a professional service. 2. a recipient of health care, regardless of the person's state of health and where the service is delivered. 3. a patient.

climacteric (klie'maktə·rik, ˌkliemək'terik) the period of the menopause in women. Also used to denote a decline in sexual drive in men.

climax ('kliemaks) 1. the stage when a disease is at its greatest intensity. 2. the stage in sexual intercourse when orgasm occurs.

clindamycin (ˌklində'miesən) an antibiotic active against Gram-positive cocci and many anaerobes.

clinic ('klinik) 1. instruction of students at the bedside. 2. a department of a hospital devoted to the treatment of a particular type of disease.

clinical ('klinikəl) relating to bedside observation and the treatment of patients. *C. nurse specialist* a qualified nurse who has acquired advanced knowledge and skills in a specific area of clinical nursing.

clip (klip) a metal device for holding the two edges of a wound together or for controlling the flow of liquid through a tube.

clitoridectomy (ˌklitə·rə'dektəmee) excision of the clitoris.

clitoris ('klitə·rəs, 'kliet-) a small organ, formed of erectile tissue, situated at the anterior junction of the labia minora in the female.

cloaca (kloh'aykə) 1. the common intestinal and urogenital opening present in many vertebrates. 2. opening through newly formed bone from a diseased area so that pus can escape. *See* INVOLUCRUM.

clofibrate (kloh'fiebrayt) a drug that lowers blood cholesterol.

clomipramine (kloh'miprəˌmeen) an antidepressant drug used to treat patients with obsessional fears.

clonazepam (kloh'nazəˌpam) an anticonvulsive drug.

clone (klohn) cells that are genetically identical to each other and have descended by asexual reproduction from the parent cell, to which they are also genetically identical.

clonic ('klonik) having the character of clonus. The second stage of a grand mal fit; also referred to as a tonic–clonic seizure. *See* EPILEPSY.

clonidine ('klohnə,deen) an antihypertensive drug which is also used to treat migraine.

clonus ('klohnəs) spasmodic muscle rigidity and relaxation. *Ankle c.* spasmodic movements of the calf muscles when the foot is suddenly pushed upwards, the leg being extended.

close-ended item question that the respondent can answer with only one of a fixed number of choices.

Clostridium (klo'stridi·əm) a genus of anaerobic spore-forming bacteria, found as commensals of the gut of animals and humans and saprophytes of the soil. Pathogenic species include *C. botulinum* (botulism), *C. tetani* (tetanus), and *C. perfringens* (also known as C. welchii) (gas gangrene).

clot (klot) a semisolid mass formed in a liquid, such as blood or lymph, by coagulation.

clotrimazole (kloh'triemə,zohl) an antifungal drug.

clotting ('kloting) coagulation. The formation of a clot. *C. time* coagulation time. The length of time taken for shed blood to coagulate.

cloxacillin (,kloksə'silən) an antibiotic drug effective against penicillin-resistant staphylococci.

clubbing ('klubing) broadening and thickening of the tips of the fingers (and toes) due to bad circulation. It occurs in chronic diseases of the heart and respiratory system, such as congenital cardiac defect and tuberculosis.

clubfoot (,klub'fuht) TALIPES. A congenital deformity of the foot.

clumping ('klumping) collecting together into clumps. The reaction of bacteria and blood cells when agglutination occurs.

CMV cytomegalovirus.

Co symbol for *cobalt.*

COAD chronic obstructive airways disease.

co-trimoxazole (,kohtrie,moksə,zohl) an antibiotic drug, taken orally and used mainly to treat urinary infections.

coagulase (koh'agyə,layz) an enzyme formed by pathogenic staphylococci that causes coagulation of plasma. Such bacteria are termed *c. positive*.

coagulation (koh,agyə'layshən) clotting.

coagulopathy (koh,agyə'lopəthee) a condition affecting the ability of the blood to coagulate.

coagulum (koh'agyələm) the mass of fibrin and cells formed when blood clots, the mass formed when other masses coagulate, e.g. milk curd.

coal tar (kohl tah) a byproduct obtained in the destructive distillation of coal; used in ointment or solution in treatment of eczema and psoriasis.

coarctation (,koh·ahk'tayshən) a condition of contraction or stricutre. *C. of aorta* a congenital malformation characterised by deformity of the aorta, causing narrowing, usually severe, of the lumen of the vessel. Surgical resection of the stricture can be performed. *See* figure p. 98.

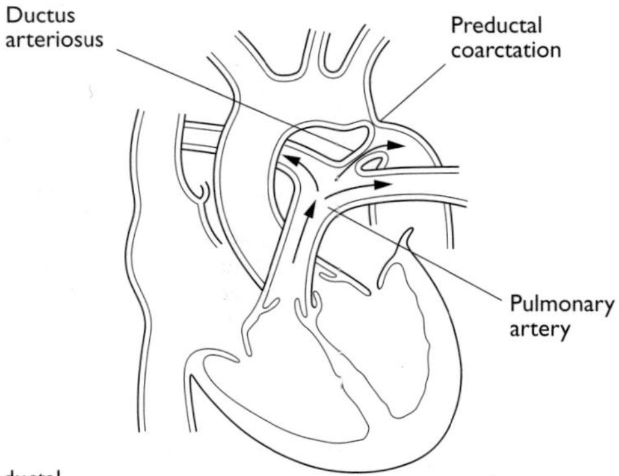

(a) Preductal

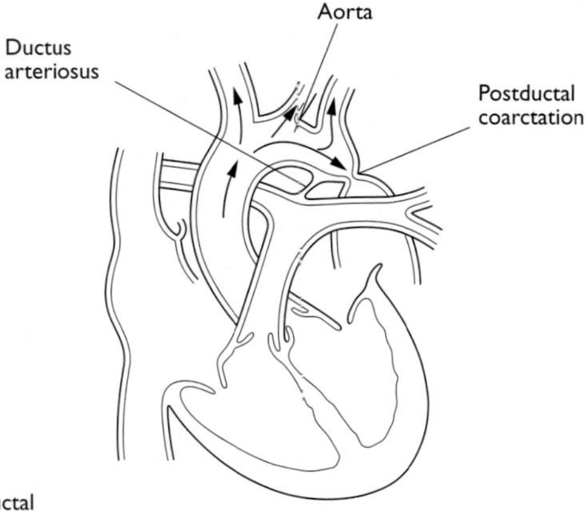

(b) Postductal

Coarctation of Aorta

cobalt ('kohbawlt) *symbol* Co. A metallic element, traces of which are necessary in the diet to prevent anaemia. *Radioactive c.* cobalt-60, used as a source of gamma irradiation in radiotherapy.

cocaine (koh'kayn) a colourless alkaloid, obtained from coca leaves, which has a powerful but brief stimulant action. Formerly used as a local anaesthetic, cocaine has been replaced by less addictive preparations such as procaine, lignocaine, and amethocaine. It is now a major recreational drug, producing euphoria with many undesirable behavioural and social effects. It is addictive and usually taken by snorting. Also known, in its various forms, as 'crack', 'coke', 'snow', 'Charlie' or 'c'.

cocainism (koh'kaynizəm) addiction to cocaine. Long-term abuse is associated with a toxic psychosis similar to that caused by amphetamines.

coccus ('kokəs) a bacterium of spheroidal shape.

coccydynia (ˌkoksə'dini·ə) persistent pain in the region of the coccyx.

coccygeal (kok'siji·əl) pertaining to the coccyx.

coccyx ('koksiks) the terminal bone of the spinal column, in which four rudimentary vertebrae are fused together to form a triangle.

cochlea ('kokli·ə) the spiral canal of the internal ear.

code (kohd) 1. a set of rules governing one's conduct. 2. a system by which information can be communicated. *Genetic c.* the arrangement of nucleotides in the polynucleotide chain of a chromosome that governs the transmission of genetic information.

codeine ('kohdeen) an alkaloid of opium. A mild analgesic and antitussive.

cod liver oil (kod livə) purified oil from the liver of the codfish; valuable sources of vitamins A and D.

coeliac ('seeleeˌak) relating to the abdomen. *C. disease* gluten ENTEROPATHY. A condition of early childhood occurring soon after the child has been weaned on to cereals, characterised by STEATORRHEA, distended abdomen, and failure to grow. The failure of carbohydrate and fat metabolism appears to be due to the gluten in wheat and rye. The condition can continue into adult life. It is managed by eating a gluten-free diet. *C. plexus* nerve complex that supplies the abdominal organs.

coenzyme (koh'enziem) an organic molecule activator to a larger protein enzyme.

cognition (kog'nishən) the mental process characterised by knowing, thinking, understanding, learning, and judging. The cognitive function of the conscious mind can be contrasted with the affective (feeling) and conative (willing) functions.

cohort ('kohˌhawt) a group of people possessing a common characteristic, such as being born in the same year or of the same sex, used in research to make generalisations derived from quantitative data. *C. study* concerning a specific group or subpopulation in a research study.

coitus ('koytəs, 'koh·itəs) sexual intercourse between male and female. *C. interruptus* a method of birth control whereby the erect penis is removed from the vagina before ejaculation occurs.

colchicine ('kolchə,seen) a drug obtained from the seeds of *Colchicum autumnale*. Used in treating gout.

cold (kohld) 1. of low temperature. 2. a viral infection affecting the membranes of the nose and throat and the bronchial tubes. *C. sore* herpes simplex. *See* HERPES.

colectomy (koh'lektəmee) the surgical excision of a portion or all of the colon.

colic ('kolik) acute paroxysmal abdominal pain. *Biliary c.* pain due to the presence of a gallstone in a bile duct. *Infantile c.* excessive crying due to pain and distress. Most common in the first three months of life. The infant might pull up his or her legs and expel gas from the anus or 'belch'. Can be due to air swallowing, milk intolerance, or natural hyperactivity. *Intestinal c.* severe griping spasmodic abdominal pain which can be a symptom of food poisoning or of intestinal obstruction. *Renal c.* pain due to the presence of a stone in the ureter. *Uterine c.* spasmodic pain originating in the uterus, as in DYSMENORRHOEA.

coliform ('kohli,fawm) resembling the bacillus *Escherichia coli*.

colistin (koh'listən) an antibiotic produced from *Bacillus polymyxa*. Used to treat gastrointestinal and other bacterial infections.

colitis (kə'lietəs, koh-) inflammation of the colon. It can be due to a specific organism, as in dysentery. The term *ulcerative c.* denotes a chronic disease, often of unknown cause, in which there are attacks of diarrhoea, with the passage of blood and mucus.

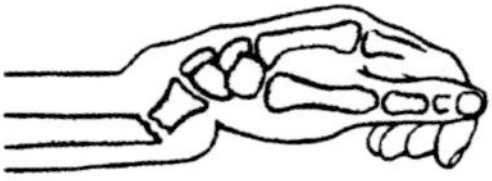

Colles' Fracture

collagen ('koləjən) a fibrous structural protein that constitutes the protein of the white (collagenous) fibres of skin, tendon, bone, cartilage, and all other connective tissues. It also occurs dispersed in a gel to provide stiffening, as in the vitreous humour of the eye. *C. diseases* a group of diseases having in common certain clinical and histological features that are manifestations of involvement of connective tissues (see connective tissues).

collapse (kə'laps) 1. a state of extreme prostration due to defective action of the heart, severe shock, or haemorrhage. 2. falling in of a structure.

collar bone ('kolə,bohn) the clavicle.

collateral (kə'latə·rəl) accessory to. *C. circulation* an alternative to the direct route for the blood when a primary vessel is blocked.

Colles' fracture ('koliz) *A. Colles, Irish surgeon, 1773–1843.* Fracture of the lower end of the radius at the wrist following a fall on the outstretched hand. Typically, it produces a 'dinner fork' deformity (*see* figure).

collimator ('kolə,maytə) a shield, shutter, or cone device used in radiotherapy machines to help in determining the limits of the treatment field.

colloid ('koloyd) 1. glue-like. 2.

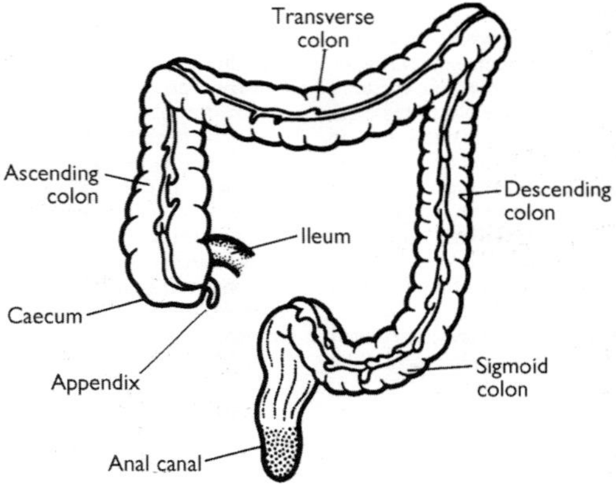

Colon

translucent, yellowish, gelatinous substance resulting from colloid degeneration. 3. a chemical system composed of a continuous medium of small particles which do not settle out under the influence of gravity and will not pass through a semi-permeable membrane, as in DIALYSIS.

coloboma (ˌkoloh'bohmə) a congenital fissure of the eye affecting the iris, ciliary body or choroid.

colon ('kohlon) the large intestine, from the caecum to the rectum (*see* figure). *Ascending c.* that part arising to the right of the abdomen to in front of the liver. *Descending c.* that part running down from in front of the spleen to the sigmoid colon. *Giant c.* megacolon. *Irritable c.* (*see* IRRITABLE bowel syndrome). *Pelvic c., sigmoid c.* that part lying in the pelvis and connecting the descending colon with the rectum. *Transverse c.* that part lying across the upper abdomen connecting the ascending and descending portions.

colonic (kə'lonik) pertaining to the colon. *C. irrigation* colonic lavage (*see* LAVAGE).

colonoscope (koh'lonəˌskohp) a fibre-optic instrument, passed through the anus, for examining the interior of the colon.

colony ('kolənee) a mass of bacteria formed by multiplication of cells when bacteria are incubated under favourable conditions.

colostomy (kə'lostəmee) an artificial opening (stoma) in the large intestine brought to the surface of the abdomen for the purpose of evacuating the bowel.

colostrum (kə'lostrəm) the fluid secreted by the breasts in the last few weeks of pregnancy and for the first 3 or 4 days after delivery, until lactation begins. Colostrum is high in protein and initially low in lactose; its fat content is equivalent to breast milk. It is an important source of passive antibody.

colour blindness ('kulə ˌbliendnəs) ACHROMATOPSIA.

colpitis (kol'pietəs) inflammation of the vagina.

colpocele ('kolpohˌseel) a hernia of either bladder or rectum into the vagina. VAGINOCELE.

colpohysterectomy (ˌkolpohˌhistə-'rektəmee) removal of the uterus through the vagina.

colpoperineorrhaphy (ˌkolpoh-ˌperini'o·frəfee) the repair by suturing of an injured vagina and torn perineum.

colpopexy ('kolpohˌpeksee) suture of a prolapsed vagina to the abdominal wall.

colpoplasty ('kolpohˌplastee) a plastic operation on the vagina.

colporrhaphy (kol'po·rəfee) repair of the vagina. *Anterior c.* repair for CYSTOCELE. *Posterior c.* repair for RETROCELE.

colposcope ('kolpəˌskohp) a speculum for examining the vagina and cervix by means of a magnifying lens; used for the early detection of malignant changes.

coma ('kohmə) a state of unconsciousness from which the patient cannot be aroused. Characterised by an absence both of spontaneous eye movements and response to painful stimuli. *See* GLASGOW COMA SCALE.

comatose (ˌkohməˌtohs, -ˌtohz) in the condition of coma.

comedo (ko'meedoh) a blackhead. A plug of keratin and sebum within the dilated orifice of a hair follicle.

commensal (kə'mensəl) living on or within another organism, and deriving benefit without harming or benefiting the host individual.

comminuted ('koməˌnyootəd) broken into small pieces, as in a comminuted fracture. *See* FRACTURE.

commissure ('komisˌyooə) a site of union of corresponding parts, as the angle of the lips or eyelids.

commode (ˌkə'mohd) a bedside chair with a cutaway seat that allows a receptacle to be fitted underneath for the collection of urine and faeces. Used by a patient who is unable to reach or use the nearest lavatory.

common bile duct ('komən biel dukt) the duct formed by the juncture of the hepatic and cystic ducts.

communicable disease (kə'myooni-kəbəl) a disease, the causative agents of which can pass (or be carried) from a person, animal, or the environment to a susceptible person either directly or indirectly.

community (kə'myoonətee) a group of individuals living in an area, having a common interest, or belonging to the same organisation. *C. nurse* a nurse who is based within the community with a responsibility for providing nursing services within the patient's own home or environment. Community nurses have a strong commitment to health promotion and the prevention of ill health. *Therapeutic c.* any treatment setting (usually psychiatric) which provides a living–learning situation through group processes emphasising social, environmental, and personal interactions.

compartment syndrome (kəm'pahtmənt) muscle ischaemia caused by increased pressure in an osteofascial compartment. Can be caused by oedema or bleeding following trauma or excessive muscle use.

compatibility (kəm,patə'bilətee) mutual suitability. Mixing together of two substances without chemical change or loss of power. *See* BLOOD GROUP.

compensation (,kompən'sayshən) 1. making good a functional or structural defect. 2. mental mechanism (unconscious) by which a person covers up a weakness by exaggerating a more desirable characteristic.

complement ('kompləmənt) a substance present in normal serum which combines with an antigen–antibody complex. (*c. fixation*) to destroy bacteria. *C. fixation test* measurement of the amount of complement with an antigen–antibody complex to destroy bacteria. Complement fixation tests are widely used to detect antibodies for infectious diseases and include the WASSERMANN test for syphilis.

complementary (,komplə'mentə·ree) pertaining to that which completes or makes perfect. *C. feed* feed given to infants to supplement breast feeding if the mother has insufficient milk. *C. therapies* a range of treatments, including yoga, reflexology, homeopathy, acupuncture, and others, which can be combined with traditional medicine.

complex ('kompleks) a grouping of various things, as of signs and symptoms, forming a syndrome. In psychology, a grouping of ideas of emotional origin which are completely or partially represented in the unconscious mind. *Inferiority c.* a feeling of inadequacy; responses can vary from assertiveness or aggression (as compensation or cover) to passivity and withdrawal (because of feelings of inadequacy). *See* ELECTRA COMPLEX and OEDIPUS COMPLEX.

complication (komplə'kayshən) an accident or second disease process arising during the course of or following the primary condition; can be fatal.

compos mentis ('kompəs 'mentəs) [L.] *of sound mind.*

compound ('kompownd) composed of two or more parts or substances. *C. fracture* a fracture in which the overlying skin has been broken.

comprehension (,komprə'henshən) mental grasp of the meaning of a situation.

compress ('kompres) folded material, e.g. lint (wet or dry), applied to a part of the body for the relief of swelling and pain.

compression (kəm'preshən) 1. the act of pressing upon or together; the state of being pressed together. 2. in embryology, the shortening or omission of certain developmental stages.

compulsion (kəm'pulshən) an overwhelming urge to perform an irrational act or ritual.

computed tomography (kəm'pyoo-,təd tə'mogrəfee) abbreviated CT. The utilisation of a computerised technique to examine a cross-section of the entire body. A CT scanner produces an image of tissue density in a complete cross-section of the part of the body being scanned.

conation (koh'nayshən) a striving in a certain direction. *See* COGNITION.

concave ('konkayv, kon'kayv) hollowed out. The opposite of convex.

concept ('konsept) an image or idea held in the mind.

conception (kən'sepshən) 1. the act of becoming pregnant, by the fertilisation of an ovum. 2. a concept.

conceptual framework (kən'sep-tyooəl, kən'sepshooəl) a group of concepts that are broadly defined and organised to provide a rationale or structure for the interpretation of information.

concretion (kən'kreeshən) a calculus or other hardened material present within an organ.

concussion (kən'kushən) a violent jarring shock. *C. of the brain* temporary loss of consciousness produced by a fall or a blow on the head. There can be amnesia, slow respiration, and a weak pulse.

conditioned response (kən'dishənd) a response that does not occur naturally but can might be developed by regular association of a physiological function with an unrelated outside event, such as ringing of a bell or flashing of a light. Eventually, the physiological function starts whenever the outside event occurs. Called also 'conditioned reflex'. *Unconditioned r.* an unlearnt response, i.e. one that occurs naturally.

conditioning (kən'dishəning) a form of learning in which a response is elicited by a neural stimulus that had previously been repeatedly presented in conjunction with the stimulus that originally elicted the response. Called also 'classical' and 'respondent' conditioning. The concept had its beginnings in experimental techniques for the study of reflexes. *Instrumental c., operant c.* learning in which a particular response is elicited by a stimulus because that response produces desirable consequences (reward). Instrumental conditioning differs from classical conditioning in that the reinforcement takes place only after the subject performs a specific act that has been previously designated. If no unconditioned stimulus is used to bring about this act, the desired behaviour is known as an operant. Once the behaviour occurs with regularity, the behaviour can be called a conditioned response. The principles and techniques related to instrumental conditioning are used clinically in behavioural therapy to help patients eliminate undesirable behaviour and substitute newly learnt behaviour that is more appropriate and acceptable (*see* BEHAVIOUR THERAPY). *Respondent c. see* CONDITIONING.

condom ('kondəm) a contraceptive sheath worn during sexual intercourse and affording some protection for both partners against sexually transmitted diseases. Now available for both males and females.

conduction system (kən'dukshən) tissue that carries electrical impulses.

conductor (kən'duktə) 1. a substance through which electricity, light, heat, or sound can pass. 2. any part of the nervous system that conveys impulses.

condyle ('kondiel, -dil) a rounded eminence occurring at the end of some bones and articulating with another bone.

condyloma (ˌkondəˈlohmə) *pl.* condylomata; an elevated wartlike lesion of the skin. *Condylomata acuminata* small, pointed PAPILLOMATA of viral origin, usually occurring on the skin or mucous surfaces of the external genitalia or perianal region. *Condylomata lata* wide, flat, syphilitic condylomata occurring on moist skin, especially about the genitals and anus.

cone (kohn) a solid figure with a rounded base, tapering upwards to a point. *Retinal c.* the cone-shaped end of a light-sensitive cell in the retina, used for acute vision and for distinguishing colours.

confabulation (kənˌfabyəˈlayshən) the production of fictitious memories and the relating of experiences which have no relation to truth, to fill in the gaps due to loss of memory. A symptom of KORSAKOFF'S SYNDROME.

confidence interval (ˈkonfədəns ˈintəvəl) quantifies the uncertainty of a statistic or the probable value range within which a population parameter is expected to lie.

confidentiality (ˌkonfəˌdenshee-ˈalətee) the nondisclosure of information except to another authorised person or assurance that a research participant's identity cannot be linked to the information that was provided to the researcher.

conflict (ˈkonflikt) a mental state arising when two opposing wishes or impulses cause emotional tension and often cannot be resolved without repressing one of the impulses into the unconscious. Conflict situations can be associated with an anxiety neurosis.

confluent (ˈkonflooənt) running together.

confusion (kənˈfyoozhən) disturbed orientation with respect to time, place, person, or situation sometimes accompanied by disordered consciousness.

congenital (kənˈjenətˈl) present at and existing from the time of birth. *C. dislocation of the hip* failure in position of the head of the femur and development of the ACETABULUM. *C. heart defect* a structural defect of the heart or great vessels or both; present at birth. *C. infection* an infection which takes place in utero. The most important congenital infections are RUBELLA, CYTOMEGALOVIRUS, HERPES SIMPLEX, human immunodeficiency virus (HIV), syphilis, and TOXOPLASMOSIS.

congestion (kənˈjeschən) an abnormal accumulation of blood in any part. *Pulmonary c.* congestion of the lung, as in pneumonia and congestive heart failure.

conisation (ˌkohnieˈzayshən) removal of a cone-shaped piece of tissue from the uterine cervix, as in cone biopsy.

conjuctiva (ˌkonjungkˈtievə) the mucous membrane covering the front of the eyeball and lining the eyelids.

conjunctivitis (kənˌjungktəˈvietəs) inflammation of the conjunctiva. 'Pink eye' ophthalmia. *Catarrhal c.* a mild form, usually due to cold or irritation. *Granular c.* trachoma. *Phlyctenular c.* marked by small vesicles or ulcers on the membrane. *Purulent c.* caused by virulent organisms, with discharge of pus.

connective (kəˈnektiv) joining together. *C. tissues* those that develop from the mesenchyme and are formed of a matrix containing fibres and cells. Areolar tissue, cartilage and bone are examples.

consanguinity (ˌkonsang·gwinətee) blood relationship.

conscious (konshəs) the state of being awake or aware. *Levels of consciousness* loosely defined states of awareness of, and response, to stimuli, essential for the assessment of an individual's neurological status. The level of consciousness is an accurate indication of the degree of brain (dys)function.

consent (kən'sent) in law, voluntary agreement with an action proposed by another. Consent is an act of reason; the person giving consent must be of sufficient mental capacity and be in possession of all essential information in order to give valid consent. *C. forms* in non-emergency situations, written consent is generally required before many clinical procedures, such as surgery (including biopsies), endoscopy, and radiographic procedures involving catheterisation. The doctor must explain to the patient the diagnosis, the nature of the procedure, including the risks involved and the chances of success, and the alternative methods of treatment that are available. It is recommended that consent forms should contain a signed declaration that the doctor has explained the nature of the procedure to the patient in non-technical words. Nurses or other members of the healthcare team might be involved in filling out the consent form and witnessing the signature of the patient (*see* INFORMED CONSENT).

conservative treatment (kən'sərvətiv) the use of non-radical methods to restore health and preserve function.

consolidation (kənˌsolə'dayshən) a state of becoming solid. *C. of lung* in pneumonia, the infected lobe becomes solid with exudate.

constipation (ˌkonstə'payshən) incomplete or infrequent action of the bowels, with consequent filling of the rectum with hard faeces. *Atonic c.* constipation due to lack of muscle tone in the bowel wall. *Spastic c.* a form of constipation in which spasm of part of the bowel wall narrows the canal.

consumption (kən'sumpshən) 1. the act of consuming, or the process of being consumed. 2. a wasting away of the body; once applied to pulmonary tuberculosis.

contact ('kontakt) 1. touching of two bodies or persons. 2. an individual known to have been in association with an infected person or animal or a contaminated environment that might have exposed him or her to infection. *C. dermatitis* a skin rash marked by itching, swelling, blistering, oozing, and scaling. It is caused by direct contact between the skin and a substance to which the person is allergic or sensitive. *C. lens* a glass or plastic lens worn under the eyelids in the front of the eye. It might be worn for therapeutic or cosmetic reasons.

contagion (kən'tayjən) 1. the communication of disease from one person to another by direct contact. 2. an infectious disease.

containment (kən'taynmənt) a term used in communicable disease control, meaning prevention of spread of disease from a focus of infection.

contamination (kən,tamə'nayshən) being soiled or exposed to harmful agents.

content analysis ('kontent ənaləsəs) a technique for the objective, systematic, and quantitative description of communications and documentary evidence.

continence ('kon,tənəns) 1. able to control urination and defecation. 2. exercising self-restraint, especially abstaining from sexual activity.

continuing care (kən'tinyooing) ongoing care of the physically, mentally, and emotionally handicapped, and those suffering from chronic incapacitating illness.

continuing education further study after the attainment of basic qualifications.

continuous ambulatory peritoneal dialysis abbreviated CAPD. The patient is ambulant while receiving peritoneal dialysis.

continuous positive airway pressure abbreviated CPAP. A process whereby medical gas is delivered to the patient at positive pressure to hold open alveoli that would normally close at the end of expiration, thereby increasing oxygenation and reducing the work of breathing.

contraception (,kontrə'sepshən) the prevention of conception and pregnancy.

contraceptive (,kontrə'septiv) an agent used to prevent conception, e.g. condom, cap that occludes the cervix, spermidical pessary or cream, intrauterine device (IUD), and oral contraceptives (hormone pills).

contraction (kən'trakshən) a shortening or drawing together, especially applied to muscle action. *Uterine c's* those occurring during labour.

contracture (kən'trakchə) fibrosis causing permanent contraction. *Dupuytren's c.* contraction of the palmar fascia causing permanent bending and fixation of one or more fingers. *Volkmann's ischaemic c.* contraction resulting from impairment of the blood supply. Can occur in upper or lower limbs.

contraindication (,kontrə,ində'kayshən) any condition that makes a particular line of treatment impracticable or undesirable.

contralateral (,kontrə'latə·rəl) occurring on the opposite side.

contrast medium ('kontrahst) a substance used in radiography to make certain organs visible or more visible.

contrecoup (,kontrə'koo) [Fr.] an injury occurring on the opposite side or at a distance from the site of the blow, e.g. brain damage on the opposite side of the skull to the blow.

control (kən'trohl) restrain or command of objects or events. *C. group* a standard for testing whereby the procedure is identical in all respects to the experimental group but the factor being studied is absent. *Birth c.* contraception.

contusion (kən'tyoozhən) a bruise.

convalescence (,konvə'lesəns) period of recovery following illness, injury, or operation.

convection (kən'vekzhən) a method of transmission of heat by the circulation of warmed molecules of a liquid or a gas.

conversion (kən'vərzhən) 1. the act of changing into something of different form or properties. 2. the transformation of emotions into physical manifestations. 3. manipulative correction of malposition of a fetal part during labour.

convex ('konveks) bowing outwards. Having an outline like a segment of a sphere.

convolution ('konvə'looshən) a fold or coil, e.g. of the cerebrum or renal tubules.

convulsion (kən'vulshən) involuntary contractions of the voluntary muscles. Convulsive seizures are symptomatic of some neurological disorder; they are not in themselves a disease entity. *Clonic c.* a convulsion marked by alternative contracting and relaxing of the muscles. *Febrile c.* a convulsion occurring almost exclusively in children aged 6 months to 5 years of age, and associated with a fever of 40°C or higher. *Tonic c.* prolonged contraction of the muscles, as a result of an epileptic discharge. *See* EPILEPSY.

Cooley's anaemia ('kooleez) *T.B. Cooley, American paediatrician, 1871–1945.* THALASSAEMIA.

Coombs' test (koomz) *R.R.A. Coombs, British immunologist, b. 1921.* A test to detect the presence of any antibody on the surface of the red blood cell. Used to detect rhesus incompatibility in maternal or fetal blood and in the diagnosis of haemolytic anaemia.

coordination (koh,awdə'nayshən) harmony of movement among several muscles or groups of muscle so that complicated manoeuvres can be made.

coping ('kohping) the process of contending with life difficulties in an effort to overcome or work through them. *C. mechanisms* conscious or unconscious strategies or mechanisms that a person uses to cope with stress or anxiety.

copper ('kopə) *symbol* Cu. A metallic element, traces of which are present in all human tissues.

coprolalia ('koprə'layli·ə) the uncontrolled use of obscene speech.

coprolith ('koprəlith) a faecalith. A hard mass of faeces in the intestinal tract.

copulation (,kopyə'layshən) coitus. Sexual intercourse between male and female.

coracoid ('ko·rə,koyd) 1. shaped like a raven's beak 2. the coracoid process of the scapula.

cord (kawd) a long cylindrical flexible structure. *Spermatic c.* that which suspends the testicle in the scrotum, and contains the spermatic artery and vein and VAS DEFERENS. *Spinal c.* the part of the central nervous system enclosed in the spinal column. *Umbilical c.* the connection between the fetus and the placenta, through which the fetus receives nourishment. *Vocal c's* folds of mucous membrane in the larynx, which vibrate to produce the voice.

cordotomy (kaw'dotəmee) *see* CHORDOTOMY.

corn (kawn) a local hardening and thickening of the skin from pressure or friction, occurring usually on the feet. CLAVUS.

cornea ('kawni·ə) the transparent portion of the anterior surface of the eyeball continuous with the sclerotic coat. *Conical c.* keratoconus.

corneal ('kawni·əl) pertaining to the cornea. *C. graft* a means of restoring sight by grafting healthy transparent cornea from a donor in place of diseased tissue. KERATOPLASTY.

corneoscleral (,kawnioh'skliə·rəl)

relating to both the cornea and sclera. *C. junction* the point where the edge of the cornea joins the sclera. The LIMBUS.

cornification (ˌkawnəfə'kayshən) keratinisation. The process whereby the skin becomes horny through the deposition of keratin.

cornu ('kawnyoo) a horn. *C. of the uterus* one of the two horn-shaped projections where the uterine tubes join the uterus at the upper pole on either side.

coronal (kə'rohn'l) relating to the crown of the head. *C. suture* the junction of the frontal and parietal bones.

coronary ('ko·rənə·ree) encircling. Crown-like. *C. arteries* the vessels that supply the heart. *C. circulation see* CIRCULATION. *C. thrombosis see* THROMBOSIS.

coroner ('ko·rənə) a public official (e.g. a barrister, solicitor, or doctor) who holds inquests concerning sudden, violent, or suspicious deaths.

coronoid ('ko·rəˌnoyd) shaped like a crow's beak. *C. process* a bony process of the mandible or of the ulna.

corpse (kawps) a dead body; cadaver.

corpulent ('kawpyələnt) obese.

corpus ('kawpəs) a body. *C. albicans* the scar tissue on the surface of the ovary which replaces the CORPUS LUTEUM before the recommencement of menstruation. *C. callosum* the mass of white matter that joins the two cerebral hemispheres together. *C. cavernosum* either of the two columns of the erectile tissue forming the body of the clitoris or the penis. *C. luteum* the yellow body left on the surface of the ovary and formed from the remains of the Graafian follicle after the discharge of the ovum. If it retrogresses, menstruation occurs, but it persists for several months if pregnancy supervenes. *C. striatum* a mass of grey and white matter in the base of each cerebral hemisphere.

corpuscle ('kawpəsəl) a small protoplasmic body or cell, as of blood or connective tissue. *See* BLOOD.

correlation (ˌko·rə'layshən) the degree of association between two variables. *C study* a type of nonexperimental research design that examines the relationship between two or more variables.

corrosive (kə'rohsiv, -ziv) a substance that erodes and destroys.

cortex ('kawteks) [L.] *an outer layer*, as the bark of the trunk or root of a tree, or the outer layer of an organ or other structure, as distinguished from its inner substance. *Adrenal c.* the tissue surrounding the medulla or core of the adrenal gland. *Cerebral c.* the grey matter covering the two cerebral hemispheres. *Renal c.* the outer covering of the kidney.

corticospinal (ˌkawtikoh'spien'l) relating to the cerebral cortex and the spinal cord. *C. tract* the pyramidal tract. The nerve fibres making up the main pathway for rapid voluntary movement.

corticosteroid (ˌkawtikoh'stiə·royd) any of the hormones produced by the adrenal cortex or their synthetic substitutes. Glucocorticoids are responsible for metabolism of carbohydrate, fat, and protein. They have powerful anti-inflammatory properties. Mineralocorticoids, e.g. aldosterone, are responsible for salt and water regulation.

corticotrophin (ˌkawtikoh'trohfən) Adrenocorticotrophic hormone (ACTH).

cortisol ('kawtəˌsol) the naturally occurring hormone of the adrenal cortex. HYDROCORTISONE.

cortisone ('kawtəˌzohn, -ˌsohn) a naturally occurring corticosteroid. Inactive in humans until converted into cortisol. *C. acetate* a synthetic preparation with anti-inflammatory and antiallergic properties.

Corynebacterium (koˌrienibak-'tie·ri·əm) a genus of slender, rod-shaped, Gram-positive and non-motile bacteria. *C. diphtheriae* Klebs–Löffler bacillus, the causative agent of diphtheria.

coryza (kə'riezə) acute infection of the upper respiratory tract, characterised by profuse discharge from nasal mucous membranes, sneezing, and watering of the eyes.

costal ('kost'l) relating to the ribs. *C. cartilages* those that connect the ribs to the sternum directly or indirectly.

cost effectiveness (ˌkost ə'fektivnəs) a concept which relates the cost of a service to its effectiveness, and thus provides value for money, e.g. screening programs to detect cervical cancer are assessed by rate of detection, cost of the service, and cost of treatment.

cot death (kot) *See* SUDDEN INFANT DEATH SYNDROME.

cotyledon (ˌkotee'leedən) A cup-shaped depression. Applied to the subdivisions of the placenta.

cough (kof) voluntary or reflex explosive expulsion of air from the lungs. Its purpose is usually to expel a foreign body or accumulations of mucus. *Dry c.* one in which no expectoration occurs. *Wet c.* expectoration or mucus or foreign body occurs. *Whooping c.* infectious disease caused by *Bordetella pertussis*.

counselling ('kownsəling) a process of consultation and discussion in which one individual (the counsellor) listens and offers guidance or advice to another who is experiencing difficulties (the client). The counsellor does not direct or make decisions for the client. The general aim is to solve problems and increase awareness. The emphasis is on clients finding their own solutions.

counterextension (ˌkowntə·rək-'stenshən) 1. the holding back of the upper fragment of a fractured bone while the lower is pulled into position. 2. the raising of the foot of the bed in such a way that the weight of the body counteracts the pull of the extension apparatus on the lower part of the limb. Used especially for fracture of the femur.

counterirritant (ˌkowntə'irətənt) a substance that produces mild inflammation of the skin when applied to it, but relieves pain and congestion.

countertraction (ˌkowntəˌtrakshən) the reduction of fractures by traction from two opposing directions at once.

coupling ('kupling) in cardiology, the frequent occurrence of a normal heartbeat followed by an extra-ventricular one. Can occur as a result of digitalis overdose.

couvade (koo'vahd) the experiencing of the symptoms of pregnancy and childbirth by the father. This psychosomatic phenomenon is common in many societies.

Cowper's glands ('koopəz) *W. Cowper,*

British surgeon and anatomist, 1666–1709. BULBOURETHRAL glands.

coxa ('koksə) the hip joint. *C. valga* a deformity of the hip in which there is an increase in the angle between the neck and the shaft of the femur. *C. vara* a deformity in which the angle between the neck and the shaft of the femur is smaller than normal.

Coxiella (ˌkoksee'elə) a genus of microorganisms of the order Rickettsiales. *C. burnetii* the causative agent of Q fever.

Coxsackie virus (kok'sakee) one of a group of enteroviruses that can give rise to a variety of illnesses, including meningitis, PLEURODYNIA, and MYOCARDITIS.

CPR cardiopulmonary resuscitation, *see* appendix 6.

crab louse ('krab ˌlows) *Phthirus pubis. See* LOUSE.

crack (krak) purified form of cocaine, produced by a technique known as 'freebasing'. *See* COCAINE.

cradle (ˌkrayd'l) 1. a frame placed over the body or limb of a bed patient to protect injured parts from coming into contact with the bed clothes. 2. infant's bed with protective sides and, in the past, often on rockers. 3. to support, hold, comfort in the arms. *C. cap* an oily crust sometimes seen on the scalp of nursing infants; also called milk crust (crusta lactea). Caused by excessive secretion of the sebaceous glands in the scalp.

cramp (kramp) a painful spasmodic muscular contraction which can result from fatigue. *Occupational c.* occurs in miners and stokers; it is associated with intense heat and dehydration.

cranial ('krayni·əl) relating to the cranium. *C. nerves* the 12 pairs of nerves arising directly from the brain.

craniopharyngioma (ˌkrayneeohfaˌrinjee'ohmə) a cerebral tumour arising in the craniopharyngeal pouch just above the SELLA TURCICA.

craniostenosis (ˌkrayneeohstə'nohsəs) premature closure of the suture lines of the skull in an infant. Surgery might be required to relieve raised intracranial pressure.

craniosynostosis (ˌkrayneeohsi'nostəsəs) premature closure of the cranial sutures.

craniotabes ('krayneeoh'taybeez) a patchy thinning of the bones of the vault of the skull of an infant; associated with rickets.

craniotomy (ˌkraynee'otəmee) a surgical opening of the skull made to relieve pressure, arrest haemorrhage or remove a tumour.

cranium ('krayni·əm) 1. the skull. 2. the bony cavity that contains the brain.

creatine ('kreeəˌteen, -tin) a nitrogenous compound present in muscle. It is also found in the urine in conditions in which muscle is rapidly broken down, e.g. acute fevers and starvation. *C. phosphate* a high-energy phosphate store in muscle.

creatinine (kree'atəˌneen) a normal constituent of urine; a product of protein metabolism.

creatinuria (kreeˌatəˌnyoo·ri·ə) increased concentration of creatine in the urine.

credentialing (krə'denshəling) review and examination of the credentials of healthcare professionals to ensure they have training and licensure necessary to deliver care.

credibility (ˌkredə'bilətee) a criterion

for evaluating the data of a qualitative study, referring to the amount of confidence in the truth of the information.

crepitation (ˌkrepə'tayshən) the grating sound caused by friction of the two ends of a fractured bone.

crepitus ('krepətəs) 1. the discharge of flatus from the bowels. 2. crepitation. 3. a crepitant râle.

cretinism ('kretəˌnizəm) congenital hypothyroidism. A condition caused by lack of thyroid secretion, characterised by arrested physical and mental development, dull facial expression, with dry skin, and lack of coordination.

Creutzfeldt–Jakob disease (ˌkroyts-felt'yakob) *H.G. Creutzfeldt, German physician, 1885–1964. A. Jakob, German physician, 1884–1931.* A rapidly progressive disease of the nervous system affecting middle-aged and elderly people; caused by a 'slow' virus. Transmission between humans is very unusual, although the disease has been reported in young people treated with human pituitary extract for short stature—now no longer used.

cribriform ('kribrəˌfawm) perforated like a sieve. *C. plate* part of the ethmoid bone. *See* ETHMOID.

cricoid ('kriekoyd) ring shaped. *C. cartilage* the ring-shaped cartilage at the lower end of the larynx.

crisis ('kriesəs) 1. a decisive point in acute disease; the turning point towards either recovery or death. *See* LYSIS. 2. a sudden paroxysmal intensification of symptoms in the course of a disease. 3. life crisis; a period of disorganisation that occurs when a person meets an obstacle to an important life goal, such as the sudden death of a family member or a difficult family conflict. *Addisonian c., adrenal c.* symptoms of fatigue, nausea and vomiting, and collapse accompanying an acute attack of adrenal failure. *Blast c.* a sudden, severe change in the course of chronic MYELOCYTIC LEUKAEMIA. The clinical picture resembles that seen in acute myelogenous leukaemia, with an increase in the proportion of myeloblasts. *Identity c.* usually occurring during adolescence, manifested by a loss of the sense of the sameness and historical continuity of one's self, and inability to accept the role the individual perceives as being expected by society. *C. intervention* counselling or psychotherapy for patients in a life crisis that is directed at supporting the patient through the crisis and helping the patient to cope with the stressful event that precipitated it.

criterion (krie'tiə·ri·ən) the basis on which a decision is made, e.g. for drug dosage, treatment plans, research trials, etc.

critique (krə'teek) the process of objectivity and critically evaluating a research report's content for scientific merit and application to practice, theory, or education.

Crohn's disease (krohnz) *B.B. Crohn, American physician, 1884–1956.* Regional ileitis. *See* ILEITIS.

Cronbach's alpha (kron'bahks) test of internal consistency that simultaneously compares each item in a scale to all other items.

cross-sectional study a non-experimental research design that looks at data at one point in time, that is, in the immediate present.

croup (kroop) a condition resulting

from acute obstruction of the larynx caused by allergy, foreign body, infection or new growth; occurs chiefly in infants and children. There is spasmodic DYSPNOEA, a harsh cough, and stridor.

crown (krown) 1. that part of the tooth that appears above the gum. 2. the top of the head or the head itself.

crowning (krowning) the stage in labour when the top of the infant's head becomes visible at the vulva.

cruciate ('krooysheeayt) resembling a cross. *C. ligament see* LIGAMENT.

crus (krus) [L.] 1. the leg, from knee to foot. 2. a leg-like part.

crush syndrome (krush) the oedema, OLIGURIA, and other symptoms of acute renal failure that follow crushing of a part, especially a large muscle mass, causing the release of MYOGLOBIN.

crutch ('kruch) appliance usually in the form of a tubular, light, metal rod with hand grips and plastic loops for the forearms, to aid walking when the patient must not weight-bear (as in fractures of lower limbs) or when a lower limb is missing.

Crutchfield tongs ('kruchfeeld) An instrument inserted into the skull to hyperextend the head and neck.

cryaesthesia (ˌkrieəs'theezi·ə) abnormal sensitiveness to cold.

cryoanalgesia (ˌkrieohˌan'l'jeezi·ə, -si·ə) the relief of pain by application of cold by cryoprobe to peripheral nerves.

cryobank ('krieohˌbank) a facility for freezing and preserving semen at low temperatures (usually –196.5°C) for future use.

cryoextractor (ˌkrieoh·ək'straktə) an instrument in which intense cold coagulates the lens of the eye for removal in cataract extraction.

cryoprecipitate (ˌkrieohprə'sipəˌtayt) any precipitate that results from cooling. Of particular therapeutic value is the cryoprecipitate from fresh plasma, which is rich in factor VIII and is used to treat haemophilia.

cryopreservation (ˌkrieohˌprezə'vayshən) maintenance of the viability of excised tissue or organs by storing at very low temperatures.

cryosurgery (ˌkrieoh'sərjə·ree) the use of extreme cold to destroy tissue.

cryotherapy (ˌkrieoh'therəpee) therapeutic use of cold.

cryptococcosis (ˌkriptohkok'ohsəs) infection caused by the fungus *Cryptococcus neoformans*, having a predilection for the brain and meninges but also invading the skin, lungs, and other parts. It particularly affects persons immunocompromised by disease or therapy.

cryptorchidism (kripˌtawkəˌdizəm) failure of the testicles to descend into the scrotum; cryptorchism.

crypts of Lieberkühn (kripts əv 'leebəˌkoon) *J.N. Lieberkühn, Germany anatomist, 1711–1756*. Glands found in the mucous membrane of the small intestine, which secrete intestinal juice.

CT *see* COMPUTED TOMOGRAPHY.

Cu symbol for *copper.*

cubitus ('kyoobətəs) 1. the forearm. 2. the elbow. *C. valgus* deformity of the elbow in which the palm of the hand is abducted and thus faces outwards. *C. varus* deformity in which there is adduction of the forearm.

culdoscope ('kuldəˌskohp) an endoscope used in CULDOSCOPY.

culdoscopy (kul'doskəpee) direct visual examination of the female viscera through an endoscope introduced into the pelvic cavity through the posterior vaginal FORNIX.

culture ('kulchə) 1. the propagation of microorganisms or of living tissue cells in special media conducive to their growth. 2. a collective noun for the symbolic and acquired aspects of human society, including convention, custom, and language. 3. a singular noun for the customs and features of an ethnic (racial, religious, or social) group.

cumulative ('kyoomyələtiv) adding to. *C. action* the toxic effects produced by prolonged use of a drug given in comparatively small doses. Usually occurs as a result of slow excretion of the drug.

cupping ('kuping) 1. the formation of a cup-shaped depression with the hand: (a) to produce a skin erythema, thereby improving local circulation; and (b) to loosen excessive secretions from air passages, and perhaps induce coughing. 2. the use of a cupping glass to stimulate skin blood flow.

curare (kyoo'rahree) an extract from a South American plant used to poison the tips of arrows. Used in surgery to produce complete muscle relaxation, it is given intravenously as TUBOCURARINE.

curative ('kyoo·rətiv) anything which promotes healing by overcoming disease.

curettage ('kyoo·rə'tahzh, kyuh-'rettij) [Fr.] the scraping of a surface with a curette for therapeutic purposes or to obtain biopsy material.

curette (kyuh'ret) a spoon-shaped instrument used for the removal of unhealthy tissues by scraping.

curietron ('kyoo·ree,tron) an apparatus used for the treatment of cancer of the cervix and body of the uterus. The applicators are placed in the patient and the radioisotope is then moved in and out of the applicators by remote control.

Curling's ulcer ('kərlingz) *T.B. Curling, English surgeon, 1811–88.* An ulcer of the duodenum seen after severe burns of the body.

curvature ('kərvəchə) the curving of a line, whether normal or abnormal. *Spinal c.* abnormal deviation of the vertebral column.

Cushingoid ('kushing,oyd) referring to symptoms resembling those of Cushing's disease, e.g. the side-effects of steroid therapy.

Cushing's disease ('kushingz) *H.W. Cushing, American surgeon, 1869–1939.* A condition of over-secretion by the adrenal cortex due to an adenoma of the pituitary gland. Symptoms include obesity, abnormal distribution of hair, and atrophy of the genital organs.

cusp (kusp) a pointed or rounded projection, such as on the crown of a tooth or a segment of a cardiac valve.

cutaneous (kyoo'taynee·əs) pertaining to the skin.

cutdown ('kut,down) an incision into a vein with insertion of a catheter for intravenous infusion. It is performed when an infusion cannot be started by venepuncture. Also used with hyperalimentation therapy when concentrated solutions need to be given into the superior VENA CAVA.

cuticle ('kyootikəl) the narrow band of epidemis extending from the nail wall on to the nail surface; called also eponychium.

CVA cerebrovascular accident.

CVP central venous pressure.

cyanocobalamin (ˌsieənohkoh'baləmən) vitamin B_{12} (anti-anaemic factor) found in liver, eggs, and fish. It combines with intrinsic factor secreted in gastric juice for absorption, and is essential for erythrocyte maturation. Administered by injection in the treatment of PERNICIOUS ANAEMIA.

cyanosis (ˌsieə'nohsəs) a bluish appearance of the skin and mucous membranes, caused by imperfect oxygenation of the blood. It indicates circulatory failure and is common in respiratory diseases. It is also seen in 'blue babies'.

cyclamate ('sieklə,mayt, 'sikləmayt) a non-nutritive sweetener.

cycle ('siekəl) a series of recurring events. *Cardiac c.* the events occurring between one heartbeat and the next. *Menstrual c.* the changes that occur each month in the female reproductive system.

cyclic ('sieklik) pertaining to or occurring in a cycle.

cyclitis (sie'klietəs) inflammation of the ciliary body of the eye.

cyclizine ('sie'klə,zeen) an antihistamine.

cyclobarbitone (ˌsiekloh'bahbəˌtohn) a short-acting barbiturate drug administered orally in cases of insomnia. Prolonged use can lead to dependence.

cyclodialysis (ˌsieklohdie'aləsəs) an operation used in glaucoma to improve drainage from the anterior chamber of the eye at the corneoscleral junction.

cyclodiathermy (ˌsiekloh,dieə'thərmee) a treatment for glaucoma without penetration of the eyeball. Diathermy is applied to the sclera to cause fibrosis around the ciliary body, so allowing the AQUEOUS HUMOUR to drain.

cyclopenthiazide (ˌsieklohpen'theeəˌzied) an oral diuretic.

cyclopentolate (ˌsiekloh'pentəˌlayt) eye drops that paralyse the ciliary muscles and dilate the pupils.

cyclophosphamide (ˌsiekloh'fosfəˌmied) a cytotoxic drug used in the treatment of LYMPHOMATA and leukaemia and as an immunosuppressant in organ transplantation.

cycloplegia (ˌsiekloh'pleeji·ə) paralysis of the ciliary muscle of the eye.

cyclopropane (ˌsiekloh'prohpayn) a gas used for general anaesthesia. It is not irritating to the respiratory tract but is highly inflammable and is therefore potentially dangerous.

cycloserine (ˌsiekloh'siə·rien) an antibiotic drug used in the treatment of tuberculosis that is resistant to first-line therapy.

cyclosporin (sieklohspo·rin, spaw·rin) an immunosuppressive agent that does not suppress the production of antibodies. Used as prophylaxis in graft-versus-host (GVH) disease and for the prevention of graft rejection in the field of organ and tissue transplantation.

cyclothymia ('siekloh'thiemi·ə) the alteration of mood seen in manic-depressive psychosis.

cyesis (sie'eesəs) pregnancy. *Pseudo-c.* signs and symptoms suggestive of pregnancy arising when no fertilisation has taken place. 'Phantom pregnancy'.

cyproterone (sie'prohtə·rohn) an antiandrogen used to treat male hypersexuality and prostatic carcinoma.

cyst (sist) 1. a cavity or sac with epithelium, containing liquid or semisolid matter. 2. a stage in the life cycle of certain protozoan parasites when they acquire tough protective coats. *Branchial c.* one formed in the neck from non-closure of the branchial cleft during development. *Chocolate c.* an ovarian cyst occurring in ENDOMETRIOSIS. *Daughter c.* a small cyst that develops from a large one. *Dermoid c.* a congenital type containing skin, hair, teeth, etc. It is due to abnormal development of embryonic tissue. *Hydatid c.* the larval cyst stage of the tapeworm, usually found in the liver. *Meibomian c.* a swelling of a MEIBOMIAN GLAND caused by obstruction of its duct. *Multilocular c.* a cyst that is divided into compartments or locules. *Ovarian c.* a cyst of the ovary, usually non-malignant, but sometimes becoming very large and requiring surgical removal. *Retention c.* any cyst caused by blockage of a duct. *Sebaceous c.* a retention cyst caused by the blockage of a duct from a sebaceous gland so that the sebum collects. *Sublingual c.* a RANULA. *Thyroglossal c.* one in the thyroglossal tract near the hyoid bone at the base of the tongue.

cystadenoma (si͵stadə'nohmə) a benign neoplasm made up of cysts containing secretions.

cystalgia (si'stalji·ə) pain in the urinary bladder.

cystathioninuria (͵sistə͵thieohnee-'nyoo·ri·ə) an hereditary disorder of cystathionine metabolism, marked by increased concentrations in the urine. Can be associated with learning difficulties.

cystectomy (si'stektəmee) complete or partial removal of the urinary bladder. The ureters are diverted into an isolated ileal segment (ileal conduit) or into the sigmoid colon.

cysteine ('sis͵teen, 'sis͵tayn) a sulphur-containing amino acid formed by the ingestion of dietary proteins.

cystic duct ('sistik duct) the duct between the gallbladder and the common bile duct.

cysticercosis (͵sistisər'kohsəs) a disease caused by infestation with the CYSTICERCUS of *Taenia solium* (pork tapeworm).

cystic fibrosis ('sistik fie'brohsəs) generalised hereditary disorder associated with accumulation of excessively thick and tenacious mucus and abnormal secretion of sweat and saliva; called also cystic fibrosis of the pancreas and MUCOVISCIDOSIS. The disease is inherited as a recessive trait. The severity of cystic fibrosis varies widely. Although it is congenital, it might not manifest itself during the early weeks of life, or it might cause intestinal obstruction and perforation in the newborn. The chief cause of complications in cystic fibrosis is the extremely thick mucus predisposing to repeated infection, leading to chronic lung disease.

cystine ('sisteen, -tin) an amino-acid closely related to cysteine. Sometimes excreted in urine in the form of minute crystals (cystinuria).

cystinosis (͵sistə'nohsəs) an inherited metabolic disorder in which cystine is deposited in the tissues.

cystisis (si'stietəs) inflammation of the urinary bladder.

cystocele ('sistoh͵seel) a prolapse of the bladder into the vagina.

cystodiathermy (ˌsistoh'dieə-ˌthərmee) the application of a high-frequency electric current to the bladder mucosa, usually for the removal of PAPILLOMATA.

cystography (si'stogrəfee) radiography of the urinary bladder after the introduction of a radio-opaque contrast medium. *Micturating c.* radiographic examination during the act of passing urine.

cystolithiasis (ˌsistohli'thieəsəs) stone or stones in the urinary bladder.

cystopexy ('sistoh'peksee) an operation for stress incontinence in which the bladder neck is fastened to the fascia at the back of the SYMPHYSIS pubis.

cystoscope ('sistəˌskohp) an endoscope for examining the interior of the urinary bladder.

cystostomy (si'stostəmee) the operation whereby a temporary or permanent opening is made into the urinary bladder.

cystotomy (si'stotəmee) incision of the urinary bladder for removal of calculi, etc. *Suprapubic c.* incision above the pubes.

cystourethrography (ˌsistohˌyoo·rə'throgrəfee) radiography of the urinary bladder and urethra.

cystourethroscope (ˌsistoh·yuhreethrəˌskohp) an instrument for examining the urethra and bladder.

cytarabine (si'tarəˌbeen) *see* CYTOSINE.

cytogenetics (ˌsietohjə'netiks) the study of cells during mitosis in order to examine the chromosomes and the relationship between chromosome abnormality and disease.

cytology (sie'toləjee) the microscopic study of the form and functions of the cells of the body. *Exfoliative c.* an aid to the early diagnosis of malignant disease. Secretions or surface cells are examined for premalignant changes.

cytolysin (sie'toləsən) a substance that causes cytolysis. *See* BACTERIOLYSIN and HAEMOLYSIN.

cytolysis (sie'toləsəs) the destruction of cells.

cytomegalic inclusion disease (ˌsietoh'megəlik in'kloozhən) an infection due to CYTOMEGALOVIRUS. In the congenital form, there is HEPATOSPLENOMEGALY with cirrhosis, and microcephaly with learning difficulties and developmental delay. Acquired disease can cause a clinical state similar to infectious MONONUCLEOSIS.

cytomegalovirus (ˌsietohˌmegəloh-'vierəs) a virus belonging to the herpes simplex group.

cytoplasm ('sietohˌplazəm) the protoplasmic part of the cell surrounding the nucleus.

cytosine ('sietohˌseen) one of the pyrimidine bases found in DEOXYRIBONUCLEIC ACID. *C. arabinoside* an antimetabolite used in the treatment of acute leukaemia. CYTARABINE.

cytotoxic (ˌsietoh'toksik) 1. having a deleterious effect upon cells. 2. an agent that destroys cells.

cytotoxin (ˌsietoh'toksən) a toxin having a specific toxic action on cells of special organs.

Dd

D symbol for *dioptre*.

dacryocystography (ˌdakreeohsi'stogrəfee) radiography of the lacrimal duct using a radio-opaque contrast medium.

dacryocystorhinostomy (ˌdakreeohˌsistohrie'nostəmee) an operation to create an opening between the lacrimal sac and the nasal cavity.

dacryolith ('dakreeohˌlith) a calculus in a lacrimal duct.

dacryoma (ˌdakree'ohmə) a benign tumour which arises from the lacrimal epithelium.

dactyl ('daktəl) a finger or toe; a digit.

dactylology (ˌdaktə'loləjee) communication between individuals by signs made with the fingers and hands.

daltonism ('dawltəˌnizəm) colour blindness; inability to distinguish red from green.

danazol ('danəˌzol) an anterior pituitary suppressant used in the treatment of, associated infertility and benign breast disease.

dander ('dandə) small scales from the hair or feathers of animals, which can be a cause of allergy in sensitive persons.

dandruff ('dandrəf) white scales shed from the scalp. If moist from serous exudate, they have a greasy appearance.

dapsone ('dapsohn) a sulphone drug used in the treatment of leprosy.

Darwinism ('dahwəˌnizəm) *C.R. Darwin, British naturalist, 1809–1882*. The theory of the evolution of species through natural selection.

data ('daytə, dahtə) *sing*. datum; facts. *Continuous d.* data that have a continuous set of values, e.g. for variables such as height, weight, and antibody titres in response to vaccination. *D. processing* the storage and analysis of data to produce statistical tabulations, often by computer. *D. saturation* A point in qualitative research when data collection can cease because no new information from participants is emerging; data from subsequent participants become repetitive and inclusion of more participants does not yield new ideas. *D. set* a collection of information made on a group and related to certain variables that are being investigated. *Discrete d.* data with a single value or characteristic, e.g. colour of hair.

database ('daytəbays, 'dahtəbays) a collection of material relating to a topic or idea organised in a systematic way; available in print, online or CD-Rom formats.

daunomycin (ˌdawnoh'miesən) a

cytotoxic antibiotic; DAUNORUBICIN.

daunorubicin (ˌdawnoh'roobəsən) DAUNOMYCIN.

dB symbol for *decibel.*

DDT dichlorodiphenyltrichloroethane; dicophane. A powerful insecticide.

deafness ('defnəs) the inability to hear. *Conduction* or *middle ear d.* deafness due to sound waves failing to reach the cochlea. *Perceptive* or *nerve d.* deafness due to damage to the cochlea or auditory nerve.

deamination (deeˌamə'nayshən) a process of hydrolysis that takes place in the liver, whereby amino acids are broken down and urea is formed.

death (deth) the cessation of all physical and chemical processes that occurs in all living organisms or their cellular components. *Brain d.* the diagnosis of clinical brain stem death. *D. certificate* certificate indicating the date and probable cause of death. Only after issue of this certificate, indicating that the death has been registered, can the body be disposed of. *Clinical d.* the absence of heartbeat (no pulse can be felt) and cessation of breathing. *Cot d.* sudden infant death syndrome (SIDS). *D. instinct* a concept, introduced by Freud, proposing a self-destructive drive opposed by the sexual instinct (which perpetually seeks a renewal of life). It can manifest itself as a repetition COMPULSION with the aim of annihilating oneself. *D. rate* the number of deaths per stated number of persons (100 or 10 000 or 100 000) in a certain region in a certain period.

debility (də'bilətee) a condition of weakness and lack of physical tone.

débridement (di'breedmonh, day-) [Fr.] the removal of foreign substances and injured tissues from a traumatic wound. Part of the immediate treatment to promote healing.

Debrisan ('debrəzan) trade name for a preparation of dextranomer beads used to assist wound cleaning and the desloughing of ulcers.

decalcification (dee'kalsəfə'kayshən) removal of calcium salts, e.g. from bone in disorders of calcium metabolism.

decannulation (deeˌkanyə'layshən) the removal of a cannula.

decapsulation (deeˌkapsyə'layshən) removal of a fibrous capsule.

decay (dee'kay, də'kay) 1. the gradual decomposition of dead organic matter. 2. the process or stage of ageing of living matter. *Radioactive d.* the process by which an unstable atom loses energy by the emission of gamma rays or beta or alpha particles and is transformed to a more stable atom.

decerebrate (dee'serəˌbrayt) a person with brain damage whose neurological reactions are severely impaired and in whom cerebral functioning has ceased.

decibel ('desəˌbel) *symbol* dB. A unit of intensity of sound, used particularly in estimating the degree of deafness.

decidua (dəˌsidyooə) the thickened lining of the uterus for the reception of the fertilised ovum to protect the developing embryo. It is shed when pregnancy terminates.

deciduoma (dəˌsidyoo'ohmə) an intrauterine tumour containing decidual cells. *D. malignum* CHORIOEPITHELIOMA.

deciduous (də'sidyooəs) falling

off; subject to being shed, as in deciduous teeth.

decompensation (ˌdeekompən-'sayshən) failure to compensate. In particular, failure of the heart to overcome disability or increased work load.

decompression (ˌdeekəm'preshən) return to normal environmental pressure after exposure to greatly increased pressure. *Cerebral d.* removal of a flap of the skull and incision of the DURA MATER for the purpose of relieving intracranial pressure. *D. sickness* a disorder characterised by joint pains, respiratory manifestations, skin lesions, and neurological signs, occurring as a result of rapid reduction in air pressure. Aviators flying at high altitudes and persons breathing compressed air in caissons and diving apparatus are particularly susceptible to this disorder. *See* BENDS.

decongestant (ˌdeekən'jestənt) 1. reducing congestion or swelling. 2. an agent that reduces congestion or swelling, usually of the nasal membranes. Decongestants can be inhaled, taken as spray or nose drops, or used orally in liquid or tablet form.

decontamination (ˌdeekənˌtamə-'nayshən) the freeing of a person or an object of some contaminating substance such as nerve gas, radioactive material, etc.

decorticate posture (de'kawtə'kayt) the rigid posture, with arms flexed across the chest, of a patient with a lesion at or above the upper brain stem.

decortication (deeˌkawtə'kayshən) an operation to strip the outer layer of an organ, e.g. the removal of the thickened pleura in the treatment of chronic emphysema.

decrudescence (ˌdeekroo'desəns) diminution or abatement of the intensity of symptoms.

decubitus (di'kyoobətəs) the position assumed when lying down. *D. ulcer* an ulcer due to interference with the local circulation from prolonged or severe pressure on the surface body tissue resulting in tissue anoxia and cell death; also called *bedsore* and *pressure sore*.

decussation (deekə'sayshən) a crossing, particularly of nerve fibres. A chiasma. *Pyramidal d.* the crossing of the pyramidal nerve fibres in the MEDULLA oblongata.

deep venous thrombosis (deep 'veenəs) a thrombus in one of the deep veins of the body.

defaecation (ˌdefə'kayshən) elimination of wastes and undigested food, as faeces, from the rectum. Also: defecation.

defence (də'fens) behaviour directed to protection of the individual from injury. *Character d.* any character trait, e.g. a mannerism, attitude, or affectation, which serves as a DEFENCE MECHANISM. *Insanity d.* a legal concept that a person cannot be convicted of a crime if he or she lacked criminal responsibility by reason of insanity at the time of commission of the crime. *D. mechanism* in psychology, an unconscious mental process or coping pattern that lessens the anxiety associated with a situation or internal conflict and protects the person from mental discomfort.

defervescence (ˌdeefə'vesəns) the period of abatement of fever.

defibrillation (deeˌfibrə'layshən) the restoration of normal rhythm to the heart in ventricular or atrial fibrillation.

defibrillator (dee'fibrə,laytə) an instrument by which normal rhythm is restored in ventricular or atrial fibrillation by the application of a high-voltage electric current.

defibrination (dee,fibrə'nayshən) the removal of fibrin from blood plasma to prevent clotting. Used in the preparation of sera.

deficiency disease (də'fishənsee) a condition caused by dietary or metabolic deficiency, including all diseases due to an insufficient supply of essential nutrients.

deficit ('de,fəsət) a deficiency or variation from that which is considered to be normal.

deglutition (,deegloo'tishən) the act of swallowing.

dehiscence (də'hisəns) splitting open, as of a wound.

dehydration (,deehie'drayshən) excessive loss of fluid from the body by persistent vomiting, diarrhoea or sweating, or from the lack of intake. Severe dehydration is a serious condition that can lead to fatal SHOCK, ACIDOSIS, and the accumulation of waste products in the body, as in URAEMIA.

deinstitutionalisation (,dee'insti-,chooshənə,liezayshən) *see* INSTITUTIONALISATION.

déjàvu (,dayzhah 'voo) [Fr.] an illusion that a new experience is a repetition of a previous experience.

deleterious (,delə'tiə·ri·əs) harmful; injurious.

delinquency (də'lingkwənsee) criminal or antisocial conduct, especially among juveniles.

delirium (də'liə·ri·əm) mental excitement. A common condition in high fever. It is marked by an irregular expenditure of nervous energy, incoherent talk, and delusions. *Traumatic d.* a possible occurrence after severe head injury. There is much confusion and disorientation. *D. tremens* an acute psychosis common in chronic alcoholism, usually following abstinence from alcohol.

delivery (də'livə·ree) childbirth; parturition.

delouse (,dee'lows) to destroy or remove lice.

Delphi technique (delfee) the technique of gaining expert opinion on a subject. It uses rounds or multiple stages of data collection, with each round using data from previous rounds.

delta wave ('deltə) the slowest of the four types of brain waves.

deltoid ('deltoyd) triangular. *D. muscle* the triangular muscle of the shoulder arising from the clavicle and scapula, with insertion into the humerus.

delusion (də'loozhən) a false idea or belief held by a person and which cannot be corrected by reasoning. *Depressive d.* a sense of unworthiness or sinfulness. *D. of grandeur* erroneous belief in one's own greatness, wealth, or position. *D. of persecution* paranoia.

dementia (də'menshə) a global and progressive deterioration of the mental faculties which is irreversible and affects memory, intellect, judgment, personality, and emotional control. Dementia is the result of an organic brain syndrome. The term 'brain failure' is gradually replacing the term 'dementia' because it conveys the fact that brain failure is a process, whereas the term 'dementia' suggests a state associated with nihilistic views on treatment and prognosis. *Arteriosclerotic d.* dementia due to insufficient blood supply to the brain caused by ARTERIOSCLEROSIS. *Presenile d.* occurs in people aged 40–60 years, and is due to early degeneration of small cerebral blood vessels. *See* ALZHEIMER'S DISEASE and CREUTZFELDT–JAKOB DISEASE. *Senile d.* dementia occurring in old age as the result of cerebral atrophy.

Demodex ('deemə͵deks) a genus of mites parasitic in the hair follicles of the host. Species of the genus cause mange in dogs and horses.

demography (də'mogrəfee) the social study of people viewed collectively with regard to race, occupation, or conditions.

demulcent (də'mulsənt) an agent that soothes and allays irritation, especially of sensitive mucous membranes.

demyelination (dee'mieələ'nayshən) destruction of the medullary or myelin sheaths of nerve fibres, such as occurs in disseminated SCLEROSIS. Demyelinisation.

dendrite ('dendriet) one of the protoplasmic filaments of a nerve cell by which impulses are transmitted from one neurone to another. Dendron.

dendritic (den'dritik) 1. appertaining to a dendrite. 2. branching. *D. ulcer* a corneal ulcer caused by the herpes simplex virus. The ulcer has a branching appearance as it spreads.

denervation (͵deenər'vayshən) severance or removal of the nerve supply to a part.

dengue ('deng·gee) a painful viral disease that occurs in tropical countries throughout the world. The virus that causes the disease, one of four types of a group B ARCOVIRUS, is carried by *Aedes* mosquitoes. Because of the intense pain in the bones, dengue is also known as 'breakbone fever'.

Denham pin (͵denəm) a steel pin with a short raised threaded length used in skeletal traction. The threaded portion engages the bony cortex, reducing the risk of the pin slipping.

denial (də'nieəl) a defence mechanism in which the existence of intolerable actions, ideas, changed circumstances, terminal illness, etc. are unconsciously denied.

dentine ('denteen) the calcified substance forming the bulk of a tooth between the pulp and the enamel.

dentition (den'tishən) the process of teething. *Primary d.* cutting of the temporary or milk teeth, beginning at the age of 6 or 7 months and continuing until the end of the second year. A full set consists of eight incisors, four canines, and eight premolars: twenty in all. Deciduous dentition. *Secondary d.* cutting of the permanent teeth, beginning in the sixth or seventh year, and complete by the 12th to 15th year except for the posterior molars or 'wisdom teeth'. There are 32 permanent teeth, eight incisors, four canines, eight premolarsor bicuspids, and twelve molars. Permanent dentition. (*See* figure.)

dentoid ('dentoyd) tooth-like.

denture ('denchə) a removable dental prosthesis, which may contain one, several, or a full set of artificial teeth.

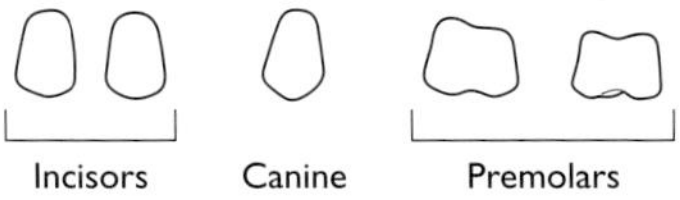

Temporary teeth

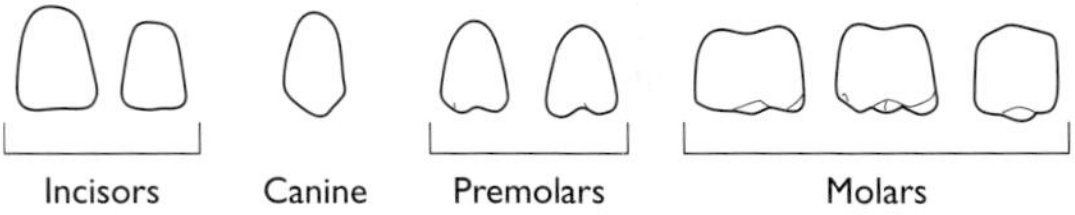

Permanent teeth

deodorant (dee'ohdə·rənt) a substance which destroys or masks an offensive odour.

deoxycortone (dee,oksee'kawtohn) a naturally occurring adrenal steroid. *D. acetate* and *d. pivalate* synthetic preparations used in the treatment of adrenocortical insufficiency.

deoxygenated (dee'oksəjə,naytəd) deprived of oxygen. *D. blood* that which has lost much of its oxygen in the tissues and is returning to the lungs for a fresh supply.

deoxyribonucleic acid (dee,oksee-,riebohnyoo'klee·ik, -'klay-) abbreviated DNA. A nucleic acid of complex molecular structure occurring in cell nuclei as the basic structure of the genes. It is responsible for the control and passing on of hereditary characteristics, and is present in all body cells of every species, including unicellular organisms and DNA viruses. The structure of DNA was described in 1953 by J.D. Watson and F.H.C. Crick.

dependence (də'pendəns) addiction; the total psychophysical state of a drug user in which the usual or increasing doses of the drug are required to prevent the onset of withdrawal symptoms (*see* WITHDRAWAL SYMPTOMS).

dependency (də'pendənsee) a state of relying on another for love, affection, mothering, comfort, security, food, warmth, shelter, protection, etc. *D. studies* the measurement of the need for care required by a patient based on the ability to carry out self-care. The main self-care activities measured are the ability to feed, the ability to carry out toilet requirements, and the level of mobility, including dressing. *D. studies for staffing ratios* studies undertaken to determine the number of staff required to provide the appropriate skills to care for specific types and numbers of patients.

depersonalisation (dee,pərsənəlie-'zayshən) a condition in which patients feel that their personality has changed so that they become onlookers of their own actions. It can occur in almost any mental illness.

depilatory (də'pilətree) an agent that will remove hair.

depressant (də'presənt) a drug that reduces functional activity of an organ. Anaesthetics, sedatives, tranquillisers, and alcohol are all depressants.

depression (də'preshən) 1. a hollow or depressed area. 2. a lowering or decrease of functional activity. 3. in psychiatry, a morbid sadness, dejection, or melancholy, distinguished from grief, which is realistic and proportionate to a personal loss. Profound depression can indicate a psychiatric disorder or it might constitute the principal manifestation of a neurosis or psychosis. *Endogenous d.* occurs sometimes without obvious cause as, for example, in the course of manic-depressive psychosis. The mood change is associated with slowing of thought and action and feelings of guilt. *Recessive d.* occurs as a result of some event, such as illness, loss of money, or bereavement.

deprivation (,deprə'vayshən) loss or absence of parts, organs, powers, or things that are needed. *Emotional d.* deprivation of adequate and appropriate interpersonal or environmental experience in the early developmental years. *Maternal d. syndrome* a group of symptoms, including stunted emotional and physical development, arising in infants who have been deprived of care and love provided by a mother or mothering figure. Deprivation of maternal care during the first 3 years of life is thought to be particularly critical because this is the optimal period for the forming of social attachments. *Sensory d.* deprivation of the usual external stimuli and the opportunity for perception.

Derbyshire neck ('dahbeeshiə) *see* GOITRE.

derealisation (,dee,riəlie'zayshən) loss of a sense of reality. Surroundings and events seem unreal.

dereism ('deeri,izəm) mental activity in which fantasy runs unhampered by logic and experience; describes autistic thinking.

dermabrasion (,dərmə'brayzhən) treatment to remove scars on the skin using wire brushes or sandpaper.

dermatitis (,dərma'tietəs) inflammation of the skin. *Contact d.* that arising from touching a substance to which the person is sensitive. *Exfoliative d.* widespread scaling and itching of the skin, sometimes occurring as a reaction to treatment by certain drugs. *Industrial d., occupational d.* that caused by exposure to chemicals or other substances met with at work. *Sensitisation d.* dermatitis due to an allergic reaction. *Traumatic d.* inflammation due to injury. *Varicose d.* dermatitis, usually of the lower portion of the leg, due to varicosities of the smaller veins. *X-ray d.* radiodermatitis; inflammatory reaction of the skin to radiotherapy.

dermatoglyphics (,dərmətoh'glifiks) study of the patterns of ridges of the skin of the fingers, palms, toes, and soles. Of interest in anthropology and law enforcement as a means of establishing identity, and in medicine, both clinically and as a genetic indicator, particularly of chromosomal abnormalities.

dermatographia (ˌdərmətoh'grafi·ə) a condition in which urticarial weals occur on the skin if a blunt instrument or fingernail is lightly drawn over it.

dermatology (ˌdərmə'toləjee) the science of skin diseases.

dermatomycosis (ˌdərmətohmie-'kohsəs) a fungal infection of the skin.

dermatomyositis (ˌdərmətoh-ˌmieoh'sietəs) a collagen disease producing inflammation of the voluntary muscles with necrosis of the muscle fibres.

dermatosis (ˌdərmə'tohsəs) any skin disease, especially one that does not produce inflammation.

dermis ('dərməs) the layer of skin just below the epidermis.

dermoid ('dərmoyd) pertaining to the skin. *D. cyst see* CYST.

descriptive/exploratory survey (də'skriptiv əks'plo·rətawree) a type of nonexperimental research design that collects descriptions of existing phenomena for the purpose of using the data to justify or assess current conditions or to make plans for improvement of conditions.

desensitisation (deeˌsensətie-'zayshən) 1. the prevention or reduction of immediate hypersensitivity reactions by the administration of graded doses of allergen; hyposensitisation. *See also* IMMUNOTHERAPY. 2. in behaviour therapy, the treatment of phobias and related disorders by intentionally exposing the patient, in imagination or in real life, to emotionally distressing stimuli.

designer drug (də'zienə) used to describe synthetic variants (drug analogues) of potent controlled drugs (including narcotics and stimulants) but which are not themselves controlled.

desipramine (də'siprəˌmeen) an antidepressant.

desquamation (ˌdeskwə'mayshən) peeling of the superficial layer of the skin, either in flakes or in powdery form.

detachment (də'tachmənt) separation. *D. of the retina* separation of the retina, or a part of it, from the CHOROID.

detergent (də'tərjənt) a cleansing and antiseptic agent.

deterioration (dəˌtiə·ri·ə'rayshən) progressive impairment of function; worsening.

detoxification (deeˌtoksəfə'kayshən) the process of neutralising toxic substances; detoxication.

detritus (də'trietəs) debris; material that has disintegrated.

detrusor (dee'troozə) muscle of the urinary bladder, the action of which is to push down.

detumescence (ˌdeetyuh'mesəns) 1. the subsidence of a swelling. 2. the subsidence of an erect penis after ejaculation.

development (də'veləpmənt) the process of growth and differentiation. *Cognitive d.* the development of intelligence, conscious thought, and problem-solving ability that begins in infancy. *Psychosexual d.* the development of the psychological aspects of sexuality from birth to maturity. *Psychosocial d.* the development of the personality, including the acquisition of social attitudes and skills, from infancy through maturity.

developmental (də,veləp'ment'l) pertaining to development. *D. anomaly* absence, deformity, or excess of body parts as the result of faulty development of the embryo. *D. milestones* significant behaviours used to mark the process of development (*see* AGE ACHIEVEMENT). Walking is a developmental milestone in locomotor development, conversation in cognitive development.

deviance ('deevi·əns) any pattern of behaviour that violates prevailing standards of morality or behaviour within a society. The term is usually qualified to indicate specific forms of deviance.

deviation (,deevee'ayshən) variation from the normal. In ophthalmology, lack of coordination of the two eyes.

devitalised (dee'vietə,liezd) devoid of vitality or life; dead.

dexamethasone (,deksə'methə-,zohn) a powerful anti-inflammatory GLUCOCORTICOID.

dextran ('dekstrən) a plasma volume expander, formed of large glucose molecules, which, given intravenously, increases the osmotic pressure of blood.

dextrin ('dekstrən) a soluble carbohydrate that is the first product in the breakdown of starch and glycogen to sugar.

dextrocardia (,dekstroh'kahdi·ə) location of the heart in the right side of the thorax.

dextromethorphan (,dekstrohmə-'thorfən) a synthetic morphine derivative used as an antitussive.

dextromoramide (,dekstroh-'mo·rə,mied) a narcotic used in the treatment of chronic pain in terminal disease.

dextrose ('dekstrohz, -trohs) an old chemical name for D-glucose, an important energy source for all tissues and the sole energy source for the brain. The term 'dextrose' continues to be used to refer to glucose solutions administered intravenously for fluid or nutrient replacement.

diabetes (,dieə'beeteez) a disease characterised by excessive excretion of urine. *See* POLYURIA. *Bronze d.* haemochromatosis. *D. insipidus* diabetes marked by an increased flow of urine of low osmolality, accompanied by great thirst. Caused by deficient production or secretion of the antidiuretic hormone (ADH) or inability of the kidney tubules to respond to ADH. *D. mellitus* A complex disorder of carbohydrate, fat, and protein metabolism that is primarily a result of a deficiency or complete lack of INSULIN secretion by the beta cells of the pancreas or resistance to insulin. It is characterised by chronic HYPERGLYCAEMIA and can present with characteristic symptoms such as thirst, polyuria, glycosuria, blurring of vision, and weight loss. In its most severe forms, ketoacidosis or a non-ketotic hyperosmolar state can develop and lead to stupor, coma and, in the absence of effective treatment, death. The diagnosis is confirmed by fasting plasma glucose and history. The various forms of diabetes have been organised into categories developed by the American Diabetes Association and the World Health Organization. *Type 1 diabetes mellitus* includes patients with diabetes caused by cellular mediated autoimmune destruction of pancreatic beta cells resulting in lack of insulin. The onset of type 1 diabetes mellitus in children is sudden. Generally individuals develop type 1 diabetes before 30 years of age, although it can occur up to the tenth decade. Individuals are prone to ketoacidosis because little or no endogenous insulin is being secreted. Type 1 diabetes mellitus is controlled by insulin, diet, and exercise, and the goal is to maintain insulin–glucose homeostasis. Patients are dependent on insulin to prevent ketosis. This group was previously called type I, insulin-dependent diabetes mellitus (IDDM), juvenile-onset diabetes, brittle diabetes, or ketosis-prone diabetes. *Type 2 diabetes mellitus* is the most common form of diabetes and includes patients with insulin resistance or with inadequate insulin secretion. Generally it occurs in individuals older than 40 years of age who have central obesity and a strong genetic predisposition. It is frequently associated with hypertension and dyslipidaemia. The onset usually begins insidiously. Patients are usually not insulin dependent but can be insulin requiring. Individuals are not ketosis prone. Type 2 diabetes mellitus is controlled by diet, exercise, and one or more oral hypoglycaemic agents, or insulin in combination with oral agents. This group was previously called type II, non-insulin-dependent diabetes mellitus (NIDDM), maturity-onset diabetes, adult-onset diabetes, ketosis-resistant diabetes, or stable diabetes. *Gestational diabetes mellitus* occurs in women who develop glucose intolerance during pregnancy resulting in hyperglycaemia of variable severity. Other types of diabetes are associated with a pancreatic disease, hormonal changes, adverse effects of drugs, or genetic or other anomalies. A fifth subclass, the impaired glucose tolerance (IGT) group, includes persons whose blood glucose levels are abnormal although not sufficiently beyond the normal range to be diagnosed as diabetic.

diabetic (ˌdieə'betik) 1. relating to diabetes mellitus. 2. a person affected with diabetes mellitus. *d. complications* include both long-term and short-term complications of diabetes mellitus. The eyes, kidneys, nervous system, skin, and circulatory system can be affected by the long-term complications of either type of diabetes; infections are common, and atherosclerosis often develops. The Diabetes Control and Complications Trial (DCCT) which studied patients with type 1 diabetes, demonstrated that tight control of blood glucose levels (i.e. frequent monitoring and maintenance at as close as possible to the level of nondiabetics) significantly reduces complications such as eye disease, kidney disease, and nerve damage. The United Kingdom Prospective Diabetes Study, which studied patients with type 2 diabetes, showed a relationship existed between improved glycaemic control and reduction in microvascular complications. *See* CATARACT, GANGRENE, MICROALBUMINURIA, NEUROPATHY, RENAL FAILURE, RETINOPATHY). Although diabetes can cause complications over time, short-term complications can arise daily due to fluctuations in blood glucose levels and can be serious if untreated; *See* HYPOGLYCAEMIA, HYPERGLYCAEMIA, KETOACIDOSIS. *D. diet* a diet prescribed in the treatment of diabetes mellitus designed to prevent wide fluctuation in the amount of glucose in the blood. *See* GLYCAEMIC INDEX FACTOR. *D. ketoacidosis* (DKA) *See* KETOACIDOSIS.

diabetogenic (ˌdieəˌbeetə'jenik) inducing diabetes. Some drugs or physical conditions, such as pregnancy or disease, precipitate the symptoms of diabetes in those prone to the disease.

diagnosis (ˌdieəg'nohsəs) determination of the nature of a disease. *Clinical d.* diagnosis made by the study of signs and symptoms. *Differential d.* the recognition of one disease among several presenting similar symptoms. *Nursing d.* a statement of a healthcare problem or the potential for one in the health status of the patient/client for which a nurse is competent to intervene and treat.

dialysate (die'aləˌsayt) the material passing through the membrane in dialysis.

dialyser ('dieəˌliezə) 1. the membrane used in dialysis. 2. the machine or 'artificial kidney' used to remove waste products from the blood in cases of renal failure.

dialysis (die'aləsəs) the process by which crystalline substances pass through a semipermeable membrane, whereas colloids do not. In medicine this process is usually employed to remove waste and toxic products from the blood in cases of renal insufficiency. *Peritoneal d.* use of the peritoneum as the semipermeable membrane. A dialysing solution is infused into the abdominal cavity and allowed to run out again when sufficient time has elapsed for dialysis to have occurred. Waste products are thus removed from the blood. *See* HAEMODIALYSIS.

diameter (die'amətə) a straight line passing through the centre of a circle to opposite points on the circumference. *Cranial d's* measurement of the skull, usually of the fetal head at term. If these are abnormal, delivery through the vagina might not be possible. *Pelvic d's* measurements between the bones and joints of the pelvis made in women to determine whether the fetus can pass through at the time of childbirth.

diamorphine hydrochloride (diə-'mawfeen) a morphine derivative similar to heroin; a powerful analgesic and drug of addiction.

diapedesis (ˌdieəpə'deesəs) the passage of blood cells through the walls of blood capillaries into the surrounding tissues.

diaphoresis (ˌdieəfə'reesəs) perspiration; particularly profuse perspiration.

diaphoretic (ˌdieəfə'retik) an agent that increases perspiration, e.g. pilocarpine.

diaphragm ('dieəˌfram) 1. the muscular dome-shaped partition separating the thorax from the abdomen. 2. any separating membrane or structure. *Contraceptive d.* a rubber cap which occludes the cervix (*see* figure).

diaphragmatocele (ˌdieəframə-'tohseel) a herniation of the diaphragm.

diaphysis (die'afəsəs) the shaft of a long bone.

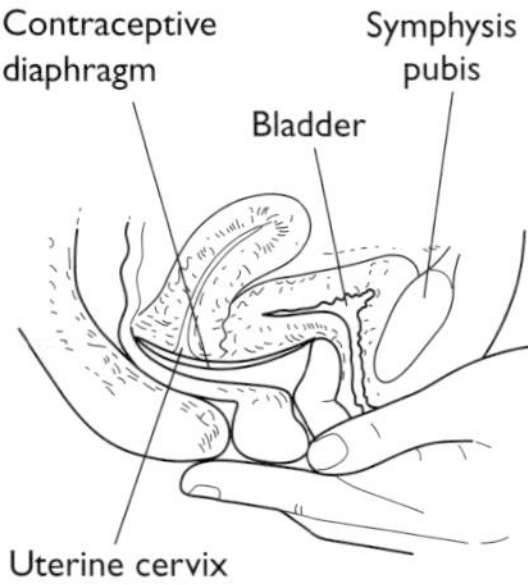

Insertion of a contraceptive diaphragm

diarrhoea (ˌdieə'reeə) rapid movement of faecal matter through the intestine resulting in poor absorption of water, nutritive elements, and electrolytes, and producing abnormally frequent evacuation of watery stools. *Summer d.* gastroenteritis of infants, probably the result of a virus infection. It is highly contagious. *Tropical d.* SPRUE.

diarthrosis (ˌdieah'throhsəs) a freely moving articulation, e.g. ball and socket joint. A synovial joint.

diastase ('dieəˌstays, stayz) 1. an enzyme, formed during germination of seeds, which converts starch into sugar. 2. one of the pancreatic enzymes excreted in the urine and the saliva. *D. test* used to estimate the excretion of diastase and therefore pancreatic function.

diastole (die'astəlee) the phase of the cardiac cycle in which the heart relaxes between contractions; specifically, the period when the two ventricles are dilated by the blood flowing into them.

diathermy ('dieəˌthərmee) production of heat in a body tissue by a high-frequency electric current. *Medical d.* sufficient heat is used to warm the tissues but not to harm them. *Short-wave d.* used in physiotherapy to relieve pain or treat infection. *Surgical d.* of very high frequency; used to coagulate blood vessels or to dissect tissues. CAUTERY.

diazepam (die'azəˌpam) a tranquilliser with muscle relaxant and anticonvulsive properties used to relieve anxiety and in the treatment of epilepsy.

diazoxide (dieaz'oksied) a vasodilator given by rapid intravenous injection in the treatment of hypertensive emergencies and orally in HYPOGLYCAEMIA due to a pancreatic tumour.

DIC disseminated intravascular coagulopathy.

dichloralphenazone (dieˌklaw·rəl'fenəˌzohn) a hypnotic drug of the chloral group well suited for children and causing fewer gastrointestinal upsets.

dichlorphenamide (ˌdieklaw'fenəˌmied) a diuretic used to reduce intraocular pressure in GLAUCOMA.

dichromatic (ˌdiekroh'matik) pertaining to colour blindness when there is ability to see only two of the three primary colours.

dicophane ('diekohˌfayn) dichlorodiphenyltrichloroethane; chlorophenothane; DDT. An insecticide.

dicrotic (die'krotik) having a double beat. *D. pulse* a small wave of distension following the normal pulse beat; occurring at the closure of the aortic valve.

dicyclomine (die'siekləˌmeen) an anticholinergic drug used in the treatment of peptic ulcer and spastic colon.

didymitis (ˌdidi'mietəs) orchitis; inflammation of a testicle.

dienoestrol (ˌdieən'eestrol) a synthetic oestrogen used to treat symptoms of atrophic vaginitis and KRAUROSIS vulvae.

diet ('dieət) the customary amount and kind of food and drink taken by a person from day to day; more narrowly, a diet planned to meet the specific requirements of the individual, including or excluding certain foods. *Bland d.* one that is free from any irritating or stimulating foods. *Elemental d.* one consisting of a well-balanced, residue-free mixture of all essential and non-essential amino acids, combined with simple sugars, electrolytes, trace elements, and vitamins. *Elimination d.* one for diagnosis of food allergy, based on omission of foods that might cause symptoms in the patient. *High-calorie d.* one that furnishes more calories than needed to maintain weight, often more than 3500–4000 kcal/day. *High-fibre d.* one relatively high in dietary fibre, which decreases bowel transit time and relieves constipation. *High-protein d.* one containing large amounts of protein, consisting largely of meats, fish, milk, legumes, and nuts. *Hospital d.* a routine diet plan, provided in a hospital, that includes general, soft, and liquid diets, and modifications of them, to suit the needs of specific patients. *Ketogenic d.* one containing large amounts of fat (see also ketogenic diet). *Liquid d.* a diet limited to liquids or to foods that can be changed to a liquid state (see also liquid diet). *Low-calorie d.* one containing fewer calories than needed to maintain weight, e.g. less than 1200 kcal/day for an adult. *Low-fat d.* one containing limited amounts of fat. *Low-residue d.* one with a minimum of cellulose and fibre and restriction of the connective tissue found in certain cuts of meat. It is prescribed for irritations of the intestinal tract, after surgery of the large intestine, in partial intestinal obstruction, or when limited bowel movements are desirable, as in colostomy patients. Called also low-fibre diet.

dietetics (ˌdieə'tetiks) the science of applying the principles of nutrition to the feeding of individuals or groups.

diethylcarbamazine (dieˌethəlkah'baməˌzeen) an anthelmintic drug used in the treatment of FILARIASIS.

diethylpropion (dieˌethəl'prohpeeon) an appetite suppressant in the treatment of obesity, similar in action to an amphetamine drug. Dependence can occur. Trade names: Apisate and Tenuate Dospan.

dietitian (ˌdieə'tishən) one who specialises in dietetics.

differential (ˌdifə'renshəl) making a difference. *D. blood count see* BLOOD COUNT. *D. diagnosis see* DIAGNOSIS.

differentiation (ˌdifəˌrenshi'ayshən) 1. the distinguishing of one thing from another. 2. the act or process of acquiring completely individual characteristics, such as occurs in the progressive diversification of cells and tissues in the embryo. 3.

increase in morphological or chemical heterogeneity.

diffuse (də'fyoos, -'fyooz) scattered or widespread, as opposed to localised.

diffusion (də'fyoozhən) 1. a process in which molecules of liquid or gas disperse, moving from regions of higher density to regions of lower density so that they become equally distributed. 2. dialysis.

diflunisal (di'floonə,sal) a salicylic acid derivative which, like aspirin, has analgesic and anti-inflammatory properties, but fewer side-effects than aspirin, does not affect bleeding time or function, and has a long half-life that permits twice-daily dosage.

digestion (die'jeschən, di-) 1. the act or process of converting food into chemical substances that can be absorbed into the blood and utilised by the body tissues. 2. the subjection of a substance to prolonged heat and moisture, so as to disintegrate and soften it.

digit ('dijət) a finger or toe. *Accessory d., supernumerary d.* an additional digit occurring as a congenital abnormality.

digitalis (,dijə'tayləs) a group of drugs used extensively for their action on the heart. They strengthen the heart-beat and slow down the conducting power of the atrioventricular bundle, thereby enabling the ventricles to beat more effectively. Particularly valuable in treating atrial fibrillation. *Digoxin* is the chief glycoside obtained from the white foxglove. The effects of digitalis are cumulative, indicated by a very slow pulse and coupling of the beats.

digitalisation (,dijətəlie'zayshən) the administration of digitalis in a dosage schedule designed to produce and maintain optimal therapeutic concentrations of its cardiotonic glycosides.

dihydrocodeine (die,hiedroh-'kohdeen) a synthetic narcotic, analgesic, and antitussive drug derived from codeine.

dihydroergotamine (die,hiedroh-·ər'gotə,meen) a drug used in the treatment of migraine. Less effective than ergotamine, but with fewer side-effects.

dihydrotachysterol (die,hiedroh-takee'stiə·rol) a preparation closely related to vitamin D. Used in cases of vitamin D deficiency and in rickets.

dilatation, dilation (,dielə'tayshən; die'layshən) 1. the act of dilating or stretching. 2. the condition, as of an orifice or tubular structure, of being dilated or stretched beyond normal dimensions. *D. and curettage* expanding of the ostium uteri to permit scraping of the walls of the uterus; also called D & C. *D. of the heart* compensatory enlargement of the cavities of the heart, with thinning of the walls.

dilator (die'laytə) 1. an instrument used for enlarging an opening or cavity such as the rectum, the male urethra or the cervix. 2. a muscle that causes dilatation. 3. a drug that causes dilatation, e.g. a vasodilator. *Hegar's d's* a series of dilators used to widen the cervical canal before examination of the uterus under anaesthesia.

diluent ('dilyooənt) 1. diluting. 2. an agent that dilutes or renders less potent or irritant.

dimenhydrinate (,diemen'hiedrə-·nayt) an antihistamine drug, useful in preventing nausea and vomiting, particularly that associated with motion sickness.

dimercaprol (ˌdiemə'kaprol) a drug which combines with heavy metals to form a stable compound, which is rapidly excreted. Used to treat poisoning by arsenic, gold, mercury, and other metals. Previously called British antilewisite or CAL.

dimethylphthalate (dieˌmethəl-'thalayt) abbreviated DIMP. An insect repellent in liquid or ointment form that is effective for several hours when applied to the skin.

diodone ('dieə dohn) a contrast medium containing iodine which is similar to iodoxyl. Used in radiology of the urinary tract.

Diogenes syndrome (die'ojəˌneez) gross self-neglect, usually in the elderly.

dioptre (die'optə) *symbol* D. The unit used in measuring lenses for spectacles. When parallel light enters a lens and focuses at a distance of 1 m, the refractive power of the lens is 1 dioptre, and from this basis abnormalities are calculated.

diphtheria (dif'thieə·ri·ə, dip-) a severe, notifiable, infectious disease, usually of children, characterised by the formation of membranes in the throat and nose and rarely the skin (in an open wound) and toxic neurological and cardiac complications; caused by the bacillus *Corynebacterium diphtheriae*. Primary prevention is provided by the routine immunisation of the population in childhood.

diphtheroid ('difthəˌroyd) resembling diphtheria. A general term applied to organisms or membranes similar to true diphtheria types.

Diphyllobothrium (dieˌfiloh-'bothri·əm) a genus of large tapeworm. *D. latum*, the broad or fish tapeworm, grows up to 10 m long and can infest humans after the consumption of uncooked infected fish.

dipipanone (die'pipəˌnohn) a potent analgesic used for the relief of severe pain.

diplegia (die'pleeji·ə) paralysis of similar parts on either side of the body.

diplococcus (ˌdiplə'kokəs) 1. any of the spherical, lanceolate or coffee-bean-shaped bacteria occurring, usually in pairs, as a result of incomplete separation after cell division in a single plane. 2. any organism of the genus *Diplococcus*.

diploid ('diployd) 1. having a pair of each chromosome characteristic of a species (in humans, 46). 2. a diploid individual or cell.

diplopia (di'plohpi·ə) double vision, in which two images are seen in place of one, due to lack of coordination of the external muscles of the eye.

diprophylline (die'prohfəleen) a theophylline derivative used in the treatment of bronchospasm or bronchial asthma associated with chronic bronchitis or asthma.

dipsomania (ˌdipsoh'mayni·ə) a morbid craving for alcohol which occurs in bouts.

disability (ˌdisə'bilətee) any restriction or lack (resulting from an impairment) of ability to perform an activity in the manner or within the range considered normal for a human being. *Developmental d.* a substantial handicap of indefinite duration, with onset before the age of 18 years, and attributable to mental handicap, autism, cerebral palsy, epilepsy, or other neuropathy.

disaccharide (die'sakə,ried) any of a class of sugars, e.g. maltose, lactose, each molecule of which yields two molecules of monosaccharide on hydrolysis. *D. intolerance* the inability to absorb disaccharides owing to an enzyme deficiency.

disarticulation (,disah,tikyə'layshən) separation; amputation at a joint.

disc (disk) a flattened circular structure. *Intervertebral d.* a fibrocartilaginous pad that separates the bodies of two adjacent vertebrae. *Optic d.* a white spot in the retina. It is the point of entrance of the optic nerve.

discharge ('dischahj) 1. a setting free, or liberation; used to describe the release of a patient from hospital, clinic, or therapy program. 2. material or force set free. 3. an excretion or substance evacuated. *D. planning* the preparation required leading to the return of a patient to the usual life at home.

disclosing solution (dis'klohzing) a topically applied preparation which reveals plaque and other deposits on teeth by staining them.

discography (dis'kogrəfee) radiographic examination after the injection of a radio-opaque contrast medium into an intervertebral disc.

discrete (də,skreet) composed of separate parts that do not become blended.

disease (də'zeez) a definite pathological process having a characteristic set of signs and symptoms. It might affect the whole body or any of its parts, and its aetiology, pathology and prognosis might be known or unknown. (For separate diseases, see under individual names.)

disimpaction (,disim'pakshən) reduction of an impacted fracture.

disinfect (,disən'fekt) to destroy microorganisms, but not usually bacterial spores, reducing the number of microorganisms to a level which is not harmful to health.

disinfectant (,disən'fektənt) an agent that destroys infection-producing organisms. Heat and certain other physical agents, such as steam, can be disinfectants, but in common usage the term is reserved for chemical substances such as glutaraldehyde, sodium hypochlorite, or phenol. Disinfectants are usually applied to inanimate objects because they are too strong to be used on living tissues. Chemical disinfectants are not always effective against spore-forming bacteria.

disinfection (disən'fekshən) the act of disinfecting. *Terminal d.* disinfection of a sick room and its contents at the termination of a disease.

disinfestation (,disinfe'stayshən) destruction of insects, rodents, or pests present on the person or the clothes or in the surroundings, and which can transmit disease.

dislocation (,dislə'kayshən) the displacement of a bone from its natural position upon another at a joint; luxation.

dismemberment (dis'membəmənt) the amputation of a limb or a part of it.

disopyramide (,diesoh'pirə,mied) a drug given orally or by slow intravenous injection to treat ventricular arrhythmia.

disorientation (dis,awreeənt-'tayshən) the loss of proper bearings, or a state of mental confusion as to time, place, or identity.

dispensary (də'spensə·ree) any place where drugs or medicines are actually dispensed.

displacement (dəs'playsmənt) removal to an abnormal location or position. *D. activity* in psychology, unconscious transference of an emotion from its original object on to a more acceptable substitute.

disposition (ˌdispə'zishən) a tendency to suffer from certain diseases.

dissect (die'sekt, di-) 1. to cut carefully in the study of anatomy. 2. during operation, to separate according to natural lines of structure.

disseminated (də'semiˌnaytəd) widely scattered or dispersed. *D. intravascular coagulopathy* abbreviated DIC. Widespread formation of microthromboses in the capillaries leading to the consumption of clotting factors, and thus resulting in the failure of the clotting mechanism at a site of bleeding. The result is a bleeding tendency—which can be catastrophic and difficult to control. It is a secondary complication of a diverse group of obstetric, surgical, haemolytic, and neoplastic disorders.

dissociation (dəˌsohsee'ayshən, -'sohshee-) separation. 1. the splitting up of molecules of matter into their component parts, e.g. by heat or electrolysis. 2. in psychology, the separation of ideas, emotions, or experiences from the rest of the mind, giving rise to a lack of unity of which the patient is unaware.

distal ('dist'l) situated away from the centre of the body or point of origin. The opposite of *proximal*.

distension (dis'tenshən) enlargement. *Abdominal d.* enlargement of the abdomen by gas in the intestines or fluid in the abdominal cavity.

distichia, distichiasis (di'stiki·ə; ˌdisti'kieəsəs) the presence of a double row of eyelashes, one or both of which are turned against the eyeball, causing irritation.

disulfiram (die'sulfəˌram) a drug used in aversion therapy in alcoholism. Antabuse is a proprietary preparation.

dithranol ('dithrəˌnol) a synthetic preparation used in the treatment of psoriasis and eczema.

diuresis (ˌdieyə'reesəs) increased excretion of urine.

diuretic (ˌdieyə'retik) 1. increasing urine excretion or the amount of urine. 2. an agent that promotes urine secretion. Diuretic drugs are classified by chemical structure and pharmacological action, although a diuretic medication can contain drugs from one or more groups, e.g. loop diuretics, osmotic and potassium-sparing diuretics, and thiazides.

diurnal (die'ərnəl) occurring during daytime or period of light. Diurnal animals have one period of rest and one of activity in 24 hours.

diverticulitis (ˌdievə'tikyə'lietəs) inflammation of a diverticulum. It is most common in the colon; lower abdominal pain with colic and constipation can occur. Intestinal obstruction or abscesses can develop as a result of collections of bacteria and irritating agents being trapped in small blind pouches formed in the intestinal walls.

diverticulosis (ˌdievəˌtikyə'lohsəs)

the presence of diverticula in the colon without inflammation.

diverticulum (dievə'tikyələm) a pouch or pocket in the lining of a hollow organ, as in the bladder, oesophagus, or large intestine. *Meckel's d.* a small sac occurring in the ileum as a congenital abnormality.

diving reflex (diev'ing) decrease in the heart rate that occurs when the face is immersed in cold water.

dizygotic, dizygous (ˌdiezie'gotik; die'ziegəs) pertaining to or derived from two separate zygotes (fertilised ova); said of twins.

dizziness ('dizeenəs) a feeling of unsteadiness or haziness, accompanied by anxiety.

DNA deoxyribonucleic acid.

dobutamine (doh'byootəˌmeen) a heart muscle stimulant administered parenterally in short-term treatment of adults with cardiac decompensation due to organic heart disease or cardiac surgical procedures.

Döderlein's bacillus ('dardəˌlienz) *A.S.G. Döderlein, German obstetrician and gynaecologist, 1860–1941.* A lactobacillus occurring normally in vaginal secretions.

dolor ('dolə, 'dohlə) [L.] *pain.*

dominant ('domənənt) in genetics, capable of expression when carried by only one of a pair of homologous chromosomes. *D. gene* one which will produce its characteristics when it is present in either a heterozygous or homozygous state, i.e. it can be inherited from one parent only.

donor ('dohnə) 1. an organism that supplies living tissue to be used in another body, as a person who furnishes blood for transfusion or an organ for transplantation. 2. a substance or compound that contributes part of itself to another substance (acceptor). *Universal d.* a person with group O blood; such blood is sometimes used in emergency transfusion. Transfusion of blood cells rather than whole blood is preferred.

dopa ('dohpə) the precursor of dopamine and an intermediate product in the biosynthesis of noradrenaline and adrenaline. It is used in PARKINSON'S DISEASE and manganese poisoning. Called also L-dopa and levodopa.

dopamine ('dohpəˌmeen) a substance allied to noradrenaline and used in the treatment of cardiogenic shock. Also occurs naturally in the adrenal medulla and the brain, where it functions as a transmitter of nervous impulses.

Doppler effect ('doplə) the relationship of the apparent frequency of waves, as of sound, light and radio waves, to the relative motion of the source of the waves and the observer.

Doppler ultrasound flowmeter a device for measuring blood flow that transmits sound at a frequency of several megaHertz along a blood vessel. Rapid pulsatile changes in flow as well as steady flow can be recorded; hence, it is helpful in assessing intermittent claudication, thrombus obstruction of deep veins and other abnormalities of blood flow in the major arteries and veins.

dorsal ('dawsəl) relating to the back or posterior part of an organ.

dorsiflexion (ˌdawsə'flekshən) bending backwards of the fingers or toes, i.e. upwards.

dorsum ('dawsəm) 1. the back. 2. the upper or posterior surface.

dosimeter (doh'simətə) one of various devices used to detect and measure exposure to radiation; worn by personnel near to radiation sources.

dothiepin (doh'thieəpən) a tricyclic antidepressant and sedative drug.

double-blind trial (dubəl bliend 'trie·əl) a test for the real effect of a new drug or treatment in clinical practice. Neither the patient nor the staff administering the treatment know which of two apparently identical treatments is the new one being tested.

douche (doosh) a stream of fluid directed to flush out a cavity of the body.

Douglas's pouch ('dugləs) *J. Douglas, British anatomist, 1675–1742*. Rectouterine pouch.

Down's syndrome (downz) *J.L.H. Down, British physician, 1828–96*. a congenital condition characterised by physical malformations and some degree of mental handicap. The disorder was formerly known as 'mongolism'. It is also called trisomy 21 syndrome because the disorder is concerned with a defect in CHROMOSOME 21. The cause of Down's syndrome is not known. There is a relatively high incidence in children of mothers who are in the older childbearing age. A particular type of Down's syndrome that occurs in children of younger mothers tends to occur in certain families. The term 'trisomy' refers to the presence of three representative chromosomes in a cell instead of the usual pair. In Down's syndrome, the 21st chromosome pair fails to separate when the germ cell (usually the ovum) is being formed. Thus the ovum contains 24 chromosomes, and when it is fertilised by a normal sperm carrying 23 chromosomes, the child is born with an extra chromosome (or total of 47) per cell.

doxapram ('doksə'pram) a respiratory stimulant used in carbon monoxide poisoning.

doxepin ('doksəpən) a tricyclic ANTIDEPRESSANT.

dracontiasis (ˌdrakon'tieəsəs) a tropical disease caused by infestation with the guinea-worm; acquired by drinking contaminated water.

Dracunculus (drə'kungkyələs) a genus of roundworms; includes the guinea-worm.

drain (drayn) 1. to withdraw liquid generally. 2. any device by which a channel or open area is established for exit of fluids or purulent material from a cavity, wound, or infected area.

drawsheet ('drawˌsheet) a narrow sheet placed across the bed under a patient to prevent soiling of the main sheet. The sheet is twice the width of the bed to enable a clean piece to be drawn under the patient without the whole sheet being changed.

dressing ('dresing) material applied to cover a wound or a diseased surface of the body.

DRG diagnostic-related groups. A system for adminstrative purposes.

drip (drip) a colloquial term used to denote intravenous infusion of fluid (blood, saline, glucose) into the body.

drive (driev) in psychology, an urge or motivating force.

droperidol (droh'perəˌdol) a major tranquilliser used to control behavioural disturbances.

droplet infection ('droplət) infection due to inhalation of respiratory pathogens suspended in liquid particles exhaled from someone already infected.

dropsy ('dropsee) an old-fashioned term used to describe excess fluid in the tissues (oedema).

drowning ('drowning) asphyxiation due to immersion in a liquid medium.

drug (drug) 1. any medicinal substance. 2. a narcotic. 3. to administer a drug. *D. abuse* the use of drugs for purposes other than those for which they are prescribed or recommended. The major groups of drugs and medicines most commonly misused are stimulants ('uppers') depressant ('downers'), psychedelics, and narcotics. *D. addiction* a state of periodic or chronic intoxication produced by the repeated consumption of a drug, characterised by: (a) an overwhelming desire or need (compulsion) to continue use of the drug and to obtain it by any means; (b) a tendency to increase the dosage; (c) a psychological (and usually a physical) dependence on its effects; and (d) a detrimental effect on the individual and on society. *D. idiosyncrasy* an individual response to a drug that is unique to that person and quite different from what is expected. *D. interaction* modification of the potency of one drug by another (or others) taken concurrently or sequentially. Some drug interactions are harmful and some can have therapeutic benefits. Present knowledge of drug interactions is limited. Drugs can also interact with various foods. In general, these interactions fall into three categories: (a) food malabsorption; (b) nutritional status; and (c) alteration of drug response by nutrients. In teaching patients self-care in the taking of prescribed medications, the need to follow directions should be emphasised, especially with respect to the intake of food and drink while the medication regimen is being followed. *D. tolerance* a progressive reduction in the effect of a drug following repeated use. To achieve the desired effect, increasingly larger doses of the medication are needed.

Duchenne dystrophy (doo,shen) *G.B.A. Duchenne, French neurologist, 1806–75*. Progressive muscular dystrophy occurring in childhood. *See* DYSTROPHY.

duct (dukt) a tube or channel for the passage of fluid, particularly one conveying the secretion of a gland.

ductless ('duktləs) without an excretory duct. *D. glands* endocrine glands. *See* ENDOCRINE.

ductus ('duktəs) a duct. *D. arteriosus* a passage connecting the pulmonary artery and aorta in intrauterine life, which normally closes soon after birth (*see* figure p. 138). When it remains open it is called persistent ductus arteriosus. *See also* PATENT DUCTUS ARTERIOSUS.

dumping ('dumping) the rapid evacuation of the contents of an organ. *D. syndrome* a feeling of fullness, weakness, sweating, and dizziness which can occur after meals following a partial gastrectomy.

duodenal (,dyooə'deenəl) pertaining to the duodenum. *D. intubation* the use of a special tube which is passed via the mouth and stomach into the

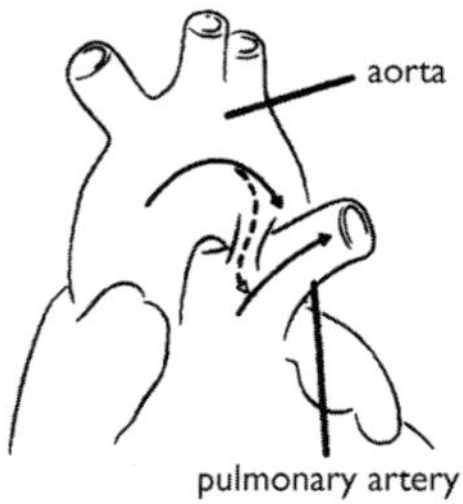

Ductus Arteriosus

duodenum. Used for withdrawal of duodenal contents for pathological examination. *D. ulcer* a peptic ulcer occurring in the duodenum near the pylorus.

duodenostomy (ˌdyooədə'nostəmee) the formation of an artificial opening into the duodenum, through the abdominal wall, for purposes of feeding in cases of gastric disease.

duodenum (ˌdyooə'deenəm) the first 20–25 cm of the small intestine, from the pyloric opening of the stomach to the JEJUNUM. The pancreatic and common bile ducts open into it.

Dupuytren's contraction or **contracture** (ˌduhpwi'trenz) *Baron G. Dupuytren, French surgeon, 1777–1835*. Contracture of the palmar fascia, causing permanent bending and fixation of one or more fingers.

dura mater ('dyoorə mahtə, -maytə) a strong fibrous membrane forming the outer covering of the brain and spinal cord.

dwarfism ('dwawfizəm) the state of being short in stature. Arrest of growth and development, e.g. due to renal rickets, cretinism, or deficient pituitary function.

dynamometer (ˌdienə'momətə) an instrument for measuring the force of muscular contracture.

dysarthrosis (ˌdisah'throhsəs) a deformed, dislocated, or false joint.

dyschondroplasia (ˌdiskondroh-'playzi·ə) a condition in which cartilage is deposited in the shaft of some bones. The affected bones become shortened and deformed.

dyscrasia (dis'krayzi·ə) a morbid condition, usually referring to an imbalance of component elements. *Blood d.* any abnormal or pathological condition of the blood.

dysdiadochokinesis (ˌdisdieˌadə-kohkə'neesəs) a sign of cerebellar disease in which the ability to perform rapid alternating movements, such as rotating the hands, is lost.

dysentery ('disəntree) inflammation of the intestine, especially of the colon, with abdominal pain, tenesmus, and frequent stools, often containing blood and mucus. The causative agent might be chemical irritants, bacteria, protozoa, viruses, or parasitic worms. *Amoebic d.* common in tropical countries; caused by the protozoon *Entamoeba histolytica*. Also called amoebiasis. *Bacillary d.* the most common and acute form of the disease, caused by bacteria of the genus *Shigella*.

dysfunction (dis'fungkshən) impairment of function.

dysgammaglobulinaemia (disˌgaməˌglobyələ'neemi·ə) an immunological deficiency state marked by selective deficiencies of one or more, but not all, classes of immunoglobulins, resulting in heightened susceptibility to infectious diseases.

dysgenesis (dis'jenəsəs) defective development.

dysgerminoma (ˌdisjərmə'nohmə) a malignant tumour derived from germinal cells that have not been differentiated to either sex, occurring in either the ovary or the testicle.

dyshidrosis (dis·hə'drohsəs) a disturbance of the sweat mechanism in which an itching vesicular rash can be present.

dyskinesia (ˌdiskə'neezi·ə) impairment of voluntary movement.

dyslalia (dis'layli·ə) impairment of speech, caused by a physical disorder.

dyslexia (dis'leksi·ə) difficulty in reading or learning to read; accompanied by difficulty in writing and spelling correctly.

dysmaturity (ˌdismə'tyoorətee) the condition of being small or immature for gestational age; said of fetuses that are the product of a pregnancy involving placental insufficiency or dysfunction. Called also 'small for dates', or 'light for gestational age'.

dysmenorrhoea (disˌmenə'reeə) painful menstruation. *Primary* (spasmodic) *d.* painful menstruation occurring without apparent cause. The onset is usually shortly after puberty and occurs with each subsequent period. Might be helped by hormonal therapy. *Secondary* (congestive) ***d.*** painful menstruation occurring in a woman who has previously had normal periods for some years. Often due to ENDOMETRITIS. The condition tends to worsen as the local congestion increases.

dysostosis (ˌdiso'stohsəs) abnormal development of bone.

dyspareunia ('dispə'rooni·ə) painful or difficult coitus in women.

dyspepsia (dis'pepsi·ə) indigestion. There can be abdominal discomfort, flatulence, nausea, and sometimes vomiting. *Nervous* ***d.*** dyspepsia in which anxiety and tension aggravate the symptoms.

dysphagia (dis'fayji·ə) difficulty in swallowing.

dysphasia (dis'fayzi·ə) difficulty in speaking as a result of a brain lesion. There is a lack of coordination and an inability to arrange words in their correct order.

dysplasia (dis'playzi·ə) abnormal development of tissue.

dyspnoea (disp'neeə) difficult or laboured breathing. *Expiratory* ***d.*** difficulty in expelling air. *Inspiratory d.* difficulty in taking in air.

dyspraxia (dis'praksi·ə) partial loss of ability to perform coordinated movements.

dysrhythmia (dis'ridhmi·ə) disturbance of a regularly occurring pattern. Often applied to an abnormality of rhythm of the brain waves, as shown in an electroencephalogram.

dystaxia (dis'taksi·ə) difficulty in controlling voluntary movements.

dystocia (dis'tohsi·ə) difficult or slow labour.

dystonia (dis'tohni·ə) a lack of tonicity in a tissue, often referring to the muscles.

dystrophia (dis'trohfi·ə) dystrophy. *D. myotonica* a rare hereditary disease of early adult life in which there is progressive muscle wasting and gonadal atrophy.

dystrophy ('distrəfee) a disorder of

an organ or tissue caused by faulty nutrition of the affected part. Dystrophia. *Muscular d.* a group of hereditary diseases in which there is progressive muscular weakness and wasting.

dysuria (dis'yoori·ə) difficult or painful micturition.

Ee

ear (iə) the organ of hearing and of equilibrium (*see* figure on p. 142). It consists of three parts: (a) the *external e.*, made up of the expanded portion, or pinna, and the auditory canal, separated from the middle ear by the drum, or tympanum; (b) the *middle e.*, an irregular cavity containing three small bones (incus, malleus, and stapes) that link the tympanic membrane to the internal ear; it also communicates with the pharyngotympanic tube and the mastoid cells; (c) the *internal e.*, which consists of a bony and a membranous labyrinth (the cochlea and semicircular canals).

EBM expressed breastmilk.

Ebola virus disease (ee'bohlə) a central African viral haemorrhagic fever with acute onset and characteristic morbilliform rash. The incubation period is 2–21 days. Outbreaks have been reported in Sudan and Zaire. It has no known source, although it is probably a ZOONOSIS. Person-to-person spread in hospitals and laboratories by accidental inoculation of blood and tissue fluids has occurred.

ecchymosis (ˌeki'mohsəs) a bruise; an effusion of blood under the skin causing discolouration.

eccrine ('ekrien, -rin) secreting externally. Applied particularly to the sweat glands, which are generally distributed over the body. *See* APOCRINE.

ECG electrocardiogram.

Echinococcus (eˌkienə'kokəs) a genus of tapeworm. *E. granulosus* infests dogs and can also infect humans. The larval form develops into cysts (hydatids), which occur in the liver, lung, brain, and other organs.

echocardiography (ˌekohˌkahdee-'ogrəfee) a method of studying the movements of the heart by the use of ultrasound.

echoencephalography (ˌekoh·en-ˌkefə'logrəfee, -ˌsef-) a method of brain investigation by ultrasonic echoes.

echolalia (ˌekoh'layli·ə) the pathological involuntary repetition of phrases or words spoken by another person.

echopraxia (ˌekoh'praksi·ə) the automatic repetition of the movements of others.

echovirus ('ekohˌvierəs) a group of viruses (enteroviruses), the name of which was derived from the first letters of the description 'enteric cytopathogenic human orphan'. At the time of the isolation of the viruses, the diseases they caused

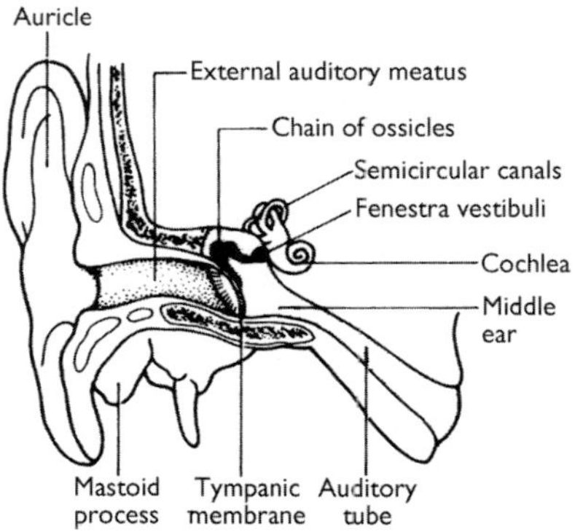

Ear

were not known, hence the term 'orphan'. It is now known that these viruses produce many types of human disease, especially aseptic meningitis, diarrhoea, and respiratory diseases.

eclampsia (ə'klampsi·ə) a severe condition of pregnancy-induced hypertension in which convulsions can occur as a result of an acute toxaemia of pregnancy.

ecmnesia (ek'neezi·ə) forgetfulness of recent events with remembrance of more remote ones.

ecology (ee'koləjee) the study of the relationship between living organisms and the environment.

economy (ee'konəmee) the management of money or domestic affairs. *Token e.* in behaviour therapy, a program of treatment in which the patient earns tokens, exchangeable for tangible rewards, by engaging in appropriate personal and social behaviour, and loses tokens for antisocial behaviour.

ecstasy ('ekstə see) 1. a feeling of exaltation. It can be accompanied by sensory impairment and lack of activity but with an expression of rapture. 2. an illegal drug that has become extremely popular since the late 1980s. It is particularly widely used as an accompaniment to modern dance music. Also known as 'MDMA', 'E', or 'ecky'.

ECT electroconvulsive therapy.

ectoderm ('ektə,dərm) the outer germinal layer of the developing embryo from which the skin and nervous system are derived.

ectogenous (ek'tojənəs) produced outside an organism. *See* ENDOGENOUS.

ectoparasite (,ektoh'parə,siet) a parasite that spends all or part of its life on the external surface of its host, e.g. a louse.

ectopia (ek'tohpi·ə) displacement or abnormal position of any part. *E. cordis* congenital malposition of the heart outside the thoracic cavity. *E. vesicae* a defect of the abdominal wall in which the bladder is exposed.

ectopic (ek'topik) 1. pertaining to or characterised by ECTOPY. 2. located away from normal position. 3. arising or produced at an abnormal site or in a tissue where it is not normally found. *E. beat* an impulse that originates at a site in the heart, other than the sinoatrial node. E. *pregnancy* pregnancy in which the fertilised ovum becomes implanted outside the uterus instead of in the wall of the uterus. Also called 'extrauterine pregnancy'.

ectopy ('ektə pee) displacement or malposition, especially if congenital.

ectropion (ek'trohpi·ən) eversion of an eyelid, often due to contraction of the skin or to paralysis. It causes a persistent overflow of tears and hypertrophy of exposed conjunctiva.

eczema ('eksimə, 'eksmə) 1. a general term for any superficial inflammatory process involving primarily the epidermis, marked early by redness, itching, minute papules, and vesicles, weeping, oozing, and crusting, and later by scaling, lichenification and often pigmentation. 2. atopic dermatitis. Eczema is a common allergic reaction in children but it also occurs in adults. Childhood eczema often begins in infancy, the rash appearing on the face, neck, and folds of elbows and knees. It can disappear by itself when an offending food is removed from the diet, or it can become more extensive and, in some instances, cover the entire surface of the body. Severe eczema can be complicated by skin infections. The cause of eczema can be exogenous (due to external or traumatic factors) or endogenous (due to internal or constitutional factors).

edema (ə'deemə) OEDEMA.

edentulous (ee'dentyələs, -'dench-) without natural teeth.

EDTA ethylenediaminetetra-acetic acid. a colourless crystalline slightly soluble organic compound used in inorganic chemistry and biochemistry.

Edwards syndrome ('edwədz) a condition due to an extra chromosome 18, characterised by mental retardation, MICROCEPHALY and other deformities. Also called TRISOMY 18.

EEG electroencephalogram.

effacement (ə'faysmənt) taking up of the cervix. The process during labour by which the internal os dilates, thus opening out the cervical canal and leaving only a circular orifice, the external os. In a PRIMIGRAVIDA, this process precedes cervical dilatation, whereas the two processes occur simultaneously in a MULTIGRAVIDA.

effector (ə'fektə) a motor or sensory nerve ending in a muscle, gland or organ.

efferent ('efə·rənt) conveying from the centre to the periphery. *E. nerves* nerves coming from the brain to supply the muscles and glands.

effleurage (ˌeflə'rahzh) [Fr.] stroking movement in massage. In NATURAL CHILDCIRTH, a light circular stroke of the lower abdomen, performed in rhythm to control breathing, to aid in relaxation of the abdominal muscles, and to increase concentration during a uterine contraction. The stroking is accomplished by moving the wrist only.

effort syndrome ('efət) a condition characterised by breathlessness, palpitations, chest pain, and fatigue, caused by an abnormal anxiety; often found in soldiers but can also occur in other individuals.

effusion (ə'fyoozhən) the escape of blood, serum or other fluid into surrounding tissues or cavities.

ego ('eegoh) in psychoanalytical theory, that part of the mind which the individual experiences as 'self'. The ego is concerned with satisfying the unconscious primitive demands of the 'id' in a socially acceptable form.

eidetic (ie'detik) the ability to visualise exactly objects or events that have previously been seen. A photographic memory.

Eisenmenger's complex ('iezən-ˌmengəz) *V. Eisenmenger, German physician, 1864–1932*. A congenital heart defect in which a ventricular septal defect is associated with increased pulmonary vascular resistance.

ejaculation (eeˌjakyə'layshən) the act of ejecting semen, a reflex action that occurs as the result of sexual stimulation.

elastic (ə'lastik) capable of stretching. *E. bandage* one that will stretch and exert continuous pressure on the part bandaged. *E. stocking* a woven rubber stocking sometimes worn for varicose veins. *E. tissue* connective tissue containing yellow elastic fibres.

elation (ə'layshən) in psychiatry, a feeling of wellbeing or a state of excitement. It occurs to a marked degree in hypomania and to an intense degree in mania. *See* EUPHORIA.

elbow ('elboh) the joint between the upper arm and the forearm. It is formed by the humerus above, and the radius and ulna below.

elective (ə'lektiv) usually pertaining to a surgical procedure that is performed by choice, as opposed to an emergency life-saving procedure.

Electra complex (ə'lektrə) libidinous fixation of a daughter towards her father. The female version of the Oedipus complex.

electrocardiogram (ə'lektroh-'kahdiəˌgram) abbreviated ECG. A tracing made of the various phases of the heart's action by means of an electrocardiograph. The normal electrocardiogram (*see* figure) is composed of a P wave, Q, R and S waves (known as the QRS COMPLEX, or QRS wave), and a T wave. The P wave occurs at the beginning of each contraction of the atria. The QRS wave occurs at the beginning of each contraction of the ventricles. The T wave seen in a normal electrocardiogram occurs as the ventricles recover electrically and prepare for the next contraction. There is a refractory period between these waves.

electrocardiograph (əˌlektroh-'kahdeeəˌgrahf, -ˌgraf) a machine that records the electrical potential of the heart from electrodes on the chest and limbs.

electrocautery (ə'lektroh'kawtə·ree) an instrument for the destruction of tissue by means of an electrically heated needle or wire loop.

electrocoagulation (əˌlektrohkoh-ˌagyə'layshən) a method of coagu-

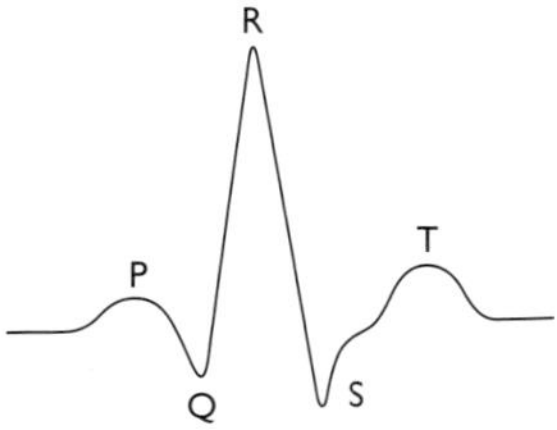

Electrocardiogram

lation using a high-frequency current. A form of surgical diathermy.

electroconvulsive therapy (əˌlektrohkən'vulsiv) abbreviated ECT. Electroplexy. The passage of an electric current through the frontal lobes of the brain, which causes a convulsion. It is used in the treatment of depression and, sometimes, of schizophrenia. A general anaesthetic and muscle relaxant are given before treatment.

electrocorticography (əˌlektrohˌkawtə'kogrəfee) electroencephalography with the electrodes applied directly to the cortex of the brain during surgery to locate a small lesion, e.g. a scar.

electrode (ə'lektrohd) the terminal of a conducting system or cell of a battery, through which electricity enters or leaves the body.

electroencephalogram (əˌlektroh·en'kefələˌgram, -'sef-) abbreviated EEG. A tracing of the electrical activity of the brain. Abnormal rhythm is an aid to diagnosis in epilepsy and cerebral tumour.

electroencephalograph (əˌlektroh·en'kefələˌgrahf, ˌ-graf, '-sef-) a machine for recording the electrical activity of the cortex of the brain. The electrodes are applied to the scalp.

electrolysis (əˌlek'troləsəs) 1. chemical decomposition by means of electricity, e.g. an electric current passed through water decomposes it into oxygen and hydrogen. 2. the destruction of tissue by means of electricity, e.g. the removal of surplus hair.

electrolyte (ə'lektrəˌliet) a compound which, when dissolved in a solution, dissociates into ions. These ions are electrically charged particles and will therefore conduct electricity. *E. balance* the maintenance of the correct balance between the different elements in the body tissues and fluids.

electron (ə'lektron) a negatively charged particle revolving round the nucleus of an atom. *See* ATOM. *E. microscope* a type of microscope employing a beam of electrons rather than a beam of light, which allows very small particles (such as viruses) to be identified.

electro-oculography (ə'lektrohˌokyəˌlogrəfee) *see* ELECTRORETINOGRAPHY.

electrophoresis (əˌlektrohfə'reesəs) a method of analysing the different proteins in blood serum by passing an electric current through the serum to separate the electrically charged particles. The particles gradually separate into bands as a result of the difference in rate of movement according to the electrical charge on the particles.

electroplexy (ə'lektrohˌpleksee, ˌelek'troplekˌsee) electroconvulsive therapy.

electroretinography (ə'lektroh,retə-,nogrəfee) a method of examining the retina of the eye by means of electrodes and light stimulation for assessment of retinal damage.

element ('eləmənt) 1. any of the primary parts or constituents of a compound. 2. in chemistry, a simple substance that cannot be decomposed by ordinary chemical means; the basic 'stuff' of which all matter is composed.

elephantiasis (,eləfən'tieəsəs) a chronic disease of the lymphatics producing excessive thickening of the skin and swelling of the parts affected, usually the lower limbs. It can be due to FILARIASIS in tropical and subtropical climates.

elevator ('elə,vaytə) an instrument used as a lever for raising bone, etc. *Periosteal e.* instrument that strips the PERIOSTEUM in bone surgery.

elimination (ə,limə'nayshən) the removal of waste matter, particularly from the body. Excretion.

ELISA abbreviation for enzyme-linked immunosorbent assay, a blood test for the detection of antibodies to the human immunodeficiency virus (HIV). First used in 1985, it can give a false-negative or false-positive result: a follow-up test should always be offered after a positive result.

elixir (ə'liksə) a sweetened spirituous liquid, used largely as a flavouring agent to hide the unpleasant taste of some drugs.

elliptocytosis (ə,liptohsie'tohsəs) an hereditary disorder in which the red blood cells are elliptical in shape. It results in increased red blood cell destruction leading to anaemia.

emaciation (ə,maysee'ayshən) excessive wasting of body tissues. Extreme thinness.

emasculation (ə,maskyə'layshən) the removal of the penis or testicles; castration.

embolectomy (,embə'lektəmee) surgical removal of an EMCOLUS, frequently arterial emboli that are cutting off the blood supply to the limbs.

embolism ('embə,lizəm) obstruction of a blood vessel by a travelling blood clot or particle of matter. *Air e.* the presence of gas or air bubbles, usually sucked into the large veins from a wound in the neck or chest. *Cerebral e.* obstruction of a vessel in the brain. *Coronary e.* the blockage of a coronary vessel with a clot. *Fat e.* globules of fat released into the blood from a fractured bone. *Infective e.* detached particles of infected blood clot from an area of inflammation which, by obstructing small vessels, results in abscess formation, i.e. PYAEMIA. *Pulmonary e.* blocking of the pulmonary artery or one of its branches by a detached clot, usually due to thrombosis in the femoral or iliac veins. *Retinal e.* blockage, due to air or a blood clot, of the central retinal artery, resulting in loss of vision.

embolus ('embələs) a substance carried by the bloodstream until it causes obstruction by blocking a blood vessel. *See* EMCOLISM.

embrocation (,embroh'kayshən) a liquid applied to the body by rubbing to treat strains. A liniment.

embryo ('embree,oh) the fertilised ovum in its earliest stages, i.e. until it shows human characteristics during the second month. After this, it is termed a FETUS.

embryology (,embree'oləjee) the

study of the growth and development of the embryo from the unicellular stage until birth.

emergency (ə'mərjənsee) a situation that arises suddenly and threatens the life or welfare of a person or group of persons, such as in a medical emergency or a disaster situation.

emesis ('eməsəs) vomiting.

emetic (ə'metik) an agent that can induce vomiting.

EMG electromyography.

emic view ('eemik) the insiders view of the world

emission (ə'mishən) involuntary ejection (of semen).

emollient (ə'moli·ənt, -'moh-) any substance used to soothe or soften the skin.

emotion (ə'mohshən) feeling or affect; a state of arousal characterised by alteration of feeling tone and by physiological behavioural changes. The physical form of emotion can be outwards and evident to others, as in crying, laughing, blushing, or a variety of facial expressions. However, emotion is not always reflected in the appearance and actions even though psychic changes are taking place. Joy, grief, fear, and anger are examples of emotions.

empathy ('empəthee) the power of projecting oneself into the feelings of another person or situation.

emphysema (ˌemfə'seemə, -fie-) the abnormal presence of air in tissues or cavities of the body. *Pulmonary e.* a chronic disease of the lungs. Distension of alveoli causes intervening walls to be broken down and bullae to form on the lung surface. It also causes distension of the bronchioles and eventual loss of elasticity so that inspired air cannot be expired, making breathing difficult. *Surgical e.* the presence of air or any other gas in the subcutaneous tissues, introduced through a wound and evidenced by crepitation on pressure.

empirical (em'pirikəl) based on observation and experiment, rather than theory; the obtaining of evidence or scientific data.

empyema (ˌempie'eemə) a collection of pus in a cavity, most commonly referring to the pleural cavity.

emulsion (ə'mulshən) a mixture in which an oil is suspended in water by the addition of an emulsifying agent.

enamel (ə'naməl) the hard outer covering of the crown of a tooth.

enarthrosis (ˌenah'throhsəs) a freely moving joint, e.g. a ball-and-socket joint.

encanthis (en'kanthəs) a small fleshy growth at the inner canthus of the eye, which can form into an abscess.

encapsulated (en'kapsyəˌlaytəd) enclosed in a capsule.

encephalin (enkephalin) (en'kefələn, -'sef-) an opiate-like substance produced by the pituitary gland that has analgesic effects. This substance can also be produced synthetically. *See* ENDORPHIN.

encephalitis (en'kefə'lietəs, -'sef-) inflammation of the brain. There are many types of encephalitis, depending on the causative agent and the structures involved. The symptoms can be mild, with headache, general malaise, and muscle ache similar to those associated with influenza. The more serious manifestations can include fever, delirium, convulsions, and coma and, in a significant number of patients, can result in death.

encephalocele (en'kefəloh,seel, -'sef-) herniation of the brain through the skull.

encephalography (en,kefə'lografee, -,sef-) radiographic examination of the ventricles of the brain after the insertion of air or a gas through a lumbar or cisternal puncture.

encephalomalacia (en,kefəlohmə-'layshi·ə, -,sef-) softening of the brain.

encephalomyelitis (en,kefəloh-,mieə'lietəs, -,sef-) inflammation of the brain and spinal cord.

encephalomyelopathy (en,kefəloh-,mieə'lopəthee, -,sef-) any disease condition of the brain and spinal cord.

encephalon (en'kefəlon, -'sef-) the brain with the spinal cord, constituting the central nervous system.

encephalopathy (en,kefə'lopəthee, -,sef-) cerebral dysfunction with diffuse disease or damage of the brain. *Dialysis e.* associated with long-term use of haemodialysis; marked by speech disorders and myoclonic fits progressing to global dementia. *Hepatic e.* a condition caused by liver failure, leading to dementia and coma. *Hypertensive e.* a transient disturbance of function associated with hypertension. Disorientation, excitability, and abnormal behaviour occur, which can be reversed if the pressure is reduced. *Wernicke's e.* A complication associated with chronic alcoholism; characterised by paralysis of the eye muscles, DIPLOPIA, NYSTAGMUS, ATAXIA, and mental changes.

enchondroma (,enkon'drohmə) a benign tumour of cartilage within the shaft of the bone.

encopresis (,enkə'preesəs) incontinence of faeces not due to organic defect or illness.

endarterectomy (,endahtə'rek-təmee) the surgical removal of the lining of an artery, usually because of narrowing of the vessel by atheromatous plaques. *Thrombo-e.* removal of a clot with the lining.

endarteritis (,endahtə'rietəs) inflammation of the innermost coat of an artery. *E. obliterans* a type that causes collapse and obstruction in small arteries.

endemic (en'demik) pertaining to a disease prevalent in a particular locality.

endemiology (en,deemeeolәgee) the study of all the factors pertaining to endemic disease.

endocarditis (,endohkah'dietəs) inflammation of the endocardium characterised by vegetations on the endocardium and heart valves. Due to infection by microorganisms, fungi, or *Rickettsia*, or to rheumatic fever.

endocardium (,endoh'kahdi·əm) the membrane lining the heart.

endocervicitis (,endoh,sərvə'sietəs) inflammation of the membrane lining the uterine cervix.

endocrine ('endə,krin, -,krien) secreting within. Applied to those glands whose secretions (hormones) flow directly into the blood and not outwards through a duct. The chief endocrine glands are the thyroid, parathyroids, suprarenals, and pituitary. The pancreas, stomach, liver, ovaries, and testes also produce internal secretions.

endocrinology (,endəkrə'noləjee) the

science of the endocrine glands and their secretions.

endoderm ('endoh,dərm) see ENTODERM.

endogenous (en'dojənəs) produced within the organism. *E. depression* one in which the disease derives from internal causes.

endolymph ('endoh,limf) the fluid inside the membranous labyrinth of the ear.

endolysin (,endoh'liesən, en'doləsən) a factor or enzyme, present in cells, that can cause dissolution of the cytoplasm.

endometriosis (,endoh,meetree-'ohsəs) the presence of endometrium in an abnormal situation, e.g. in the ovaries, the intestines, or the urinary bladder. The ectopic tissue undergoes the same hormonal changes as normal endometrium (*see* figure p. 150). Because there is no outlet for bleeding when menstruation occurs, the woman suffers severe pain.

endometritis (,endohmə'trietəs) inflammation of the endometrium.

endometrium (,endoh'meetri·əm) the mucous membrane lining the uterus.

endomyocarditis (,endoh,mieohkah-'dietəs) inflammation of the lining membrane and muscles of the heart.

endoparasite (,endoh'parə,siet) a parasite that lives within the body of its host.

endophthalmitis (,endof'thal-'mietəs) inflammation of the ocular cavity and adjacent structures.

endorphin (en'dawfən) one of a group of opiate-like peptides produced naturally by the body at neural synapses at various points in the central nervous system, where they modulate the transmission of pain perceptions. Endorphins raise the pain threshold and produce sedation and euphoria; the effects are blocked by naloxone, a narcotic antagonist.

endoscope ('endə,skohp) an instrument used for direct visual inspection of a hollow organ or cavity.

endosteitis (,endostee'ietəs) inflammation of the endosteum.

endosteoma (en,dostee'ohmə) a neoplasm in the medullary cavity of a bone.

endosteum (en'dostee·əm) the lining membrane of bone cavities.

endothelioma (,endoh,theelee-'ohmə) a malignant growth originating in the endothelium.

endothelium (,endoh'theeli·əm) the membranous lining of serous, synovial, and other internal surfaces.

endotoxin (,endoh'toksən) a poison produced by, and retained within, a bacterium, which is released only after the destruction of the bacterial cell. *See* EXOTOXIN.

endotracheal (,endohtrə'keeəl) within the trachea. *E. tube* an airway catheter which is inserted into the trachea when a patient requires ventilatory support (*see* figure on p. 151). It also allows for the removal of secretions by suction.

enema ('enəmə) 1. introduction of fluid into the rectum. 2. a solution introduced into the rectum to promote evacuation of faeces or as a means of administering nutrient or medicinal substances. 3. introduction of a radio-opaque material in a radiological examination of the colon (barium e.), or via a tube inserted into the JEJUNUM in a radiological examination of the small bowel (small bowel e.).

enervation (,enə'vayshən) 1. general

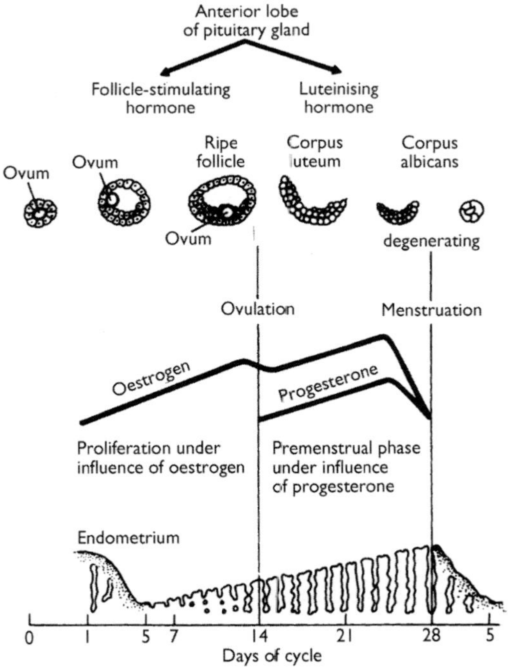

Endometrial and Follicular Changes During the Menstrual Cycle

weakness and loss of strength. 2. removal of a nerve.

en face (ˌonh 'fahs) [Fr.] a position in which the mother's face and that of her infant are on the same plane and approximately 20 cm apart; a position usually held during breastfeeding.

engagement (ən'gayjmənt) the entry of the presenting part of the fetus, normally the head, into the true pelvis. Occurs in the last stage of pregnancy.

enkephalin (en'kefələn) one of two pain-relieving pentapeptides produced in the body.

(a)

(b)

(c)

(d)

(e)

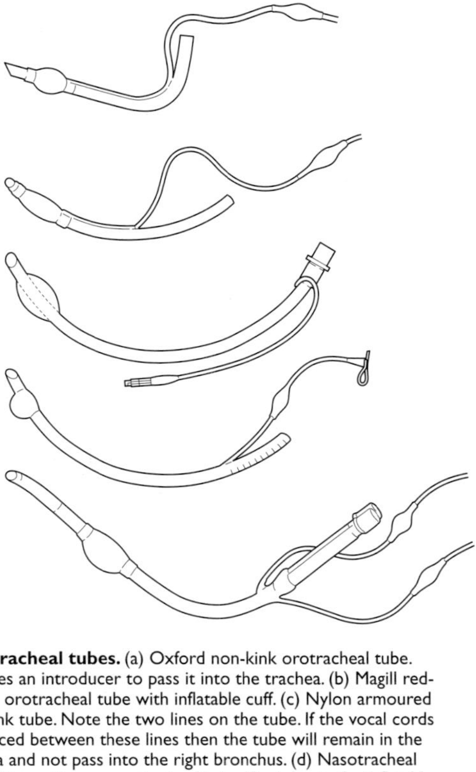

Endotracheal tubes. (a) Oxford non-kink orotracheal tube. Requires an introducer to pass it into the trachea. (b) Magill red-rubber orotracheal tube with inflatable cuff. (c) Nylon armoured non-kink tube. Note the two lines on the tube. If the vocal cords are placed between these lines then the tube will remain in the trachea and not pass into the right bronchus. (d) Nasotracheal tube. Thinner than an orotracheal tube, the tube to the inflatable cuff is attached further back and is buried in the main tube to prevent damage to the nasal mucosa. (e) Robertshaw double-lumen tube that allows one-lung ventilation during thoracic surgery. Note the individual inflatable cuffs for the trachea and the left brochus.

Endotracheal Tubes

enophthalmos (ˌenof'thalməs) a condition in which the eyeball is abnormally sunken into its socket.

ensiform ('ensəˌfawm) xiphoid; sword shaped. *E. cartilage* the lowest portion of the sternum.

Entamoeba (ˌentə'meebə) a genus of protozoa, some of which are parasitic in man. *E. histolytica* the cause of amoebic dysentery.

enteral ('entə·ral) within the gastrointestinal tract. *E. diets* or *e. feeding* diets taken by mouth or through a nasogastric tube.

enterectomy (ˌentə'rektəmee) excision of a portion of the intestine.

enteric (en'terik) pertaining to the intestine. *E.-coated* a special coating applied to tablets or capsules which prevents release and absorption of their contents until they reach the intestine.

enteritis (ˌentə'rietəs) inflammation of the small intestine.

Enterobacteriaceae (ˌentə·roh-baktiə·ree'aysee·ee) a family of Gram-negative, rod-shaped bacteria, many of which are normally found in the human intestine.

enterobiasis (ˌentə·roh'bieəsəs) infestation by threadworms.

Enterobius (ˌentə'rohbi·əs) a genus of nematode worms. *E. vermicularis* the threadworm or pinworm, a small white worm parasitic in the upper part of the large intestine. Gravid females migrate to the anal region to deposit their eggs, sometimes causing severe itching. Infection is frequent in children.

enterocele (ˌentə·rohˌseel) a hernia of the intestine.

enterococcus (ˌentə·roh'kokəs) any streptococcus of the human intestine. An example is *Streptococcus faecalis*, only harmful out of its normal habitat, when it can cause a urinary infection or endocarditis.

enterocolitis (ˌentə·rohkə'lietəs, -koh-) inflammation of both the large and the small intestine.

enterokinase (ˌentə·roh'kienayz) an intestinal enzyme that converts trypsinogen into trypsin; enteropeptidase.

enterolith ('entə·rohˌlith) a concretion in the intestines.

enterospasm ('entə·rohˌspazəm) intestinal colic.

enterostomy (ˌentə'rostəmee) the formation of an external opening into the small intestine. It can be: (a) temporary, to relieve obstruction; or (b) permanent, in the form of an ileostomy in cases of total COLECTOMY.

enterotomy (ˌentə'rotəmee) any incision of the intestine.

enterotoxin (ˌentə·roh'toksən) a toxin that is produced by one of the many organisms that cause food poisoning. Such toxins frequently prove more resistant to destruction than the bacteria themselves.

enterovirus (ˌentə·roh'vierəs) a virus that infects the gastrointestinal tract and then attacks the central nervous system. This group includes Coxsackie, polio, and echoviruses, and are now known, together with rhinoviruses, as PICORNAVIRUSES.

enterozoon (ˌentə·roh'zoh·on) an animal parasite infesting the intestines.

entoderm ('entohˌdərm) the innermost of the three germ layers of the embryo. It gives rise to the lining of most of the respiratory tract and to the intestinal tract and its glands. Also called 'endoderm'.

Entonox ('entə,noks) trade name for a mixture of nitrous oxide and oxygen, 50% of each, premixed in one cylinder, and used as an analgesic.

entropion (en'trohpi·ən) inversion of an eyelid, so that the lashes rub against the eyeball.

enucleation (ən,nyooklee'ayshən) removal of an organ or other mass intact from its supporting tissues, as of the eyeball from the orbit.

enuresis (,enyə'reesəs) involuntary passing of urine, usually during sleep at night (bed-wetting).

environment (en'vierənmənt) the surroundings of an organism which influence its development and behaviour.

enzyme ('enziem) a protein that will catalyse a biological reaction. *See* CATALYST.

eosin ('eeohsən) a red dye used to stain biological specimens. A derivative of bromine and fluorescein.

eosinophil (eeə'sinəfil) a cell having an affinity for eosin. A type of white blood cell containing eosin-staining granules.

eosinophilia (,eeə,sinə'fili·ə) excessive numbers of eosinophils present in the blood.

ependyma (e'pendəmə) the membrane lining the cerebral ventricles and the central canal of the spinal cord.

ependymoma (e,pendə'mohmə) a neoplasm arising from the lining cells of the ventricles or central canal of the spinal cord. It gives rise to signs of HYDROCEPHALUS and is treated by surgery and radiotherapy.

ephedrine ('efə,dreen, -drin) a drug that relieves spasm of the bronchi, having a similar action to adrenaline but can be taken orally. Widely used in asthma and chronic bronchitis.

ephidrosis (,efə'drohsəs) profuse sweating; hyperhidrosis.

epiblepharon (,epee'blefə·ron) a congenital condition in which an excess of skin of the eyelid folds over the lid margin so that the eyelashes are pressed against the eyeball.

epicanthus (,epee'kanthəs) a vertical fold of skin on either side of the nose, sometimes covering the inner canthus; a normal characteristic in persons of certain races, but anomalous in others.

epicardium (,epee'kahdi·əm) the visceral layer of the pericardium.

epicondyle (,epee'kondiel) a protuberance on a long bone above its condyle.

epicritic (,epee'kritik) pertaining to sensory nerve fibres in the skin which give the appreciation of touch and temperature.

epidemic (,epə'demik) the presence in a population of disease or infection in excess of that usually expected.

epidemiology (,epə,deemee'oləjee) the study of the distribution of diseases.

epidermis (,epee'dərməs) the non-vascular outer layer or cuticle of the skin. It consists of layers of cells which protect the dermis.

epidermoid (,epee'dərmoyd) pertaining to certain tumours which have the appearance of epidermal tissue.

Epidermophyton (epee,dərmə-'fietən) a genus of fungi that attacks skin and nails, but not hair. The cause of ringworm and athlete's foot.

epididymis (,epee'didəməs) [Gr.] an elongated, cord-like structure along the posterior border of the testis; its coiled duct provides for the storage, transport, and maturation of spermatozoa.

epididymitis (ˌepeeˌdidə'mietəs) inflammation of the epididymis.

epididymo-orchitis (ˌepeeˌdidəmoh-·aw'kietəs) inflammation of the epididymis and the testis.

epidural (ˌepee'dyoorəl) outside the DURA MATER. *E. analgesia* also known as extradural or peridural anaesthesia. A form of pain relief for labour and chronic pain, obtained by the injection of a local analgesic into the epidural space in order to block the spinal nerves. It can be approached by two routes: (1) caudal, through the sacro-coccygeal membrane covering the sacral hiatus; or (2) lumbar, through the intervertebral space and ligamentum flavum.

epigastrium (ˌepee'gastri·əm) that region of the abdomen situated over the stomach.

epiglottis (ˌepee'glotəs) a cartilaginous structure which covers the opening from the pharynx into the larynx during swallowing and prevents food from passing into the trachea.

epilation (ˌepə'layshən) removal of hairs with their roots. It can be effected by pulling out the hairs or by electrolysis.

epilatory (eˌpilətə·ree) an agent that produces epilation.

epilepsy ('epəˌlepsee) convulsive attacks due to disordered electrical activity of the brain cells. In a major attack of 'grand mal', the patient falls to the ground unconscious, following an 'aura' or unpleasant sensation. There are tonic contractions, and then clonic contractions, from which stage the patient passes into a deep sleep. A minor attack of 'petit mal' is a momentary loss of consciousness only. Both these types of epilepsy are idiopathic and are not caused by any damage to the brain. *Focal* or *Jacksonian e.* a symptom of a cerebral lesion. The convulsive movements are often localised and close observation of the onset and course of the attack assists diagnosis. *Temporal lobe e.* characterised by hallucinations of sight, hearing, taste, and smell, paroxysmal disorders of memory, and automatism. Caused by temporal or parietal lobe disease.

epileptiform (ˌepee'leptəˌfawm) resembling an epileptic fit.

epiloia (ˌepee'loyə) tuberous SCLEROSIS. A congenital disorder with areas of hardening in the cerebral cortex and other organs, characterised clinically by mental handicap and epilepsy.

epinephrine (ˌepee'nefrən) adrenaline.

epineurium (ˌepee'nyoori·əm) the sheath of tissue surrounding a nerve.

epiphora (ə'pifə·rə) persistent overflow of tears, often due to obstruction in the lacrimal passages or to ectropion.

epiphysis (ə'pifəsəs) the end of a long bone, developed separately from, but attached by cartilage to, the diaphysis (the shaft), with which it eventually unites. Growth in length takes place from the line of junction.

episcleritis (ˌepee·sklə'rietəs) inflammation of the outer coat of the eyeball. It is seen as a slightly raised bluish nodule under the CONJUNCTIVA.

episiorrhaphy (ˌepee'so·rəfee) the

repair of a laceration of the peritoneum.

episiotomy (ə'peezee'otəmee) an incision made in the perineum when it will not stretch sufficiently during the second stage of labour (*see* figure).

epispadias (ˌepee'spaydi·əs) a malformation in which there is an abnormal opening of the urethra on to the dorsal surface of the penis. *See* HYPOSPADIAS.

epistaxis (ˌepee'staksəs) bleeding from the nose.

epithelioma (ˌepeeˌtheelee'ohmə) any tumour originating in the epithelium.

epithelium (ˌepee'theeli·əm) the surface layer of cells of the skin or lining tissues.

epithelisation (ˌepeeˌtheelie'zayshən) development of epithelium. The final stage in the healing of a surface wound. Epithelialisation.

epizoon (ˌepee'zoh·on) any external animal parasite.

Epstein–Barr virus (ˌepstien'bah) *M.A. Epstein, British pathologist, b. 1921; Y. Barr, English virologist, b. 1932*. A herpes virus that causes infectious MONONUCLEOSIS. It has been isolated from cells cultured from BURKITT'S LYMPHOMA, and has been found in certain cases of nasopharyngeal cancer. Called also EB virus.

Erb's palsy (airps) *W.H. Erb, German physician, 1840–1921*. Paralysis of the arm, often due to birth injury causing pressure on the brachial plexus or lower cervical nerve roots.

erectile (ə'rektiel) having the power of becoming erect. *E. tissue* vascular tissue which, under stimulus, becomes congested and swollen, causing erection of that part. The

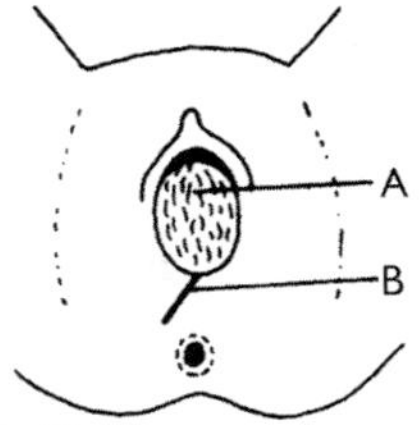

A. Fetal head;
B. Mediolateral incision

Episiotomy

penis consists largely of erectile tissue.

erection (ə'rekshən) the enlarged and rigid state of the sexually aroused penis. Erection can also occur in the clitoris and the nipples of the female.

erepsin (ə'repsən) the enzyme of succus entericus, secreted by the intestinal glands, which splits peptones into amino acids.

ergometrine (ˌərgoh'metreen) an alkaloid of ergot which stimulates contraction of the uterine muscle.

ergonomics (ˌərgə'nomiks) the scientific study of human beings in relation to their work and the effective use of human energy.

ergosterol (ər'gostə·rol) a sterol occurring in animal and plant tissues which, on ultraviolet irradiation, becomes a potent antirachitic substance, vitamin D_2 (ergocalciferol).

ergot ('ərgot) a drug from a fungus that grows on rye. Used chiefly to contract the uterus and decrease the risk of haemorrhage at childbirth.

ergotamine (ər'gotəˌmeen) an alkaloid of ergot used in the treatment of migraine.

ergotism ('ərgəˌtizəm) the effects of poisoning from ergot, which can lead to gangrene of the fingers and toes.

erogenous (ə'rojənəs) arousing erotic feelings. *E. zones* areas of the body, stimulation of which produces erotic desire, e.g. the genitalia, the oral and anal orifices, and the nipples.

erosion (ə'rohzhən) the breaking down of tissue, usually by ulceration. *Cervical e.* a covering of columnar epithelium on the vaginal part of the uterine cervix, arising from erosion of the squamous epithelium, which normally covers it.

erotic (ə'rotik) pertaining to sexual love or lust.

eroticism, erotism (ə'rotəˌsizəm; 'erəˌtizəm) a sexual instinct or desire; the expression of instinctual energy or drive, especially the sex drive.

eructation (ˌiruk'tayshən) belching; the escape of gas from the stomach through the mouth.

eruption (ə'rupshən) a breaking out, e.g. of a skin lesion, or the cutting of teeth.

erysipelas (ˌerə'sipələs) a febrile disease characterised by inflammation and redness of the skin and subcutaneous tissues, and caused by group A haemolytic streptococci.

erysipeloid (ˌerə'sipəˌloyd) an infective dermatitis or cellulitis due to infection with *Erysipelothrix insidiosa*; it usually begins in a wound (often the result of a prick by a fish bone) and remains localised, rarely becoming generalised and septicaemic.

erythema (ˌerə'theemə) redness of the skin caused by congestion of the capillaries in its lower layers. It occurs with any skin injury, infection, or inflammation. *E. induratum* a manifestation of VASCULITIS. *E. multiforme* an acute eruption of the skin, which can be due to an allergy or to drug sensitivity. *E. nodosum* a painful disease in which bright-red, tender nodes occur below the knee or on the forearm; it can be associated with tuberculosis.

erythematous (ˌerə'theemətəs) characterised by erythema.

erythrasma (ˌerə'thrazmə) a skin disease due to infection by *Corynebacterium minutissimum* in the armpits or groins. It causes no irritation but is contagious.

erythroblast (ə'rithrohˌblast) originally, any nucleated erythrocyte, but now more generally used to designate the nucleated precursor from which an erythrocyte develops.

erythroblastosis (əˌrithrohblas'tohsəs) the presence of erythroblasts in the blood. *E. fetalis* a severe haemolytic anaemia with an excess of erythroblasts in the newly born. Due to rhesus incompatibility between the child's and the mother's blood.

erythrocyanosis (ə'rithrohˌsieə'nohsəs) swelling and blueness of the legs and thighs occurring mainly in young women and during cold weather.

erythrocyte (ə'rithrəˌsiet) a mature red blood cell. The cells contain haemoglobin and serve to transport oxygen. They are developed in the red bone marrow found in the cancellous tissue of all bones (*see* figure). The haemopoietic

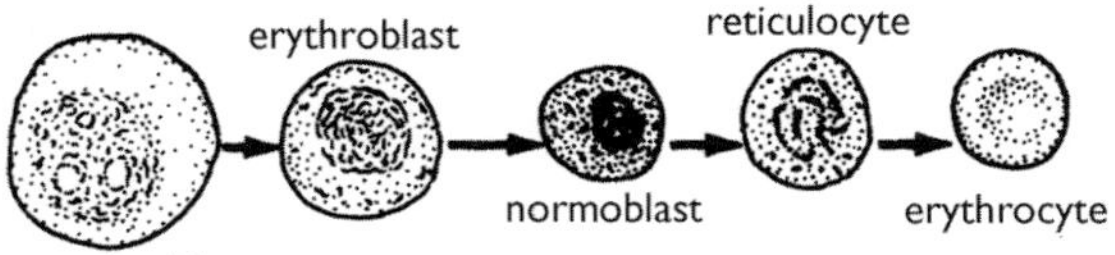

Erythrocyte Development in Bone Marrow

factor vitamin B_{12} is essential for the change from proerythroblast to normoblast, and iron, thyroxine and vitamin C are also necessary for its perfect structure. *E. sedimentation rate* (abbreviated ESR). The rate at which the cells of citrated blood form a deposit in a graduated 200 mm tube (Westergren method). The rate is much increased in severe infection and acute rheumatism.

erythrocythaemia (ə,rithrohsie'theemi·ə) increase in numbers of red blood cells due to overactivity of the bone marrow; Vazquez' disease; POLYCYTHAEMIA vera.

erythrocytopaenia (ə,rithroh,sietoh'peeni·ə) erythropaenia; deficiency in the number of red blood cells.

erythrocytosis (ə'rithrohsie'tohsəs) ERYTHROCYTHAEMIA.

erythroderma (ə,rithrə'dərmə) abnormal redness of the skin, usually over a large area.

erythroedema polyneuropathy (ə,rithrə'deemə ,polee,nyoo'ropəthee) a disease of infancy and early childhood. Marked by pain, swelling, and pink colouration of the fingers and toes, and by listlessness, irritability, failure to thrive, profuse perspiration and, sometimes, scarlet colouration of the cheeks and tip of the nose. Called also 'acrodynia', 'pink disease'.

erythromycin (ə,rithroh'miesən) a broad-spectrum antibiotic produced by a strain of *Streptomyces erythreus*. It is effective against a wide variety of organisms, including Gram-negative and Gram-positive bacteria.

erythropoiesis (ə,rithrohpoy'eesəs) the manufacture of red blood cells.

erythropoietin (ə,rithroh'poyətən, -poy'ee-) a hormone produced by the kidney which stimulates the production of red blood cells in the bone marrow.

erythropsia (,eri'thropsi·ə) a defect of vision in which all objects appear red. Can occur after a cataract operation.

eschar ('eskar) a slough or scab which forms after the destruction of living tissue by gangrene, infection or burning.

escharotomy (,eskə'rotəmee) a surgical incision into necrotic tissue, resulting from burns, to prevent oedema building up and impairing the blood supply.

Escherichia (,esh·ə'riki·ə) a genus of Enterobacteriaceae. *E. coli* an organism normally present in the intestines of humans and other vertebrates. Although not generally pathogenic, it can cause infections of the gallbladder, bile ducts, and urinary tract. It was formerly called *Bacillus coli*.

Esmarch's tourniquet ('ezmahks) *J.F.A. von Esmarch, German surgeon, 1823–1908.* A rubber bandage used in surgery to express blood from a limb and render it less vascular.

esophoria (ˌeesə'faw·ri·ə) latent convergent STRACISMUS. The eyes turn inwards only when one is covered up.

esotropia (ˌeesoh'trohpi·ə) convergent STRACISMUS. One or other eye turns inwards, resulting in double vision.

ESR erythrocyte sedimentation rate.

ESRD end-stage renal disease. *See* RENAL.

essence ('esəns) 1. an indispensable part of anything. 2. a volatile oil dissolved in alcohol.

essential (ə'senshəl) indispensable. *E. amino acids* those amino acids that must be obtained in the diet and are necessary for the maintenance of tissue growth and repair. *See* AMINO ACID. *E. fatty acids* unsaturated fatty acids that are necessary for body growth. *E. oils* specially prepared aromatic oils which are obtained from the different parts of plants including flowers, leaves, seeds, wood, roots, and bark. Used in aromatherapy.

ester ('estə) a compound formed by the combination of an acid and an alcohol, with the elimination of water.

esterase ('estəˌrayz) an enzyme that causes the hydrolysis of esters into acids and alcohol.

ethambutol (e'thambyəˌtol) a drug used in combination with other drugs in the treatment of tuberculosis.

ethanol ('ethə'nol, 'eethə-) alcohol.

ethanolamine (ˌethə'noləˌmeen) an intravenous sclerosing agent used to inject varicose veins.

ether ('eethə) a volatile inflammable liquid formerly used as a general anaesthetic agent.

ethics ('ethiks) a code of moral principles. *Nursing e.* the code governing a nurse's behaviour with patients and their relatives, and with colleagues.

etic view ('etik) an outsider's view of the other's world.

ethmoid ('ethmoyd) a sieve-like bone separating the cavity of the nose from the cranium. The olfactory nerves pass through its perforations.

ethmoidectomy (ˌethmoy'dektəmee) surgical removal of a portion of the ethmoid bone.

ethnic ('ethnik) pertaining to a social group, members of which share cultural bonds or physical (racial) characteristics. *E. minority* a social grouping of people who share cultural or racial factors but who constitute a minority within the greater culture or society.

ethnocentrism (ˌethnoh'sentriz'm) involves the belief that one's own group, community, society, or way of doing things is superior to those of others, leading to mistrust or doubt about others' values and beliefs.

ethnology (eth'noləjee) the science dealing with the human races, their descent, relationship, etc.

ethnography (eth'nogrəfee) a qualitative research approach designed to produce cultural theory.

ethoglucid (ˌethoh'gloosəd) an

antineoplastic agent which can be used to treat bladder cancers by intravesical instillations.

ethoheptazine (ˌethoh'heptəzeen) an analgesic related to pethidine. It relieves pain and muscle spasm.

ethopropazine (ˌethoh'prohpəzeen) an antispasmodic drug used in the treatment of PARKINSONISM.

ethosuximide (ˌethoh'suksəˌmied) an anticonvulsant used in the treatment of petit mal epilepsy.

ethyl biscoumacetate (ˌethəl-ˌbiskoomasətayt, ˌeethəl-, -thiel-) an anticoagulant of the coumarin group.

ethyl chloride (ˌethəl'klor·ried) a volatile liquid used as a local anaesthetic. When sprayed on intact skin, it causes local insensitivity through freezing.

ethylene oxide (ˌethəleen oksied) a gas which is sporicidal and viricidal and capable of penetrating relatively inaccessible parts of an apparatus during sterilisation. It is used for equipment which is too delicate to be sterilised by other methods.

ethylenediaminetetra–acetic acid (ˌethəleenˌdieəmeenˌtetrə·ə'seetik) abbreviated EDTA. A chelating agent used in the treatment of lead poisoning.

ethyloestrenol (ˌethəl'eestrəˌnol) an anabolic steroid that can be used to treat severe weight loss, debility, and OSTEOPOROSIS.

etiolation (ˌeetee·ə'layshən) paleness of the skin due to lack of exposure to sunlight.

etiology (ˌeetee'oləjee) *see* AETIOLOGY.

eucalyptus oil (ˌyookə'liptəs) an oil derived from the leaves of the eucalyptus tree; it has mild antiseptic properties and is used in the treatment of nasal catarrh.

eugenics (yoo'jeniks) the study of measures that can be taken to improve future generations, both physically and mentally.

eugenol ('yoojəˌnol) a local anaesthetic and antiseptic, derived from oil of cloves and cinnamon, used in dentistry.

eukaryote (yoo'kareeˌoht) a cell with a true nucleus. Also eucaryote.

eunuch ('yoonək) a castrated male.

euphoria (yoo'for·ri·ə) an exaggerated feeling of wellbeing, often not justified by circumstances. Less than ELATION.

euplastic (yoo'plastik) capable of being transformed into healthy tissue. The term can be applied to a wound that is healing well.

eurhythmics (yoo'ridhmiks) gentle body exercises performed to music.

Eustachian tube (yoo'stayshən) *B. Eustachio, Italian anatomist, 1520–74.* the PHARYNGOTYMPANIC TUBE.

euthanasia (ˌyoothə'nayzi·ə, -zhə) 1. an easy or good death. 2. the deliberate ending of life of a person suffering from an incurable disease; this can be voluntary or involuntary.

euthyroid (yoo'thieroyd) normally functioning thyroid gland.

evacuant (ee'vakyooənt) 1. promoting evacuation. 2. an agent that promotes evacuation.

evacuation (eeˌvakyoo'ayshən) 1. an emptying or removal, especially the removal of any material from the body by discharge through a natural or artificial passage. 2. material discharged from the body, especially the discharge from the bowels.

evacuator (ee'vakyooˌaytə) an instrument that produces evacuation, e.g. one designed to wash out small particles of stone from the bladder after lithotrity.

evaluation (ee,valyoo'ayshən) a critical appraisal or assessment; a judgment of the value, worth, character, or effectiveness of that which is being assessed. In the healthcare field, this includes assessment of the patient's position on the health–illness continuum, and evaluation of the effectiveness of patient care activities in bringing about a change in his or her position. Accepted as the fourth phase of the nursing process.

eventration (,eevən'trayshən) 1. the protrusion of the intestines through the abdominal wall. 2. removal of abdominal viscera.

eversion (ee'vərzhən) turning outwards. *E. of the eyelid* ECTROPION. The upper eyelid can be everted for examination of the eye or for the removal of a foreign body.

evidence-based practice the conscious and judicious use of the current 'best' evidence in the care of patients and delivery of healthcare services. Research studies are categorised according to the weight of the evidence based on the following classification system.

Levels of evidence

- Level I: A systematic review of all relevant randomised controlled trials (RCTs).
- Level II: At least one properly designed randomised controlled trial.
- Level III.1: Controlled trials without randomisation.
- Level III.2: Well-controlled cohort or case study control studies, preferably from more than one study group or centre.
- Level III.3: Multiple-time series studies with or without intervention.
- Level IV: Opinions of respected authorities, based on clinical experience, descriptive studies or reports of experts.

evisceration (ee,visə'rayshən) removal of internal organs. *E. of the eye* removal of the contents of the eyeball, but not the SCLERA.

evolution (,eevə'looshən) the development of living organisms which change their characteristics during succeeding generations.

evulsion (ee'vulshən) extraction by force.

Ewing's tumour ('yooingz) *J. Ewing, American pathologist, 1866–1943.* A form of sarcoma usually affecting the shaft of a long bone in young adults.

exacerbation (ek'sasə'bayshən, ig,zasə-) an increase in the severity of the symptoms of a disease.

exanthem (eg'zanthəm, ek's-) an infectious disease characterised by a skin rash.

exanthematous (,egzan'themətəs, eks-) pertaining to any disease associated with a skin eruption.

excavation (,ekskə'vayshən) scooping out. *Dental e.* the removal of decay from a tooth before inserting a filling.

excision (ek'sizhən) the cutting out of a part.

excitation (,eksie'tayshən) the act of stimulating.

excitement (ək'sietmənt) a physiological and emotional response to a stimulus.

excoriation (ek,skor·ree'ayshən) an abrasion of the skin.

excrement ('ekskrəmənt) faecal

matter; waste matter from the body.

excrescence (ek'skresəns) abnormal outgrowth of tissue, e.g. a wart.

excreta (ek'skreetə) the natural discharges of the excretory system: faeces, urine, and sweat.

excretion (ek'skreeshən) the discharge of waste from the body.

exercise ('eksəˌsiez) performance of physical exertion for improvement of health or correction of physical deformity. *Active e.* motion imparted to a part by voluntary contraction and relaxation of its controlling muscles. *Isometric e.* active exercise performed against stable resistance, without change in the length of the muscle. No movement occurs at any joints over which the muscle passes. *Passive e.* motion imparted to a segment of the body by another individual, machine or other outside force, or produced by voluntary effort of another segment of the patient's own body. *Range of movement (ROM) e's* exercises that move each joint through its full range of movement, that is, to the highest degree of movement of which each joint is normally capable.

exfoliation (eksˌfohlee'ayshən) the splitting off from the surface of dead tissue in thin flaky layers.

exhalation (ˌeks·hə'layshən) 1. the giving off of a vapour. 2. the act of breathing out.

exhibitionism (ˌeksə'bishəˌnizəm) 1. showing off; a desire to attract attention. 2. exposing the genitals to persons of the opposite sex in socially unacceptable circumstances.

exocrine ('eksə'krin, -ˌkrien) pertaining to those glands that discharge their secretion by means of a duct, e.g. salivary glands. *See* ENDOCRINE.

exogenous (ek'sojənəs) of external origin.

exomphalos (ek'somfələs) 1. hernia of the abdominal viscera into the umbilical cord. 2. congenital umbilical hernia.

exophthalmometer (ˌeksofthal'momətə) an instrument for measuring the extent of protrusion of the eyeball.

exophthalmos (ˌeksof'thalməs) abnormal protrusion of the eyeball which results in a marked stare. Can be due to injury or disease and is often associated with THYROTOXICOSIS.

exostosis (ˌekso'stohsəs) a bony outgrowth from the surface of a bone.

exotoxin (ˌeksoh'toksən) a poison produced by a bacterial cell and released into the tissues surrounding it. *See* ENDOTOXIN.

exotropia (ˌeksoh'trohpi·ə) divergent strabismus; the eyes turn outwards.

expectorant (ək'spektə·rənt) a remedy that promotes and facilitates expectoration.

expectoration (əkˌspektə'rayshən) sputum; secretions coughed up from the air passages. Its characteristics are a valuable aid in diagnosis and note should be taken of the quantity ejected, its colour, and the amount of effort required. Frothiness denotes that it comes from an air-containing cavity; fluidity indicates oedema of the lungs.

experiment (əks'perəmənt) a scientific investigation in which observations are made and data collected by means of the characteristics of control, randomisation, and manipulation.

experimental group (aks,perə-'ment'l) the group in an experimental investigation which receives an intervention or treatment.

expiration (,ekspə'rayshən) 1. the act of breathing out. 2. termination or death.

exploration (,eksplə'rayshən) the operation of surgically investigating any part of the body.

expression (ək'spreshən) 1. the aspect or appearance of the face as determined by the physical or emotional state. 2. the act of squeezing out or evacuating by pressure, e.g. the removal of breast milk by hand. 3. the manifestation of a heritable trait in an individual carrying the gene or genes that determine it.

exsanguination (ək,sang·gwə-'nayshən) extensive blood loss due to internal or external haemorrhage.

extension (ək'stenshən) 1. the straightening out of a flexed joint, such as the knee or elbow. 2. the application of traction to a fractured or dislocated limb by means of a weight.

extensor (ek'stensə, -saw, ək-) a muscle that extends or straightens a limb.

exterior (ek'stiə·ri·ə, ək-) on the outside.

exteriorise (ek'stiə·ri·ə,riez, ək-) 1. to bring an organ or part of one to the outside of the body by surgery. 2. in psychiatry, to turn one's interests outwards.

external fixators (ek'stərnəl, ək-) a type of skeletal fixation in which the bone fragments are held by metal pins which transfix the fragments, and are themselves held by a strong external frame.

extirpation (,ekstər'payshən) complete removal of an organ or tissue.

extracapsular (,ekstrə'kapsyələ) outside the capsule. Can refer to a fracture occurring at the end of the bone, but outside the joint capsule, or to cataract extraction.

extracellular (,ekstrə'selyələ) outside the cell. *E. fluid* tissue fluid that surrounds the cells.

extract ('ekstrakt) a concentrated preparation of a drug made by extracting its soluble principles by steeping in water or alcohol and then evaporating the fluid.

extraction (ek'strakshən, ək-) 1. the process or act of pulling or drawing out. 2. the preparation of an extract. *Breech e.* extraction of an infant from the uterus in cases of breech presentation. *Vacuum e.* removal of the uterine contents by application of a vacuum. An alternative to the forceps method of delivering a baby.

extradural (,ekstrə'dyoorəl) outside the DURA MATER.

extrahepatic (,ekstrəhəpatik) outside the liver. Relating to a condition affecting the liver in which the cause is outside the liver.

extrapyramidal (,ekstrəpə'raməd'l) outside the pyramidal (cerebrospinal) tract. *E. system* the nerve tracts and pathways which are not within the pyramidal tracts.

extrasensory (,ekstrə'sensə·ree) outside or beyond any of the known senses. *E. perception* abbreviated ESP. Appreciation of the thoughts of others or of current or future events without any normal means of communication.

extrasystole (,ekstrə'sistəlee) premature contraction of the atria or ventricles. *See* SYSTOLE.

extrauterine (,ekstrə'yootə,rien)

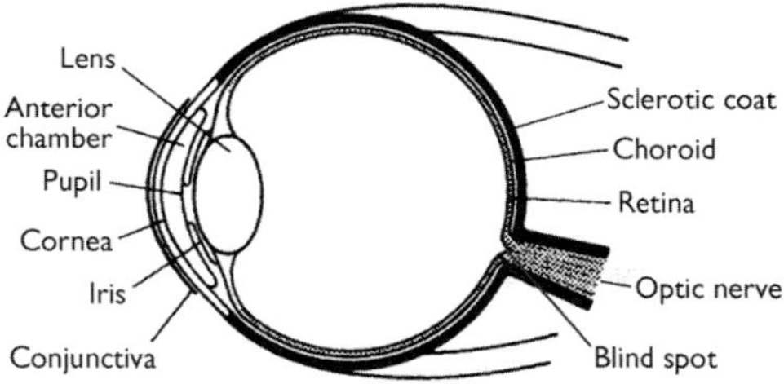

Eye

occurring outside the uterus. *E. pregnancy* ectopic gestation; development of a fetus outside the uterus.

extravasation (ək,stravə'sayshən) effusion or escape of fluid from its normal course into surrounding tissues. *E. of blood* a bruise.

extremity (ək'stremətee) distal part; a hand or foot.

extrinsic (ək'strinsik, -zik) originating externally. *E. factor* a substance present in meat and other foodstuffs. Called also CYANOCOCALAMIN (vitamin B_{12}), it is necessary for the manufacture of red blood cells. The intrinsic factor produced in the stomach is necessary for the absorption of vitamin B_{12}. *E. muscle* a muscle originating away from the part that it controls, such as those controlling the movements of the eye.

extroversion (,ekstrə'vərzhən) turning inside out, e.g. of the uterus, as sometimes occurs after labour.

extrovert ('ekstrə,vərt) a person who is sociable, a good mixer and interested in what goes on around him or her. A personality type first described by Jung. *See* INTROVERT.

extubation (,ekstyə'bayshən) removal of a tube used in intubation.

exudation (,eksyə'dayshən) the slow discharge of serous fluid through the walls of the blood cells and its deposition in or on the tissues.

eye (ie) the organ of sight. A globular structure with three coats. The nerve tissue of the retina receives impressions of images via the pupil and lens. From this, the optic nerve conveys the impressions to the visual area of the CEREBRUM (*see* figure).

eyelid ('ie,lid) a protective covering of the eye, composed of muscle and dense connective tissue covered with skin, lined with conjunctiva, and fringed with eyelashes. Eyelids contain the MEICOMIAN GLANDS.

eyetooth (ie'tooth) an upper canine tooth.

Ff

F symbol for *Fahrenheit* and *fluorine*.

f waves waves that represent fibrillation or flutter on an ECG.

face (fays) the front of the head from the forehead to the chin. *F. presentation* the appearance of the face of the fetus first at the cervix during labour.

facet ('fasət) a small flat area on the surface of a bone. *F. syndrome* a slight dislocation of the small facet joints of the vertebrae giving rise to pain and muscle spasm.

facial ('fayshəl) pertaining to the face or lower anterior portion of the head. *F. nerve* the seventh cranial nerve, which supplies the salivary glands and superficial face muscles. A local anaesthetic can be injected into this nerve before an operation when a general anaesthetic is contraindicated. *F. paralysis see* PARALYSIS.

facies ('fayseeˌeez, 'fayshee-) facial expression; it often gives some indication of the patient's condition. *Adenoid f.* The open mouth and vacant expression associated with mouth breathing and nasal obstruction. *Parkinson f.* fixed expression, due to paucity of movement of facial muscles, characteristic of PARKINSONISM.

factor analysis ('faktə ə'naləsəs) a type of validity that uses a statistical procedure for determining the underlying dimensions or components of a variable.

faecalith ('feekəlith) a hard stony mass of faecal material which can obstruct the lumen of the appendix and be a cause of inflammation. A coprolith.

faeces ('feeseez) waste matter excreted by the bowel, consisting of indigestible cellulose, food which has escaped digestion, bacteria (living and dead), and water.

Fahrenheit scale ('farənˌhiet) *D.G. Fahrenheit, German physicist, 1686–1736.* A scale of heat measurement. It registers the freezing-point of water at 32°, the normal heat of the human body at 98.4°, and the boiling point of water at 212°.

failure ('faylyə) inability to perform or to function properly. *Heart f.* inability of the heart to maintain a circulation sufficient to meet the body's needs. *Kidney f.*, *renal f.* inability of the kidney to excrete metabolites at normal plasma levels under normal loading, or inability to retain electrolytes when intake is normal; in the acute form, marked by uraemia and usually by oliguria, with hyperkalaemia and pulmonary oedema. *Respiratory f.*, *ventilatory* *f.* a life-threatening condition in which respiratory function is inadequate to maintain the body's needs for oxygen supply and carbon dioxide removal while at rest. *F. to thrive* retardation of normal growth and development in an infant. Causes are numerous but malnutrition or difficulty in absorbing essential nutrients are main factors, as well as those that are psychosocial in origin, e.g. maternal deprivation syndrome.

fainting ('faynting) *see* SYNCOPE.

falciform ('falsə,fawm) sickle shaped. *F. ligament* a fold of peritoneum which separates the two main lobes of the liver and connects it with the anterior abdominal wall and the diaphragm.

fallopian tube (fə'lohpi·ən) *G. Fallopius, Italian anatomist, 1523–63.* Uterine tube. One of a pair of tubes, about 10–14 cm long, arising out of the upper part of the uterus. The distal end of each tube is fimbriated and lies near an ovary. Their function is to conduct the ova from the ovaries to the interior of the uterus. An oviduct.

Fallot's tetralogy ('fahlohz te'traləjee) *E.L.A. Fallot, French physician, 1850–1911.* A congenital heart disease with four characteristic defects: (a) pulmonary artery stenosis; (b) interventricular defect of the septum; (c) overriding of the aorta, i.e. opening into both right and left ventricles; (d) hypertrophy of the right ventricle. *See* figure on p. 166.

falx (falks) a sickle-shaped structure. *F. cerebri* the fold of DURA MATER that separates the two cerebral hemispheres.

familial (fə'mili·əl) occurring in or affecting members of a family more than would be expected by chance.

family ('famәlee) 1. a group of people related by blood or marriage, such as parents, children, and siblings. 2. a taxonomic category below an order and above a genus. *Blended f.* a family unit composed of a married couple and their offspring, including some from previous marriages. *Extended f.* a nuclear family and their close relatives, such as the children's grandparents, aunts, and uncles. *Extended nuclear f.* a nuclear family who nevertheless make frequent social contacts with the extended family group despite geographical distance. *Nuclear f.* a couple and their children, by birth or adoption, who are living together and are more or less isolated from their extended family. *F. planning* the arrangement, spacing, and limitation of the children in a family, depending upon the wishes and social circumstances of the parents. *Single parent f.* a lone parent and offspring living together as a family unit. *F. therapy* a therapeutic process whereby the psychotherapist treats several members of the family simultaneously.

Fanconi's syndrome (fan'kohneez) *G. Fanconi, Swiss paediatrician, 1892–1979.* A rare inherited disorder of metabolism in which reabsorption of phosphate, amino acids, and sugar by the renal tubules is impaired. The kidneys fail to produce acid urine, and the resulting features are thirst, POLYURIA, and rickets, leading to chronic renal failure.

fang (fang) the root of a tooth.

fantasy ('fantəsee) an imagined sequence of events or mental images

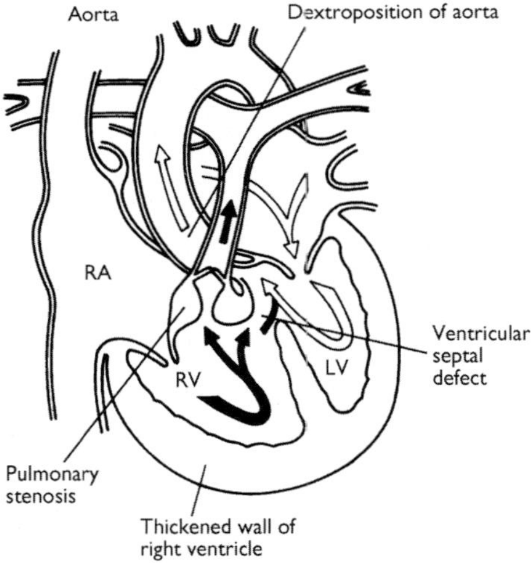

Fallot's Tetralogy

that serves to satisfy unconscious wishes or to express unconscious conflicts.

farinaceous (ˌfarə'nayshəs) starchy or containing starch. Refers to foods such as wheat, oats, barley, and rice.

farmer's lung ('fahməz) a disease occurring in those in contact with mouldy hay. It is thought to be due to a hypersensitivity, with widespread reaction in the lung tissue. It causes excessive breathlessness.

FAS fetal alcohol syndrome.

fascia ('fashi·ə) a sheath of connective tissue enclosing muscles or other organs.

fasciculation (fəˌsikyə'layshən) isolated fine muscle twitching which gives a flickering appearance.

fasciculus (fə'sikyələs) a small bundle of nerve or muscle fibres; a fascicle.

fasciotomy (ˌfashee'otəmee) a surgical incision into the fascia.

fast (fahst) 1. resistance to change. 2. abstaining from food.

fat (fat) 1. the adipose or fatty tissue of the body. 2. neutral fat; a triglyceride which is an ester of fatty acids and glycerol. *Wool-f.* lanolin. *See also* BROWN FAT.

fatigue (fə'teeg) a state of weariness which can range from mental disinclination for effort to profound exhaustion after great physical and mental effort. *Muscle f.* can occur during prolonged effort owing to oxygen lack and accumulation of waste products.

fatty ('fatee) containing or similar to fat. *F. acid see* ESSENTIAL. *F. degeneration* a degenerative change in tissue cells due to the invasion of fat and consequent weakening of the organ. The change occurs as a result of incorrect diet, shortage of oxygen in the tissues, or excessive consumption of alcohol.

fauces ('fawseez) the opening from the mouth into the pharynx. *Pillars of the f.* the two folds of muscle covered with mucous membrane that pass from the soft palate on either side of the fauces. One fold passes into the tongue, the other into the pharynx, and between them is situated the tonsil.

favism ('fayvizəm) an acute haemolytic anaemia caused by ingestion of fava beans or inhalation of the pollen of the plant, usually occurring in certain individuals as a result of a genetic abnormality with a deficiency in an enzyme, glucose-6-phosphate dehydrogenase, in the erythrocytes. Called also fabism.

favus ('fayvəs) a type of ringworm infection, with formation of scabs, in appearance like a honeycomb. It usually affects the scalp and is due to a fungus infection. (Trichophyton schoenleini).

Fe symbol for *iron* (L. ferrum).

fear (fiə) a normal emotional response, in contrast to anxiety and phobia, to consciously recognised external sources of danger; it is manifested by alarm, apprehension, or disquiet. *Obsessional f.* a recurring irrational fear that is not amenable to ordinary reassurance; a phobia.

febrile ('feebriel, 'feb-) characterised by, or relating to, fever. *F. convulsion* a convulsion which occurs in childhood and is associated with PYREXIA.

fecundation (ˌfekən'dayshən, fee-) fertilisation.

fecundity (fə'kundətee) the ability to produce offspring frequently and in large numbers. In demography, the physiological ability to reproduce, as opposed to fertility.

feedback ('feedˌbak) a method of control in which some of the output is returned as input for monitoring purposes. Feedback mechanisms are important in the regulation of such physiological processes as hormone and enzyme reactions. *Negative f.* a rise in the output of a substance is detected and further output is thus inhibited. *Positive f.* a rise in output causes either a direct or indirect rise in the output of another substance.

felon ('felən) an abscess of the distal phalanx of a finger; a whitlow.

Felty's syndrome ('felteez) *A.R. Felty, American physician, 1895–1963*. The triad of rheumatoid arthritis, SPLENOMEGALY, and LEUKOPAENIA. Often associated with anaemia, LYMPHADENOPATHY, and VASCULITIC CUTANEOUS ULCERATION.

feminisation ('femənie'zayshən) 1. the normal induction or development of female sexual characteristics. 2. the induction or development of female secondary sexual characteristics in the male. *Testicular f.* a condition in which the subject is phenotypically female, but lacks nuclear sex chromatin and is of XY chromosomal sex.

femoral ('femə·rəl) pertaining to the

femur. *F. artery* that of the thigh from groin to knee. *F. canal* the opening below the inguinal ligament through which the femoral artery passes from the abdomen to the thigh.

femur ('feemə) the thigh bone.

fenbufen (fen'byoofen) a non-steroidal anti-inflammatory drug (NSAID) that acts as a PRODRUG. It is associated with a lower incidence of gastrointestinal haemorrhage but a higher incidence of skin rashes than some other NSAIDS.

fenestra (fə'nestrə) a window-like opening. *F. ovalis* the oval opening between the middle and the internal ear.

fenoprofen (ˌfeenoh'prohfən) an anti-inflammatory drug used in the treatment of arthritic conditions.

fentanyl ('fentəˌnil) a short-acting narcotic analgesic, widely used during anaesthesia.

ferritin ('ferətən) a complex formed of an iron and protein molecule; one of the forms in which iron is stored in the body.

ferrous ('ferəs) containing iron. *F. fumarate*, *f. gluconate*, *f. succinate*, and *f. sulphate* are iron salts which are given orally to treat iron-deficiency anaemia.

ferrule ('ferool, -rəl) a rubber cap placed on the ends of walking sticks, frames and crutches to prevent slipping.

fertilisation (ˌfərtəlie'zayshən) the impregnation of the female sex cell, the ovum, by a male sex cell, a spermatozoon. *In vitro f.* artificial fertilisation of the ovum in laboratory conditions. The timing and conditions for implantation into a uterus have to be perfect if successful pregnancy is to ensue.

fester ('festə) to become superficially inflamed and to suppurate.

festination (ˌfestə'nayshən) an involuntary tendency to take short accelerating steps in walking; seen in conditions such as PARKINSON'S DISEASE.

fetal ('feet'l) pertaining to the fetus. *F. alcohol syndrome* abbreviated FAS. Physical and mental abnormalities due to maternal alcohol intake during pregnancy. Abnormalities can include MICROCEPHALY, growth deficiencies, mental handicap, hyperactivity, heart murmurs, and skeletal malformation. The exact amount of alcohol consumption that will produce fetal damage is unknown. *F. assessment* determination of the wellbeing of the fetus. Assessment techniques and procedures include: (a) medical and family histories and physical examination of the mother; (b) ULTRASONOGRAPHY; (c) assessment of fetal activity using the Cardiff kick chart; (d) chemical assessment of placental function; (e) assays of amniotic fluid obtained by AMNIOCENTESIS; and (f) electronic and ultrasonic fetal heart rate monitoring.

fetishism ('fetiˌshizm) a state in which an object is regarded with an irrational fear, or an erotic attraction which can be so strong that the object is necessary for achieving sexual excitement.

fetor ('feetə, -taw) an offensive smell.

fetoscope ('feetəˌskohp) 1. an endoscope for viewing the fetus in utero. 2. a type of stethoscope designed for listening to the fetal heartbeat.

fetus-, foetus-, ('feetəs) the developing baby between the eighth week and the end of pregnancy.

fever ('feevə) 1. an abnormally high body temperature; PYREXIA. 2. any disease characterised by marked increase of body temperature.

fibre ('fiebə) a thread-like structure.

fibre optics (ˌfiebə'roptiks) the transmission of light rays along flexible tubes by means of very fine glass or plastic fibres. Use is made of this in endoscopic instruments such as the gastroscope.

fibrescope ('fiebəˌskohp) an endoscope in which fibre optics are used.

fibrillation (ˌfibrə'layshən, ˌfie-) a quivering, vibratory movement of muscle fibres. *Atrial f.* rapid contractions of the atrium causing irregular contraction of the ventricles in both rhythm and force. *Ventricular f.* fine rapid twitchings of the ventricles leading to circulatory arrest. Rapidly fatal unless it can be controlled.

fibrin ('fiebrən) an insoluble protein that is essential to CLOTTING of blood, formed from fibrinogen by action of THROMBIN.

fibrinogen (fie'brinəjən) a soluble protein which is present in blood plasma and is converted into fibrin by the action of thrombin when the blood clots.

fibrinolysin (ˌfiebri'noləsən) a proteolytic enzyme that dissolves fibrin.

fibrinolysis (ˌfiebrə'noləsəs) the dissolution of fibrin by the action of fibrinolysin. The process by which clots are removed from the circulation after healing has taken place.

fibrinopaenia (ˌfiebrənoh'peeni·ə) a deficiency of fibrinogen in the blood. There is a tendency to bleed because the coagulation time is increased.

fibroadenoma (ˌfiebrohˌadə'nohmə) a benign tumour of glandular and fibrous tissue. *See* ADENOMA.

fibroangioma (ˌfiebrohˌanjee'ohmə) a benign tumour containing both fibrous and vascular tissue.

fibroblast ('fiebrohˌblast) a connective tissue cell.

fibrocartilage (ˌfiebroh'kahtəlij) cartilage with fibrous tissue in it.

fibrochondritis (ˌfiebrohkon'drietəs) inflammation of fibrocartilage.

fibrocyst ('fiebrohˌsist) a fibroma that has undergone cystic degeneration.

fibrocystic (ˌfiebroh'sistik) fibrous and cystic. *F. disease of the pancreas* an inherited disease affecting the mucus-secreting glands, the sweat glands, and the pancreas. It is characterised by fatty stools and repeated lung infections. MUCOVISCIDOSIS; cystic fibrosis.

fibroid ('fiebroyd) 1. having a fibrous structure. 2. a FICROMA or a fibromyoma, usually one occurring in the uterus.

fibroma (fie'brohmə) a benign tumour of connective tissue. *Cystic f.* fibrocyst.

fibromyoma (ˌfiebrohmie'ohmə) a tumour consisting of fibrous and muscle tissue; frequently found in or on the uterus (*see* figure p. 170).

fibroplasia (ˌfiebrohmie'playzi·ə) the formation of fibrous tissue when a wound heals. *Retrolental f.* a condition characterised by the presence of fibrous tissue behind the lens, leading to detachment of the retina and blindness, attributed to use of excessively high concentrations of oxygen in the care of preterm infants.

fibrosarcoma (ˌfiebrohsah'kohmə)

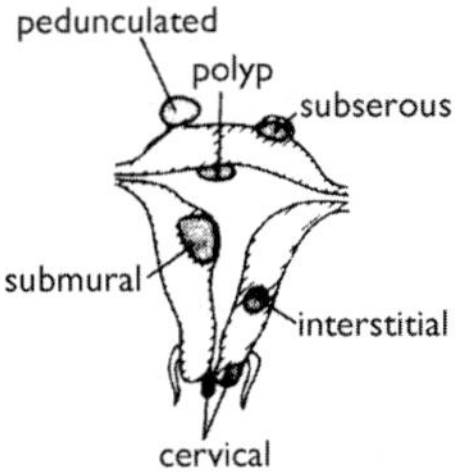

Fibromyomata of Uterus

a malignant tumour arising in fibrous tissue.

fibrosis (fie'brohsəs) fibrous tissue formation, such as occurs in scar tissue or as the result of inflammation. It is the cause of adhesions of the peritoneum or other serous membranes. *F. of the lung* condition that can precede BRONCHIECTASIS and EMPHYSEMA.

fibrositis (ˌfiebrə'sietəs) inflammation of fibrous tissue. The term is loosely applied to pain and stiffness, particularly of the back muscles, for which no other cause can be found.

fibula ('fibyələ) the slender bone from knee to ankle, on the outer side of the leg.

field of vision (ˌfeeld əv 'vizhən) the area within view, as for the fixed eye, a camera or in an operation. *Visual f.* the area within which stimuli will produce the sensation of sight with the eye in a straight-ahead position.

filament ('filəmənt) a small thread-like structure.

Filaria (fi'lair·ri·ə) a genus of nematode worms which can be found in the connective tissues and lymphatics, having been transmitted to man by mosquitoes. Found mainly in the tropics and subtropics.

filariasis (ˌfilə'rieəsəs) an infection by filaria, particularly by *Wuchereria bancrofti*, resulting in blockage of the lymphatics, which causes swelling of the surrounding tissues. ELEPHANTIASIS can occur.

filiform ('filəˌfawm, 'fie-) thread-like. *F. papillae* the fine thread-like processes that cover the anterior two-thirds of the tongue.

filter ('filtə) a device for eliminating certain elements, as (a) particles of certain size from a solution, or (b) rays of certain wavelength from a stream of radiant energy. *Millipore f.* trade name for a device used to filter nutrient solutions as they are administered intravenously.

filtrate ('filtrayt) the fluid that passes through a filter.

filtration (fil'trayshən) 1. the removal of precipitate from a liquid by means of a filter. 2. the removal of rays of a certain wavelength from an electromagnetic beam. *F. angle* the angle of the anterior chamber of the eye through which the aqueous humour drains; blockage of this channel gives rise to glaucoma.

fimbria ('fimbri·ə) a fringe. *F. of the uterine tube* the thread-like projections that surround the pelvic opening of the uterine tube.

finger ('fing·gə) a digit of the hand. *Clubbed f.* one with enlargement of the terminal phalanx with constant osseous changes; occurs in many heart and lung diseases. *Hammer f.*, *mallet f.* permanent flexion of the distal phalanx of a finger due to avulsion of the extensor tendon. *Trigger f.* temporary flexion of a finger which is overcome in a sudden jerk by active or passive extension of the finger. It is caused by thickening of the flexor tendon in a narrowed tendon sheath. *Webbed f's* fingers more or less united by strands of tissue; syndactyly.

first aid (ˌfərst 'ayd) emergency care and treatment of an injured person before complete medical and surgical treatment can be secured.

fission ('fishən) a form of asexual reproduction by dividing into two equal parts, as in bacteria. *Binary f.* the splitting in two of the nucleus and the protoplasm of a cell, as in protozoa. *Nuclear f.* the splitting of the nucleus of an atom, with the release of a great quantity of energy.

fissure ('fishə) a narrow slit or cleft. *Anal f.* a painful crack in the mucous membrane of the anus. *F. of Rolando* a furrow in the cortex of each cerebral hemisphere, dividing the sensory from the motor area; the central sulcus.

fistula ('fistyələ) an abnormal passage between two epithelial surfaces, usually connecting the cavity of one organ with another or a cavity with the surface of the body. *Anal f.* the result of an ischiorectal abscess where the channel is from the anus to the skin. *Biliary f.* a leakage of bile to the exterior, following operation on the gallbladder or ducts. *Blind f.* one which is open at only one end. *Faecal f.* one in which the channel is from the intestine through the wound caused by an operation on the intestines when sepsis is present. *Rectovaginal f.* fistula from the rectum to the vagina which can result from severe perineal tear during childbirth. *Tracheo-oesophageal f.* an opening from the trachea into the oseophagus; a congenital deformity. *Vesicovaginal f.* an opening from the bladder to the vagina, either from error during operation or from ulceration, as can occur in carcinoma of the cervix.

fit (fit) a commonly used term for paroxysmal motor discharges leading to sudden convulsive movements, as in epilepsy, ECLAMPSIA and hysteria. The term is sometimes applied to apoplexy.

fittingness ('fitingnəs) answers the question in qualitative research studies: Are the findings applicable outside the study situation? Are the results meaningful to the individuals not involved in the research?

fixation (fik'sayshən) 1. the process of rendering something immovable, such as a joint or a fractured bone. 2. in psychology, a term used to describe a failure to progress wholly or in part through the normal stages of psychological development to a fully developed personality. 3. in ophthalmology, directing the sight straight at an object.

flaccid ('flaksəd, 'flasəd) soft, flabby. *F. paralysis see* PARALYSIS.

flail (flayl) exhibiting abnormal or pathological mobility, as flail chest or flail joint. *F. chest* a loss of stability of the chest wall due to multiple rib fractures or detachment of the sternum from the ribs as a result of a severe crushing chest injury. The loose chest segment moves in a direction that is the reverse of normal. *F. joint* an unusually movable joint.

flap (flap) a mass of tissue, used for grafting in plastic surgery, which is left attached to its blood supply and used to repair defects either adjacent to it or at some distance from it.

flare (flair) the response of the skin to an allergic or hypersensitivity reaction. Reddening of the skin that spreads outwards.

flatfoot ('flat,fuht) a condition due to absence or sinking of the medial longitudinal arch of the foot, caused by weakening of the ligaments and tendons. Pes planus.

flatulence ('flatyələns) excessive formation of gases in the stomach or intestine.

flatulent ('flatyələnt) suffering from flatulence. *F. distension* swelling due to gas in the stomach or intestines. It is a common complication after abdominal operations and is caused by intestinal stasis.

flatus ('flaytəs) gas in the stomach or intestine.

flea (flee) a small, wingless blood-sucking insect parasite. The common human flea, *Pulex irritans*, rarely transmits disease. Cat and dog fleas, *Ctenocephalides*, are also relatively harmless. The rat fleas *Xenopsylla* and *Nosopsyllus* are the vectors of bubonic plague.

flexibilitas cerea (,fleksə,bilətəs 'seeə·ri·ə) waxy flexibility; a cataleptic state in which the limbs retain any position in which they are placed. A symptom of some forms of schizophrenia; also occurs occasionally in hysteria.

flexion ('flekshən) bending; moving a joint so that the two or more bones forming it draw towards each other. *Dorsi-f.* bending the fingers or toes backwards. *Plantar f.* bending the fingers or toes downwards.

Flexner's bacillus ('fleksnəz) *S. Flexner, American bacteriologist, 1863–1946*. One of the group of pathogenic bacteria which cause bacillary dysentery; *Shigella flexneri*.

flexor ('fleksə) any muscle causing flexion of a limb or other part of the body.

flexure ('flekshə) a bend or curve.

flight of ideas (fliet əv iediəz) the rapid movement of ideas and speech from one fragmentary topic to another that occurs in mania.

floaters ('flohtəz) wisps or strands within the eye that are visible to the patient. Usually caused by detachment and collapse of the vitreous humour and the normal ageing process.

flooding ('fluding) 1. excessive loss of blood from the uterus. 2. a form of desensitisation for the treatment of phobias and related disorders. The patient is repeatedly exposed, in imagination or in real life, to emotionally distressing aversive stimuli of high intensity. Called also IMPLOSION.

florid ('flo·rid) a flushed facial appearance.

flowmeter ('floh,meetə) an instrument used to measure the flow of liquids or gases.

flucloxacillin (,flookloksə'silən) an antibiotic drug used in the treatment of infection by penicillin-resistant bacteria.

fluctuation (,fluktyoo'ayshən, -chyoo-) a wave-like motion felt on palpation of the abdomen.

fludrocortisone (,floodroh'kawtə-,sohn, -,zohn) a synthetic CORTICOSTEROID used in the treatment of adrenal disorders.

fluid ('flooəd) 1. a liquid or gas; any liquid of the body. 2. composed of molecules which freely change their

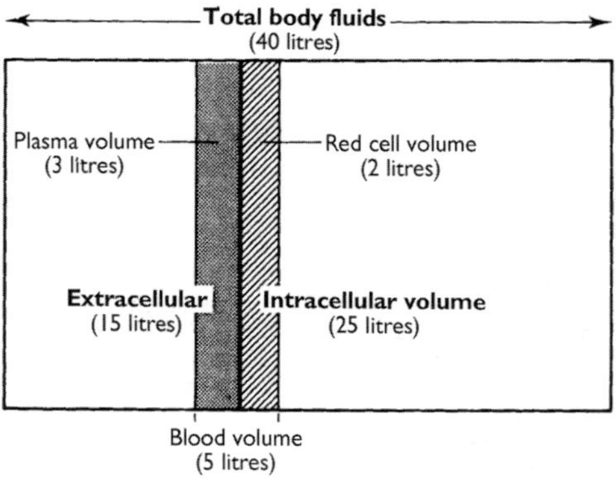

Total Body Fluids

relative positions without separation of the mass. *Amniotic f.* the fluid within the amnion that bathes the developing fetus and protects it from mechanical injury. *Body f's* the fluids within the body, composed of water, electrolytes, and non-electrolytes. The volume and distribution of body fluids vary with age, sex, and amount of adipose tissue (*see* figure). *Cerebrospinal f.* the fluid contained within the ventricles of the brain, the subarachnoid space, and the central canal of the spinal cord. *Interstitial f.* the extracellular fluid bathing most tissues, excluding the fluid within the lymph and blood vessels.

fluid balance a state in which the volume of body water and its solutes (electrolytes and non-electrolytes) is within normal limits and there is normal distribution of fluids within the intracellular and extra-cellular compartments. The total volume of body fluids should be about 60% of the body weight.

fluke (flook) one of a group of parasitic flatworms (Trematoda). Different varieties can affect the blood, the intestines, the liver, or the lungs.

fluorescein (ˌfloo'rəsee·ən) a dye used to detect corneal ulceration. When it is dropped on the eye, the ulcer stains green.

fluorescence (ˌfloo'resəns) the property of reflecting back light waves, usually of a lower frequency than that absorbed, so that invisible light (e.g. ultraviolet) becomes visible.

fluorescent (ˌfloo'resənt) capable of producing fluorescence. *F. screen* a screen that becomes fluorescent when exposed to X-rays. *F. treponemal antibody test* a serological test for syphilis; the first to become positive after infection.

fluoridation (ˌfloo·rəˈdayshən) the adding of fluorine to water, in those areas where it is lacking, in order to reduce the incidence of dental caries.

fluorine (ˈfloo·reen) *symbol* F. Any binary compound of fluorine.

fluoroscope (ˌfloo·rəˌskohp) an instrument for the study of moving internal organs and contrast medium in motion using X-rays.

fluorouracil (ˌfloo·rohˈyoo·rəsil) an antimetabolite cytotoxic drug used particularly in the treatment of solid tumours.

fluphenazine (flooˈfenəˌzeen) a major tranquilliser.

flurandrenolone (ˌfloo·ranˈdrenə-lohn) a topical steroid used for eczema and other inflammatory skin conditions that have not responded to weaker steroids.

flurbiprofen (ˌflərbi·prohfən) a non-steroidal anti-inflammatory drug.

flush (flush) a redness of the face and neck. *Hectic f.* one occurring in conditions such as septic poisoning and pulmonary tuberculosis. *Hot f.* one occurring during the menopause, accompanied by a feeling of heat.

flutter (ˈflutə) an irregularity of the heartbeat.

focus (ˈfohkəs) 1. the point of convergence of light or sound waves. 2. the local seat of a disease.

focusing (ˈfohkəsing) the ability of the eye to alter its lens power to focus correctly at different distances.

foetus (ˈfeetəs) for words beginning with thus, s*ee* FETUS

Foley catheter (ˈfohlee ˈkathətə) *F.E.B. Foley, American physician 1891–1966.* Rubber catheter with a balloon tip that is filled with sterile water after it is placed in the bladder. Used for continuous drainage of the bladder.

folic acid (ˈfohlik) one of the VITAMINS of the B complex. Folic acid is involved in the synthesis of amino acids and DNA; its deficiency causes MEGALOBLASTIC anaemia. Green vegetables, liver, and yeast are major sources. *F. a. antagonist* any antimetabolite cytotoxic drug that inhibits the action of the folic acid enzyme.

folie à deux (foˈlee) [Fr.] the occurrence of identical psychoses simultaneously in two closely associated persons.

follicle (ˈfolikəl) a very small sac or gland. *Graafian f.* a vesicular ovarian follicle. *See* GRAAFIAN FOLLICLE. *Hair f.* The sheath in which a hair grows. *F.-stimulating hormone* abbreviated FSH. A hormone, produced by the anterior pituitary gland, which controls the maturation of the Graafian follicles in the ovary.

follicular (fəˈlikyələ) pertaining to a follicle. *F. conjunctivitis* inflammation occurring in the lower conjunctival fornix. *F. tonsillitis* tonsillitis arising from infection of the tonsillar follicles.

folliculosis (fəˌlikyəˈlohsəs) an abnormal increase in the number of lymph follicles. *Conjunctival f.* a benign non-inflammatory overgrowth of follicles of the conjunctiva of the eyelids.

fomentation (ˌfohmenˈtayshən) treatment by warm, moist applications; also, the substance thus applied.

fomes (ˈfohmeez) *See* FOMITES.

fomites (fəˈmieteez, ˈfohmə-) [L.]

sing. fomes; inanimate objects or material on which disease-producing agents can be conveyed.

fontanelle (ˌfontə'nel) a soft membranous space between the cranial bones of an infant (*see* figure). *Anterior f.* that between the parietal and frontal bones, which closes at about the age of 18 months. Rickets causes delay in this process. *Posterior f.* the junction of the occipital and parietal bones, at the sagittal suture, which closes within 3 months of birth.

food (food) anything which, when taken into the body, serves to nourish or build up the tissues or to supply body heat. *F. poisoning* a group of notifiable acute illnesses caused by ingestion of contaminated food. It can result from toxaemia from foods, such as those inherently poisonous or those contaminated by poisons, foods containing poisons formed by bacteria, or foodborne infections. Food poisoning usually causes inflammation of the gastrointestinal tract (gastroenteritis). This can occur quite suddenly, soon after the food has been eaten. The symptoms are acute, and include tenderness, pain, or cramps in the abdomen, nausea, vomiting, diarrhoea, weakness, and dizziness. *See* BOTULISM.

foot (fuht) the terminal part of the lower limb. *Athlete's f.* ringworm of the foot; tinea pedis. *F. drop* inability to keep the foot at the correct angle owing to paralysis of the flexors of the ankle. *F. presentation* the presentation of one or both legs instead of the head during labour.

foramen (fə'raymən) an opening or hole, especially in a bone. *F. magnum* the hole in the occipital bone through which the spinal cord passes. *F. ovale* the hole between the left and right atria in the fetus. *Obturator f.* the large hole in the innominate bone. *Optic f.* the opening in the posterior part of the orbit through which the optic nerve and the ophthalmic artery pass.

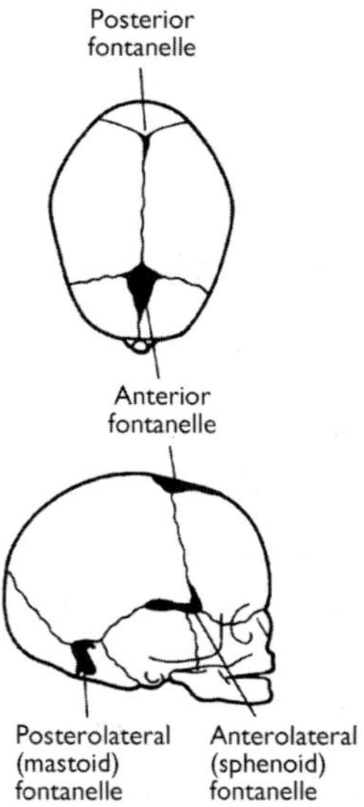

The Fontanelles

forceps ('fawseps) surgical instruments used for lifting or compressing an object. *Artery f.* (*Spencer Wells f.*) compress bleeding points during an operation. *Cheatle f.* long forceps for lifting utensils. *Obstetric f.* of various patterns are used in difficult labour to facilitate delivery. *Vulsellum f.* have claw-like ends for exerting traction.

forensic (fə'renzik, -sik) pertaining to or applied in legal proceedings. *F. medicine* the branch that is concerned with the law and has a bearing on legal problems. It includes the investigation of unexplained death or injury.

foreskin ('faw,skin) the PREPUCE.

formaldehyde (faw'maldə,hied) a gaseous compound with strongly disinfectant properties. It is used in solution (formol) for disinfection of excreta and utensils and also in the preparation of toxoids from toxins.

formula ('fawmyələ) [L] 1. an expression (incorporating numbers or symbols) of the composition of a compound, or an expression of directions for preparing such a compound, such as a medicine; or an expression of the procedure to follow to obtain a desired result; or an expression of a single concept. 2. a mixture for feeding an infant, composed of milk and/or other ingredients.

formulary ('fawmyələ·ree) a prescriber's handbook of drugs.

fornix ('fawniks) an arch. *F. cerebri* an arched structure at the back and base of the brain. *Conjunctival f.* the reflection of the conjunctiva from the eyelids on to the eyeball. *F. of the vagina* the recesses at the top of the vagina in front (anterior f.), back (posterior f.), and sides (lateral f.) of the cervix uteri.

fossa ('fosə) a small depression or pit. Usually applied to fossae in bones. *Cubital f.* the triangular depression at the front of the elbow. *Iliac f.* the depression on the inner surface of the iliac bone. *Pituitary f.* the depression in the sphenoid bone. *See* SELLA TURCICA.

Fothergill's operation ('fodhə,gilz) *W.E. Fothergill, British gynaecologist, 1865–1926.* Amputation of the cervix, with anterior and posterior COLPORRHAPHY for prolapse of the uterus.

fourchette (faw'shet) [Fr.] the fold of membrane at the perineal end of the vulva.

fovea ('fohvi·ə) a fossa; a small depression. *f. centralis* an area at the centre of the retina which contains a large number of cones giving form and colour to vision; the area of most accurate vision.

Fowler's position ('fowləz) *G.R. Fowler, American surgeon 1848–1906.* The position of a patient lying face up with the head of the bed elevated 45 to 60 degrees and with the knees slightly elevated.

fracture ('frakchə) 1. to break a part, especially a bone. 2. a break in the continuity of bone. The signs and symptoms are pain, swelling, deformity, shortening of the limb, loss of power, abnormal mobility, and CREPITUS. Fractures are usually caused by trauma, by either direct or indirect force on the bone. Fractures can also be caused by muscle spasm or by disease that results in decalcification of the bone. The different types and classification of fractures are shown in the figure. *Pathological f.* one due to weakening of the bone structure by pathological processes, such as NEOPLASIA, OSTEOMALACIA, or OSTEOMYELITIS. *Pott's f.* a fracture dislocation of the ankle involving

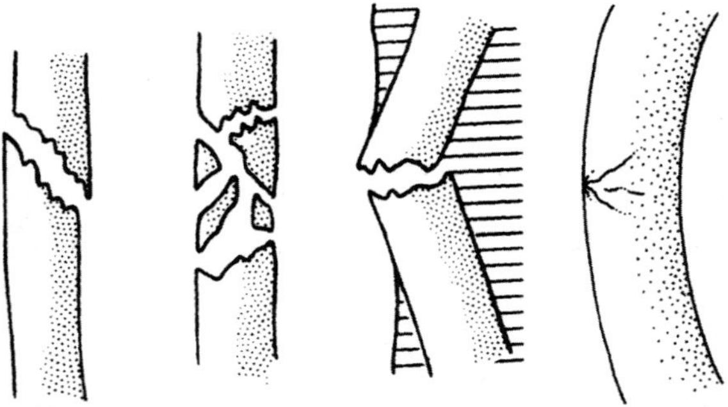

Fractures of Bones

the lower end of the fibula and sometimes the internal malleolus of the tibia. *Spontaneous f.* one that occurs as a result of little or no violence, usually of a bone weakened by disease.

frame (fraym) a rigid supporting structure or a structure for immobilising a part. *Balkan f. see* BALKAN FRAME. *Braun f.* a metal frame used to elevate the lower limb in fractures of the tibia and fibula. *Quadriplegic standing f.* a device for supporting in the upright position a patient whose four limbs are paralysed. *Stryker f.* one consisting of canvas stretched on anterior and posterior frames, on which the patient can be rotated around the longitudinal axis. *Walking f.* a walking aid with three or four legs.

framycetin (ˌframə'seetən) an aminoglycoside antibiotic, similar to neomycin. Used for topical application or to reduce bacterial population of the colon before bowel surgery.

freckle ('frekəl) a brown pigmented spot on the skin. *Hutchinson's melanotic f.* a non-invasive malignant melanoma which occurs mainly on the face of middle-aged women.

free association (free əˌsohsee'ayshən) in psychoanalysis, a spontaneous mental process whereby words used in a non-logical chain suggest ideas, thoughts, or feelings without selection or repression.

Freiberg's disease (friebərgz) *A.H. Freiberg, American surgeon, 1868–1940.* OSTEOCHONDRITIS of the second metatarsal bone, in which there is pain on walking and standing.

Frei's test (friez) *W.S. Frei, German dermatologist, 1885–1943.* An intradermal test to aid the diagnosis of LYMPHOGRANULOMA venereum.

fremitus ('fremitəs) a thrill or vibration, e.g. that produced in the chest by speaking and felt on palpation.

frenotomy (frə'notəmee) the cutting of the frenulum of the tongue to cure tongue-tie.

frenulum ('frenyələm) frenum; a fold of mucous membrane which limits the movement of an organ. *F. of the tongue* the fold under the tongue.

Freudian ('froydee·ən) *S. Freud, Austrian psychiatrist, 1856–1939.* Relating to the theories of Freud, who was the originator of psychoanalysis and the psychoanalytical theory of the cause of neurosis.

friable ('frieəbəl) easily crumbled.

friction ('frikshən) the act of rubbing one object against another. *F. massage* a circular or transverse pressure applied by fingertip or thumb to a localised area. Used for the relief of pain. *F. murmur* the grating sound heard in auscultation when two rough surfaces rub together, as in dry pleurisy.

Friedländer's bacillus ('freed,lendəz) *K. Friedländer, German pathologist, 1847–87.* The cause of a rare form of pneumonia. *Klebsiella friedländeri.*

Friedreich's ataxia or **disease** ('freedrieks) *N. Friedreich, German physician, 1825–82.* A rare form of hereditary ATAXIA.

frigidity (frə'jidətee) an absence of normal sexual desire, usually refers to women.

Frölich's syndrome ('frərliks) *A. Frölich, Austrian neurologist, 1871–1953.* A group of symptoms associated with disease of the pituitary body: increased adiposity, atrophy of the genital organs, and development of feminine characteristics.

frontal ('frunt'l) 1. relating to the forehead. 2. relating to the front or anterior aspect of a structure.

frostbite ('frost,biet) impairment of circulation chiefly affecting the fingers, the toes, the nose, and the ears due to exposure to severe cold. The first stage is represented by chilblains. Advanced cases show thrombosis and dry gangrene.

frottage (fro'tahzh) [Fr.] 1. a rubbing movement in massage. 2. sexual gratification by rubbing against another person's body.

frozen shoulder ('frohzən) a stiff and painful shoulder; capsulitis. Treatment can include stretching under anaesthesia, combined with exercises. The cause is unknown.

fructose ('fruktohs, -tohz, 'fruhk-) fruit sugar, a monosaccharide.

frusemide ('froozəmied) a diuretic with a rapid and powerful action used in the treatment of oedema and of acute renal failure.

FSH follicle-stimulating hormone.

fugue (fyoog) a period of altered awareness during which a person can wander for hours or days and perform purposive actions although memory for the period might be lost. It can follow an epileptic fit or can occur in hysteria or schizophrenia.

fulguration (,fulgyə'rayshən) the destruction by diathermy of papillomata (warts), particularly inside the urinary bladder.

fulminating ('fuhlmə,nayting, 'ful-) sudden in onset and rapid in course.

fumigation (,fyoomə'gayshən) disinfection by exposure to the fumes of a vaporised germicide.

function ('fungk,shən) 1. the natural

action or intended purpose of a person, organ, or structure. 2. to perform special work or an action.

fundus ('fundəs) the base of an organ or the part farthest removed from the opening. *F. of the eye* the posterior part of the inside of the eye as shown by an ophthalmoscope. *F. of the stomach* that part above the cardiac orifice. *F. of the uterus* the top of the uterus; that part farthest from the cervix.

fungate ('fung·gayt) to grow rapidly and produce fungus-like growths. Often occurs in the late stages of malignant tumours.

fungicide ('funjə,sied) a preparation that destroys fungal infection.

fungiform ('funjə,fawm) shaped like a fungus or mushroom.

fungus ('fung·gəs) a low form of vegetable life which includes mushrooms and moulds. Some varieties cause disease, such as ACTINOMYCOSIS and ringworm.

funis ('fyoonəs) the umbilical cord.

funnel chest ('fun'l) a developmental deformity in which there is a depression in the sternum and an inwards curvature of the ribs and costal cartilages.

furor ('fyoo·raw) a state of intense excitement during which violent acts can be performed. This can occur after an epileptic fit.

furuncle ('fyoo·rungkəl) a boil.

furunculosis (fyə,rungkyə'lohsəs) a staphylococcal infection represented by many, or crops of, boils.

furunculus (fyə'rungkyələs) a furuncle. *F. orientalis* a protozoal infection, mainly of the tropics, which causes a chronic ulceration. Cutaneous LEISHMANIASIS.

fusidic acid (fyoo'sidik) an antibiotic used to treat penicillin-resistant staphylococci. It is usually used in combination with another antibiotic effective against staphylococci.

fusiform ('fyoozə,fawm) shaped like a spindle.

fusion ('fyoozhən) 1. the union between two adjacent structures. 2. the coordination of separate images of the same object in the two eyes into one image.

Fusobacterium (,fyoozohbak'tiə·ri·əm) a genus of anaerobic Gram-negative bacteria found as normal flora in the mouth and large bowel, and often in necrotic tissue, probably as secondary invaders.

Gg

g symbol for *gram*.
G symbol for *guanine*.
Ga symbol for *gallium*.
gag (gag) 1. an instrument placed between the teeth to keep the mouth open. 2. the reflex action that occurs when the back of the throat is stimulated.
gait (gayt) manner of walking. *Ataxic g.* the foot is raised high, descends suddenly, and the whole sole strikes the ground. *Cerebellar g.* a staggering walk indicative of cerebellar disease. *Four-point g.* a method that can be adopted when using sticks or crutches, which allows maximum stability. *Spastic g.* stiff, shuffling walk, the legs being kept together.
galactocele (gə'laktəˌseel) 1. a milk-containing cyst in the breast. 2. a HYDROCELE containing a milky fluid.
galactorrhoea (ˌgaləktə'reeə) 1. an excessive flow of milk. 2. secretion of milk after breastfeeding has ceased.
galactosaemia (gə'laktə'seemi·ə) an inborn error of metabolism in which there is inability to convert galactose to glucose. The disorder becomes manifest soon after birth and is characterised by feeding problems, vomiting and diarrhoea, abdominal distension, enlargement of the liver, and mental handicap. Treatment consists of exclusion from the diet of milk and all foods containing galactose or lactose.
galactose (gə'laktohz, -ohs) a monosaccharide derived from lactose. D-galactose is found in lactose or milk sugar and cerebrosides of the brain. *G. tolerance test* a laboratory test to determine the liver's ability to convert the sugar galactose into glycogen.
gall (gawl) bile, a digestive fluid secreted by the liver and stored in the gallbladder. *G.-bladder* the sac under the lower surface of the liver which acts as a reservoir for bile. *G.-stone* a concretion formed in the gallbladder or bile ducts. Gallstones are often multiple and faceted. *G. -stone colic see* BILIARY (colic).
gallamine ('galəˌmeen) a synthetic muscle relaxant, chemically related to curare but less potent and shorter acting.
gallipot ('galəˌpot) a small receptacle for lotions.
gallium ('gali·əm) *symbol* Ga. A radioisotope used in detecting some soft-tissue disorders.
gallop rhythm ('galəp) heart rhythm that can occur when there is ventricular overload.
galvanometer (ˌgalvə'nomətə) an instrument for detecting or measur-

ing the strength of a current of electricity.

gamete ('gameet) a sex cell which combines with another to form a zygote, from which a complete organism develops. A SPERMATOZOON or an ovum.

gametocyte (gə'meetoh,siet) a cell that is undergoing gametogenesis.

gametogenesis (,gamitoh'jenəsəs) the production of the gametes by the gonads.

gamma ('gamə) the third letter in the Greek alphabet, γ. *G.-benzene hexachloride* a drug used as a cream, lotion, or shampoo to treat head lice. *G. camera* an apparatus for depicting a part of the body into which radioactive isotopes emitting gamma rays have been introduced. *G. encephalography* a method of localising a brain tumour by using radioactive isotopes emitting gamma rays. *G.-globulin* a class of plasma proteins composed almost entirely of IgG, an IMMUNOGLOBULIN protein that contains most antibody activity. *G. rays* electromagnetic rays, of shorter wavelength and with greater penetration than X-rays, which are given off by certain radioactive substances and which are used in radiotherapy. Also used in the sterilisation of articles that would be destroyed by the heat and moisture required in autoclaving.

ganglion ('gang·glee·ən) 1. a collection of nerve cells and fibres forming an independent nerve centre, as is found in the sympathetic nervous system. 2. a cystic swelling on a tendon.

ganglionectomy (,gang·glee·ə'nektəmee) excision of a ganglion.

gangrene ('gang·green) death of body tissue, generally in considerable mass, due either to loss of blood supply or to the effects of certain infections. *Dry g.* occurs gradually and results from slow reduction of the blood flow in the arteries. There is no subsequent bacterial decomposition; the tissues become dry and shrivelled. It occurs only in the extremities, and can occur with ARTERIOSCLEROSIS and DIACETES mellitus. *Gas g.* results from dirty lacerated wounds infected by anaerobic bacteria, especially species of *Clostridium*. It is an acute, severe, painful condition in which muscles and subcutaneous tissues become filled with gas and a serosanguineous exudate. *Moist g.* is caused by sudden stoppage of blood, resulting from burning by heat or acid, severe freezing, physical accident that destroys the tissue, or a clot or other embolism. At first, tissue affected by moist gangrene has the colour of a bad bruise, is swollen, and often blistered. The gangrene is likely to spread with great speed. Toxins are formed in the affected tissues and absorbed.

Ganser's syndrome (state) ('ganzəz) *S.J.M. Ganser, German psychiatrist, 1853–1931.* Amnesia, disturbance of consciousness and hallucinations, associated with senseless answers to questions, and absurd acts. Usually a transient response to a troublesome situation, e.g. prisoners on remand (prison psychosis).

gargle ('gahgəl) 1. a solution for rinsing the mouth and throat. 2. to rinse the mouth and throat by holding a solution in the open mouth and agitating it by expulsion of air from the lungs.

gargoylism ('gahgoy·lizəm) *See* HURLER'S SYNDROME.

gas (gas) molecules of a substance very loosely combined; a vapour. *G. and air analgesia* an authorised form of analgesia using nitrous oxide and air, by which the pains of labour are lessened without affecting uterine contractions. *G. gangrene* the result of infection of a wound by anaerobic organisms, especially *Clostridium perfringens* (also known as *C. welchii*). *Laughing g.* nitrous oxide. *Marsh g.* methane. *Sternulatory g.* one which causes sneezing. *Tear g.* one that is irritating to the eyes and causes excessive lacrimation.

Gasser's ganglion ('gasəz) *J.L. Gasser, Austrian anatomist, 1723–65.* The trigeminal ganglion. The ganglion of the sensory root of the fifth cranial nerve.

gastrectomy (ga'strektəmee) excision of part or whole of the stomach. *Billroth g.* removal of most of the lesser curvature and pyloric portion and joining of the duodenum to the refashioned stomach. This cuts down the production of secretin and acid. *Partial g.* removal of a part, usually the distal portion, of the stomach. Commonly performed in the surgical treatment of peptic ulcer. *Polya g.* removal of the first part of the duodenum and the greater part of the stomach, and anastomosis of the stomach to the JEJUNUM. The blind portion of the duodenum supplies the bile and pancreatic and duodenal secretions.

gastric ('gastrik) pertaining to the stomach. *G. analysis* analysis of the stomach contents by microscopy and tests to determine the amount of acid present. *G. bypass* surgical creation of a small gastric pouch that empties directly into the JEJUNUM through a gastrojejunostomy, thereby causing food to bypass the duodenum; performed for the treatment of gross OBESITY. *G. flu* a popular term for any of several disorders of the stomach and intestinal tract. The symptoms are nausea, diarrhoea, abdominal cramps, and fever. *G. juice* the clear fluid secreted by the glands of the stomach to assist digestion. It contains an enzyme called pepsin, which acts upon proteins in the presence of weak hydrochloric acid. *G. lavage* a treatment for some types of poisoning whereby the stomach contents are washed out through a stomach tube. *G. ulcer* ulceration of the gastric mucosa, associated with hyperacidity; often precipitated by stress.

gastrin ('gastrin) a hormone, secreted by the walls of the stomach, which excites continued secretion of digestive juice while food is in the stomach.

gastritis (ga'strietəs) inflammation of the lining of the stomach.

gastrocnemius (ˌgastrok'neemee·əs) the principal muscle of the calf of the leg. It flexes both the ankle and the knee.

gastrocolic (ˌgastroh'kolik) pertaining to the stomach and colon. *G. reflex* after a meal, increased peristalsis causes the colon to empty into the rectum. This gives rise to a desire to defaecate.

gastroduodenostomy (ˌgastrohˌdyooədee'nostəmee) a surgical anastomosis between the stomach and the duodenum.

gastroenteritis (ˌgastrohˌentə'rietəs) inflammation of the lining of the stomach and intestine. Psychological causes of gastroenteritis include fear, anger, and other emotional upset. Allergic reactions to certain foods can cause gastroenteritis, as can irritation by excessive use of alcohol. Severe gastroenteritis, with such symptoms as headache, nausea, vomiting, weakness, diarrhoea and gas pains, can result from various viral and bacterial infections, such as INFLUENZA.

gastroenterology (ˌgastrohˌentə'roləjee) the study of diseases of the gastrointestinal tract.

gastroenteropathy (ˌgastrohˌentə'ropəthee) any disease condition affecting both the stomach and the intestine.

gastroenterostomy (ˌgastrohˌentə'rostəmee) a surgical anastomosis between the stomach and small intestine.

gastroileac (ˌgastroh'ileeak) pertaining to the stomach and ileum. *G. reflex* food entering the stomach sets up powerful peristalsis in the ileum and opening of the ILEOCAECAL VALVE.

gastrointestinal (ˌgastroh·in'testən'l) pertaining to the stomach and intestine. *G. tract* the alimentary tract.

gastrojejunostomy (ˌgastrohˌjejə'nostəmee) a surgical anastomosis between the stomach and the JEJUNUM.

gastro-oesophagostomy (ˌgastroh·əˌsofə'gostəmee) a surgical anastomosis between the stomach and the oesophagus.

gastroscope ('gastrəˌskohp) an endoscope especially designed for passage into the stomach to permit examination of its interior. The gastroscope is a hollow, cylindrical tube fitted with special lenses and lights, which acts by reflecting light and creating a mirror effect, making it possible to 'go around corners' and facilitating visualisation of the curvature of the stomach.

gastrostomy (ga'strostəmee) the creation of an opening into the stomach. This procedure is done to provide for the administration of food and liquids when stricture of the oesophagus or other conditions make swallowing impossible. *See* ARTIFICIAL (feeding).

gastrotomy (ga'strotəmee) a surgical incision of the stomach.

gastrula ('gastrələ) an early stage in the development of the fertilised ovum.

gatekeepers ('gaytˌkeepəz) the individuals or groups in an organisation who regulate access to goods and services, e.g. a doctor's receptionist.

Gaucher's disease (gho'shayz) *P.C.E. Gaucher, French physician, 1854–1918.* A rare familial disease in which fat is deposited in the reticuloendothelial cells, causing an enlarged spleen and anaemia.

gauze (gawz) a thin open-meshed material used for dressing wounds.

gavage ('gavahzh) forced feeding; the giving of fluids and nourishment by oesophageal or other type of tube directly into the stomach.

gay (gay) 1. any person who is homosexual. 2. pertaining to homosexuality.

Geiger counter ('giegə) *H. Geiger, German physicist, 1882–1945.* An instrument for detecting and registering radioactivity. The apparatus is sensitive to the rays emitted.

gelatin ('jelətən) an albuminoid,

obtained from connective tissue or bone. Used in pharmacy for suppositories and capsules, and in bacteriology as a culture medium. In absorbable film and sponge, it is used in surgical procedures.

gender ('jendə) sex; the category to which an individual is assigned on the basis of sex. *G. identity* the concept that a person has of being male and masculine or female and feminine. Differentiation of gender identity begins in infancy, continues throughout childhood, and is reinforced during adolescence. Includes parental attitudes and expectations as well as psychological and social pressures. *G. identity disorder* a psychiatric label for those disorders marked by a sense of inappropriateness and attendant discomfort concerning one's sexual anatomy and sex role. This category usually includes transvestism, transsexualism, and gender identity disorders in childhood.

gene (jeen) a hereditary unit that is composed of a sequence of DNA and occupies a specific position or locus on a particular chromosome. *Dominant g.* one that is capable of transmitting its characteristics irrespective of the genes from the other parent. *Recessive g.* one that can pass on its characteristics only if it is present with a similar recessive gene from the other parent. *See* MENDEL'S THEORY. *G. therapy* the use of 'healthy' genes to cure or treat a hereditary disease.

genetic (jə'netik) 1. pertaining to reproduction or to birth or origin. 2. inherited. *G. code* the arrangement of genetic material stored in the DNA molecule of the chromosome. *G. counselling* supportive service for prospective parents who can receive advice as to the likelihood of their children being born with a genetically transmitted disorder.

genetics (jə'netiks) the study of heredity and natural development.

genitalia (ˌjenə'taylee·ə) the organs of reproduction visible on the outside of the body.

genome ('jeenohm) the complete set of genes in the chromosomes of each cell of a specific organism.

genitourinary (ˌjenitoh'yoo·rənə·ree) referring to both the reproductive organs and the urinary tract.

genotype ('jenohˌtiep, 'jeenoh-) the genetic characteristics of an individual.

gentamicin (ˌjentə'miesən) an antibiotic effective against many Gram-negative bacteria, especially *Pseudomonas* species, as well as certain Gram-positive bacteria, especially *Staphylococcus aureus*.

genu ('jenyoo) [L.] the knee. *G. valgum* knock-knee. *G. varum* bowleg.

genupectoral (ˌjenyoo'pektə·rəl) relating to the knee and chest. *G. position* the knee–chest position. *See* POSITION.

geriatrics (ˌjeree'atriks) the branch of medicine covering older people, the ageing process, and the disorders arising from it.

germ (jərm) 1. a microbe. 2. that from which something might develop; a seed.

German measles ('jərmən 'meezəlz) *see* RUBELLA.

germicide ('jərməˌsied) an agent capable of destroying pathogenic microorganisms.

germinoma (ˌjərmə'nohmə) a neoplasm of the testis or ovum.

gerontology (ˌjeron'toləjee) the

study of older people and the ageing processes.

gestaltism (gə'shtaltizəm) a theory of holism in psychology which claims that ideas come as a whole and are not subdivisible.

gestation (je'stayshən) the period of development of the young in mammals, from the time of fertilisation of the ovum to birth. *See also* PREGNANCY. *Ectopic g.* fetal development in some part other than the uterus, usually the uterine tube (*see* figure). *G. period* the duration of pregnancy; in the human female about 280 days when measured from the first day of the last menstrual period.

Ghon focus (gon) *A. Ghon, Czechoslovakian pathologist, 1866–1936.* The primary lesion of pulmonary tuberculosis, as seen on chest radiograph, after it has healed by fibrosis and calcification.

giardiasis (ˌjiah'dieəsəs) *A. Giard, French biologist, 1846–1908.* An infection with *Giardia lamblia*, a pear-shaped protozoon that causes a persistent diarrhoea, often resulting in intestinal malabsorption.

gigantism ('jiegan,tizəm, jie'gantizəm) abnormal excessive growth of the body, often due to overactivity of the anterior lobe of the pituitary gland.

Gilles de la Tourette's syndrome (disease) (ˌzheel də lah too'rets) *G. Gilles de la Tourette, French neurologist, 1857–1904.* Multiple tics, especially of the face and upper part of the body, often associated with involuntary obscene utterances. The condition usually has its onset in childhood and often becomes chronic. The cause is unknown.

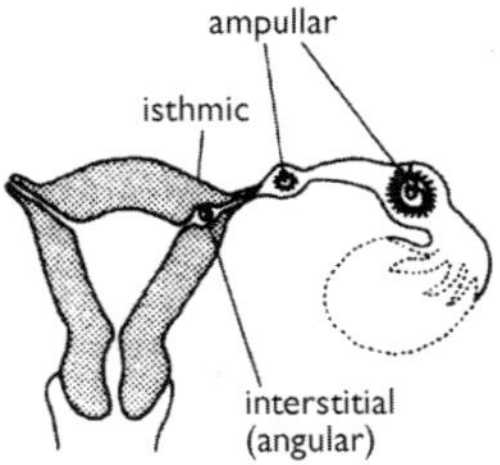

Ectopic Gestation

gingiva ('jinjəvə, jin'jievə) the gum; connective tissue surrounding the necks of the teeth.

gingivectomy (ˌjinjə'vektəmee) the surgical removal of the gum margins to remove pockets and improve the shape of the gums.

gingivitis (ˌjinjə'vietəs) inflammation of the gums.

gland (gland) an organ composed of cells which secrete fluid prepared from the blood, either for use in the body, or for excretion as waste material. *Ductless* (endocrine) *g.* one that produces an internal secretion but has no canal (duct) to carry the secretion away, e.g. the thyroid gland. *Exocrine g.* one that discharges its secretion through a duct, e.g. the parotid gland. *Lymph g. see* LYMPH nodes. *Mucous g.* one that secretes mucus.

glanders ('glandəz) a disease of horses communicable to humans and caused by the glanders bacillus, *Pseudomonas mallei*.

glandular ('glandyələ) pertaining to a gland. *G. fever see* INFECTIOUS mononucleosis.

glans (glanz) an acorn-shaped body,

such as the rounded end of the penis or the clitoris.

Glasgow coma scale (ˌglazgoh ˈkohmə ˌskayl) a standardised system for quickly evaluating the level of consciousness in the critically ill. Measures include: (a) eye opening according to 4 criteria; (b) verbal response against 5 criteria; and (c) motor response using 6 criteria. Scores of 7 or less qualify as 'coma'. Coma is defined as no response and no eye opening.

glaucoma (glawˈkohmə) raised intraocular pressure. *Closed-angle g.* one that occurs when there is a mechanical defect in the drainage angle; can be primary or secondary. It can be acute, in which there is pain and blurring of vision, or chronic, in which there can be no pain, but a gradual loss of vision. *Open-angle g.* chronic primary glaucoma in which the angle remains open but drainage becomes gradually diminished. *Primary g.* one that occurs without any previous disease. It is a common cause of blindness, partial or complete, in the elderly. *Secondary g.* one that occurs when some ocular disease is complicated by an increase in intraocular pressure.

gleet (gleet) chronic gonococcal URETHRITIS marked by a transparent mucous discharge.

glenoid (ˈgleenoyd) resembling a hollow. *G. cavity* the socket of the shoulder joint.

glia (ˈglieə) neuroglia; the connective tissue of the brain and spinal cord.

glibenclamide (glieˈbengkləˌmied) an oral hypoglycaemic agent of the sulphonylurea group used in the treatment of type 2 DIABETES mellitus.

glioblastoma (ˌglieohblaˈstohmə) a malignant GLIOMA arising in the cerebral hemispheres.

glioma (glieˈohmə) a malignant tumour composed of neuroglial cells affecting the brain and spinal cord; seldom metastasises.

Glisson's capsule (ˈglisənz) *F. Glisson, British physician and anatomist, 1597–1677.* The connective tissue capsule of the liver which envelops the portal vein, hepatic artery, and hepatic ducts.

globin (ˈglohbən) a protein used in the formation of haemoglobin.

globulin (ˈglobyələn) a protein constituent of the blood (serum g.) and cerebrospinal fluid.

globus (ˈglobəs) a ball or globe. *G. hystericus* a symptom of hysteria whereby a patient feels unable to swallow because there is a lump in the throat. *G. pallidus* the pale medial part of the lentiform nucleus of the brain.

glomerulitis (gloˌmeryəˈlietəs) inflammation of the glomeruli of the kidney.

glomerulonephritis (gloˌmeryəlohnəˈfrietəs) a bilateral, non-infectious inflammation of the kidneys. The cause is unknown but the condition is associated with immunological disturbance. It can be acute, presenting rapidly but reversibly, or it can be chronic, presenting slowly and irreversibly.

glomerulosclerosis (gloˌmeryəlohskləˈrohsəs) degenerative changes in the glomerular capillaries of the renal tubule, leading to renal failure.

glomerulus (gloˈmeryələs) the tuft of capillaries within the nephron, which filters urine from the blood.

glossal (ˈglosəl) relating to the tongue.

Glossina (glo'sienə) a genus of biting flies, the tsetse flies.

glossitis (glo'sietəs) inflammation of the tongue.

glossolalia (ˌglosə'layli·ə) unintelligible speech. The patient speaks in an imaginary or unknown language.

glossopharyngeal (ˌglosohfə'rinji·əl, -ˌfarən'ji·əl) pertaining to the tongue and pharynx. *G. nerve* the ninth cranial nerve.

glossoplegia (ˌglosoh'pleeji·ə) paralysis of the tongue.

glottis ('glotəs) the space between the vocal cords. The term is sometimes used for that part of the larynx which is associated with voice production.

glucagon ('glookəˌgon) a polypeptide produced by the pancreas. It stimulates glycogen breakdown to glucose in the liver and raises the blood sugar level. Glycogen secretion is stimulated by hypoglycaemia and by growth hormone in the anterior pituitary gland. A crystallised glucagon preparation is used in the treatment of severe hypoglycaemia.

glucocorticoid (ˌglookoh'kawtəˌkoyd) any corticoid substance that raises the concentration of liver glycogen and blood sugar, i.e. cortisol (hydrocortisone), cortisone, and corticosterone.

glucometer ('glookomətə) trade name for a battery-operated instrument used to monitor blood glucose levels. A single drop of blood is required to calculate the level.

gluconeogenesis (ˌglookohˌneeoh'jenəsəs) the production of glucose from the non-nitrogen portion of the amino acids after deamination. It occurs in the liver and kidneys.

glucose ('glookohs, -kohz) a simple sugar, a monosaccharide in certain foodstuffs, especially fruit, and in normal blood; the chief source of energy for living organisms. *See also* DEXTROSE. *G.-6-phosphate dehydrogenase* a red-cell enzyme. Inherited deficiency causes a tendency to haemolytic anaemia. *See* FAVISM. *G. tolerance test* test in which a quantity of glucose is given and the concentration of glucose in the blood is estimated at intervals afterwards. Used mainly when DIABETES mellitus is suspected.

glue ear ('gloo iə) the accumulation of sticky material in the middle ear resulting in impaired hearing, most common in young schoolchildren.

glue sniffing ('gloo ˌsnifing) solvent abuse.

glutamic acid (gloo'tamik) one of the 22 amino acids formed by the digestion of dietary protein. *g.a. decarboxylase* (gad) *autoantibody* an antibody found in patients with type 1 diabetes mellitus.

glutamic–oxaloacetic transaminase (glooˌtamikˌoksəloh·ə'seetik tranz'aməˌnayz) an enzyme found in cardiac muscle and the liver. Raised serum levels (SGOT) can indicate an acute MYOCARDIAL infarction or the presence of liver disease.

glutamic–pyruvic transaminase (glooˌtamikpie'roovik tranz'aməˌnayz) an enzyme found in the liver. Measurement of serum levels (SGPT) is used in the study and diagnosis of liver diseases.

glutaraldehyde (ˌglootə'raldəˌhied) a disinfectant active against all viruses, fungi, vegetative bacteria, and spores. Used in aqueous solution for sterilisation of non-heat-resistant equipment.

gluteal ('glooti·əl, gloo'ti·əl) relating to the buttocks. *G. muscles* three muscles which form the fleshy part of the buttocks.

gluten ('glootən) the protein of wheat and other grains. *G.-induced enteropathy* COELIAC disease.

Glycaemic Index (GI) factor (glie'seemik) the classification of carbohydrate foods based on their overall effects on blood glucose levels. Foods are ranked from 1 to 100. Food with a low GI factor raise blood glucose levels a little, whereas those with a high GI raise blood glucose levels dramatically.

glycerin ('glisə͵rin) a colourless syrupy substance obtained from fats and fixed oils. It has a hygroscopic action. As an emollient, it is an ingredient of many skin preparations. *G. suppository* one composed of glycerin and gelatin, used as an evacuant. *G. of thymol* an antiseptic mouthwash and gargle.

glyceryl trinitrate (͵glisə·ril trie'nietrayt) nitroglycerin. Glyceryl trinitrate is a vasodilator used to relieve certain types of pain, especially in the prophylaxis and treatment of ANGINA (pectoris). It is administered sublingually or by transdermal patch or gel.

glycine ('glieseen) a non-essential amino acid.

glycogen ('gliekəjən) the form in which carbohydrate is stored in the liver and muscles. Animal starch. *G. storage disease* inherited disease in which there is a deficiency in the synthesis of glycogen. This accumulates in the liver, causing enlargement.

glycogenesis (͵gliekoh'jenəsəs) the process of glycogen formation from the blood glucose.

glycogenolysis (͵gliekəjə'noləsəs) the breakdown of glycogen to glucose in the body so that it can be utilised.

glycoside ('gliekə͵sied) a crystalline body in plants which, when acted on by acids or ferments, produces sugar. If the sugar is glucose, it can be termed a glucoside. *See* DIGITALIS.

glycosuria (͵gliekoh'syoo·ri·ə) the abnormal presence of glucose in the urine, a symptom of DIABETES mellitus. *Renal g.* sugar in the urine in an otherwise healthy person, due to an inherited inability to reabsorb glucose normally.

glycosylated haemoglobin (GHb or HbA1c) (glie'kohsəlaytəd ͵heemə'glohbən) a haemoglobin A molecule with a glucose group on the terminal amino acid unit of the beta chain. The HbA1c concentration represents the average blood glucose level over the previous three months. It is used to assess the level of blood glucose control of people with DIABETES mellitus.

glymidine ('gliemə͵deen) a drug of the sulphonylurea group used in the treatment of DIABETES mellitus.

gnathic ('nathik) pertaining to the jaw.

gnathoplasty ('nathoh͵plastee) a plastic operation on the jaw.

goblet cell ('goblət ͵sel) a goblet-shaped cell, found in the intestinal epithelium, which produces mucus.

goitre ('goytə) enlargement of the thyroid gland causing a swelling in the front of the neck. Simple endemic goitre, sometimes referred to as Derbyshire neck, is usually caused by lack of iodine in the diet. *Colloid g.* an enlarged but soft thyroid gland with no signs of HYPERTHYROIDISM. *Exophthalmic g.* hyperthyroidism with marked protrusion of the eyeballs (exophthalmos). Graves' disease. *Intrathoracic g.* enlargement of the gland mainly in the thorax, so the swelling might not be easily visible. *Sporadic g.* a simple non-toxic enlargement. *Substernal g.* enlargement of the gland behind the sternum so that swelling in the neck might not be apparent. *Toxic g.* signs of excess of thyroxine in the blood, but with no enlargement of the thyroid. The patient complains of weight loss and is generally nervous. EXOPHTHALMOS can be present.

gold (gohld) *symbol* Au. A metallic element used in treating rheumatoid arthritis. Gold salts are among the most toxic of therapeutic agents. Toxic reactions can vary from mild to severe kidney or liver damage, and blood DYSCRASIAS. *Radioactive g.* an isotope which gives off beta rays and gamma rays. Used in the form of small grains or seeds, it can be implanted into malignant tissues. In colloidal form, it can be instilled into a serous cavity to treat malignant effusions.

Golgi apparatus ('goljee, 'golgee) *C. Golgi, Italian histologist, 1844–1926.* Specialised structures seen near the nucleus of a cell on microscopic examination.

Golgi's organ the sensory end-organs in muscle tendons that are sensitive to stretch.

gonad ('gohnad, 'gonad) a reproductive gland; the testicle or ovary.

gonadotrophic (ˌgonədə'trohfik) having influence on the gonads. *G. hormones* GONADOTROPHIN.

gonadotrophin (ˌgonədə'trohfən) any hormone having a stimulating effect on the gonads. Two such hormones are secreted by the anterior pituitary: follicle-stimulating hormone (FSH) and luteinising hormone (LH), both of which are active, but with differing effects, in the two sexes. *Chorionic g.* a gonad-stimulating hormone produced by CYTOTROPHOBLASTIC cells of the placenta; used in treatment of underdevelopment of the gonads and to induce ovulation in infertile women.

gonion ('gohni·ən) [Gr.] the midpoint of the mandible (lower jaw).

gonioscope ('gohneeohˌskohp) an apparatus for examining the angle of the anterior chamber of the eye.

goniotomy (ˌgohnee'otəmee) an operation for glaucoma; it consists in opening Schlemm's canal under direct vision.

gonococcus (ˌgonə'kokəs) *Neisseria gonorrhoeae*, a diplococcus which causes GONORRHOEA.

gonorrhoea (ˌgonə'reeə) a common sexually transmitted disease caused by *Neisseria gonorrhoeae* which infects the genital tract of either sex causing a discharge and pain on micturition, although the disease is often asymptomatic in females. Spread by the bloodstream, it can give rise to IRITIS or arthritis. Scar tissue formation can bring about urethral stricture or infertility by occlusion of the uterine tubes. The eyes of babies can be infected at birth during passage through the birth canal of an infected mother. The condition is called OPHTHALMIA neonatorum, and is a notifiable disease. In the past, it was a major cause of blindness in babies.

gonorrhoeal (ˌgonə'reeəl) relating to gonorrhoea. *G. arthritis* intractable infection of joints, causing great pain and disability.

Goodpasture's syndrome ('guhd-ˌpahschəz) *E.W. Goodpasture, American pathologist, 1886–1960.* A rare haemorrhagic lung disorder associated with GLOMERULONEPHRITIS.

gouge (gowj) a curved chisel used for scooping out diseased bone or other hard substances.

gout (gowt) an hereditary form of arthritis with an excess of uric acid in the blood. It is characterised by painful inflammation and swelling of the smaller joints, especially those of the big toe and thumb. Inflammation is accompanied by the deposit of urates around the joints.

GPI general paralysis of the insane; dementia paralytica. *See* PARALYSIS.

Graafian follicle ('grahfi·ən) *R. de Graaf, Dutch physician and anatomist, 1641–73.* A follicle which is formed in the ovary and contains an ovum (*see* figure). A follicle matures during each menstrual cycle, ruptures and releases the ovum (ovulation), which is then picked up by the fimbriated end of the uterine tube.

graft (grahft) 1. any tissue or organ for implantation or transplantation. 2. to implant or transplant such tissue. *Autogenous g.* a graft taken from and given to the same individual. *Bone g.* a portion of bone transplanted to repair another bone. *Corneal g.* a portion of cornea, usually from a recently dead person, used to repair a diseased cornea. *Homologous g.* tissue obtained from the body of another animal of the same species but with a genotype differing from that of the recipient; a homograft or allograft. *Pedicle g.* a skin graft, one end of which remains attached to its original site until the grafting has become established.

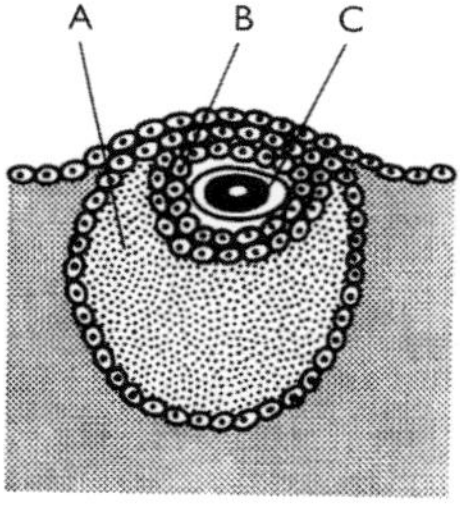

A Follicular fluid
B Granulosa cells
C Ovum

Graafian Follicle

graft-versus-host disease (reaction) (ˌgrahftvərsəz'hohst) abbreviated GVH disease. A condition that occurs when immunologically competent cells or their precursors are transplanted into an immunologically incompetent recipient (host) that is not histocompatible with the donor. Characteristic signs include skin lesions, ulceration, alopecia, painful joints, and haemolytic anaemia. GVH disease is a frequent complication of bone marrow transplants. Human leukocyte antigen (HLA) matching of the donor and recipient reduces the possibility of GVH disease.

gram (gram) *symbol* g. The fundamental SI unit of weight, equal to one thousandth of a kilogram.

Gram's stain (gramz) *H. Gram, Danish physician, 1853–1938.* A method of staining bacteria which is used to classify them into Gram-negative and Gram-positive.

grand mal (ˌgronh ˈmal) [Fr.] major epilepsy. *See* EPILEPSY.

granular (ˈgranyələ) containing small particles. *G. casts* the degenerated cells from the lining of renal tubules excreted in the urine in certain kidney disorders.

granulation (ˌgranyəˈlayshən) 1. the division of a hard solid substance into small particles. 2. the growth of new tissue by which ulcers and wounds heal when the edges are not in apposition. It consists of new capillaries and fibroblasts which fill in the space and later form fibrous tissue. The resulting scar is often unsightly.

granule (ˈgranyool) a small particle or grain.

granulocyte (ˈgranyələˌsiet) any cell containing granules in its cytoplasm, especially POLYMORPHONUCLEAR LEUKOCYTES which contain neutrophilic, basophilic and eosinophilic granules in their cytoplasm.

granulocytopaenia (ˌgranyəlohˌsietəˈpeeni·ə) a marked reduction in the number of granulocytes in the blood. The condition can precede AGRANULOCYTOSIS.

granuloma (ˌgranyəˈlohmə) a tumour composed of granulation tissue, usually due to chronic infection or invasion by a foreign body.

granulomatosis (ˌgranyəˌlohməˈtohsəs) an infection producing GRANULOMATA. *Lipoid g.* xanthomatosis; Hand–Schüller–Christian disease; *Malignant g.* lymphadenoma; Hodgkin's disease.

gravel (ˈgravəl) small 'sandy' calculi formed in the kidneys and bladder, and sometimes excreted with the urine. They can also form in the gallbladder where they can accumulate or cause low-grade CHOLECYSTITIS.

Graves' disease (grayvz) *R.J. Graves, Irish physician, 1796–1853.* Exophthalmic goitre; THYROTOXICOSIS.

gravid (ˈgravəd) pregnant.

gravity (ˈgravətee) weight. *Specific g.* the weight of a substance compared with that of an equal volume of water.

gray (gray) *symbol* Gy. The SI unit used to denote the absorbed dose in radiation therapy.

grey-scale display (ˈgrayˌskayl) a method to show the texture of tissue on ULTRASOUND display. The amplitude of each echo is represented by varying shades of grey. A bright-white outline is seen from specular surfaces, a mottled-grey outline from various tissue areas, and a black outline from collections of fluid, such as the bladder and AMNIOTIC SAC.

grief (greef) a pattern of physical and emotional responses to bereavement, separation, or loss.

griseofulvin (ˌgrizeeohˈfuhlvən) an oral antifungal antibiotic that is used in the treatment of infections of the skin, hair, and nails.

grounded theory (ˈgrowndəd) theory that is constructed inductively on the basis of observations of the world as it is lived by a selected group of people.

group therapy (groop) a form of psychotherapy in which a group of patients meets frequently with a therapist to discuss and share problems, anxieties, and fears in a psychotherapeutic setting. The group also provides emotional support for self-revelation and a structured environment for trying out new ways of relating to people.

growing pains ('groh·ing) recurrent quasi-rheumatic limb pains peculiar to early youth, once believed to be caused by the growing process. It is now recognised that growth does not cause pain and that these pains can be a symptom of many different disorders.

growth (grohth) 1. the progressive development of a living thing, especially the process by which the body reaches its point of complete physical development. 2. an abnormal formation of tissue, such as a tumour. *G. hormone* a substance that stimulates growth, especially a secretion of the anterior lobe of the PITUITARY gland that directly influences protein, carbohydrate, and lipid metabolism, and controls the rate of skeletal and visceral growth.

guanethidine (gwah'nethə͵deen) a drug used in the treatment of hypertension. It is an adrenergic blocking agent.

guanine ('gwahneen) a purine base, one of the constituents of all nucleic acids.

Guillain–Barré syndrome (͵giyanh-'bara)Y *G. Guillain, French neurologist, 1876–1961; J.A. Barrè, French neurologist, 1880–1967.* Acute infective POLYNEURITIS. After an infection, usually respiratory, there is a general weakness or paralysis which frequently affects the respiratory muscles as well as the peripheral muscles.

guillotine ('gilə͵teen) a surgical instrument used for excising tonsils.

guinea-worm ('ginee͵wərm) a nematode worm, *Dracunculus medinensis*, which burrows into human tissues, particularly into the legs or feet.

gumboil ('gum͵boyl) the opening on the gum of an abscess at the root of a tooth.

gumma ('gummə) a soft, degenerating tumour characteristic of the tertiary stage of syphilis. It can occur in any organ or tissue.

gustatory (gu'staytə·ree) relating to taste.

gut (gut) the intestine.

Guthrie test ('guthree ͵test) a blood test carried out on a neonate between the 6th and 14th days of life to diagnose PHENYLKETONURIA.

gutta ('gutə) a drop. *G. percha* the juice of a tropical tree which, when dried, forms an elastic semisolid substance. Used in dentistry as a root filler.

GVH disease graft-versus-host disease.

Gy symbol for GRAY.

gynaecologist (͵gienə'kolə͵jəst) a physician who specialises in the diseases of the female reproductive organs and breasts.

gynaecology (͵gienə'kolәjee) the science of those diseases that are peculiar to the female reproductive organs and breasts.

gynaecomastia (͵gienәkoh'masti·ә) excessive growth of the male breast.

gypsum ('jipsəm) plaster of Paris (calcium sulphate).

gyrus ('jierəs) a convolution, as of the cerebral cortex.

Hh

H symbol for *hydrogen*.

habituation (hə,bichoo'ayshən) the gradual adaptation to a stimulus or to the environment. The acquisition of a habit, e.g. a condition resulting from the repeated consumption of a drug, but with little or no tendency to increase the dose; there can be psychic dependence without physical dependence on the drug.

haemangioblastoma (hee,man-jeeohbla'stohmə) a tumour of the brain or spinal cord consisting of proliferated blood vessel cells.

haemangioma (,heemanjee'ohmə) a benign tumour formed by dilated blood vessels. *Strawberry h.* a birthmark, which can become very large, but frequently disappears in a few years.

haemarthrosis (,heemah'throsəs) an effusion of blood into a joint.

haematemesis (,heemə'teməsəs) vomiting of blood. If it has been in the stomach for some time and become partially digested by gastric juice, it is of a dark colour and contains particles resembling coffee grounds.

haematin ('heemətən) the iron-containing part of haemoglobin.

haematocele ('heemətoh,seel) a swelling produced by effusion of blood, e.g. in the sheath surrounding a testicle or a broad ligament.

haematocolpos (,heemətoh'kolpos) an accumulation of blood or menstrual fluid in the vagina. *See* CRYPTOMENORRHOEA.

haematocrit ('heemətoh,krit, hi'matə-) the volume of red cells in the blood. Usually expressed as a percentage of the total blood volume.

haematology (,heemə'toləjee) the science dealing with the nature, functions, and diseases of blood.

haematoma (,heemə'tohmə) a swelling containing clotted blood.

haematometra (,heemətoh'meetrə) an accumulation of blood or menstrual fluid in the uterus.

haematomyelia (,heemətohmie-'eeli·ə) an effusion of blood into the spinal cord.

haematosalpinx (,heemətoh'sal-pingks) an accumulation of blood in the uterine tubes; haemosalpinx.

haematuria (,heemə'tyoo·ri·ə) the presence of blood in the urine due to injury or disease of any of the urinary organs.

haemochromatosis (,heemoh-,krohmə'tohsəs) a condition in which there is high absorption and deposition of iron leading to a high serum level, pigmentation of

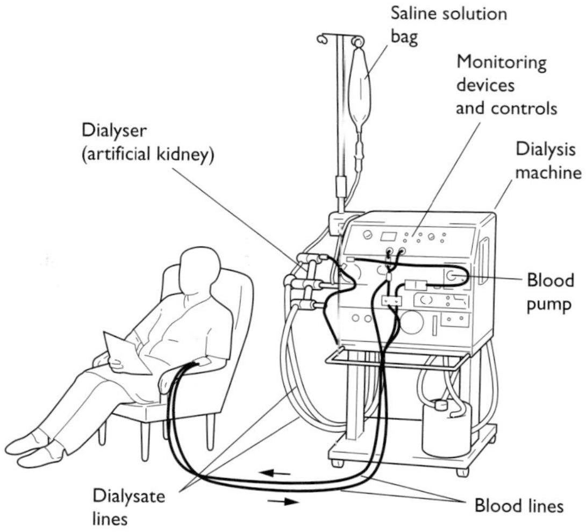

Haemodialysis

the skin, and liver failure. Bronze diabetes.

haemoconcentration (ˌheemohˌkonsən'trayshən) a loss of circulating fluid from the blood resulting in an increase in the proportion of red blood cells to plasma. The viscosity of the blood is increased.

haemocytology (ˌheemohsie'toləjee) the study of the cellular contents of blood.

haemocytometer (ˌheemohsie'tomətə) an apparatus for counting the blood corpuscles in a specific volume of blood.

haemodialysis (ˌheemohdie'aləsəs) the removal of waste material from the blood of a patient with acute or chronic renal failure by means of a dialyser or artificial kidney. The apparatus is coupled to an artery and dialysis is achieved by the blood and rinsing fluid (dialysate) passing through a semipermeable membrane. Blood is returned through a vein. (*See* figure).

haemoglobin (ˌheemə'glohbən) the complex protein molecule contained within the red blood cells which gives them their colour and by which oxygen is transported.

haemoglobinaemia (ˌheeməˌglohbə'neemi·ə) the presence of haemoglobin in the blood plasma.

haemoglobinometer (ˌheemə-ˌglohbə'nomətə) an instrument for estimating the haemoglobin content of the blood.

haemoglobinopathy (ˌheemə-ˌglohbə'nopəthee) any one of a group of hereditary disorders, including sickle-cell ANAEMIA and THALASSAEMIA, in which there is an abnormality in the production of haemoglobin.

haemolysin (hee'moləsən) a substance that destroys red blood cells. It can be an antibody, a bacterial toxin, or a component of a virus.

haemolysis (hee'moləsəs) the disintegration of red blood cells. Excessive haemolysis, which can produce anaemia; can be caused by poisoning or by bacterial infection.

haemolytic (ˌheemə'litik) having the power to destroy red blood cells. *H. disease of the newborn* a condition associated with rhesus incompatibility. *See* RHESUS FACTOR.

haemophilia (ˌheemoh'fili·ə) a condition characterised by impaired coagulability of the blood and a strong tendency to bleed. More than 80% of all patients with haemophilia have haemophilia A (classic haemophilia), which is characterised by a deficiency of clotting factor VIII. Haemophilia B (Christmas disease), which affects about 15% of all haemophiliac patients, results from a deficiency of factor IX. Inherited as an X-linked recessive trait, it is transmitted by females only, to their male offspring. To avoid the debilitating and crippling effects of haemophilia, treatment must raise the level of the deficient clotting factor and maintain it. The patient must learn to avoid trauma and to obtain prompt treatment for bleeding episodes. Before surgery or dental treatment, the patient must be given an infusion of the appropriate clotting factor.

Haemophilus (hee'mofələs) a genus of Gram-negative rod-like bacteria. *H. ducreyi* the cause of soft chancre. *H. influenzae* a species once thought to be the cause of epidemic influenza; it produces a highly fatal form of meningitis, especially in infants. *H. pertussis* the cause of whooping cough; Bordet–Gengou bacillus.

haemophthalmia (ˌheemof'thalmi·ə) bleeding into the vitreous of the eye, usually the result of trauma; haemophthalmos.

haemopneumothorax (ˌheemoh-ˌnyoomoh'thaw·raks) the presence of blood and air in the pleural cavity, usually the result of injury.

haemopoiesis (ˌheemohpoy'eesəs) the formation of red blood cells, which normally takes place in the bone marrow and continues throughout life. *Extramedullary h.* the formation of blood cells other than in the bone marrow, e.g. in the liver or spleen.

haemopoietic (ˌheemohpoy'etik) relating to red blood cell formation. *H. factors* those necessary for the development of red blood cells, e.g. vitamin B_{12} and folic acid.

haemoptysis (hee'moptəsəs) the coughing up of blood from the lungs or bronchi. Being aerated, it is bright-red and frothy.

haemorrhage ('hemə·rij) an escape of blood from a ruptured blood vessel, externally or internally. *Arterial h.* bright-red blood which escapes in rhythmic spurts, corresponding to the beats of the heart. *Venous h.* dark-red blood which escapes in an even flow. Haemorrhage can also be classified as: (a) primary, at the time of operation or injury; reactionary or recurrent, occurring later when the blood pressure rises and a ligature slips or a vessel opens up; or (b) secondary, usually about 10 days after injury, and usually due to sepsis. Special types are as follows. *Antepartum h.* that which occurs before labour starts. *See* PLACENTA (praevia). *Cerebral h.* an episode of bleeding into the cerebrum; one of the three main forms of STROKE. *Concealed h.* collection of the blood in a cavity of the body. *Intracranial h.* bleeding within the cranium, which can be extradural, subdural, subarachnoid, or cerebral. *Intradural h.* bleeding beneath the dura mater. It can be due to injury and causes signs of compression. The cerebrospinal fluid is bloodstained. *Postpartum h.* that which occurs within 12–24 h of delivery, from the genital tract, and which either measures 500 mL or more or adversely affects the woman's condition. Secondary postpartum haemorrhage is excessive bleeding more than 24 hours after delivery.

haemorrhagic (ˌhemə'rajik) pertaining to or characterised by haemorrhage. *H. disease of the newborn* a self-limited haemorrhagic disorder of the first days of life, caused by deficiency of vitamin K-dependent blood clotting factors II, VII, IX, and X. It should be prevented by the prophylactic administration of vitamin K to all newborn babies. *Viral h. fevers* a group of notifiable virus diseases of diverse aetiology but with similar characteristics of fever, headache, myalgia, prostration, and haemorrhagic symptoms. They include dengue haemorrhagic fever, Marburg disease, Ebola virus disease, Lassa fever, and yellow fever.

haemorrhoid ('heməˌroyd) a 'pile' or locally dilated rectal vein. Piles can be either external or internal to the anal sphincter. Pain is caused on defecation and bleeding can occur.

haemorrhoidectomy (ˌhemə·roy-'dektəmee) the surgical removal of haemorrhoids.

haemosalpinx (ˌheemo'salpingks) haematosalpinx.

haemosiderosis (ˌheemohˌsidə-'rohsəs) iron deposits in the tissues resulting from excessive haemolysis of red blood cells.

haemostasis (ˌheemoh'staysəs, hee'mostəsis) the arrest of bleeding or the slowing up of blood flow in a vessel.

haemostatic (ˌheemoh'statik) a drug or remedy for arresting haemorrhage; a styptic.

haemothorax (ˌheemoh'thor·raks) blood in the thoracic cavity, e.g. from injury to soft tissues as a result of fracture of a rib.

Hageman factor ('haygəmən) factor XII, which facilitates the clotting of blood (called after the first person found to be suffering from a deficiency of it).

hair (hair) a delicate keratinised epidermal filament growing out of the skin. The root of the hair is enclosed beneath the skin in a tubular follicle (*see* figure).

halibut oil ('haləbat ˌoyl) a vitamin-rich (A and D) oil derived from the liver of halibut.

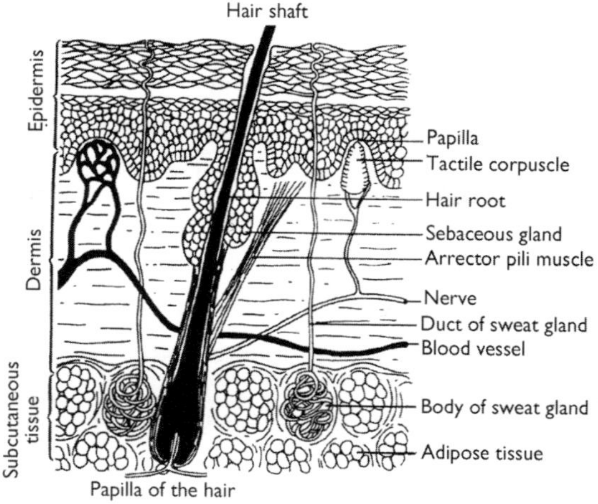

Structure of Hair

halitosis (ˌhalə'tohsəs) foul-smelling breath.

hallucination (həˌloosə'nayshən) a sensory impression (sight, touch, sound, smell, or taste) that has no basis in external stimulation. Hallucinations can have psychological causes, as in mental illness, or they can result from drugs, alcohol, organic illnesses (such as brain tumour), or exhaustion.

hallucinogen (hə'loosənəˌjen) an agent that causes hallucinations, e.g. LSD or cannabis.

hallux ('haləks) the big toe. *H. valgus* a deformity in which the big toe is bent towards the other toes of the same foot. *H. varus* a deformity in which the big toe is bent away from the other toes of the same foot.

halo ('hayloh) a circular structure, such as a luminous circle seen surrounding an object or light. *Glaucomatous h., h. glaucomatosus* a narrow light zone surrounding the optic disc in glaucoma.

halo effect a beneficial effect noted after a healthcare intervention, visit, or research project. The halo effect cannot be attributed to the content of the interview, visit, or project, but is the outcome of indefinable factors as a result of the intervention.

halo splint an orthopaedic device used to immobilise the head and neck to assist in the healing of cervical injuries and postoperatively after cervical surgery.

halogen ('haləjən, 'heil-) one of the

non-metallic elements: chlorine, iodine, bromine, and fluorine.

haloperidol (ˌhaloh'perəˌdol) a sedative and tranquilliser used in the treatment of schizophrenia and other psychiatric disorders, particularly mania.

halothane ('halohˌthayn) a widely used anaesthetic; used as an inhalation to induce and maintain anaesthesia.

hamamelis (ˌhamə'meeləs) a soothing agent prepared from witch-hazel and used in suppository form in the treatment of haemorrhoids.

hamartoma (ˌhamə'tohmə) a benign nodule which is an overgrowth of mature tissue.

hammer ('hamə) the malleus. *H.-toe* a deformity in which there is permanent plantar flexion *H.-toe* a deformity in which there is permanent plantar flexion of the distal phalanx or of the distal and middle phalanges.

hamstring ('hamˌstring) the flexors of the knee joint that are situated at the back of the thigh.

hand (hand) the terminal part of the arm below the wrist. *Claw h.* a paralytic condition in which the hand is flexed and the fingers contracted, caused by injury to nerves or muscles. *Cleft h.* a congenital deformity in which the cleft between the third and fourth fingers extends into the palm. *H., foot and mouth disease* a mild infectious disease in children, caused by Coxsackie virus, which results in vesicle formation on all three sites. Not the same as foot and mouth disease.

Hand–Schüller–Christian disease (ˌhandˌshoolə'krischən) *A. Hand, American paediatrician, 1868–1949; A. Schüller, Austrian neurologist, 1874–1958; H.A. Christian, American physician, 1876–1951.* A disease of the reticuloendothelial system in which GRANULOMATA containing cholesterol are formed, chiefly in the skull.

handicap ('handeeˌkap) a disadvantage for a given individual, resulting from an impairment or a disability that limits or prevents the fulfilment of a role that is normal (depending on age, sex, and social and cultural factors) for that individual.

Hansen's disease ('hansənz) *G.H.A. Hansen, Norwegian physician, 1841–1912.* Leprosy, caused by Hansen's bacillus, *Mycobacterium leprae.*

haploid ('haployd) having one set of chromosomes after division instead of two.

Harrison's groove or **sulcus** ('harisənz) *E. Harrison, British physician, 1789–1838.* A horizontal groove along the lower border of the thorax corresponding to the costal insertion of the diaphragm; seen in rickets.

Hartnup disease ('hahtnup) an hereditary defect in amino acid metabolism which can produce learning difficulties (named after the first person found to suffer from it).

Hashimoto's disease (ˌhashi'mohtohz) *H. Hashimoto, Japanese surgeon, 1881–1934.* A lymphoadenoid goitre caused by the formation of antibodies to thyroglobulin. It is an autoimmune condition giving rise to HYPOTHYROIDISM.

hashish ('hasheesh, -ish) Indian hemp. *See* CANNABIS.

haustration (haw'strayshən) a

HAUSTRUM, pouches that give the colon a puckered appearance.

haustrum ('hawstrəm) any one of the pouches formed by the sacculations of the colon.

Haversian canal (hə'vərsi·ən, -shən) *C. Havers, British physician and anatomist, 1650–1702*. One of the minute canals that permeate compact bone, containing blood and lymph vessels to maintain its nutrition. *See* CONE.

Hawthorne effect ('hawthawn) the term given to the usual beneficial effect of a study on the persons participating in the study. It was named after an industrial management study in the USA, where the effect was first identified.

hayfever ('hayfeevə) an atopic ALLERGY characterised by sneezing, itching, and watery eyes, running nose and a burning sensation of the palate and throat. It is a localised reaction to an extrinsic allergen, most commonly pollens and the spores of moulds. When the allergen comes in contact with mast cell-bound IgE immunoglobulin in the tissues of the conjunctiva, nasal mucosa, and bronchial tree, the cells release mediators such as histamine which produce the characteristic symptoms of hayfever, including swelling of tissues, itching, and sneezing. ATOPY.

hazard ('hazəd) something that has the potential to cause injury or disease to people, damage to property, or disruption to work practices.

HCG human chorionic gonadotrophin. *See* GONADOTROPHIN.

head (hed) the anterior or superior part of a structure or organism, in vertebrates containing the brain and the organs of special sense. *H. injury* traumatic injury to the head resulting from a fall or violent blow. Such an injury can be open or closed and can involve a brain CONCUSSION, skull fracture, or contusions of the brain. All head injuries are potentially dangerous because there can be a slow leakage of blood from damaged blood vessels into the brain, or the formation of a blood clot which gradually increases pressure against brain tissue. Long-term effects of head injury can include chronic headache, disturbances in mental and motor function, and a host of other symptoms that might or might not be psychogenic. Organic brain damage and post-traumatic epilepsy resulting from scar formation are possible sequelae to head injury.

headache ('hed,ayk) a pain or ache in the head. A symptom rather than a disorder. It accompanies many diseases and conditions, including emotional distress. *See also* MIGRAINE.

Heaf test (heef) *F.G.R. Heaf, British physician, 1894–1973*. A form of tuberculin testing. A drop of tuberculin solution on the skin is injected by means of a number of very short needles mounted on a spring-loaded device (Heaf's gun).

healing ('heeling) the process of return to normal function after a period of disease or injury. *H. by first intention* signifies union of the edges of a clean incised wound without visible granulations, and leaving only a faint linear scar. *H. by second intention* is union of the edges of an open wound by the formation of granulations from the bottom and sides. *H. by third* *intention* is union of a wound that is closed surgically several days after the injury.

health (helth) the World Health Organization (WHO) states that 'Health is a state of complete physical, mental and social wellbeing and not merely the absence of disease or infirmity'. *H. assessment* an evaluation made by a healthcare professional of an individual's health status, which takes account of the health history and lifestyle together with the findings of a physical examination. *H. centre* a community health organisation for providing ambulatory health care and coordinating the efforts of all health agencies, commonly focused around a general practitioner's services. *H. culture* a system that attempts to explain and treat health problems and illness and to maintain health. Part of the wider culture to which people belong, it might be a traditional or a biomedical system. *Holistic h.* a system of preventative medicine that takes into account the whole individual, his or her own responsibility for wellbeing, and the total influences (social, psychological, spiritual, environmental) that affect health, including nutrition, exercise, and mental relaxation. *Public h.* the field of medicine that is concerned with safeguarding and improving the health of the community as a whole. *H. services* the term is usually employed to connote the system or program by which health care is made available to the population and financed by government or private enterprise, or both. *H. statistics* summated data on any aspect of the health of populations; for example, mortality, morbidity, use of health services, treatment outcome, and costs of health care.

health education various methods of education aimed at the prevention of disease; includes the changing of behaviours that have been identified as risk factors for particular diseases. All nurses, midwives, and health visitors have particular responsibilities and opportunities to promote good health.

healthcare system an organised plan of health services. The term is usually employed to denote the system or program by which health care is made available to the population and financed by government or private enterprise or both. *H.C. facilities* employ health professionals to manage and treat health-related problems. Can include community care, private and public hospitals, home care, day-stay centres, and residential aged-care services.

hearing ('hiə·ring) the reception of sound waves and their transmission onwards to the brain in the form of nerve impulses. *H. aid* an apparatus, usually electronic, to amplify sounds before they reach the inner ear.

heart (haht) a hollow, muscular organ which pumps the blood throughout the body, situated behind the sternum slightly towards the left side of the thorax (*see* figure). *H. attack* MYOCARDIAL INFARCTION. *H. block* impairment of conduction in heart excitation; often applied specifically to atrioventricular heart block. *H. failure* can be acute, as sometimes occurs after coronary thrombosis, or chronic. *H. –lung*

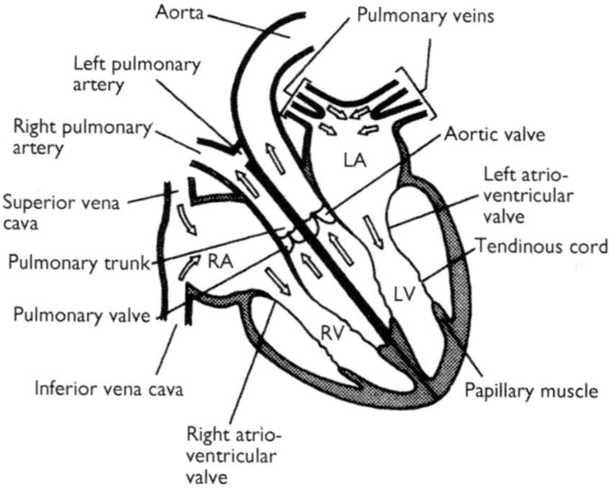

Heart

machine an apparatus used to perform the functions of both the heart and the lungs during heart surgery. *H. murmur* an abnormal sound heard in the heart, frequently caused by disease of the valves. Occurs when the blood flow through the heart exceeds a certain velocity. *H. sounds* the sound heard when listening to the heartbeat. They are caused by the closure of the valves.

heartburn ('haht,bərn) indigestion marked by a burning sensation in the oesophagus, often with regurgitation of acid fluid. PYROSIS.

heat (heet) warmth. A form of energy, which can cause an increase in temperature or a change of state, e.g. the conversion of water into steam. *H. exhaustion* a rapid pulse, anorexia, dizziness, cramps in arms, legs, or abdomen, and sometimes followed by sudden collapse, caused by loss of body fluids and salts under very hot conditions. *Prickly h.* MILIARIA; heat rash. Acute itching caused by blocking of the ducts of the sweat glands following profuse sweating. *H.-stroke* a severe life-threatening condition resulting from prolonged exposure to heat. *See* SUNSTROKE.

hebephrenia (,hebi'freeni·ə) a form of schizophrenia characterised by thought disorder and emotional incongruity. Delusions and hallucinations are common.

Heberden's nodes ('hebə,dənz) *W. Heberden, British physician, 1710–1801.* Bony or cartilaginous outgrowths causing deformity of the terminal finger joints in OSTEOARTHRITIS.

hebetude ('hebətyood) emotional dullness. A common symptom in dementia and schizophrenia.

hectic ('hektik) occurring regularly. *H. fever* a regularly occurring increase in temperature; it is frequently observed in pulmonary tuberculosis. *H. flush* a redness of the face accompanying a sudden rise in temperature.

hedonism ('heedə,nizəm, 'hed-) excessive devotion to pleasure.

Hegar's dilators ('haygahz) *A. Hegar, German gynaecologist, 1830–1914.* A series of graduate dilators used to dilate the uterine cervix.

Heimlich manoeuvre ('hiemlik) A technique for removing foreign matter from the trachea of a choking person. Wrap the arms around the person and allow his or her torso to hang forwards. Make a fist with one hand and grasp it with the other, then with both hands against the victim's abdomen (above the navel and below the rib cage), forcefully press into the abdomen with a sharp upwards thrust. The manoeuvre can be repeated several times if necessary to clear the air passages. If unconscious or prone, turn the victim on to back, kneel astride the torso and, with both hands, use the manoeuvre as described.

Heine–Medin disease (,hienə-'maydin) the major form of POLIOMYELITIS.

heliotherapy (,heeleeoh'therəpee) treatment of disease by exposure of the body to sunlight.

helium ('heelee·əm) *symbol* He. An inert gas sometimes used in conjunction with oxygen to facilitate respiration in obstructional types of DYSPNOEA and for decompressing deep-sea divers.

helix ('heeliks) 1. a spiral twist. Used to describe the configuration of certain molecules, e.g. deoxyribonucleic acid (DNA). 2. the outer rim of the auricle of the ear.

Heller's operation ('heləz) *E.Heller, German surgeon, 1877–1964.* An operation for the relief of cardiospasm by dividing the muscle coat at the lower end of the oesophagus.

helminthiasis (,helmin'thieəsəs) an infestation with worms.

hemeralopia (,hemə·rə'lohpi·ə) day blindness. Poor vision in a bright light, but comparatively good vision when the light is dim. *See* NYCTALOPIA.

hemianopia (,hemi·ə'nohpi·ə) partial blindness, in which the patient can see only half of the normal field of vision. It arises from disorders of the optic tract and of the occipital lobe.

hemiballismus (,hemeebə'lizməs) involuntary chorea-like movements on only one side of the body.

hemicolectomy (,hemeekoh'lektəmee) the removal of the ascending and part of the transverse colon with an ileotransverse colostomy (*see* figure).

hemiparesis (,hemeepə'reesəs) paralysis on one side of the body; HEMIPLEGIA.

hemiplegia (,hemee'pleeji·ə, -jə) paralysis of one half of the body, usually due to cerebral disease or injury. The lesion is on the side of the brain opposite to the side paralysed.

hemisphere ('heməs,fiə) a half sphere. In anatomy, one of the

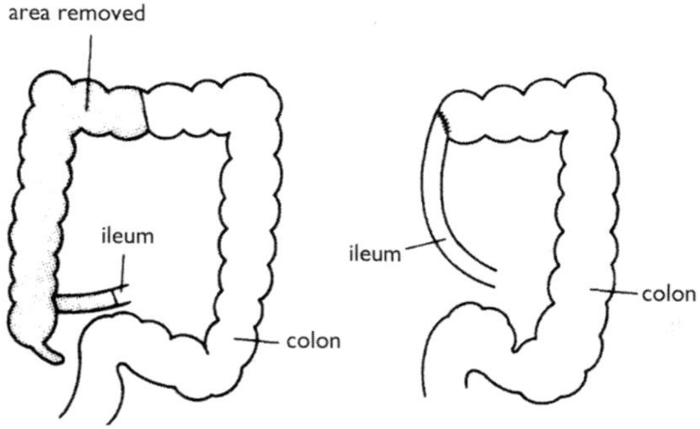

Hemicolectomy and Transverse Ileocolostomy

two halves of the cerebrum or CEREBELLUM.

hemp (hemp) *see* CANNABIS.

henbane ('henbayn) *see* HYOSCYAMUS.

Henle's loop ('henleez) *F.G.J. Henle, German anatomist, 1809–1885*. The U-shaped loop of the uriniferous tubule of the kidney.

Henoch's purpura (henokhs) *E.H. Henoch, German paediatrician, 1820–1910*. Allergic purpura. *See* PURPURA.

heparin ('hepə·rən) an anticoagulant formed in the liver and circulated in the blood. Injected intravenously, it prevents the conversion of prothrombin into thrombin, and is used in the treatment of THROMBOSIS.

hepatectomy (ˌhepə'tektəmee) excision of a part or the whole of the liver.

hepatic (hi'patik) relating to the liver. *H. flexure* the angle of the colon that is situated under the liver.

hepaticojejunostomy (hiˌpatikoh-ˌjejə'nostəmee) the anastomosis of the hepatic duct to the JEJUNUM, usually created after extensive excision for carcinoma of the pancreas.

hepaticostomy (hiˌpati'kostəmee) a surgical opening into the hepatic duct.

hepatitis (ˌhepə'tietəs) inflammation of the liver. Acute inflammation can be caused by viral infections; drug reactions, e.g. halothane; carbon tetrachloride poisoning; paracetamol poisoning; alcohol; ischaemia; mushroom poisoning; Wilson's disease; and eclampsia. Chronic inflammation of the liver is defined as inflammation continuing for at least 6 months, without improvement; it is caused by a range of chronic diseases, drugs, or alcohol, and can lead to cirrhosis and end-stage liver disease. *Fulminant h.* a clinical syndrome resulting from massive necrosis of the liver cells, or sudden and severe impairment of liver function. *Hepatitis A* (formerly called viral or infective h.) is usually a relatively mild illness with spontaneous recovery, and does not usually cause chronic hepatitis. Risk factors include eating shellfish, overseas travel, family contact, and sexual lifestyle. A preventative vaccine is available. *Hepatitis B* (formerly called serum h.) causes both acute and chronic inflammation, and is transmitted by exposure to infected blood or bodily secretions. A preventative vaccine is available. *Hepatitis C* (formerly called non-A, non-B h.) causes both acute and chronic inflammation, and is transmitted by exposure to infected blood. The most common risk is injecting drug use; less commonly sexual transmission. No preventative vaccine. *Hepatitis D* is a coinfection with hepatitis B. Rare in Australia. *Hepatitis E* causes acute inflammation, transmitted enterically, and rare in Australia. *Hepatitis G* is a newly discovered virus, similar to hepatitis C.

hepatisation (ˌhepətie'zayshən) the alteration of lung tissue into a solid mass resembling liver, which occurs in acute lobar pneumonia.

hepatocele ('hepətohˌseel) herniation of the liver through the abdominal wall or the diaphragm.

hepatocellular (ˌhepətoh'selyələ) referring to the cells of the liver.

hepatocirrhosis (ˌhepətohsə'rohsəs) cirrhosis of the liver.

hepatogenous (ˌhepətoh'jenəsəs) arising in the liver. Applied to jaundice in which the disease arises in the parenchymal cells of the liver.

hepatolenticular ('hepətohlen'tikyələ) pertaining to the liver and the lentiform nucleus. *H. degeneration* Wilson's disease; a progressive condition, usually occurring between the ages of 10 and 25 years. There are tremors of the head and limbs, pigmentation of the cornea, and sometimes defective twilight vision.

hepatolithiasis (ˌhepətohli'thieəsəs) calculi formation in the liver.

hepatoma (ˌhepə'tohmə) a primary malignant tumour arising in the liver cells.

hepatomegaly (ˌhepətoh'megəlee) an enlargement of the liver.

hepatorenal syndrome (ˌhepətoh-'reen'l) a gradual loss of renal function related to liver disease.

hepatosplenomegaly (ˌhepətohˌspleenoh'megəlee) enlargement of the liver and spleen, such as can be found in KALA-AZAR.

hepatotoxic (ˌhepətoh'toksik) applied to drugs and substances that cause destruction of liver cells.

herd immunity (hərd) the immunity of a population. When there are enough persons in a population immune to a particular infection, the infection fails to spread because of the absence of enough susceptibles. For example, in measles, this can be achieved by vaccination of 90–95% of the population.

hereditary (hə'redətree) derived from ancestry; inherited.

heredity (hə'redətee) the transmission of both physical and mental characteristics to the offspring from the parents. Recessive characteristics can miss one or two generations and reappear later.

hermaphrodite (hər'mafrəˌdiet) an individual whose gonads contain both testicular and ovarian tissue. These can be combined as an ovotestis or there can be a testis on one side and an ovary on the other. The external genitalia can be indeterminate or of either sex. *Pseudo-h.* one whose gonads are histologically of one sex but in whom the genitalia have the appearance of the opposite sex. *True h.* one who possesses both male and female gonads.

hernia ('hərni·ə) a protrusion of any part of the internal organs through the structures enclosing them. *Cerebral h.* a protrusion of brain through the skull. *Diaphragmatic h.* and *hiatus h.* a protrusion of a part of the stomach through the oesophageal opening in the diaphragm. *Femoral h.* a loop of intestine protruding into the femoral canal. More common in females. *Incisional h.* a hernia occurring at the site of an old wound. *Inguinal h.* protrusion of the intestine through the inguinal canal. This can be congenital or acquired, and is commoner in males. A rupture. *Irreducible h.* a hernia that cannot be replaced by manipulation. *Reducible h.* a hernia that can be returned to its normal position by manipulative measures. *Strangulated h.* a hernia of the bowel in which the neck of the sac containing the bowel is so constricted that the venous circulation is impeded, and gangrene will result if not treated promptly (*see* figure). *Umbilical h.* protrusion of bowel through the umbilical ring. This can be congenital or acquired. *Vaginal h.* RECTOCELE or CYSTOCELE.

hernioplasty ('hərneeoh,plastee) a surgical repair of the abdominal wall performed after reduction of a hernia.

herniorrhaphy (,hərnee'o·rəfee) removal of a hernial sac and repair of the abdominal wall.

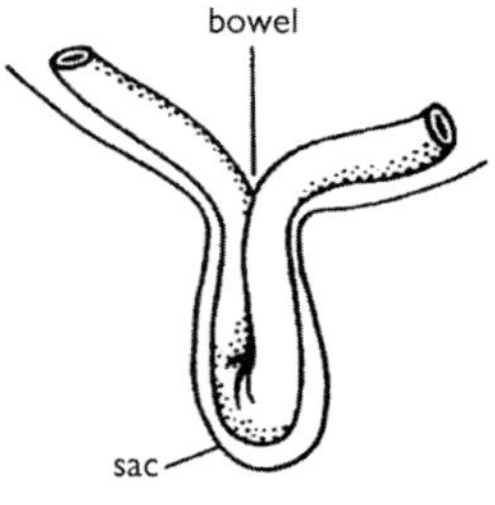

Strangulated Hernia

herniotomy (,hərnee'otəmee) an operation to remove a hernial sac.

heroin ('heroh·ən) a diacetate of morphine used as an analgesic and abused illicitly for its euphoriant effects. The drug readily induces physical dependence and can be sniffed, smoked ('chasing the dragon'), or injected subcutaneously or intravenously ('shooting up' or 'mainlining'). Slang terms for heroin include 'smack', 'H', and 'brown sugar'.

herpes ('hərpeez) an inflammatory skin eruption of small vesicles caused by a herpes virus. *H. simplex* a viral infection which gives rise to localised vesicles in the skin and mucous membranes and is characterised by latency and subsequent recurrence. It is caused by herpes simplex viruses types 1 and 2. Type 1 infection is common in children and is often symptomless. Type 2 infection is common in older age groups and is associated with sexual activity. Lesions appear on the cervix, vulva, and surrounding skin in women and on the penis in men. In homosexual men, rectal lesions are common. Recurrent genital herpes can follow primary infection. Type 2 virus can cause aseptic meningitis. *H. zoster* is a local manifestation of reactivation of infection of the varicella-zoster virus, the causative agent of chickenpox, characterised by a vesicular rash in the area of distribution of a sensory nerve. Called also shingles.

herpes virus ('hərpeez ˌvierəs) one of a group of DNA-containing viruses. They include the causative agents of herpes simplex, herpes zoster, chickenpox, cytomegalic inclusion disease, and infective mononucleosis.

Hess's test ('hesəz) *A.F. Hess, American physician, 1875–1933.* A test used to diagnose PURPURA. An inflated blood pressure cuff causes an increase in capillary pressure and rupture of the walls, causing purpuric spots to develop.

heterochromia (ˌhetə·roh'krohmi·ə) a difference in colour in the irises of the two eyes or in different parts of one iris. It can be congenital or can be secondary (due to inflammation).

heterogeneous (ˌhetə·roh'jeeni·əs) composed of diverse constituents.

heterogenous (ˌhetə'rojənəs) derived from different sources.

heterophoria (ˌhetə·roh'faw·ri·ə) a tendency to squint when FUSION is interrupted. It occurs mainly when a person is tired or in poor health.

heterosexual (ˌhetə·roh'seksyooəl) 1. pertaining to, characteristic of, or directed towards the opposite sex. 2. a person with erotic interests directed towards the opposite sex.

heterotropia (ˌhetə·roh'trohpi·ə) a marked deviation of the eyes; STRACISMUS or squint.

heterozygous (ˌhetə·roh'ziegəs) possessing dissimilar alternative genes for an inherited characteristic, one gene coming from each parent. One gene is dominant and the other is recessive. *See* HOMOZYGOUS.

hexachlorophane (ˌheksə'klor-·rə'feen) a detergent and germicidal compound commonly incorporated in soaps and dermatological agents. Topical preparations have been associated with severe neurotoxicity and should not be used on children under 2 years of age except on medical advice. Avoid use on large raw areas.

hexamine ('heksəˌmeen) methenamine; a urinary antiseptic which releases formaldehyde in an acid urine.

Hg symbol for *mercury* (*L. hydrargyrum*).

hiatus (hie'aytəs) a space or opening. *H. hernia* a protrusion of a part of the stomach through the oesophageal opening in the diaphragm.

hiccup ('hikup) hiccough; a spasmodic contraction of the diaphragm causing an abrupt inspiratory sound.

Hickman line ('hikmən ˌlien) trade name for a central venous line catheter.

hidrosis (hi'drohsəs) the excretion of sweat.

high-altitude sickness (hie'altə-tyood) a condition resulting from difficulty in adjusting to diminished oxygen pressure at high altitudes. It can take the form of mountain sickness, high-altitude pulmonary oedema, or cerebral oedema.

hilum ('hieləm) hilus; a recess in an organ by which blood vessels, nerves, and ducts enter and leave.

hindbrain ('hiend,brayn) that part of the brain consisting of the MEDULLA oblongata, the PONS and the CEREBELLUM.

hip (hip) 1. the region of the body at the articulation of the femur and the innominate bone at the base of the lower trunk. These bones meet at the hip joint. Called also *coxa*. 2. loosely, the hip joint. *Total h. replacement* replacement of the femoral head and acetabulum with prostheses that are cemented into the bone; called also *total h. arthroplasty*. The procedure is done to replace a severely damaged arthritic hip joint.

hippus ('hipəs) alternate contraction and dilatation of the pupils. This occurs in various diseases of the nervous system, e.g. MULTIPLE SCLEROSIS.

Hirschsprung's disease ('hərsh-spruhngz) *H. Hirschsprung, Danish physician, 1831–1916. See* MEGACOLON.

hirsute ('hərsyoot) hairy.

hirsutism ('hərsyoo,tizəm) excessive hairiness.

hirudin (hi'roodin) the active principle in the secretion of the leech and certain snake venoms that prevents clotting of blood.

Hirudo (hi'roodoh) a genus of leeches. *H. medicinalis* the medical leech.

histamine ('histəmeen) an enzyme that causes local vasodilatation and increased permeability of the blood vessel walls. Readily released from body tissues, it is a factor in allergy response, greatly increases gastric secretion of hydrochloric acid, and increases the heart rate. *H. test* 1. subcutaneous injection of 0.1% solution of histamine to stimulate gastric secretion in order to measure maximal acid output. 2. after rapid intravenous injection of histamine phosphate, normal persons experience a brief fall in blood pressure; in those with PHAEOCHROMOCYTOMA, after the fall in blood pressure, there is a marked rise.

histidinaemia (,histidə'neemi·ə) an hereditary metabolic defect marked by excessive histidine in the blood and urine due to deficient histidase activity; many affected persons show mild mental handicap and disordered speech development.

histidine ('histə,deen) one of the 9 essential amino acids formed by the digestion of dietary protein. Histamine is derived from it.

histiocyte ('histeeoh,siet) a stationary macrophage of connective tissue. Derived from the reticulo-endothelial cells, it acts as a scavenger, removing bacteria from the blood and tissues.

histiocytoma (,histeeohsie'tohmə) a tumour containing histiocytes, causing a vascular nodule.

histiocytosis (,histeeohsie'tohsəs) a group of diseases of bone in which granulomata containing HISTIOCYTES and eosinophil cells appear. *See* LETTERER–SIWE DISEASE and HAND–SCHÜLLER–CHRISTIAN DISEASE.

histocompatibility (,histohkəm-,patə'bilətee) the ability of cells to be accepted and to function in a new situation. Tissue typing reveals this and ensures a higher success rate in organ transplantation.

histogram ('histə,gram) a bar-chart. Statistical values are expressed as blocks on a graph.

histology (hi'stoləjee) the science dealing with the minute structure, composition and function of tissues.

histolysis (hi'stoləsəs) the disintegration of tissues.

histoplasmosis (ˌhistohplaz'mohsəs) infection caused by inhalation of the spores of a yeast-like fungus, *Histoplasma capsulatum*. Usually symptomless, the infection can progress and produce a condition resembling tuberculosis.

HIV human immunodeficiency virus.

hives (hievz) URTICARIA.

Hodge pessary (ˌhoj 'pesə·ree) *H.L. Hodge, American gynaecologist, 1796–1873*. A pessary used to maintain the position of the uterus after correction of a retroversion. *See* PESSARY.

Hodgkin's disease ('hojkənz) *T. Hodgkin, British physician, 1798–1866*. LYMPHADENOMA, a malignant condition of the reticuloendothelial cells. There is progressive enlargement of lymph nodes and lymph tissue all over the body. Treated by radiotherapy and cytotoxic drugs. This disease has a good prognosis.

Hofmann reaction ('hofmən riˌakshən) chemical inactivation, without the activity of enzymes, of compounds that occur spontaneously in the blood.

holism ('hohlizəm) a philosophy in which the person is considered as a functioning whole rather than as a composite of several systems.

holistic (hə'listik) pertaining to holism. *H. health care* a comprehensive approach to health care that implies body–mind–spirit consideration in all actions and interventions for the patient, while recognising the concept of the uniqueness of the individual and the influence of external and internal environmental factors on health.

Homans' sign ('hohmənz) *J. Homans, American surgeon, 1877–1954*. Pain elicited in the calf when the foot is dorsiflexed. Indicative of venous thrombosis.

homatropine (hoh'matrəˌpin) a short-acting mydriatic used in ophthalmology to dilate the pupil and so allow a better view of the fundus of the eye.

homeopathy (ˌhohmee'opəthee) a system of medicine promulgated by C.F.S. Hahnemann (German physician, 1755–1843) and based upon the principle that 'like cures like'. Remedies are given which can produce in the patient the symptoms of the disease to be cured, but they are administered in minute doses.

homeostasis (ˌhohmeeoh'staysəs, ˌhom-) a tendency of biological systems to maintain stability while continually adjusting to conditions that are optimal for survival.

homogeneity (ˌhohməjə'neeətee) similarity of conditions. Also called INTERNAL CONSISTENCY.

homogeneous (ˌhohmə'jeeni·əs) uniform in character. Similar in nature and characteristics.

homogenise (hə'mojəˌniez) to make homogeneous. To reduce to the same consistency.

homogenous (hə'mojənəs) derived from the same source.

homograft ('homəˌgrahft, 'homoh-) a tissue or organ transplanted from one individual to another of the same species. An ALLOGRAFT.

homolateral (ˌhomə'latə·rəl, ˌhoh-moh-) on the same side; ipsilateral.

homologous (hə'moləgəs) 1. in anatomy, having the same embryological origin although performing a different function. 2. in chemistry, possessing a similar structure. *H.*

chromosomes those that pair during meiosis and contain an identical arrangement of genes in the DNA pattern.

homologue ('homə,log) a part or organ which has the same relative position or structure as another.

homoplasty ('homoh,plastee, 'hohm-) surgical replacement of defective tissues with a homograft.

homosexual (,homoh'sekshooəl, ,hohm-) 1. of the same sex. 2. a person who is sexually attracted to a person of the same sex.

homosexuality (,homoh,sekshoo'alətee, ,hohm-) sexual and emotional orientation towards persons of the same sex.

homozygous (,homoh'ziegəs) possessing an identical pair of genes for an inherited characteristic. *See* HETEROZYGOUS.

hookworm ('huhk,wərm) *see* ANCYLOSTOMA.

hordeolum (hordee'ohləm) a stye; inflammation of the sebaceous glands of the eyelashes.

hormone ('hawmohn) a chemical substance that is generated in one organ and carried by the blood to another, in which it excites activity. *H. replacement therapy* the giving of prepared hormones as a substitute for those hormones that the body no longer produces or that have been lost as a result of surgery. A combination of oestrogenic hormones that can be given to women for the relief of menopausal symptoms and the prevention of osteoporosis. Known as HRT.

Horner's syndrome ('hawnəz) *J.F. Horner, Swiss ophthalmologist, 1831–86.* A condition in which there is a lesion on the path of sympathetic nerve fibres in the cervical region. The symptoms include ENOPHTHALMOS, PTOSIS, a contracted pupil, and a decrease in sweating.

Horton's syndrome ('hawtənz) *B.T. Horton, American physician, 1895–1980.* Severe headache caused by the release of histamine in the body or by its administration. Histamine CEPHALALGIA.

hospice ('hospəs) the concept of a hospice is that of a caring community of professional and non-professional people, together with the family. Emphasis is on dealing with emotional and spiritual problems as well as the medical problems of the terminally ill. Of primary concern is control of pain and other symptoms, keeping the patient at home for as long as possible or desirable, and making the remaining days as comfortable and meaningful as possible. After the patient dies, family members are given support throughout their period of bereavement.

hospital ('hospət'l) a health facility for the care, diagnosis and treatment of the sick and injured. *H.-acquired infection see* hospital-acquired INFECTION.

host (hohst) the animal, plant, or tissue on which a parasite lives and multiplies. *Definitive* or *final h.* one that harbours the parasite during its adult sexual stage. *Intermediate h.* one that shelters the parasite during a non-reproductive period.

hourglass contraction ('owə,glahs kən,trakshən) a contraction near the middle of a hollow organ, such as the stomach or uterus, producing an outline resembling that shape.

housemaid's knee ('howsmaydz) prepatellar CURSITIS; inflammation of the prepatellar bursa, which becomes distended with serous fluid.

humidity (hyoo'midətee) the degree of moisture in the air. *H. therapy* the therapeutic use of water to prevent or correct a moisture deficit in the respiratory tract. The principal reasons for employing humidity therapy are: (a) to prevent drying and irritation of the respiratory mucosa; (b) to facilitate ventilation and diffusion of oxygen and other therapeutic gases being administered; and (c) to aid in the removal of thick and viscous secretions that obstruct the air passages. Another important use of water aerosol therapy is to aid in obtaining an induced sputum specimen.

humour ('hyoomə) any fluid of the body, such as lymph or blood. *Aqueous h.* the fluid filling the anterior chamber of the eye. *Vitreous h.* the jelly-like substance that fills the chamber of the eye between the lens and the retina.

Huntington's chorea (disease) ('huntingtənz) *G.S. Huntington, American physician, 1851–1927.* A rare, degenerative inherited disorder of the brain in which there is progressive CHOREA and mental deterioration (dementia).

Hurler's syndrome ('hərləz) *G. Hurler, Austrian paediatrician.* An inherited disorder in which learning difficulties are caused by excess MUCOPOLYSACCHARIDES being stored in the brain and reticuloendothelial system. Gargoylism.

Hutchinson's teeth ('hutchənsənz) *Sir J. Hutchinson, British surgeon, 1828–1913.* Typical notching of the borders of the permanent incisor teeth occurring in congenital syphilis.

hyaline ('hieə,lien) resembling glass. *H. degeneration* a form of deterioration that occurs in tumours and is due to deficiency of blood supply. It precedes cystic degeneration. *H. membrane disease see* RESPIRATORY (distress syndrome of newborn).

hyaluronidase (,hieəlyə'roni,dayz) an enzyme that facilitates the absorption of fluids in subcutaneous tissues. It is found in the testes of mammals, and a preparation of it is particularly used with subcutaneous infusions to promote absorption.

hydatid ('hiedətəd) a cystic swelling containing the embryo of *Echinococcus granulosus*. It can be found in any organ of the body, e.g. in the liver. 'Daughter cysts' are produced from the original. Infection is from contaminated foods, e.g. salads. *H. disease* the result of the presence of hydatids in the lungs, liver, or brain.

hydatidiform (,hiedə'tidə,fawm) resembling a hydatid cyst. *H. mole see* MOLE.

hydraemia (hie'dreemi·ə) a modification of the blood in which there is an excess of plasma in relation to the cells. A degree of hydraemia is physiological in pregnancy.

hydralazine (hie'dralə,zeen) a vasodilator and antihypertensive agent used to lower blood pressure.

hydramnios (hie'dramneeəs) an excessive amount of amniotic fluid in the uterus in the later months of pregnancy.

hydrarthrosis (,hiedrah'throhsəs) a collection of fluid in a joint.

hydrate ('hiedrayt) a compound of an element with water.

hydroa (hie'droh·ə) a childhood hypersensitivity of the skin to sunlight, resulting in the formation of a vesicular eruption on the exposed parts, with intense irritation.

hydrocarbon (ˌhiedroh'kahbən) a compound of hydrogen and carbon. Fats are of this type.

hydrocele ('hiedrəˌseel) a swelling caused by accumulation of fluid, especially in the TUNICA VAGINALIS surrounding the testicle.

hydrocephalus (ˌhiedroh'kefələs, -'sef-) 'water on the brain'. Enlargement of the skull due to an abnormal collection of cerebrspinal fluid around the brain or in the ventricles. It can be congenital, or can be acquired from inflammation of the meninges during infancy. The most effective treatment is surgical correction employing a shunting technique. It frequently accompanies SPINA BIFIDA.

hydrochloric acid (ˌhiedrə'klo·rik, -'klaw·rik) HCl, a colourless compound of hydrogen and chlorine. It is present (in 0.2% solution) in gastric juice, and aids digestion.

hydrochlorothiazide (ˌhiedrəˌklaw-·roh'thieəˌzied) an oral diuretic similar to, but more potent than, chlorothiazide. It is used in the treatment of oedema and hypertension.

hydrocortisone (ˌhiedroh'kawti-ˌzohn) cortisol, the principal GLUCOCORTICOID secreted by the adrenal gland; it is used in the treatment of inflammations, allergies, pruritus, collagen diseases, adrenocortical insufficiency, severe status asthmaticus, shock, and certain neoplasms.

hydroflumethiazide (ˌhiedroh-ˌfloomə'thieəˌzied) an oral thiazide diuretic used in the treatment of oedema and hypertension.

hydrogen ('hiedrəjən) *symbol* H. A combustible gas, present in nearly all organic compounds, which, in combination with oxygen, forms water. *H. ion concentration* the amount of hydrogen in a liquid, which is responsible for its acidity. The degree of acidity is expressed in pH values: the higher the hydrogen ion concentration, the greater the acidity, and the lower the pH value. The concentration in the blood is of importance in acidosis. *H. peroxide* H_2O_2, a strong disinfectant, cleansing, and bleaching liquid used, diluted in water, for cleansing wounds.

hydrolysis (hie'droləsəs) the process of splitting up into smaller molecules by uniting with water.

hydrometer (hie'dromətə) an instrument for estimating the specific gravity of fluids, e.g. a urinometer.

hydromyelia ('hiedrohmie'eeli·ə) a dilatation of the central canal of the spinal cord caused by an accumulation of cerebrospinal fluid.

hydronephrosis (ˌhiedrohnə'frohsəs) an accumulation of urine in the pelvis of the kidney, resulting in atrophy of the kidney structure due to an obstruction to the flow of urine from the kidney. The condition can be: (a) congenital, due to malformation of the kidney or ureter; or (b) acquired, due to an obstruction of the ureter by tumour or stone, or to back pressure from stricture of the urethra or an enlarged prostate gland.

hydropathy (hie'dropəthee) the treatment of disease by the use of water internally and externally; HYDROTHERAPY.

hydropericarditis (ˌhiedrohˌperee-kah'dietəs) inflammation of the pericardium resulting in serous fluid in the pericardial sac.

hydroperitoneum (ˌhiedrohˌperitə-'neeəm) *see* ASCITES.

hydrophobia (ˌhiedrə'fohbi·ə) 1. rabies. 2. irrational fear of water.

hydropneumothorax (ˌhiedroh-ˌnyoomoh'thor·raks) the presence of fluid and air in the pleural space.

hydrops ('hiedrops) [L.] abnormal accumulation of serous fluid in the tissues or in a body cavity; called also dropsy. *Fetal h., h. fetalis* gross oedema of the entire body of the newborn infant, occurring in haemolytic disease of the newborn.

hydrosalpinx (ˌhiedroh'salpingks) distension of the fallopian tubes by fluid.

hydrotherapy (ˌhiedroh'therəpee) the treatment of disease by means of water.

hydrothorax (ˌhiedroh'thor·raks) fluid in the pleural cavity due to serous effusion, as in cardiac, renal, and other diseases.

hydroureter ('hiedroh·yə'reetə) an accumulation of water or urine in a ureter.

hydroxytryptamine (hieˌdroksee-'triptəˌmeen) SEROTONIN.

hydroxyurea (hieˌdrokseeyə'reeə) an orally active cytotoxic agent used mainly in the treatment of melanoma, resistant chronic MYELOCYTIC LEUKAEMIA and recurrent, metastatic, or inoperable ovarian carcinoma.

hygiene ('hiejeen) 1. the science of health and its preservation. 2. a condition of practice, such as cleanliness, that is conducive to preservation of health. *Communal h.* the maintenance of the health of the community by the provision of a pure water supply, efficient sanitation, good housekeeping, etc. *Industrial h.* (occupational health) care of the health of workers in an industry. *Mental h.* the science dealing with development of healthy mental and emotional reactions and habits. *Oral h.* the proper care of the mouth and teeth. *Personal h.* individual measures taken to preserve one's own health.

hygroma (hie'grohmə) a swelling caused by fluid. *Cystic h.* a cystic LYMPHANGIOMA of the neck. *Subdural h.* a collection of clear fluid in the subdural space.

hygrometer (hie'gromətə) an instrument for measuring water vapour in the air.

hygroscopic (ˌhiegrə'skopik) readily absorbing moisture. An example is glycerin, which is used in suppositories as a means of aiding evacuation by moistening the faeces.

hymen ('hiemen) a fold of mucous membrane partially closing the entrance to the vagina. *Imperforate h.* a membrane which completely occludes the vaginal orifice.

hymenectomy (ˌhieməˌnektəmee) surgical removal of the hymen.

hymenotomy (ˌhiemə'notəmee) surgical incision of the hymen.

hyoid ('hieoyd) shaped like a U, *H. bone* a U-shaped bone above the thyroid cartilage, to which the tongue is attached.

hyoscine ('hieəˌseen) scopolamine; an anticholinergic drug used as an anaesthetic premedicant, antispasmodic, and in the treatment of motion sickness. Should be avoided in the elderly because of its tendency to cause restlessness and confusion (central cholinergic syndrome).

hypaesthesia (ˌhiepəs'theezi·ə) impairment of the sense of touch.

hypalgesia (ˌhiepal'jeezi·ə) a decrease in sensitivity to pain.

hypamnios (hiep'amneeəs) a deficiency of fluid in the amniotic sac.

hyperacidity (ˌhiepə·ə'sidətee) excessive acidity. *Gastric h.* HYPERCHLORHYDRIA.

hyperactive (ˌhiepə'raktiv) exhibiting hyperactivity; hyperkinetic.

hyperactivity (ˌhiepə·rak'tivətee) abnormally increased activity. Developmental hyperactivity of children (hyperkinesia) is characterised by very restless, impulsive behaviour. These children are usually inattentive and have a poor concentration span. Other features that can be associated with hyperactivity include aggression, anxiety, poor eating and sleeping patterns, and social and learning difficulties.

hyperaemia (ˌhiepə'reemi·ə) excess of blood in any part.

hyperaesthesia (ˌhiepə·rəs'theezi·ə) excessive sensitiveness to touch or to other sensations, e.g. taste or smell.

hyperalgesia (ˌhiepə·ral'jeezi·ə) excessive sensibility to pain.

hyperalimentation (ˌhiepəˌraləmen'tayshən) a program of parenteral administration of all nutrients for patients with gastrointestinal dysfunction; also called total parenteral alimentation (TPA) and total parenteral nutrition (TPN). Although the term 'hyperalimentation' is commonly used to designate total or supplementary nutrition by intravenous feedings, it is not technically correct inasmuch as the procedure does not involve an abnormally increased or excessive amount of feeding. *See* NUTRITION (parenteral).

hyperasthenia (ˌhiepə·rəs'theeni·ə) extreme weakness.

hyperbaric (ˌhiepə'barik) at a greater pressure than normal; applied to gases under greater than atmospheric pressure. *H. oxygenation* exposure to oxygen under conditions of greatly increased pressure. The patient is placed in a sealed enclosure, called a hyperbaric chamber. Compressed air is introduced; at the same time, the patient is given pure oxygen through a face mask. Patients suffering from tetanus and gas gangrene (infections caused by bacteria that are resistant to antibiotics but vulnerable to oxygen) are helped by hyperbaric oxygenation. The technique is also useful in radiotherapy for cancer. When full of oxygen, cancer cells seem more vulnerable to radiation. Carbon monoxide poisoning can be treated by hyperbaric oxygenation. Carbon monoxide molecules, displacing the oxygen in the erythrocytes, usually cause asphyxiation, but hyperbaric oxygenation can often keep the patient alive until the carbon monoxide has been eliminated from his or her system. The technique is also increasingly used in an attempt to accelerate the healing of injuries (especially sports injuries).

hyperbilirubinaemia (ˌhiepəˌbileeˌroobə'neemi·ə) an excess of bilirubin in the blood.

hypercalcaemia (ˌhiepəkal'seemi·ə) an excess of calcium in the blood. Can be caused by over-administration of vitamin D, HYPER-

PARATHYROIDISM, THYROTOXICOSIS, breakdown of bone by malignant disease, or impaired renal function.

hypercalciuria (ˌhiepəˌkalsee'yoo-·ri·ə) a high level of calcium in the urine leading to renal stone formation.

hypercapnia (ˌhiepə'kapni·ə) an increased amount of carbon dioxide in the blood, causing overstimulation of the respiratory centre. Hypercarbia.

hypercatabolism (ˌhiepəkə'tabəˌlizəm) an excessive rate of catabolism leading to wasting or destruction of a part of tissue.

hyperchloraemia (ˌhiepəˌklaw'reemi·ə) an excess of chloride in the blood.

hyperchlorhydria (ˌhiepəklaw'hiedri·ə) an excess of hydrochloric acid in the gastric juice.

hypercholesteraemia, hypercholesterolaemia (ˌhiepəkəˌlestə'reemi·ə; ˌhiepəkəˌlestə·rə'leemi·ə) excess of cholesterol in the blood. Predisposes to ATHEROMA and gallstones.

hypercusis (ˌhiepə'kyoosəs) excessive sensitivity to sound.

hyperdynamia (ˌhiepədie'nami·ə) excessive muscle activity. *H. uteri* excessive uterine contractions in labour.

hyperemesis (ˌhiepə'reməsəs) excessive vomiting. *H. gravidarum* an uncommon, serious complication of pregnancy, characterised by severe and persistent vomiting, the aetiology of which is not fully understood.

hyperextension (ˌhiepə·rek'stenshən) the forcible extension of a limb beyond the normal. It can be used to correct orthopaedic deformities.

hyperflexion (ˌhiepə'flekshən) the forcible bending of a joint beyond the normal.

hypergalactia, hypergalactosis (ˌhiepəgə'lakti·ə; ˌhiepəˌgalək'tohsəs) excessive secretion of milk.

hypergammaglobulinaemia (ˌhiepəˌgaməˌglobyələ'neemi·ə) increased gamma-globulins in the blood.

hyperglycaemia (ˌhiepəglie'seemi·a) excess of sugar in the blood (normal 3.0–5.8 mmol/litre when fasting); a sign of DIABETES mellitus.

hyperhidrosis (ˌhiepəhi'drohsəs) excessive perspiration; hyperidrosis.

hyperinsulinism (ˌhiepə'insyələˌnizəm) 1. excessive secretion of insulin. 2. shock produced by an overdose of insulin.

hyperkalaemia (ˌhiepəkə'leemi·ə) an excess of potassium in the blood. If untreated, causes cardiac arrest.

hyperkeratosis (ˌhiepəˌkerə'tohsəs) hypertrophy of the horny layers of the skin.

hyperkinesis (ˌhiepəkə'neesəs) a condition in which there is excessive motor activity. *See* HYPERACTIVITY.

hyperlipaemia (ˌhiepəli'peemi·ə) an excess of fat or lipids in the blood.

hypermastia (ˌhiepə'masti·ə) 1. the presence of one or more supernumerary breasts. 2. overdevelopment of one or both breasts.

hypermetropia (ˌhiepəme'trohpi·ə) hyperopia; long-sightedness. The light rays entering the eye converge beyond the retina. Clear vision can be obtained by the wearing of spectacles or contact lenses.

hypermotility (ˌhiepəmoh'tilətee) excessive movement. *Gastric h.* increased muscle action of the stomach wall, associated with increased secretion of hydrochloric acid.

hypernatraemia (ˌhiepənə'treemi·ə) an excess of sodium in the blood, usually diagnosed when the plasma sodium is above 150 mmol/litre. It is the result of loss of water and electrolytes from the body caused by diarrhoea, POLYURIA, excessive sweating, or inadequate fluid intake. Can also occur in infants if excessive salt has been added to feeds, resulting in convulsions and brain damage.

hypernephroma (ˌhiepəne'frohmə) a malignant tumour of the kidney; renal cell carcinoma.

hyperostosis (ˌhiepə·ro'stohsəs) a thickening of bone; a bony outgrowth; exostosis.

hyperparathyroidism (ˌhiepəˌparə-'thieroyˌdizəm) excessive activity of the parathyroid glands, causing drainage of calcium from the bones, with consequent fragility and liability to spontaneous fracture.

hyperphagia (ˌhiepə'fayji·ə) overeating.

hyperphasia (ˌhiepə'fayzi·ə) excessive talkativeness.

hyperphenylalaninaemia (ˌhiepə-ˌfeenəlˌalənə'neemi·ə) an excess of phenylalanine in the blood, as in PHENYLKETONURIA.

hyperpituitarism (ˌhiepəpə-'tyooətəˌrizəm) overactivity of the pituitary gland.

hyperplasia (ˌhiepə'playzi·ə) excessive formation of normal cells in a tissue or organ, which increases in size.

hyperpnoea (ˌhiepə'neeə, -pəp'neeə) overbreathing; hyperventilation; an abnormal increase in the rate and depth of breathing.

hyperprolactinaemia (ˌhiepəproh-ˌlaktə'neemi·ə) increased levels of prolactin in the blood; in women, it is associated with infertility and can lead to GALACTORRHOEA; has been reported to cause impotence in men.

hyperpyrexia (ˌhiepəpie'reksi·ə) an excessively high body temperature, i.e. over 41°C.

hypersensitivity (ˌhiepəˌsensə-'tivətee) abnormal sensitivity, especially to a particular antigen. The reactions include allergies (such as asthma) and ANAPHYLAXIS. *Contact h.* produced by contact of the skin with a chemical substance having the properties of an antigen or hapten; it includes CONTACT dermatitis. *Delayed h.* a slowly developing increase in cell-mediated immune response (involving T lymphocytes) to a specific antigen, as occurs in graft rejection, autoimmune disease, etc. *Immediate h.* antibody-mediated hypersensitivity characterised by lesions resulting from release of histamine and other mediators of hypersensitivity from reagin-sensitised mast cells, causing increased vascular permeability, oedema, and smooth muscle contraction; it includes ANAPHYLAXIS and ATOPY.

hypersplenism (ˌhiepə'splenizəm) overactivity of an enlarged spleen resulting in the destruction of blood cells and platelets.

hypertelorism (ˌhiepə'teləˌrizəm) abnormally increased distance between two organs or parts. *Ocular h., orbital h.* increase in the interocular distance, often associated with craniofacial DYSOSTOSIS and sometimes with mental handicap.

hypertension (ˌhiepə'tenshən)

persistently high BLOOD PRESSURE. In adults, it is generally agreed that a blood pressure is abnormally high when the resting, supine arterial systolic pressure is equal to or greater than 140 mm Hg and the diastolic pressure is equal to or greater than 90 mm Hg. A diagnosis of hypertension should be based on a series of readings rather than a single measurement. *Essential h.* high blood pressure with no apparent cause; primary hypertension. *Malignant h.* severe, fulminant, life-threatening high blood pressure. *Portal h.* raised pressure in the portal system. *Pulmonary h.* increased pressure in the arteries of the lung, usually as a result of EMPHYSEMA or FIBROSIS.

hyperthermia (ˌhiepə'thərmi·ə) an exceedingly high body temperature. *Malignant h.* a serious condition, sometimes arising during general anaesthesia.

hyperthyroidism (ˌhiepə'thieroyˌdizəm) excessive activity of the thyroid gland. *See* THYROTOXICOSIS.

hypertonic (ˌhiepə'tonik) 1. showing excessive tone or tension, as in a blood vessel or muscle. 2. describing a solution that has greater osmotic pressure than normal physiological tissue fluid.

hypertrichosis (ˌhiepətri'kohsəs) excessive growth of hair on any part of the body.

hypertrophy (hie'pərtrəfee) an increase in the size of a tissue or a structure caused by an increase in the size of the cells that compose it (as opposed to an increase in the number of cells). *See* HYPERPLASIA.

hyperuricaemia (ˌhiepəˌyoo·rə'seemi·ə) an excess of uric acid in the blood. *See* GOUT.

hyperventilation (ˌhiepəˌventə'layshən) 1. increase of air in the lungs above the normal amount. 2. abnormally prolonged and deep breathing, usually associated with acute anxiety or emotional tension.HYPERPNOEA.

hypervitaminosis (ˌhiepəˌvitəmə'nohsəs) a condition caused by the intake of an excessive quantity of vitamins, particularly vitamins A and D.

hypervolaemia (ˌhiepəvo'leemi·ə) abnormal increase in the volume of circulating fluid (plasma) in the body.

hyphaema (hie'feemi·ə) haemorrhage into the anterior chamber of the eye.

hypnosis (hip'nohsəs) an artificially induced passive state in which there is increased amenability and responsiveness to suggestions and commands. In hypnosis, a drowsy phase is followed by a sleep. It can also be used to produce painless childbirth and tooth extraction.

hypnotherapy (ˌhipnoh'therəpee) treatment by hypnosis or by the induction of prolonged sleep.

hypnotic (hip'notik) an agent that causes sleep; a soporific.

hypnotism ('hipnəˌtizəm) the practice of hypnosis.

hypoaesthesia (ˌhiepoh·əs'theezi·ə) HYPAESTHESIA.

hypoalgesia (ˌhiepoh·al'jeezeeə) HYPALGESIA.

hypobaric (ˌhiepoh'barik) at a pressure lower than normal.

hypocalcaemia (ˌhiepohkal'seemi·ə) a deficiency of calcium in the blood.

hypocapnia (ˌhiepoh'kapni·ə) a deficiency of carbon dioxide in the blood.

hypochloraemia (ˌhiepohklo-

'reemi·ə) a deficiency of chloride in the blood.

hypochlorhydria (ˌhiepohklaw-'hiedri·ə) a less than normal amount of hydrochloric acid in the gastric juice.

hypochlorite (ˌhiepoh'klaw·riet) any salt of hypochlorous acid used in solution to yield chlorine, a disinfecting and germicidal agent. Milton, a proprietary preparation, is used in solution for the disinfection of equipment and infant feeding utensils.

hypochondria (ˌhiepə'kondri·ə) a morbid preoccupation or anxiety about one's health. The sufferer feels that first one part of the body and then another part is the site of some serious disease.

hypochondriac (ˌhiepə'kondriˌak) one affected by hyponchondria. *H. region* the hypochondrium.

hypochondrium (ˌhiepoh'kondri·əm) the upper region of the abdomen on each side of the EPIGASTRIUM.

hypochromic (ˌhiepoh'krohmik) deficient in pigmentation or colouring.

hypodermic (ˌhiepə'dərmik) beneath the skin; applied to subcutaneous injections and to the syringes used for such injections.

hypofibrinogenaemia (ˌhiepohfieˌbrinəjə'neemi·ə) a lack of fibrinogen in the blood. This can occur in severe trauma or haemorrhage or as an inherited condition.

hypogammaglobulinaemia (ˌhiepohˌgaməˌglobyəli'neemi·ə) a deficiency of gamma-globulin in the blood, rendering the person susceptible to infection.

hypogastrium (ˌhiepoh'gastri·əm) the lower middle area of the abdomen, immediately below the umbilical region.

hypoglossal (ˌhiepoh'glosəl) under the tongue. *H. nerve* the 12th cranial nerve.

hypoglycaemia (ˌhiepohglie-'seemi·ə) a condition in which the blood sugar level is less than normal. Usually arising in diabetic patients as a result of insulin overdosage, delay in eating or a rapid combustion of carbohydrate. *See* HYPERGLYCAEMIA.

hypokalaemia (ˌhiepohkə'leemi·ə) a low potassium level in the blood. This is likely to be present in dehydration and with the prolonged use of certain diuretics.

hypomania (ˌhiepoh'mayni·ə) a degree of elation, excitement, and activity higher than normal but less severe than that present in mania.

hypometropia (ˌhiepohme'trohpi·ə) myopia; short-sightedness.

hypomotility (ˌhiepohmoh'tilətee) deficient power of movement in any part.

hyponatraemia (ˌhiepohnə'treemi·ə) a deficiency of sodium in the blood.

hypoparathyroidism (ˌhiepohparə'thieroy·dizəm) a lack of parathyroid secretion, leading to a low blood calcium and tetany.

hypophysis (hie'pofəsəs) an outgrowth. *H. cerebri* the PITUITARY gland.

hypopituitarism (ˌhiepohpi'tyooətəˌrizəm) deficiency of secretion from the anterior lobe of the pituitary gland, causing excessive deposition of fat in children. *See* FRÖLICH'S SYNDROME. Dwarfism can result. In adults, asthenia, drowsiness, and adiposity can occur, together with an impairment of sexual activity and premature senility.

hypoplasia (ˌhiepoh'playzi·ə) imperfect development of a part or organ.

hypopnoea (ˌhiepoh'neeə, -'popni·ə) shallow breathing.

hypoproteinaemia (ˌhiepohˌprohtə'neemi·ə) a deficiency of serum proteins in the blood.

hypoprothrombinaemia (ˌhiepohprohˌthrombə'neemi·ə) a deficiency of prothrombin in the blood, leading to a tendency to bleed. *See also* HAEMOPHILIA.

hypopyon (hie'pohpi·ən) an accumulation of pus in the anterior chamber of the eye.

hyposecretion (ˌhiepohsə'kreeshən) a deficiency in secretion from any glandular structure or secreting cells.

hyposensitivity (ˌhiepohˌsensə'tivətee) a lack of sensitivity, especially to a particular allergen with which the patient might have been overdosed over a period of time.

hypospadias (ˌhiepə'spaydi·əs) a developmental anomaly in the male in which the urethra opens on the underside of the penis or on the perineum. *Female h.* a developmental anomaly in the female in which the urethra opens into the vagina.

hypostasis (ˌhie'postəsəs) 1. a sediment or deposit. 2. congestion of blood in a part, due to slowing of the circulation.

hypostatic (ˌhiepoh'statik) relating to hypostasis. *H. pneumonia see* PNEUMONIA.

hypotension (ˌhiepoh'tenshən) abnormally low arterial blood pressure; hypopiesis. *Controlled* or *induced h.* an artificially produced lowering of the blood pressure so that an operation field is rendered practically bloodless. *Orthostatic* or *postural h.* temporary hypotension when the patient stands up, producing giddiness and sometimes a faint.

hypotensive (ˌhiepoh'tensiv) producing a reduction in tension, especially pertaining to a drug that lowers the blood pressure.

hypothalamus (ˌhiepə'thaləməs) the portion of the DIENCEPHALONS lying beneath the THALAMUS at the base of the CEREBRUM and forming the floor and part of the lateral wall of the third ventricle. It influences peripheral autonomic mechanisms, endocrine activity, and many somatic functions, e.g. a general regulation of water balance, body temperature, sleep, thirst, hunger, and the development of secondary sexual characteristics. It plays an important role in the regulation of protein, fat, and carbohydrate metabolism, body fluid volume and electrolyte content, and internal secretion of endocrine hormones.

hypothermia (ˌhiepoh'thərmi·ə) 1. a severe reduction in the body temperature. The condition usually arises gradually and can be fatal if untreated. It is most common among babies and elderly people. 2. artificial cooling of the body to reduce the oxygen requirements of the tissues. *Mild h.* a reduction of the body temperature to 34°C, which can be induced by surface cooling with cold air. Generalised lowering of the body temperature is used in three main situations: (a) to control fever, as in malignant HYPERTHERMIA; (b) to enable certain cardiac and neurological operations to be carried out; and (c) to protect the brain from raised intracranial pressure in patients with head injuries or following drowning.

hypothesis (hie'pothəsəs) a supposition that appears to explain a group of phenomena and is assumed as a basis of reasoning and experimentation. A starting point for further investigations from known facts. *Null h.* a statement that there is no relationship between the variables and that any relationship observed is a function of chance or fluctuation in sampling.

hypothrombinaemia (ˌhiepoh-ˌthrombə'neemi·ə) a diminished amount of thrombin in the blood, with a consequent tendency to bleed.

hypothyroidism (ˌhiepoh'thieroy-dizəm) an insufficiency of thyroid secretion. In children, it can produce cretinism. In adults, it leads to MYXOEDEMA.

hypotonia (ˌhiepoh'tohni·ə) 1. deficient muscle tone. 2. deficient tension in the eyeball.

hypotonic (ˌhiepoh'tonik) describing a solution that has a lower osmotic pressure than another one. *See* HYPERTONIC.

hypoventilation (ˌhiepohˌventə-'layshən) hypopnoea; shallow breathing, usually at a very slow rate. It can cause a build-up of carbon dioxide in the blood.

hypovolaemia (ˌhiepohvo'leemi·ə) a reduction in the circulating blood volume due to external loss of body fluids or to loss from the blood into the tissues, as in shock.

hypoxaemia (ˌhiepok'seemi·ə) an insufficient oxygen content in the blood.

hypoxia (hie'poksi·ə) a diminished amount of oxygen in the tissues. *Anaemic h.* low oxygen content due to deficiency of haemoglobin in the blood.

hystera (hi'sterə) [Gk.] *the uterus.*

hysteralgia (ˌhistə'ralji·ə) pain in the uterus.

hysterectomy (ˌhistə'rektəmee) removal of the uterus. *Abdominal h.* removal via an abdominal incision. *Subtotal h.* removal of the body of the uterus only. *Total h.* removal of the body of the uterus and the cervix. *Vaginal h.* removal through the vagina. *Wertheim's h.* additional excision of the PARAMETRIUM, upper vagina, and lymph glands. Radical abdominal hysterectomy.

hysteria (his'tiə·ri·ə) a psychoneurosis in which the individual converts anxiety created by emotional conflict into physical symptoms, e.g. tics, mutism, or paralysis of an arm or leg, that have no organic basis; called also conversion reaction or conversion hysteria. The term 'hysteria' is also used to describe a state of tension or excitement in which there is a temporary loss of control over the emotions.

hysterical (hi'sterikəl) relating to hysteria.

hysterocele (ˌhistə·rohseel) a hernia containing part of the uterus.

hysteromyoma (ˌhistə·rohmie-'ohmə) a FIBROMYOMA of the uterus.

hysteromyomectomy (ˌhistə·roh-ˌmieə'mektəmee) excision of a hysteromyoma.

hystero-oöphorectomy (ˌhistə·roh-ˌoh·əfə'rektəmee) excision of the uterus and the ovaries.

hysterosalpingography (ˌhistə·roh-ˌsalping'gogrəfee) radiographic examination of the uterus and uterine tubes after the injection of a radio-opaque dye. Utero-salpingography. This procedure has been replaced with laparoscopy and subsequent hysteroscopic procedures. *See* HYSTEROSCOPY.

hysterosalpingostomy (ˌhistə·roh-ˌsalping'gostəmee) the establishment of an opening between the distal portion of the uterine tube and the uterus in an effort to overcome infertility when the medial portion is occluded or excised.

hysteroscopy (ˌhistə'roskəpee) inspection of the interior of the uterus with an endoscope.

hysterotomy (ˌhistə'rotəmee) incision of the uterus, usually in order to remove a fetus in mid pregnancy when it is too late to perform a therapeutic abortion. *See* CAESAREAN SECTION.

Ii

I symbol for *iodine*.

iatrogenic (ie,atroh'jenik) brought about by surgical or medical treatment, e.g. unwanted effects of drugs.

ibuprofen (ie,byooproh,fen) a nonsteroidal anti-inflammatory analgesic and antipyretic drug used in the treatment of mild rheumatic and arthritic conditions.

ice (ies) water in a solid state, at or below freezing point. *I. bag* a rubber or plastic bag half-filled with pieces of ice and applied near or to a part to relieve pain or swelling. *Dry i.* carbon dioxide snow.

ichthammol ('ikthə,mol) an ammoniated coal tar product, used in ointment form for certain skin diseases.

ichthyosis (,ikthee'ohsəs) a congenital abnormality of the skin in which there is dryness and roughness, the horny layer is thickened and large scales appear.

ICM International Confederation of Midwives.

ICN International Council of Nurses.

ICP intracranial pressure.

ICSH interstitial cell stimulating hormone.

icterus (iktə·rəs) jaundice. *I. gravis* a fatal form of jaundice occurring in pregnancy. Acute yellow atrophy. *I. gravis neonatorum* haemolytic disease of the newborn. *See* RHESUS FACTOR.

id (id) that part of the personality, containing the instinctive drives, which leads to gratification of primitive needs and which exists in the unconscious.

IDDM insulin dependent diabetes mellitus.

idea (ie'diə) a mental impression or conception. *Autochthonous i.* a strange idea that comes into the mind in some unaccountable way, but is not an hallucination. *Compulsive i.* an idea that persists despite reason and will and that drives one to action, usually inappropriate. *Dominant i.* a morbid or other impression that controls or colours every action and thought. *Fixed i.* a persistent morbid impression or belief that cannot be changed by reason. *I. of reference* the incorrect idea that the words and actions of others refer to one's self, or the projection of the causes of one's own imaginary difficulties upon someone else.

identical (ie'dentikəl) exactly alike. *I. twins* twins of the same sex developing from a single fertilised ovum.

identification (ie,dentəfə'kayshən)

a mental mechanism by which an individual adopts the attitudes and ideas of another, often admired, person.

identity (ie'dentətee) part of the 'self concept' of being distinguishable and separate from others. *I. crisis* one in which the individual loses their sense of self-distinctiveness and role in society. Occurs most commonly in the transition from one phase of life to the next, e.g. during adolescence.

ideomotion (ˌiedeeoh'mohshən) the association of ideas and muscle action, as in involuntary acts.

idiopathic (ˌideeoh'pathik) self-originated; applied to a condition with no known cause.

idiosyncrasy (ˌideeoh'singkrəsee) 1. a habit or quality of body or mind peculiar to any individual. 2. an abnormal susceptibility to an agent (e.g. a drug) that is peculiar to the individual.

idoxuridine abbreviated **IDU** (ˌie-doks'yoo·rədeen) an iodine-containing drug used to treat infections caused by herpes virus, particularly keratitis and corneal dendritic ulcer.

ileal ('ili·əl) referring to the ileum. *I. conduit* a surgical procedure in which the ureters are transplanted into the ileum, an isolated loop of which is then brought to the surface of the abdomen to allow the urine to drain into a bag.

ileitis (ˌil'ietəs) inflammation of the ILEUM. *Regional i.* Crohn's disease. A chronic condition of the terminal portion of the ileum in which granulation and oedema can give rise to obstruction.

ileocolitis (ˌileeohkə'lietəs) inflammation of the ileum and colon.

ileocolostomy (ˌileeohkə'lostəmee) the making of a permanent opening between the ileum and some part of the colon.

ileocystoplasty (ˌileeoh'sistoh-ˌplastee) repair of the wall of the urinary bladder with an isolated segment of the ileum.

ileoproctostomy (ˌileeohprok-'tostəmee) surgical anastomosis between the ileum and the rectum; ILEORECTAL anastomosis.

ileorectal (ˌileeoh'rekt'l) referring to the ileum and rectum. *I. anastomosis* ILEOPROCTOSTOMY.

ileostomy (ˌilee'ostəmee) an artificial opening (stoma) created from the ileum and brought to the surface of the abdomen for the purpose of evacuation. Ileostomy is an inevitable part of PROCTOCOLECTOMY. An ileostomy can be temporary or permanent. *I. bags* disposable bags to collect the liquid faecal matter discharged from an ileostomy. The bags can be adhesive or worn on a belt.

ileum ('ili·əm) the last part of the small intestine, terminating at the caecum.

ileus ('ili·əs) a failure of intestinal peristalsis that can cause intestinal obstruction if it does not resolve. The failure of peristalsis results from disturbances in neural stimulation of the bowel, and can be due to a variety of causes including handling of the bowel during abdominal surgery, peritonitis, mesenteric ischaemia, retroperitoneal or intra-abdominal hematomata, and metabolic disturbances (e.g., hypokalemia). The principal signs and symptoms of intestinal obstruction due to ileus are abdominal pain and distension, vomiting (the vomitus can contain faecal material), and constipation. If the intestinal obstruction does not resolve or is not relieved, the patient becomes extremely ill with SHOCK and DEHYDRATION.

iliac ('ilee,ak) pertaining to the ilium. *I. artery* the right and left iliac arteries are the terminal branches of the abdominal aorta and supply blood to the pelvic region and the lower limbs. *I. crest* the crest of the hip bone. *I. fossa* the depression on the concave surface of the iliac bone. *I. vein* the right and left veins join to form the inferior VENA CAVA and drain the blood from the lower limbs and pelvis.

ilium ('ili·əm) the haunch bone; the upper part of the hip bone.

illness ('ilnəs) a condition marked by pronounced deviation from the normal healthy state; sickness. *I. behaviour* the way in which ill individuals regard the structure and function of their own bodies, interpret symptoms, and seek treatment for their conditions. *I experience* the process of being ill

illusion (i'loozhən) a mistaken perception due to a misinterpretation of a sensory stimulus; believing something to be what it is not.

image ('imij) 1. the mental recall of a former precept. 2. the optical picture transferred to the brain cells by the optic nerve.

imago (i'maygoh, i'mahgoh) [L.] 1. in psychoanalysis, a childhood memory or fantasy of a loved person that persists in adult life. 2. the adult or definitive form of an insect.

imbalance (im'baləns) lack of balance, e.g. of endocrine secretions, between water and electrolytes, or of muscles.

imipramine (i'miprə,meen) a drug, chemically related to chlorpromazine, that can be effective in relieving depression. *See* ANTIDEPRESSANT. Also used to treat nocturnal ENURESIS in children.

immature (,imə'tyooə, -chyooə) unripe; not fully developed, as a cataract when only a part of the lens is opaque.

immiscible (i'misəbəl) incapable of being mixed, e.g. oil and water.

immobilise (i'mohbə,liez) to render incapable of being moved, as by a plaster of Paris cast.

immune (i'myoon) protected against a particular infection or allergy. *I. reaction, i. response* 1. the reaction to and interaction with substances interpreted by the body as not-self which causes a body to reject a transplanted organ. 2. formation of a papule and AREOLA without development of a vesicle after smallpox vaccination.

immunity (i'myoonətee) the resistance possessed by the body to infectious diseases, foreign tissues, foreign non-toxic substances, and other ANTIGENS. *Acquired i.* is produced specifically in response to an ANTIGEN. It involves a change in the behaviour of cells and in the production of antibody. Antibody is produced as a primary response and, after a short time, the body becomes sensitised. The secondary response is produced more quickly and is more marked. *Active i.* this can be (a) natural, i.e. from infectious diseases, or (b) artificial, i.e. from injection of living or dead organisms or their products in the form of toxins and toxoids. *Passive i.* this can be: (a) natural, e.g.

maternal IMMUNOGLOBULIN G (IgG) via the placenta protects the infant from various infectious diseases for a few months, but undesirable antibodies such as anti-D immunoglobulin can also be transmitted to the fetus; or (b) acquired, e.g. the temporary immunity that follows the injection of antibodies of human origin (gamma globulin) or, more rarely, animal origin. *Natural* or *innate i.* is mainly non-specific. It is provided by intact cellular barriers of epithelium and by humoral substances such as COMPLEMENT and LYSOZYME. It is affected by genetic factors, age, race, and hormone levels.

immunisation (ˌimyənie'zayshən) the act of creating immunity by artificial means. *I. schedule* a standard schedule for immunisation against infectious diseases (*see* Appendix 8).

immunoassay (ˌimyənoh'asay) a quantitative estimate of the proteins contained in the blood serum.

immunodeficiency (ˌimyənohdə'fishənsee) a deficiency of the immune response, either that mediated by humoral antibody or that mediated by immune lymphoid cells. *I. disorders* acquired or congenital conditions in which the body's immune system fails to protect against infection, foreign material, and some forms of cancer.

immunoglobulin (ˌimyənoh'globyələn) antibody. A variety of chemical compounds found mainly in gamma-globulin (*see* GAMMA GLOBULIN). Types are as follows: (a) immunoglobulin G (IgG) is small and crosses the placental barrier; (b) immunoglobulin M (IgM) is composed of large molecules; (c) immunoglobulin A (IgA) is produced in secretions, colostrum, and breast milk. It lines the gut and, with LACTOFERRIN, promotes the growth of non-pathogenic lactobacilli and inhibits pathogens; (d) immunoglobulin D (IgD), the function of which is not yet known; (e) immunoglobulin E (IgE), responsible for atopic hypersensitivity, often called allergy.

immunology (ˌimyə'noləjee) the study of immunity and the body's defence mechanisms.

immunosuppression (ˌimyənohsə'preshən) inhibition of the formation of antibodies to antigens; used in transplantation procedures to prevent rejection of the transplanted organ or tissue.

immunosuppressive (ˌimyənohsə'presiv) 1. pertaining to or inducing immunosuppression. 2. an agent that induces immunosuppression.

immunotherapy (ˌimyənoh'therəpee) 1. treatment by immunisation. Sometimes used in the treatment of leukaemia. 2. the establishing of passive immunity.

immunotransfusion (iˌmyoonoh-trans'fyoozhən, -trahns-) transfusion of blood from a donor previously rendered immune to the disease affecting the patient.

Imodium (i'mohdeeəm) trade name for preparations of loperamide hydrochloride, an antidiarrhoeal.

impaction (im'pakshən) a state of being wedged. *Dental i.* the condition in which a tooth, usually a molar, is unable to erupt through the gum because it is lodged in position by bone or the other teeth. *Faecal i.* a collection of putty-like or hardened faeces in the rectum or sigmoid.

impairment (im'pairmənt) any loss

or abnormality of psychological, physiological, or anatomical structure or function.

impalpable (im'palpəbəl) incapable of being felt by manual examination. Can apply to an organ or a tumour.

imperforate (im'pərfə·rət) without an opening. *I. anus* a congenital defect in which this opening is closed. *I. hymen* complete closure of the vaginal opening by the hymen. *See* CRYPTOMENORRHOEA.

impermeable (im'pərmi·əbəl) not permitting the passage of fluid or molecules.

impetigo (ˌimpə'tiegoh) an acute contagious inflammation of the skin marked by pustules and scabs; of streptococcal or staphylococcal origin. It occurs mainly on the face and limbs, particularly those of children.

implant (im'plahnt, 'implahnt, -ant) any substance grafted into the tissues. *Hormone i.* a hormonal pellet which can be implanted subcutaneously. *Intraocular lens **i.*** a plastic lens which can be implanted in the eye after lens extraction. *Plastic **i.*** a silicone implant can be used in plastic surgery, e.g. to reshape the breast.

implantation (ˌimplahn'tayshən, -plan-) the act of planting or setting in. 1. the embedding of the fertilised ovum in the wall of the uterus. 2. the placing of a drug within the tissues. 3. the surgical introduction of healthy tissue to replace tissue that has been damaged.

implementation (ˌimpləmen'tayshən) the third phase of the nursing process signifying the giving of care in relation to defined nursing interventions and goals. During implementation, the nursing care plan is tested for effectiveness and accuracy. Data gathering continues and plans can change on the basis of new information obtained. The implementation phase concludes with the recording of the activities performed and the response of the patient. *See* ASSESSMENT and EVALUATION.

implosion (im'plohzhən) in behavioural therapy, a form of desensitisation used in the treatment of phobias and related disorders. *See* FLOODING.

impotence ('impətəns) inability in a man to carry out sexual intercourse as a result of psychological or physical causes.

impregnation (ˌimpreg'nayshən) insemination; rendering pregnant.

impulse ('impuls) 1. a sudden pushing force. 2. a sudden uncontrollable act. 3. nerve impulse. *Cardiac i.* movement of the chest wall caused by the heartbeat. *Nerve i.* the electrochemical process propagated along nerve fibres.

IMV intermittent mandatory ventilation.

in situ (in'sityoo) [L.] *in the original position.*

in vitro (in'veetroh, -'vit-) [L.] *in a glass.* Refers to observations made outside the body. For example in an artificial environment such as a laboratory. *Compare* IN VIVO.

in vitro fertilisation (IVF) a method of fertilisating human ova outside the body by collecting the mature ova and placing them in a dish with a sample of spermatozoa. After fertilisation the ova are injected into the uterus via the cervix.

in vivo (in'veevoh) [L.] *within the living body. Compare* IN VITRO.

inaccessibility (ˌinəkˌsesə'bilətee) state of unresponsiveness characteristic of certain psychiatric patients, e.g. schizophrenics.

inarticulate (ˌinah'tikyələt) 1. without joints. 2. unable to speak intelligibly.

incarcerated (in'kahsəˌraytəd) held fast. Applied to: (a) a hernia that is immovable, and therefore curable only by operation; and (b) a pregnant uterus held under the sacral brim.

incest ('insest) sexual intercourse between close blood relatives, e.g. brothers and sisters; marriage between them is legally or culturally prohibited. Some form of incest taboo is found in all known societies, although the relationships that are prohibited vary.

incident ('insədənt) undesirable event that results in injury to people, or loss or damage of property.

incidence ('insədəns) the number of particular new events which occur in a population in a given period of time. For example, the number of new cases of a disease, such as measles, expressed per 1000 of population per year.

incipient (in'sipi·ənt) beginning to exist.

incision (in'sizhən) 1. in surgery, a cut into soft tissue. 2. the act of cutting.

incisor (in'siezə) one of the four front teeth in the centre of each jaw.

inclusion (ing'kloozhən) something that is enclosed or the act of enclosing. *I. bodies* particles that are temporarily enclosed in the cytoplasm of a cell. For example, in trachoma, virus particles can be seen in the conjunctival epithelial cells.

incoherent (ingkoh'hiə·rənt) 1. unconnected; inconsistent. 2. uttering speech that is disconnected and rambling.

incompatibility (ˌingkəmpatə'biliətee) the state of two or more substances being antagonistic, or destroying the efficiency of each other. Applied to mixtures of drugs, and to blood. *See* BLOOD GROUP.

incompetence (ing'kompətəns) inefficiency. *Aortic i.* failure of the aortic valves to regulate the flow of blood. *Mitral i.* failure of the mitral valve to close properly.

incontinence (ing'kontənəns) inability to control natural functions or discharges. *Faecal i.* inability to control the movements of the bowels. *Overflow i.* that from an overfull bladder, most common in elderly men with urinary obstruction. *Paralytic i.* loss of control of anal and urethral sphincters due to injury to nerve centres. *Stress i.* that which is due to a defect in the urethral sphincters and is liable to occur when intra-abdominal pressure is increased, as in coughing or lifting heavy weights; most common in women with weak pelvic muscles. *Urinary i.* inability to control the outflow of urine.

incoordination (ˌingkohˌawdə-nay'shən) inability to adjust harmoniously various muscle movements.

incrustation (ˌinkru'stayshən) the formation of a crust or scab on a wound.

incubation (ˌingkyə'bayshən) the development and growth of microorganisms and animal embryos. *I. period* the period between the date of infection and the appearance of symptoms of an infectious disease.

incubator ('ingkyəˌbaytə) 1. a warmed servo-controlled Perspex box for nursing ill and preterm babies. 2. an apparatus used to develop bacteria at a uniform temperature suitable to their growth.

incus ('ingkəs) the small anvil-shaped bone of the middle ear. The second auditory ossicle.

indicator ('ində,kaytə) 1. the index finger, or the extensor muscle of the index finger. 2. any substance that indicates the appearance or disappearance of a chemical by a colour change or attainment of a certain pH.

indigenous (in'dijənəs) occurring naturally in a certain locality.

indigestion (,indi'jeschən) *See* DYSPEPSIA.

indolent ('indələnt) slow growing. Reluctant to heal. Largely painless. *I. ulcer* a chronic ulcer of the skin or mucous membrane.

indomethacin (,indoh'methəsən) an anti-inflammatory analgesic used in the treatment of arthritis and of acute attacks of gout.

induction (in'dukshən) the act of initiating something. *I. of abortion* the intentional bringing about of an abortion. *I. of anaesthesia* the start of the administration of a general anaesthetic. *Electromagnetic i.* the production of an electric current in a body because of its nearness to an electrified (or magnetised) body. *I. of labour* the artificial starting of the process of childbirth.

induration (,indyə'rayshən) the abnormal hardening of a tissue or organ.

inebriation (i,neebree'ayshən) the condition of being intoxicated by alcohol; drunkenness.

inert (i'nərt) having no action. *I. gas* a gas that does not react with other elements, e.g. neon.

inertia (i'nərshə) sluggishness; inability to move except when stimulated by an external force. *Uterine i.* lack of muscle contraction during the first and second stages of labour.

infant ('infənt) a child under 1 year of age. Educationally, a child under 7 years of age. *I. feeding* the supplying of nutrition to an infant. Breast milk is the ideal food for a baby, and if breastfeeding is established satisfactorily for the first few months, it can aid physical and emotional development. If breast-feeding is not possible, an infant food formula can be given. *Floppy i., floppy i. syndrome* a congenital myopathy of infants, marked clinically by MYOTONIA and muscle weakness. *I. mortality rate* the number of deaths of children under 1 year of age per 1000 live births in any one year. *Premature i.* one born before the state of maturity. *See* PRETERM INFANT.

infanticide (in'fantə,sied) the killing of a child during the first year of its life.

infantile ('infən,tiel) concerning an infant; childish. *I. paralysis* POLIOMYELITIS.

infantilism (in'fantə,lizəm) persistence of the characters of childhood into adult life, marked by under-development of the reproductive organs, and often short stature.

infarct ('infahkt) the wedge-shaped area of necrosis in an organ produced by the blocking of a blood vessel, usually due to an embolus. *Red i.* a haemorrhage infarct. Red blood cells infiltrate the area. *White i.* an anaemic infarct. The area is suddenly deprived of blood and is pale.

infarction (in'fahkshən) the formation of an infarct. *Myocardial i.* an infarct of the heart muscle following a coronary THROMBOSIS. *Pulmonary i.* an infarct resulting from obstruction of a branch of the pulmonary artery by EMBOLISM or thrombosis.

infection (in'fekshən) 1. invasion and multiplication of microorganisms in body tissues, especially that causing local cellular injury due to competitive metabolism, toxins, intracellular replication, or antigen–antibody response. 2. an infectious disease. *Airborne i.* infection by inhalation of organisms suspended in air on water droplets, droplet nuclei, or dust particles. *Anaerobic i.* infection caused by an ANAEROBE. *I. control* the utilisation of procedures and techniques in the surveillance, investigation, and compilation of statistical data in order to reduce the spread of infection, particularly hospital-acquired infections. *Cross i.* infection transmitted between patients infected with different pathogenic microorganisms. *Droplet i.* infection due to inhalation of respiratory pathogens suspended on liquid particles exhaled by someone already infected. *Dustborne i.* infection by inhalation of pathogens that have become affixed to particles of dust. *Hospital-acquired i's* those acquired during hospitalisation; called also nosocomial infections. The most common causative agents are *Escherichia coli*, *Proteus*, *Pseudomonas*, and *Klebsiella*, among the Gram-negative organisms, and *Staphylococcus* and *Enterococcus* among the Gram-positive organisms. *See also* INFECTION control. *Mixed i.* infection with more than one kind of organism at the same time. *Secondary i.* infection by a pathogen superimposed upon an infection by a pathogen of another kind. *Subclinical i.* infection associated with no detectable symptoms but caused by microorganisms capable of producing easily recognisable diseases, such as poliomyelitis or mumps; it is detected by the production of antibody, or by delayed hypersensitivity exhibited in a skin test reaction to such antigens as TUBERCULOPROTEIN.

infectious (in'fekshəs) caused by or capable of being communicated by infection (*see* table). *I. disease* disease resulting from multiplication of microorganisms in the body. Most are communicable, but not all. *See also* COMMUNICABLE DISEASE. *I. mononucleosis* (glandular fever) an acute virus infection, characterised by sore throat and glandular enlargement, caused by the Epstein–Barr (EB) virus. Worldwide common infection particularly prevalent in older children and young adults in Western countries. The source of infection is human and spread is by oropharyngeal secretions, for example, during kissing. The incubation period is 4–6 weeks and infectivity after the disease can be prolonged.

infective (in'fektiv) infectious, capable of producing infection; pertaining to or characterised by the presence of pathogens.

inferior (in'fiə·ri·ə) lower. *I. vena cava* the lower large vein.

inferiority (in,fiə·ri'orətee) lesser

Common Infectious Diseases

Disease	*Incubation period (days)*	*Period of infectivity*
Chickenpox (varicella)	14–21	Up to 5 days before until 5 days after onset of rash
Diphtheria	2–7	Until culture of three consecutive nose swabs proves negative
Enteric fevers Typhoid Paratyphoid	6–21	Until at least 1 month after onset of disease and stool cultures are negative
Measles (morbilli)	6–12	4 days before until 4 days after onset of rash
Mumps (parotitis)	12–25	6 days before until up to 9 days after onset of swelling
Whooping cough (pertussis)	7–14	7 days before until 3 weeks after onset of cough
German measles (rubella)	14–21	During incubation period until 2 days after resolution of symptoms

rank, stature, position or ability. *I. complex see* COMPLEX.

infertility (ˌinfər'tilətee) inability of a woman to conceive or of a man to bring about conception.

infestation (ˌinfe'stayshən) the presence of animal parasites, e.g. mites, ticks or worms, in or on the body, in clothing or in a house.

infiltration (ˌinfəl'trayshən) the entrance and diffusion of some substance not usually found there, either fluid or solid, into tissues or cells. *I. analgesia* the injection into tissues of a local analgesic solution.

inflammation (ˌinflə'mayshən) a localised protective response elicited by injury or destruction of tissues, which serves to destroy, dilute, or wall off both the injurious agent and the injured tissue. The cardinal signs are heat, swelling, pain, and redness. *Acute i.* sudden onset of inflammation, with marked and progressive symptoms. *Catarrhal i.* inflammation in which mucous surfaces are attacked, with stimulation of exudation. *Chronic i.* inflammation that develops slowly. Granulation tissue forms and tends to localise the infection. *Diffuse i.* extensive inflammation, as in NEPHRITIS and CELLULITIS. *Suppurative i.* one marked by pus formation. *Traumatic i.* that which follows an injury.

influenza (ˌinfloo'enzə) an acute viral infection of the respiratory tract, occurring in isolated cases, epidemics, and pandemics. Called also 'flu. Transmission is by droplet inhalation and the period of infectivity lasts from 1 day before the onset of symptoms until up to 7 days later. Most cases occur in winter. There is fever, headache, pain in the back and limbs, anorexia and, sometimes, nausea and vomiting. The fever subsides in 2–3 days, leaving a feeling of lassitude. There is no specific drug cure for influenza, but an influenza vaccine is available, the formulation of which is changed annually to include recently circulating strains of viruses on recommendation of the WHO. Annual vaccination is advised for persons with chronic heart, lung, or renal disease, those with diabetes, patients on immunosuppressive therapy, and for elderly people living in residential and nursing homes.

informed consent (in'fawmd kən'sent) an ethical principle that requires a researcher to obtain voluntary participation of subjects in research, or a healthcare practitioner to obtain voluntary consent from a patient before undergoing a clinical or surgical procedure. In both cases, the person providing consent must be given full advice regarding the nature of the research or procedure, the risks involved, the chances of success, and the alternative methods of research or treatment that are available. *See also* CONSENT.

infra-red (ˌinfrə'red) rays of a lower wavelength than those in the visible spectrum. They can produce radiant heat which is used in the treatment of rheumatic conditions. *See* ULTRAVIOLET RAYS.

infusion (in'fyoozhən) 1. the process of extracting the soluble principles of substances (especially drugs) by soaking in water. 2. the solution thus produced. 3. the slow therapeutic introduction by gravity of fluid other than blood into a vein.

infundibulum *pl* **infundibula** (ˌinfuhn'dibyələm; -ələ) a general anatomical term for a funnel-shaped structure or passage, such as the cavity formed by the fimbriae tubae at the distal end of the fallopian tube; the stalk that extends from the hypothalamas to the posterior lobe of the pituitary gland; passage connecting the middle meatus of the nose with the frontal sinus.

ingestion (in'jeschən) the taking in of food and drugs by mouth.

inguinal ('ing·gwin'l) relating to the groin. *I. canal* the channel through the abdominal wall, above POUPART'S LIGAMENT, through which the spermatic cord and vessels pass to the testis in the male, and which contains the round ligament of the uterus in the female. *I. ligament* Poupart's ligament; that connecting the anterior superior spine of the ilium to the tubercle of the pubis.

inhalation (ˌinhə'layshən) 1. the drawing of air or other substances into the lungs. 2. any drug or solution of drugs, administered (as by means of nebulisers or aerosols) by the nasal or oral respiratory route.

inhaler (in'haylə) an apparatus used for administering an inhalation.

inherent (in'hiə·rənt -'her-) a characteristic that is innate or natural and essentially a part of the person.

inheritance (in'herətəns) the acquisition of qualities and characteristics from parents and ancestors.

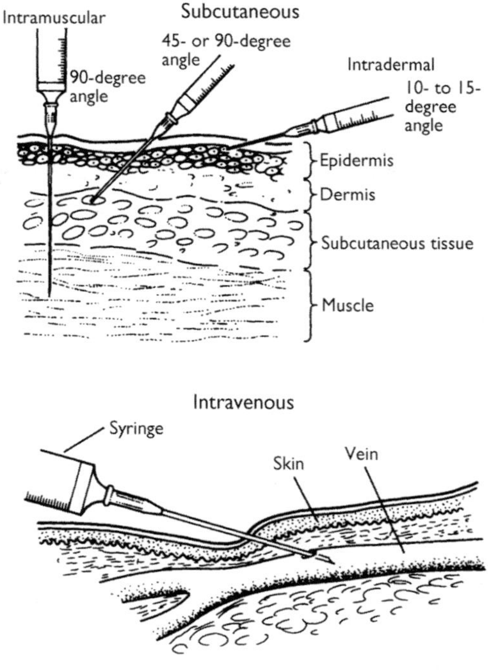

Intramuscular, Subcutaneous, Intradermal and Intravenous Injections

inhibition (ˌinhəˈbishən) arrest or restraint of a process. In psychiatry, the unconscious restraining of an instinctual drive.

injection (inˈjekshən) 1. the forcing of a liquid into a part, as into the subcutaneous tissues, the vascular tree or an organ (*see* figure). 2. a substance so forced or administered; in pharmacy, a solution of a medicament suitable for injection. 3. prominence of small blood vessels on the surface of an organ or tissue, frequently indicating the vascular phase of an inflammatory response. *Hypodermic i.* that made just below the skin; a subcutaneous injection. *Intramuscular* *i.* that made into a muscle. *Intrathecal i.* that made into the subarachnoid space of the spinal cord. *Intravenous i.* that made into a vein. *Subcutaneous i.* that made into the subcutaneous tissues; a hypodermic injection.

inlay ('in͵lay) material inserted to replace a defect in a tissue, for example, a bone graft or a filling cast in metal to fit a hole in a tooth.

innate (i'nayt) inborn; present in the individual at birth.

innervation (͵inə'vayshən) nerve supply to a part.

innocent ('inəsənt) as applied to a tumour, benign or non-malignant.

innocuous (i'nokyooəs) harmless.

innominate (i'nomənət) unnamed. *I. artery* a branch of the aorta, now termed the brachiocephalic trunk. *I. bone* the hip bone, formed by the union of the ilium, ischium, and pubis.

inoculation (i͵nokyə'layshən) 1. introduction of pathogenic micro-organisms, injected material, serum, or other substances into tissues of living organisms or into culture media. 2. introduction of a disease agent (usually a live infectious agent) into a healthy individual to produce a mild form of the disease, followed by IMMUNITY.

inorganic (͵inaw'ganik) of neither animal nor vegetable origin.

inositol (i'nohsə͵tol) a form of muscle or plant carbohydrate that has the same formula as simple sugar but not its other properties. *I. nicotinate* a vasodilator used in peripheral vascular disease.

inotropic (͵ienə'trohpik, -tropik) affecting the force or energy of muscular contractions, particularly the heart muscle. Beta-blocking drugs are said to be inotropic.

inquest (͵ingkwest) a legal inquiry held by a coroner, with or without a jury, into the cause of sudden or unexpected death.

insanity (in'sanətee) a legal term for mental illness, roughly equivalent to PSYCHOSIS and implying inability to be responsible for one's acts.

insecticide (in'sektə͵sied) one of a large group of chemical compounds that kill insect pests.

insemination (in͵semə'nayshən) 1. fertilisation of an ovum by a SPERMATOZOON. 2. introduction of semen into the vagina. *Artificial i.* insemination by means other than sexual intercourse. The semen can be either the husband's (AIH) or some other donor's (AID).

insensible (in'sensəbəl) 1. unable to perceive with the senses. 2. unconscious. 3. imperceptible to the senses.

insertion (in'sərshən) 1. the act of implanting. 2. something that is implanted. 3. the attachment of a muscle to the bone that it moves.

insidious (in'sidi·əs) describing a gradual or subtle development. A term applied to a disease (for example, glaucoma) in which symptoms develop gradually and are undetected by the person until the disease is well established.

insight ('in͵siet) mental awareness. The capacity of individuals to estimate a situation or their own behaviour, or the connection between their present attitudes and past experiences. In psychiatry, a recognition by the patient that he or she is ill. Insight in this connection can be complete, partial, or absent, and can alter during the course of the illness.

insoluble (in'solyəbəl) not capable of being dissolved in a liquid.

insomnia (in'somni·ə) inability to sleep.

inspiration (inspə'rayshən) the act of drawing in the breath.

inspissated (in'spisaytəd) thickened, through evaporation or absorption of fluid.

instillation (ˌinstə'layshən) the act of pouring a liquid into a cavity drop by drop, e.g. into the eye.

instinct ('instingkt) a complex of unlearnt responses characteristic of a species. *Death i.* in psychoanalysis, the latent instinctive impulse towards death; the drive to reduce tensions by reaching the ultimate tensionless state of death. *Herd i.* the instinct or urge to be one of a group and to conform to its standards of conduct and opinion.

institutionalisation (instəˌtyoo-shənəlie'zayshən) a condition of apathy and withdrawal occurring in residents of long-stay institutions, prisons, etc., as a result of rigid routines and lack of independence. The person might resist leaving because the routine has become predictable and familiar, making minimal demands.

insufficiency (ˌinsə'fishənsee) inadequacy. Used to describe the failure of function of an organ, such as the heart, stomach, liver, or muscles.

insufflation (ˌinsə'flayshən) the act of blowing air, gas, or powder into a cavity of the body.

insulin ('insyələn) a protein hormone formed in the beta cells of the pancreatic ISLETS OF LANGERHANS. The major fuel-regulating hormone, it is secreted into the blood in response to a rise in concentration of blood glucose or amino acids. A deficiency results in DIABETES mellitus. Various types of commercially prepared insulin are available. There are three main groups: rapid acting, intermediate acting, and long acting. Diabetic patients react differently in the rate at which they absorb and utilise insulin, and the duration of action therefore varies from patient to patient. Insulin is measured in units. The concentration used is 100 units/mL. This strength allows for accurate measurement of dosage and reduces the possibility of error in calculating an individual dose. *I. pump* a device consisting of a syringe filled with a predetermined amount of short-acting insulin, a plastic cannula and a needle, and a pump that periodically delivers the desired amount of insulin.

insulin dependent diabetes mellitus (IDDM) an inability to metabolise carbohydrate that requires insulin replacement by injection.

insulin sensitivity test a test used to determine the body's response to HYPOGLYCAEMIA induced by a small intravenous dose of insulin. It is used to test anterior pituitary function, particularly the ability to secrete growth hormone.

insulinase ('insyələˌnayz) an enzyme that destroys the action of insulin.

insulinoma (ˌinsyələ'nohmə) a benign adenoma of the islet cells of the pancreas, causing HYPOGLYCAEMIA.

insult ('insult) any trauma, irritation, poisoning, or injury to the body.

integument (in'tegyəmənt) 1. the skin. 2. a layer of tissue covering a part or organ of the body.

intellect ('intə'lekt) the mind, thinking faculty, or understanding.

intelligence (in'teləjəns) 1. the capacity to understand. 2. general mental ability. *I. quotient* abbreviated IQ. The ratio of the mental age to the chronological age expressed as a percentage. *I. test* a test designed to measure the level of intelligence, usually expressed as an IQ.

intensive care unit (in'tensiv) abbreviated ICU. A hospital unit in which is concentrated special equipment and specially trained personnel for the care of seriously ill patients requiring immediate and continuous monitoring and treatment. Called also critical care unit (CCU) or intensive therapy unit (ITU). *Neonatal icu* (NICU) an intensive care unit that is designated solely for small, preterm neonates and those neonates requiring surgery or other specialised care.

intention (in'tenshən) a process of healing.

intercellular (ˌintə'selyələ) between the cells of a structure. Can be applied to the connective tissue or to fluid bathing the cells.

intercostal (ˌintə'kost'l) between the ribs. *I. muscles* muscles situated between the ribs and controlling their movements during inspiration and expiration.

intercourse ('intəˌkaws) 1. social exchange. 2. COITUS.

intercurrent (ˌintə'kurənt) occurring at the same time. Describes a disease occurring during the course of another disease in the same person.

interdisciplinary (ˌintə'disəplənəree) joint working between professional disciplines.

interferon (ˌintə'fie·ron) a protein, produced by cells infected by a virus, which has an inhibitory effect on the multiplication of the invading viruses.

interlobular (ˌintə'lobyələ) between lobules. *I. veins* branches of the portal vein in the liver.

intermenstrual (ˌintə'menstrooəl) occurring between two menstrual periods.

intermission (ˌintə'mishən) a temporary interruption, particularly of a feverish condition.

intermittent (ˌintə'mitənt) occurring at intervals. *I. claudication See* CLAUDICATION. *I. fever* one in which the temperature drops to normal or lower, at times. *I. mandatory ventilation* abbreviated IMV. A type of mechanical ventilation in which the VENTILATOR is set to deliver a prescribed tidal volume at specified intervals and a high-flow gas system permits the patient to breathe spontaneously between cycles. *I. positive airway ventilation* abbreviated IPAV. A method of assisted ventilation in which oxygen or air is used under pressure to inflate the lungs when the patient is unable to breathe spontaneously.

internal (in'tərn'l) situated on the inside. *I. haemorrhage* one occurring in a cavity or into the tissues. *I. secretion* one in which the hormones pass directly into the bloodstream from the secreting gland. *I consistency* the extent to which items within a scale reflect or measure the same concept.

interphase ('intəˌfayz) the period between two cell divisions during which the chromosomes are not easily visible.

intersex ('intəˌseks) 1. a congenital abnormality in which anatomical features of both sexes are evident. 2. a person displaying INTERSEXUALITY.

intersexuality (ˌintəˌseksyoo'alətee, -seksh-) an intermingling of the characters of each sex (including physical form, reproductive tissue, and sexual behaviour) in one individual, as a result of some flaw in embryonic development.

interstitial (ˌintə'stishəl) situated within the tissue spaces or between the tissues. *I. cell stimulating hormone* abbreviated ICSH, luteinising hormone. *I. fluid* the fluid in which body cells are bathed. It acts as an intermediary between the cells and the blood. Extracellular fluid. *I. keratitis see* KERATITIS. *I. nephritis* chronic NEPHRITIS associated with fibrosis and hypertension.

intertrigo (ˌintə'triegoh) an irritating, eczematous skin eruption caused by chafing of two moist skin surfaces.

intervention (ˌintə'venshən) in health care, any act carried out to prevent harm to patients or to improve, promote, or enhance their physical, mental, or spiritual wellbeing.

intervertebral (ˌintə'vərtəbrəl) between the vertebrae. *I. disc* the pad of fibrocartilage between the bodies of the vertebrae. Protrusion of the contents of the disc can cause SCIATICA by exerting pressure on the nerve roots.

interview ('intəˌvyoo) a method of data collection in which a researcher questions a participant verbally. Interviews can: (a) be face to face or performed over the telephone; (b) consist of open-ended or semi-structured questions; and (c) permit a researcher–participant relationship to develop in which questions can be clarified or explored.

intestinal (ˌinte'stienəl, in'testən'l) referring to the INTESTINE.

intestine (in'testən) that part of the alimentary canal that extends from the stomach to the anus. *Small i.* the first 6 m from the pylorus to the caecum, consisting of the duodenum, the jejunum, and the ileum. *Large i.* the final 2 m, consisting of the caecum, ascending colon, transverse colon, descending colon, and rectum.

intima ('intəmə) the innermost coat of an artery or vein.

intolerance (in'tolə·rəns) lack of power to endure. Applied to the effect of some drugs on individuals, e.g. iodine and quinine. *See* IDIOSYNCRASY.

intoxication (inˌtoksə'kayshən) 1. poisoning by drugs or harmful substances. 2. the condition produced by excessive use of alcohol.

intra-abdominal (ˌintrə·əb'domən'l) within the abdomen.

intra-articular (ˌintrə·ah'tikyələ) within a joint capsule. *I-a. injection* injection into a joint capsule, for example, injection of hydrocortisone into a joint.

intra-atrial (ˌintrə'aytri·əl) within the atrium. *I-a. thrombosis* a blood clot formed in the atrium of the heart.

intracapsular (ˌintrə'kapsyələ) within a capsule, usually of a joint. *I. extraction* the removal of the whole lens with its capsule in the treatment of cataract. *I. fracture see* FRACTURE.

intracellular (ˌintrə'selyələ) within a cell. *I. fluid* the water and its dissolved salts found within the cells.

intracerebral (ˌintrə'serəbrəl) within the brain substance. *I. haemorrhage* an escape of blood in the CEREBRUM, most often arising from the middle cerebral artery or from an ANEURYSM.

intracranial (ˌintrə'krayni·əl) within the skull. *I. abscess* one arising within the brain or meninges. *I. aneurysm* dilatation of one of the cerebral vessels. It can be congenital or acquired. *I. pressure* abbreviated ICP. The pressure exerted by the cerebrospinal fluid within the subarachnoid space and ventricles of the brain.

intractable (in'traktəbəl) not able to be relieved, controlled, or cured.

intradermal (ˌintrə'dərməl) between the layers of the skin.

intradural (ˌintrə'dyoo·rəl) within the DURA MATER. *I. haemorrhage see* HAEMORRHAGE.

intragastric (ˌintrə'gastrik) within the stomach.

intrahepatic (ˌintrəhə'patik) within the liver. Referring to a condition of the liver cells or connective tissue.

intralobular (ˌintrə'lobyələ) within a lobule. *I. veins* veins which collect blood from within the lobules of the liver.

intramedullary (ˌintrəmə'dulə·ree) 1. within the MEDULLA oblongata. 2. within the bone marrow. *I. nail* a metal pin used for the internal fixation of fractures.

intramuscular (ˌintrə'muskyələ) within muscle tissue.

intranasal (ˌintrə'nayzəl) within the nose.

intraocular (ˌintrə'okyələ) within the eyeball.

intraorbital (ˌintrə'awbət'l) within the orbit of the eye.

intraosseous (ˌintrə'osi·əs) within a bone.

intraperitoneal (ˌintrəˌperətə'neeəl) within the peritoneal cavity.

intrathecal (ˌintrə'theekəl) within the meninges of the spinal cord, usually in the subarachnoid space.

intratracheal (ˌintrə'traki·əl, -trə'keeəl) endotracheal; within the trachea. *I. anaesthesia* inhalation anaesthesia. *See* ANAESTHESIA.

intrauterine (ˌintrə'yootə·rien) within the uterus. *I. contraceptive device* a contraceptive device introduced into the uterine cavity. *I. douche* irrigation of the uterine cavity. A special grooved nozzle is used, so that the fluid can return and is not forced into the uterine tubes. *I. growth retardation* associated with poor blood supply to the placenta or with maternal disease. Other factors include infection during pregnancy, maternal smoking, or drug addiction. The infant at birth is 'small for dates' and falls below the tenth centile appropriate gestational age for infants. *I. life* fetal development in the uterus.

intravenous (ˌintrə'veenəs) within a vein. *I. flow rate* the rate at which fluids, medications, and blood products flow into the bloodstream during intravenous infusion. The flow rate is usually ordered by the doctor as total volume (mL) per total hours or, in the case of drugs, total dose per total hours. *I. infusion* the therapeutic introduction of a fluid, such as saline, into a vein. The infusion works by gravity, in that the container of fluid is higher than the blood vessel into which the fluid is being introduced. *I. urography* radiographic examination of the urinary tract after the injection of a radio-opaque contrast medium into a vein.

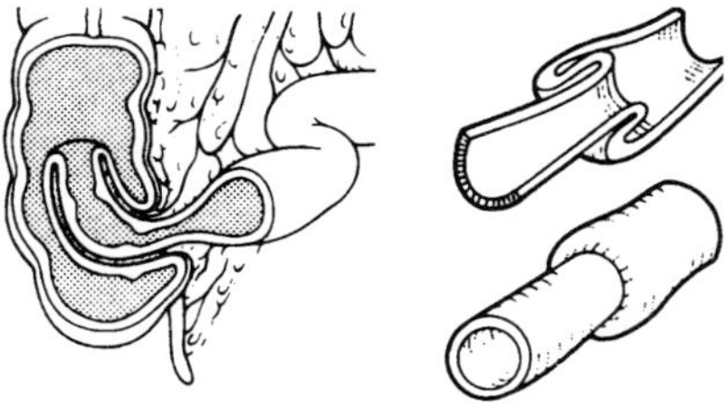

Intussusception

intraventricular (ˌintrəvenˈtrikyələ) within a ventricle; can apply to a cerebral or a cardiac ventricle.

intrinsic (inˈtrinsik, -zik) particular to or contained within an organ. I. factor a glycoprotein, contained in the gastric juices, which is necessary for the absorption of the EXTRINSIC factor (vitamin B_{12}).

introitus (inˈtroh·itəs) [L.] an opening or entrance into a hollow organ or cavity. *I. vaginae* the vulva.

introjection (ˌintrəˈjekshən) a mental process by which an individual takes into himself or herself the personal characteristics of another person, usually those of someone much loved or admired.

introspection (ˌintrəˈspekshən) a subjective study of the mind and its processes, in which an individual studies his or her own reactions.

introversion (ˌintrəˈvərzhən) 1. a turning inwards within itself of a hollow organ. 2. preoccupation with oneself, with reduction of interest in the outside world.

introvert (ˈintrəˌvərt) a person whose interests are turned inwards upon himself or herself. *See* EXTROVERT.

intubation (ˌintyəˈbayshən) the introduction of a tube into a part of the body, particularly into the air passages to allow air to enter the lungs.

intumescence (ˌintyooˈmesəns) a swelling or increase in bulk, as of nasal mucous membrane in catarrh.

intussusception (ˌintəsəˈsepshən) prolapse of one part of the intestine into the lumen of an immediately adjacent part, causing OBSTRUCTION (intestinal) (*see* figure).

inunction (inˈungkshən) 1. rubbing an oily or fatty preparation containing a medicinal ingredient into the skin, with absorption of the drug. 2. any preparation so applied.

invagination (inˌvajəˈnayshən) 1. the folding inwards of a part, thus forming a pouch. 2. INTUSSUSCEPTION.

invasion (inˈvayzhən) 1. the entry of bacteria into the body. 2. the entrance of parasites into the body of a host.

invasive (inˈvaysiv, -ziv) 1. having the quality of invasiveness. 2. involving puncture or incision of the skin or insertion of an instrument or foreign material into the body;

said of diagnostic or therapeutic techniques.

invasiveness (in'vaysivnəs) 1. the ability of microorganisms to enter the body and spread in the tissues. 2. the ability to infiltrate and actively destroy surrounding tissue, a property of malignant tumours.

inversion (in'vərshən) a turning upside down or inside out. *Sexual i.* homosexuality. *Uterine i.* the condition of the uterus after parturition when a part of its upper segment protrudes through the cervix.

invertebrate (in,vərtə'brət, -brayt) 1. without a spinal column. 2. an animal without a spinal column.

involucrum (,invo'lookrəm) new bone which forms a sheath around necrosed bone, as in chronic OSTEOMYELITIS.

involuntary (in'voləntree) independent of the will. *I. muscle* one that acts without conscious control, forexample, the heart and stomach muscles.

involution (,invə'looshən) 1. turning inwards; describes the contraction of the uterus after labour. The process whereby the uterus returns to its normal size. 2. the progressive degeneration occurring naturally with advancing age, resulting in shrivelling of organs or tissues.

iodine ('ieə,deen, -ien) symbol I. A nonmetallic element with a distinctive odour obtained from seaweed. Iodine is essential in nutrition, being especially prevalent in the colloid of the THYROID (gland). It is used in the treatment of HYPOTHYROIDISM and as a topical antiseptic. It is a frequent cause of poisoning. Iodine is opaque to X-rays and can be combined with other compounds for use as contrast media in diagnostic radiology.

iodopsin (,ieə'dopsən) a violet pigment found in the retinal cones of the eyes.

iodoxyl (,ieə'doksəl) a radio-opaque contrast medium. *See* INTRAVENOUS urography.

ion ('ieən) an atom or group of atoms having a positive (cation) or negative (anion) electric charge by virtue of having gained or lost one or more electrons. Substances forming ions are ELECTROLYTES. *See* HYDROGEN.

ionisation (,ieənie'zayshən) the breaking up of molecules into electrically charged particles or ions when an electric current is passed through an elecrolytic solution.

iontophoresis (ie,ontohfə'reesəs) the introduction through the skin of therapeutic ions by ionisation.

ipecacuanha (,ipə,kakyoo'ahnə) the dried root of a Brazilian shrub, given in small doses as an expectorant and, in larger doses, as an emetic.

IPPV intermittent positive-pressure ventilation.

ipsilateral (,ipsee'latə,rəl) occurring on the same side. Applied particularly to paralysis or other symptoms occurring on the same side as the cerebral lesion causing them.

IQ intelligence quotient. *See* INTELLIGENCE.

IRDS infant respiratory distress syndrome.

iridectomy (,irə'dektəmee) excision of a part of the iris, usually for the treatment of GLAUCOMA.

iridencleisis (,irəden'kliesəs) an operation to make a drain out of a part of the iris, used in the treatment of GLAUCOMA.

iridium (i'ridi·əm) *symbol* Ir. A radioactive metal often used in the form of wires or hairpins to treat superficial malignancies, e.g. those of the tongue, cheek, or breast.

iridocele (iˌridoh'seel) herniation of a part of the iris through a corneal wound.

iridocyclitis (ˌiridohsie'klietəs) inflammation of the iris and ciliary body.

iridodonesis (ˌiridohdə'neesis) trembling of the iris due to lack of support from the lens in dislocation of the lens or after a cataract extraction.

iridoptosis (ˌirədop'tohsəs) prolapse of the iris.

iridotomy (ˌirə'dotəmee) the making of a hole in the iris to form an artificial pupil.

iris ('ierəs) the coloured part of the eye, made of two layers of muscle, the contraction of which alters the size of the pupil and so controls the amount of light entering the eye. *I. bomb* a bulging forwards of the iris due to pressure of the AQUEOUS HUMOUR when its passage into the anterior chamber is obstructed.

iritis (ie'rietəs) inflammation of the iris, causing pain, photophobia, contraction of the pupil, and discolouration of the iris. *See* UVEITIS.

iron ('ieən) *symbol* Fe. A metallic element, present in the body in small quantities and essential to life. A deficiency can produce ANAEMIA.

irradiation (iˌraydee'ayshən) the treatment of disease by electromagnetic radiation.

irreducible (ˌirə'dyoosəbəl) incapable of being replaced in a normal position. Applied to a fracture or a hernia.

irrigation (ˌirə'gayshən) the washing out of a cavity or wound with a stream of lotion or water.

irritable ('irətəbəl) reacting excessively to a stimulus. *I. bowel syndrome* mucous COLITIS; spastic colon. The patient complains of disordered bowel function with abdominal pain, but no organic disease can be found.

irritant ('irətənt) an agent causing stimulation or excitation.

irritation (ˌirə'tayshən) 1. a condition of undue nervous excitement resulting from abnormal sensitiveness. *Cerebral i.* a stage of excitement present in many brain conditions and typical of the recovery stage of concussion. 2. itching of the skin.

ischaemia (is'keemi·ə) a deficiency in the blood supply to a part of the body. *Myocardial i.* ischaemia of the heart muscles, which causes ANGINA PECTORIS.

ischiorectal (ˌiskeeoh'rekt'l) concerning the ischium and the rectum. *I. abscess* a collection of pus in the ischiorectal connective tissue. An anal fistula can result.

ischium ('iski·əm) the lower posterior bone of the pelvic girdle.

Ishihara colour charts (ˌishee'hahrə) *S. Ishihara, Japanese ophthalmologist, 1879–1963*. Patterns of dots of the primary colours on similar backgrounds which make numbers or patterns. The numbers or patterns can be seen by a normal-sighted person, but a person who is colour blind will be able to identify only some of them, depending on the type of colour blindness.

islet of Langerhans (ˌielet əv 'langəˌhanz) *P. Langerhans, German pathologist, 1847–88*. One of a group of cells in the pancreas that produce insulin and glucagon; islet of the pancreas.

isocarboxazid (ˌiesohkah'boksəˌzid) a monoamine oxidase inhibitor used in the treatment of depressive illness.

isograft ('iesohˌgrahft) a tissue graft from one identical twin to another.

isoimmunisation (ˌiesohˌimyənie-'zayshən) the development of antibodies against an antigen derived from an individual of the same species, e.g. a rhesus-negative woman can immunise herself against her fetus, if it is rhesus-positive, by forming specific ANTIBODY.

isolation (ˌiesə'layshən) the separation of a person with an infectious disease from those non-infected. *I. period* quarantine; the length of time during which a patient with an infectious fever is considered capable of infecting others by contact.

ieoleucine (ˌiesoh'looseen) one of the 9 essential amino acids that are vital for health in the adult.

isometric (ˌiesə'metrik) having equal dimensions. *I. exercises* the contraction and relaxation of muscles without producing movement; used to maintain muscle tone after a fracture.

isoniazid (ˌiesoh'nieəzid) INH. A drug given orally in combination with streptomycin or para-aminosalicylic acid (PAS), which is effective in treating tuberculosis. Combined therapy reduces the risk of bacterial resistance.

isoprenaline (ˌiesoh'prenəlin) a sympathomimetic drug which has an action like adrenaline and can be used to treat asthma.

isosorbide dinitrate (ˌiesohˌsorbied die'nietrayt) a short-acting vasodilator similar in action to glyceryl trinitrate and used in the treatment of ANGINA PECTORIS.

isotonic (ˌiesə'tonik) having uniform tension. *I. solution* is of the same osmotic pressure as the fluid with which it is compared. Normal saline (0.9% solution of salt in water) is isotonic with blood plasma.

isotope ('iesəˌtohp) one of the several forms of an element with the same atomic number but different atomic weights. *Radioactive i.* an unstable isotope which decays and emits alpha, beta, or gamma rays. Can be used in the diagnosis and treatment of malignant disease.

isthmus ('isməs) a narrow connection between two larger bodies or parts, e.g. the band of tissue between the two lobes of the thyroid gland.

itch (ich) a skin eruption with irritation. *Baker's i.* eczema of the hands due to the proteins of flour. *Barber's i.* sycosis; tinea barbae. *Dhobie i.* TINEA cruris. The name is derived from the belief in India that the spread of infection was due to washermen (dhobies) wearing their clients' clothes. *I. mite* the cause of scabies, *Sarcoptes scabiei*. *Washer-women's i.* dermatitis of the hands due to the constant use of detergents.

ITP idiopathic thrombocytopenic purpura.

IUCD intrauterine contraceptive device.

IVF in vitro fertilisation. *See* FERTILISATION.

IVP intravenous pyelography.

IVU intravenous urography.

Jj

J symbol for *joule*.

Jacksonian epilepsy (jak'sohni·ən) *J.H. Jackson, British neurologist, 1835–1911*. Focal motor EPILEPSY.

Jacquemier's sign ('zhahkmi-·ayz,sien) *J.M. Jacquemier, French obstetrician, 1806–79*. Blueness of the lining of the vagina seen from the early weeks of pregnancy.

jactitation (,jaktə'tayshən) the extreme restlessness of a severely ill patient.

Jakob–Creutzfeldt disease (yakob-'kroytsfelt də,zeez) *A.M.Jakob, German psychiatrist, 1884–1931; H.G.Creutzfeldt, German psychiatrist, 1885–1964*. Pre-senile dementia due to a slow virus.

jargon ('jahgən) 1. the terminology used and generally understood only by those who have knowledge of that speciality, e.g. medical jargon, legal jargon. 2. gibberish talked by insane persons.

Jarvic-7 ('jahvik) *R.K.Jarvic, American physician, b. 1946.* An artifical heart designed for use in humans.

jaundice ('jawndəs) icterus; a yellow discolouration of the skin and conjunctivae, due to the presence of bile pigment in the blood. It can be one of the following types. (1) *Haemolytic j.* due to excessive destruction of red blood cells, causing increase of BILIRUBIN in the blood. The liver is not involved. *Acholuric j.* is of this type. It is characterised by increased fragility of the red blood cells. (2) *Hepatocellular j.* in which the liver cells are damaged by either infection or drugs. (3) *Obstructive j.* in which the bile is prevented from reaching the duodenum owing to obstruction by a gallstone, a growth, or a stricture of the common bile duct. (4) *Physiological j.* (icterus neonatorum) which occurs within the first few days of life, and is caused by the breakdown of the excessive number of red blood cells present in the newborn.

jaw (jor) a bone of the face in which the teeth are embedded. *Lower j.* the mandible. *Upper j.* the two maxillae.

jejunectomy (,jejə'nektəmee) excision of a part or the whole of the JEJUNUM.

jejunoileostomy (jə,joonoh,ilee-'ostəmee) the making of an anastomosis between the JEJUNUM and the ILEUM.

jejunostomy (,jejə'nostəmee) the making of an opening into the jejunum through the abdominal wall.

jejunotomy (ˌjejəˈnotəmee) an incision into the JEJUNUM.

jejunum (jəˈjoonəm) the portion of the small intestine from the DUODENUM to the ILEUM; about 2.4 m in length.

jelly (ˈjelee) a soft, coherent, resilient substance; generally, a colloidal semisolid mass. *Contraceptive j.* a non-greasy jelly used in the vagina for prevention of conception (*see also* CONTRACEPTION). *Petroleum j.* a purified mixture of semisolid hydrocarbons obtained from petroleum (called also 'petrolatum'). *Wharton's j.* the soft, jelly-like intracellular substance of the umbilical cord which insulates the vein and arteries, preventing occlusion and fetal hypoxia.

jerk (jərk) a sudden muscular contraction. *Knee j.* a kicking movement produced by tapping the tendon below the patella. Used with other jerks such as the ankle jerk to test the nervous reflexes.

jigger (ˈjigə) a sand flea, found in the tropics, which burrows into the soles of the feet and causes severe irritation.

Jobst suit (jobst) a pressure wrap applied to control hypertrophic scar formation.

joint (joynt) an articulation; the point of junction of two or more bones, particularly one which permits movement of the individual bones relative to each other.

Jordan's frame (jawˈdəns) a type of stretcher used to lift and transport patients with suspected or actual spinal injuries.

joule (jool) *symbol* J. The SI unit of energy and heat that is the work being done by a force of 1 newton acting over a distance of I metre.

judgment (ˈjujmənt) the ability of an individual to estimate a situation, to arrive at reasonable conclusions, and to decide on a course of action.

jugular (ˈjugyələ) relating to the neck. *J. veins* several veins in the neck which drain the blood from the head.

Jung (yuhng) *Carl Gustav Jung, Swiss psychologist and psychiatrist, 1875–1961.*

juvenile (ˈjoovəˌniel) relating to young people.

juxta-articular (ˌjukstə·ahˈtikyələ) near a joint.

juxtaglomerular (ˌjukstəgloˈmeryələ) near to a GLOMERULUS of the kidney. *J. cells* specialised cells found in the kidney which appear to play an important part in the control of aldosterone release.

juxtaposition (ˌjukstəpəˈzishən) adjacent; side by side.

Kk

K symbol for *potassium*.

Kahn test (kahn) *R.L. Kahn, American bacteriologist, 1887–1979.* An agglutination test for syphilis.

kala-azar (ˌkahlə·ə'zah) visceral LEISHMANIASIS. A tropical disease caused by the protozoan parasite *Leishmania donovani* which is carried by the sandfly. Symptoms include enlargement of the liver and spleen, anaemia, and wasting. The disease is often fatal.

kanamycin (ˌkanə'miesən) a broad-spectrum antibiotic for use against severe infections with Gram-negative organisms if penicillin is ineffective.

kaolin ('kayələn) powdered clay containing aluminium silicate. It is taken orally in the treatment of diarrhoea and is also used as a dusting powder and for poultices.

Kaposi's sarcoma ('kapohˌzeez) *M.K. Kaposi, Austrian dermatologist, 1837–1902.* A multifocal, metastasising, malignant RETICULOSIS with angiosarcoma-like features, involving chiefly the skin. Rarely seen in the developed world until the outbreak of AIDS. Kaposi's sarcoma is a major feature of this disease.

Kaposi's spots a serious complication of infantile eczema occurring as a result of exposure to HERPES simplex virus infection. Also known as Kaposi's varicelliform eruption.

karaya (kə'rie·ə) a gum made from certain species of *Sterculia*, a genus of tropical trees and shrubs. Used as an aid to applying ostomy bags to the skin.

karyotype ('kareeohˌtiep) 1. the chromosomal constitution and arrangement of a cell of an individual. 2. the pattern that is seen when human chromosomes are photographed during metaphase. The pictures are then enlarged and paired according to the length of the short arm of the chromosome.

Kegel exercises ('kaygəl) specific exercises named after Dr Arnold H. Kegel, a gynaecologist who first developed the exercises to strengthen the pelvic–vaginal muscles as a means of controlling stress incontinence in women.

Keller's operation ('keləz) *W.L. Keller, American surgeon, 1874–1959.* An operation for correcting HALLUX valgus.

keloid ('keeloyd) hard, raised scar tissue in the skin, common in people with dark skins. A type occurs in a healed wound due to overgrowth of fibrous tissue, causing the scar to be raised above the skin level.

Kennedy's syndrome ('kenədeez) *F. Kennedy, American neurologist, 1884–1952*. Ipsilateral optic atrophy caused by a frontal lobe tumour which involves one of the optic nerves.

keratectasia (ˌkerətek'tayzi·ə) protrusion of the cornea following inflammation.

keratectomy (ˌkerə'tektəmee) excision of a portion of the cornea.

keratic (kə'ratik) 1. horny. 2. relating to the cornea. *K. precipitates* inflammatory exudates adhering to the back of the cornea; a sign of IRITIS and CYCLITIS.

keratin ('kerətən) an albuminoid substance which forms the principal constituent of all horny tissues.

keratinise (kə'ratəˌnayz) to make or become horny.

keratitis (ˌkerə'tietəs) inflammation of the cornea. The causes can be physical (trauma, exposure to dust or vapours or to ultraviolet light) or infectious conditions such as corneal and dendritic ulcers. *Interstitial k.* deep chronic keratitis, usually arising in congenital syphilis. *Striate k.* inflammation that appears in lines due to the folding over of the cornea after injury or operation, particularly one for cataract.

keratocele ('kerətohˌseel) DESCEMETOCELE; protrusion of Descemet's membrane through the base of a corneal ulcer. A horny growth of the skin.

keratoconjunctivitis (ˌkerətohkənˌjungktə'vietəs) inflammation of both the cornea and the conjunctiva of the eye.

keratoiritis (ˌkerətoh·ie'rietis) inflammation of both the cornea and the iris.

keratoma (ˌkerə'tohmə) KERATOSIS a hard thick epidermal growth caused by hyperthropy of the horny layer of the shin also called callus

keratomalacia (ˌkerətohmə'layshi·ə) ulceration and softening of the cornea due to a deficiency of vitamin A.

keratome ('keraˌtohm) a knife for incising the cornea.

keratometer (kerə'tomətə) ophthalmometer. An instrument by which the amount of corneal astigmatism can be measured accurately.

keratophakia (ˌkerətoh'fayki·ə) KERATOPLASTY in which a slice of donor's cornea is shaped to a desired curvature and inserted between layers of the recipient's cornea to change its curvature.

keratoplasty ('kerətohˌplastee) a plastic operation on the cornea, including corneal grafting.

keratoscope ('kerətohˌskohp) an instrument for examining the eye to detect keratoconus.PLACIDO's DISC.

keratosis (ˌkerə'tohsəs) a skin disease marked by excessive growth of the epidermis or horny tissue.

keratotomy (ˌkerə'totəmee) incision of the cornea.

kerion ('keeri·ən) a complication of ringworm of the scalp, with formation of pustules.

kernicterus (kər'niktə·rəs) a condition in the newborn marked by severe neural symptoms, associated with high levels of BILIRUBIN in the blood; it is commonly a sequela of ICTERUS gravis neonatorum.

Kernig's sign ('kərnigz) *V.M. Kernig, Russian physician, 1840–1917*. A sign of meningitis. When the thigh is supported at right angles to the trunk with the knee bent, the knee cannot be fully straightened (either actively or passively).

ketamine ('ketə,meen) a rapidly acting, non-barbiturate, general anaesthetic which is given by intramuscular or intravenous injection.

ketoacidosis (,keetoh,asə'dohsəs) an acute life-threatening complication of uncontrolled diabetes mellitus. In this condition urinary loss of water, potassium, ammonium, and sodium results in hypovolaemia, electrolyte imbalance, extremely high blood glucose levels, and breakdown of free fatty acids, causing acidosis, often with coma.

ketogenic (,keetə'jenik) forming or capable of being converted into ketone bodies. *K. diet* one containing large amounts of fat, with minimal amounts of protein and carbohydrate. The object of such a diet is to produce KETOSIS; it is occasionally used in the treatment of certain types of epilepsy in young children.

ketone ('keetohn) an organic compound containing the carbonyl group (CO) attached to two hydrocarbon groups. Ketones are produced by the CATABOLISM of fats.

ketonuria (,keetə'nyoo·ri·ə) the presence of ketones in urine; ACETONURIA.

ketoprofen (,keetoh'profen) non-steroidal anti-inflammatory drug used in the treatment of mild rheumatic and arthritic conditions.

ketosis (kee'tohsəs) the condition in which ketones are formed in excess in the body and accumulate in the blood. Severe ACIDOSIS can occur.

ketosteroid (,keetoh'stiə·royd) a steroid hormone which contains a ketone group attached to a carbon atom. *17-K's* are excreted in the urine and formed from the adrenal corticosteroids, testosterone and, to a lesser extent, oestrogens.

kidney ('kidnee) one of two organs situated in the lumbar region which purify the blood and secrete urine. It secretes renin and renal erythropoietic factor. *Articial k.* the apparatus used to remove retained waste products from the blood when kidney function is impaired. *K. failure* the condition in which renal function is severely impaired and the organs are unable to maintain the fluid and electrolyte balance of the body. *Granular k.* the small fibrosed kidney of chronic NEPHRITIS. *Horseshoe k.* a congenital defect in which there is a fusion of the two kidneys into a horseshoe shape. *Polycystic k.* a congenital bilateral condition of multiple cysts replacing kidney tissue. *K. transplant* the surgical implantation of a kidney taken from a live donor or from one who has recently died. Used in the treatment of renal failure.

kilocalorie ('kilə,kalə·ree) *Symbol* kcal. One thousand calories; a unit of food energy.

kilojoule ('kilə,jool) *symbol* kJ. One thousand joules; a unit of food energy (1 kcal = 4.184 kJ).

Kimmelstiel–Wilson syndrome (,kiməlsteel'wilsən) A degenerative complication of DIABETES mellitus, with ALBUMINURIA, OEDEMA, hypertension, renal insufficiency, and RETINOPATHY. Also called 'intercapillary GLOMERULOSCLEROSIS'.

kinaesthesia (,kinəs'theezi·ə) the combined sensations by which position, weight, and muscular position are perceived.

kinanaesthesia (,kinanəs'theezi·ə) an

inability to perceive the sensation of movements of parts of the body.

kinase ('kienayz) an enzyme activator; *see* ENTEROKINASE and THROMBOKINASE.

kineplasty ('kinə,plastee) plastic amputation; amputation in which the stump is so formed as to be utilised for producing motion of the prosthesis.

kinetic (kə'netik) producing or pertaining to motion.

kinin ('kienən) a polypeptide which occurs naturally and is a powerful vasodilator.

kinship ('kin,ship) relationship. *K. studies* (anthropological term) the study of kin (relatives) and their patterns of marriage, descent, inheritance, habitation, social values, and economics.

Kirschner wire ('kiəshnə) *M. Kirschner, German surgeon, 1879–1942.* A thin wire that can be passed through a bone to apply skeletal traction.

kiss of life (,kis əv 'lief) the expired air method of artificial respiration, by either mouth-to-nose or mouth-to-mouth breathing.

Klebsiella (,klebsee'elə) a genus of Gram-negative bacteria (family Enterobacteriaceae).

Klebs–Löffler bacillus (,klebz'lərflə) *T.A.E. Klebs, German bacteriologist, 1834–1913; F.A.J. Löffler, German bacteriologist, 1852–1915. Corynebacterium diphtheriae*, the causative agent of diphtheria.

Kleihauer test ('kliehowə) a microscopic test to detect fetal cells in the maternal circulation, usually done immediately after delivery so that, if the mother is rhesus-negative and the fetus rhesus-positive, anti-D immunoglobulin can be given to prevent ISOIMMUNISATION.

kleptomania ('kleptəmayni·ə) an irresistible urge to steal when there is often no need and no particular desire for the objects. Often associated with depression.

Klinefelter's syndrome ('klienfeltəz) *H.F. Klinefelter, American physician, b. 1912.* A congenital chromosome abnormality in which each cell has three sex chromosomes, XXY, rather than the usual XX or XY, making a total of 47 (normal is 46). Affected men have female breast development and small testes, and are infertile.

Klippel–Feil syndrome (,klipəl'fiel) A congenital abnormality in which the neck is very short as a result of the absence or fusion of several vertebrae in the cervical region.

knee (nee) the joint between the femur and the tibia. *K. cap* the patella. *Housemaid's k.* prepatellar BURSITIS. *K. jerk* an upwards jerk of the leg obtained by striking the patellar tendon when the knee is passively flexed. *Knock-k.* a condition in which the knees turn inwards towards each other; GENU valgum.

Koch's bacillus (,koks bə'siləs) *R. Koch, German bacteriologist, 1843–1910. Mycobacterium tuberculosis*, the causative organism of tuberculosis.

Köhler's disease ('kərləz) *A. Köhler, German physician and radiologist, 1874–1947.* OSTEOCHRONDRITIS of the navicular bone of the foot, occurring in children.

koilonychia (,koylə'niki·ə) the development of brittle, spoon-shaped nails which can occur in iron-deficiency anaemia.

Koplik's spots ('kopliks) *H. Koplik,*

American paediatrician, 1858–1927. Small pink-to-red spots with a bluish-white centre that sometimes appear on the mucous membranes inside the mouth in measles on the second day of onset, before the general rash.

Korotkoff's method (ko'rotkofs) *N.S. Korotkoff, Russian physician, 1874–1920.* A method of finding the systolic and diastolic blood pressures by listening to the sounds produced in an artery while the pressure in a previously inflated cuff is gradually reduced.

Korsakoff's syndrome or **psychosis** ('kawsəkofs) *S.S. Korsakoff, Russian neurologist, 1854–1900.* A chronic condition in which there is impaired memory, particularly for recent events, and the patient is disorientated in time and place. It can be present in psychosis of infective, toxic, or metabolic origin, or in chronic alcoholism.

kraurosis (kraw'rohsəs) dryness and shrinking of a part of the body. *K. vulvae* a degenerative condition of the vulva. Can be treated by giving oestrogen preparations.

Kreb's cycle (krebz) *Sir H.A. Krebs, German–British biochemist, 1900–1981.* A series of reactions during which the aerobic oxidation of pyruvic acid takes place. This is part of carbohydrate metabolism. *K. urea c.* the way in which urea is formed in the liver.

Küntscher nail ('koontshə) *G. Küntscher, German orthopaedic surgeon, 1902–72.* An intramedullary nail used in treating fractures of long bones, especially the shaft of the femur. *See* figure.

Kupffer's cells (kuhpfəz) *K.W. von Kupffer, German anatomist, 1829–1902.* Phagocytic reticuloendothelial cells of the liver which form bile from haemoglobin released by disintegrated ERYTHROCYTES.

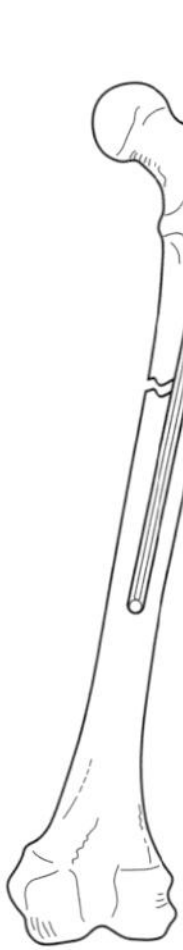

Küntscher Intramedullary Nail

kuru ('kooroo) (New Guinea shivering) a slow progressive fatal infection of the central nervous system found only in natives of New Guinea. The disease was transmitted by eating brain tissue during funeral rites. No new cases have been reported since cessation of cannibalism.

Kussmaul breathing ('kuhsmowl) Deep, rapid, and sighing respirations, associated with diabetic acidosis.

Kveim test ('kvaym) *M.A. Kveim, Norwegian physician, 1892–1966*. A test for SARCOIDOSIS in which antigen from the lymph nodes or spleen of a patient with sarcoidosis is injected intradermally.

kawashiorkor (ˌkawshee'awkə) a condition of protein malnutrition occurring in children in underprivileged populations. Fatty infiltration of the liver arises and can cause cirrhosis.

kymograph ('kieməˌgrahf, -ˌgraf) an instrument for recording variations or undulations, arterial or other.

kyphoscoliosis (ˌkiefohˌskohlee'ohsəs) an abnormal curvature of the spine in which there is forwards and sideways displacement.

kyphosis (kie'fohsəs) posterior curvature of the spine; humpback.

Ll

L symbol for litre.
labetalol (lə'beetəlol) an alpha- and beta-adrenergic receptor blocker used in the treatment of hypertension.
labial ('laybi·əl) pertaining to the lips or labia.
labile ('laybiel) unstable. Applied to those chemicals that are subject to change or readily altered by heat.
lability (lə'bilətee) instability. *L. of mood* the tendency to sudden changes of mood of short duration.
labium ('laybi·əm) a lip. *L. majus pudendi* the large fold of flesh surrounding the vulva. *L. minus pudendi* the lesser fold within the labium majus.
labor *see* LABOUR.
labour ('laybə) parturition or childbirth, which takes place in three stages: (a) dilatation of the cervix uteri; (b) passage of the child through the birth canal; and (c) expulsion of the placenta. *Induced l.* labour brought on by artificial means before term, as in cases of contracted pelvis or if overdue. *Obstructed l.* labour in which there is a mechanical hindrance. *Precipitate l.* labour in which the baby is delivered extremely rapidly. *Premature l.* labour which occurs before term. *Spurious l.* ineffective labour pains which sometimes precede true labour pains.
labyrinth ('labə·rinth) the structures forming the internal ear, i.e. the cochlea, vestibule, and semicircular canals. *Bony l.* the bony canals of the internal ear. *Membranous l.* the soft structure inside the bony canals.
labyrinthectomy (ˌlabə·rin'thektəmee) excision of the labyrinth.
labyrinthitis (ˌlabə·rin'thietəs) inflammation of the labyrinth, causing vertigo.
laceration (ˌlaesə'rayshən) a wound with torn and ragged edges.
lacrimal ('lakrəməl) relating to tears. *L. apparatus* the structures secreting the tears and draining the fluid from the conjunctival sac (*see* figure on p. 250). *L. gland* a gland that secretes tears, which drain through two small openings in the eyelids (l. puncta) into a pair of ducts (l. canaliculi) into the sac and finally into the nasal cavity through the nasolacrimal duct. Situated in the outer and upper corner of the orbit.
lacrimation (ˌlakrə'mayshən) an excessive secretion of tears.
lacrimator ('lakrəˌmaytə) a substance that causes excessive secretion of tears, e.g. tear gas.
lactagogue ('laktəˌgog) any agent

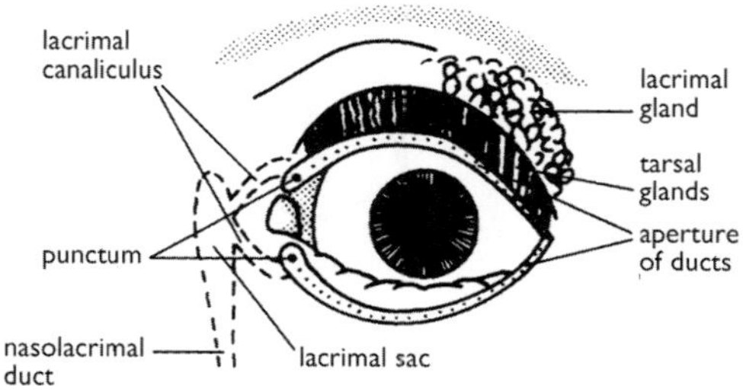

Lacrimal Apparatus

that promotes the secretion or flow of milk; galactagogue.

lactalbumin (lak'talbyəmən) an albumin of milk.

lactase ('laktayz) an enzyme produced in the small intestine, which converts lactose into glucose and galactose.

lactate ('laktayt) 1. any substance given to promote lactation. 2. any salt of lactic acid. 3. to secrete milk. *L. dehydrogenase* abbreviated LD, LDH. An enzyme that catalyses the interconversion of lactate and pyruvate. Widespread in tissues and particularly abundant in kidney, skeletal muscle, liver, and MYOCARDIUM. It has five isoenzymes denoted LD_1 to LD_5. The 'flipped' pattern, in which the serum LD_1 level is greater than the LD_2 level, is indicative of an acute myocardial infarction. This pattern occurs within 12–24 hours after the attack.

lactation (lak'tayshən) 1. the period during which the infant is nourished from the breast. 2. the process of milk secretion by the mammary glands.

lacteal ('lakti·əl) 1. consisting of milk. 2. a lymphatic duct in the small intestine which absorbs CHYLE

lactic ('laktik) pertaining to milk. *L. acid* an acid formed by the fermentation of lactose or milk sugar. It is produced naturally in the body as a result of glucose metabolism. An excess of the acid accumulating in the muscles can cause cramp.

lactiferous (lak'tifə·rəs) conveying or secreting milk.

lactifuge ('laktəfyooj) a drug or agent that retards the secretion of milk.

Lactobacillus (ˌlaktohbə'siləs) a genus of Gram-positive, rod-shaped bacteria, many of which produce fermentation.

lactoferrin (ˌlaktoh'ferən) an iron-binding protein found in neutrophils and bodily secretions (milk, tears, saliva, bile, etc.), having bactericidal activity and acting as an inhibitor of colony formation by GRANULOCYTES and MACROPHAGES.

lactogenic (ˌlaktə'jenik) stimulating the production of milk. *See* LUTEOTROPHIN.

lactometer (lak'tomətə) an instrument for measuring the specific gravity of milk.

lactose ('laktohz, -tohs) milk sugar consisting of glucose and galactose.

lactosuria (ˌlaktə'syoo·ri·ə) lactose in the urine.

lactovegetarian (ˌlaktohˌvejə'tair·ri·ən) 1. a person who subsists on a diet of milk or milk products and vegetables. 2. pertaining to such a diet.

lactulose ('laktyəlohz) a synthetic disaccharide which is used as a laxative.

lacuna (lə'kyoonə) a small cavity or depression in any part of the body.

Laënnec's disease (ˌla·e'nek) *R.T.H. Laënnec, French physician, 1781–1826.* The most common type of cirrhosis of the liver, frequently attributable to high alcohol consumption.

laevulose ('levyəˌlohz) fruit sugar; fructose.

laking ('layking) haemolysis of the red blood cells. The cells swell and burst and the haemoglobin is released.

lallation (la'layshən) a babbling, infantile form of speech.

Lamaze method (la'mayz) *F. Lamaze, French obstetrician, 1890–1957.* A method of preparing for NATURAL CHILDBIRTH based on the technique of training the mind and body for the purpose of modifying perception of pain during labour and delivery.

lambdoid ('lamdoyd) shaped like the Greek letter lambda Λ or λ. *L. suture* the junction of the occipital bone with the parietals.

lambliasis (lam'blieəsəs) GIARDIASIS.

lamella (lə'melə) 1. a thin layer, membrane or plate, as of bone. 2. a thin medicated disc of gelatin used in applying drugs to the eye. The gelatin dissolves and the drugs are absorbed.

lamina ('lamənə) a bony plate or layer.

laminectomy (ˌlamə'nektəmee) excision of the posterior arch of a vertebra, sometimes performed to relieve pressure on the spinal cord or nerves.

Lancefield's groups ('lansfeeldz) *R.C. Lancefield, American bacteriologist, 1895–1981.* Divisions of β-haemolytic streptococci, which are classified on the basis of serological action into groups A–R. Most human infections are due to group A.

Landry's paralysis (lan'dreez) *J.B.G. Landry, French physician, 1826–65.* Guillain–Barr syndrome; acute ascending POLYNEURITIS.

Landsteiner's classification ('landstienəz) *K. Landsteiner, Austrian biologist, 1868–1943.* A system of blood groups; the ABO system, consisting of groups A, B, AB, and O.

Lange colloidal gold test ('langə) *C.F.A. Lange, German physician, 1883–1953.* A test made on cerebrospinal fluid to detect syphilis, disseminated sclerosis, meningitis, and other neurological conditions.

Langerhans, islet of ('langəˌhanz) *P. Langerhans, German pathologist, 1847–88.* One of the group of cells in the pancreas that produce insulin.

Langhans' cell ('langhanz) *T. Langhans, Swiss pathologist, 1834–1915.* A deep cell of a CHORIONIC VILLUS.

lanolin ('lanələn) a fat obtained from

sheep's wool and used as a basis for ointments, salves, creams, and cosmetics.

lanugo (lə'nyoogoh, -noo-) the fine hair that covers the body of the fetus and newly born infants, especially those who are premature. Called also *down*.

laparoscopy (ˌlapə'roskəpee) viewing of the abdominal cavity by passing an endoscope through the abdominal wall.

laparotomy (ˌlapə'rotəmee) incision of the abdominal wall for exploratory purposes.

laryngeal (lə'rinji·əl, ˌlarən'jeeəl) pertaining to the larynx.

laryngectomy (ˌlarən'jektəmee) excision of the larynx.

laryngismus (ˌlarən'jizməs) a spasmodic contraction of the larynx. *L. stridulus* a crowing sound on inspiration, following a period of apnoea, due to spasmodic closure of the glottis. It occurs in children, particularly those suffering from rickets. Croup.

laryngitis (ˌlarən'jietəs) inflammation of the larynx causing hoarseness or loss of voice due to acute infection or irritation by gases.

laryngoscope (lə'ring·gəˌskohp) an endoscopic instrument for examining the larynx or for aiding the insertion of endotracheal tubes or the bronchoscope.

laryngospasm (lə'ring·gohˌspazəm) a reflex, prolonged contraction of the laryngeal muscles that is liable to occur on insertion or withdrawal of an intratracheal tube.

laryngostenosis (ləˌring·gohstə'nohsəs) contraction or stricture of the larynx.

laryngostomy (ˌlaring'gostəmee) the making of an opening into the larynx to provide an artificial air passage.

laryngotomy (ˌlaring'gotəmee) an incision into the larynx to make a temporary opening in an emergency when the larynx is obstructed. TRACHEOSTOMY.

laryngotracheal (ləˌring·goh'traki·əl) referring to both the larynx and trachea.

laryngotracheitis (ləˌring·ohˌtrakee'ietəs) inflammation of both the larynx and trachea.

laryngotracheobronchitis (ləˌring·gohˌtrakeeohbrong'kietəs) an acute viral infection of the respiratory tract which occurs particularly in young children.

larynx ('laringks) [Gr.] the muscular and cartilaginous structure, lined with mucous membrane, situated at the top of the trachea and below the root of the tongue and the hyoid bone. The larynx contains the vocal cords and is the source of the sound heard in speech; also called the 'voice box'.

laser ('layzə) light amplification by stimulated emission of radiation. An apparatus producing an extremely concentrated beam of light that can be used to cut metals. Used in the treatment of neoplasms, detached retina, diabetic RETINOPATHY and macular degeneration, and some skin conditions.

Lassa fever ('lasə) a West African viral haemorrhagic fever with insidious onset and an incubation period of 6–21 days. It is a ZOONOSIS, the reservoir of infection of which is the multimammate rat. Devastating outbreaks of person-to-person transmission have occurred in hospitals in West Africa by accidental inoculation of blood and tissue fluid from infected patients.

Lassar's paste ('lasəz) *G. Lassar, German dermatologist, 1849–1908.* A soothing paste used in skin diseases, containing salicylic acid, zinc oxide, starch, and soft paraffin.

lassitude ('lasə,tyood) a feeling of extreme weakness and apathy.

latent ('laytənt) temporarily concealed; not manifest. *L. heat* the heat absorbed by a substance during a change in state, e.g. from water into steam. When condensation occurs, this heat is released. *L. period* 1. the incubation period of an infectious disease. 2. the time between the application of a nerve stimulus and the reaction.

lateral ('latə·rəl) situated at the side; therefore, away from the centre.

lateroversion (,latə·roh'vərshən, -zhən) a turning to one side, such as can occur of the uterus.

laudanum ('lawd'nəm) tincture of opium; a preparation formerly used as a narcotic.

laughing gas ('lahfing) nitrous oxide.

lavage ('lavij, la'vahzh) the washing out of a cavity. *Colonic l.* the washing out of the colon. *Gastric l.* the washing out of the stomach.

laxative ('laksətiv) a medicine that loosens the bowel contents and encourages evacuation. A laxative with a mild or gentle effect on the bowels is also known as an aperient; one with a strong effect is referred to as a cathartic or a purgative.

LE lupus erythematosus. *LE cell* a mature neutrophilic POLYMORPHONUCLEAR LEUKOCYTE that has phagocytised a large, spherical inclusion derived from another neutrophil; a characteristic of lupus erythematosus but also found in analogous connective tissue disorders.

lead (led) *symbol* Pb. A metallic element, many of the compounds of which are highly poisonous. *L. lotion* lead subacetate solution used externally on bruises. *L. poisoning* a condition that usually occurs in children as the result of excessive lead in the atmosphere, or from chewing objects covered with paint containing lead. The symptoms and signs include malaise, diarrhoea and vomiting, and sometimes ENCEPHALITIS. There is often pallor and a blue line around the gums.

Leber's disease (laybərz) *T.B. Leber, German ophthalmologist, 1840–1917.* Hereditary optic atrophy.

Leboyer method ('leboyə) A method of delivering an infant designed to minimise trauma and encourage maternal–infant bonding.

lecithin ('lesəthən) one of a group of phospholipids that are found in the cell tissues and are concerned in the metabolism of fat.

leech (leech) *Hirudo medicinalis*, an aquatic worm which sucks blood and secretes hirudin (an anticoagulant) in its saliva. On rare occasions, used to withdraw blood from patients.

leg (leg) the lower limb, from knee to ankle. *Barbados l.* ELEPHANTIASIS. *Bow-l.* genu varum. *Scissor l.* condition in which the patient is cross-legged, such as occurs in CEREBRAL DIPLEGIA. *White l.* PHLEGMASIA alba dolens.

Legionella pneumophila (,leejə'nelə nyoo'mofələ) a species of Gram-negative, non-acid-fast, rod-shaped bacteria which require both cysteine and iron for growth; it is the causative agent of LEGIONNAIRES' DISEASE and PONTIAC FEVER.

legionellosis (ˌleejəne'lohsəs) disease caused by infection with *Legionella* species, such as *L. pneumophila*.

legionnaires' disease (ˌleejən'airz) a pulmonary form of legionellosis, resulting from infection with *Legionella pneumophila*. It is contagious and symptoms include fever, pain in the muscles and across the chest, a dry cough, and a partial loss of kidney function.

leiomyoma (ˌlieohmie'ohmə) a benign smooth muscle tumour (fibroid) most commonly found in the uterus.

leiomyosarcoma (ˌlieohˌmieoh-sah'kohmə) a malignant muscle tumour.

Leishmania (leesh'mayni·ə) a genus of parasitic flagellated protozoa which infect the blood of humans and are the cause of LEISHMANIASIS.

leishmaniasis (ˌleeshmə'nieəsəs) a group of diseases caused by one of the protozoan *Leishmania* parasites. *See* KALA-AZAR.

Lembert's suture (lanh'bairz) *A. Lembert, French surgeon, 1802–51.* A series of stitches used for wounds of the intestine. So arranged that the edges are turned inwards and the peritoneal surfaces are in contact.

lens (lenz) 1. a piece of glass or other material shaped to transmit light rays in a particular direction. 2. the transparent crystalline body situated behind the pupil of the eye. It serves as a refractive medium for rays of light. *Contact l.* a thin sheet of glass or plastic moulded to fit directly over the cornea. Worn instead of spectacles.

lentigo (len'tiegoh) a brownish or yellowish spot on the skin. A freckle. *L. maligna* Hutchinson's melanotic freckle. *See* FRECKLE.

leontiasis (ˌlien'tieəsəs) an osseous deformity of the face which produces a lion-like appearance. It occurs sometimes in leprosy and rarely in OTEITIS deformans.

lepidosis (ˌlepə'dohsəs) any scaly eruption of the skin.

leprosy ('leprəsee) HANSEN'S DISEASE. An incurable, chronic infection of the skin, mucous membrane, and nerves with *Mycobacterium leprae*. It is predominantly a tropical disease which is transmitted by direct contact. There is an insidious onset of symptoms, mainly involving the skin and nerves, after an incubation period of between 1 and 30 years. The disease can be classified into three types: (a) lepromatous, which is a steadily progressive form, often resulting in paralysis, disfigurement and deformity; this form is often complicated by tuberculosis; (b) tuberculoid, which is often self-limiting and generally runs a more benign course; and (c) indeterminate, in which there are skin symptoms representative of both lepromatous and tuberculoid forms. Leprosy can be controlled by the use of sulphone drugs.

leptomeningitis (ˌleptohˌmenən-'jietəs) inflammation of the PIA MATER and arachnoid membranes of the brain and spinal cord.

Leptospira (ˌleptoh'spierə) a genus of spirochaetes. *L. icterohaemorrhagiae* the cause of spirochaetal jaundice WEIL'S DISEASE).

leptospirosis (ˌleptohspie'rohsəs) any of a group of notifiable infectious diseases due to serotypes of

Leptospira. The best known is WEIL'S DISEASE, or leptospiral jaundice; others are mud fever, autumn fever, and swineherd's disease. The aetiological agent is a spiral organism that is common in water. Initially, the symptoms include fever, rigors, vomiting, headache and, often, jaundice. Diagnosis can be difficult because the symptoms resemble those of several other diseases. Jaundice is a key symptom. Sanitation measures can reduce the spread of the disease in both humans and animals.

Leriche's syndrome (lə'reeshiz) *R. Leriche, French surgeon, 1879–1955*. A condition in which ATHEROSCLEROSIS of peripheral arteries is accompanied by obstruction of the lower end of the aorta.

lesbianism ('lezbi·ənizəm) sexual attraction of one woman to another; female homosexuality.

Lesch–Nyhan syndrome (ˌlesh-'niehan) *M. Lesch, American physician, b. 1939; W.L. Nyhan Jr, American physician, b. 1926*. A hereditary disorder of purine metabolism transmitted as an X-linked recessive trait with physical and mental handicap, compulsive self-mutilation of fingers and lips by biting, choreoathetosis, spastic cerebral palsy, and impaired renal function.

lesion ('leezhən) any pathological or traumatic discontinuity of tissue or loss of function of a part. Lesion is a broad term, including wounds, sores, ulcers, tumours, cataracts, and any other tissue damage. Lesions range from the skin sores associated with eczema to the changes in lung tissue that occur in tuberculosis.

lethargy ('lethəjee) a condition of drowsiness or stupor that cannot be overcome by the will.

Letterer–Siwe disease (ˌletə·rə-'seevə) *E. Letterer, German physician, 1895–1982; S.A. Siwe, Swedish physician, 1897–1966*. Reticuloendotheliosis of early childhood, marked by a haemorrhagic tendency, eczematoid skin eruption, HEPATOSPLENOMEGALY with lymph node involvement, and progressive anaemia.

leucine ('looseen) a naturally occurring essential amino acid, vital for growth in infants and for nitrogen equilibrium in adults.

leuco- for words beginning thus, *see* LEUKO-.

leukaemia (loo'keemi·ə) a progressive, malignant disease of the blood-forming organs, marked by abnormal proliferation and development of leukocytes and their precursors in the blood and bone marrow. It is accompanied by a reduced number of ERYTHROCYTES and blood platelets, resulting in anaemia and increased susceptibility to infection and haemorrhage. Other typical symptoms include fever, pain in the joints and bones, and swelling of the lymph nodes, spleen, and liver. Leukaemia is classified clinically on the basis of: (a) the duration and character of the disease (acute or chronic); and (b) the cell line involved, i.e. myeloid (myelocytic, myeloblastic, granulocytic) or lymphoid (lymphatic, lymphoblastic, lymphocytic). A widely used classification of acute leukaemia based on cell type is the French American British (FAB) classification. The incidence of the disease is growing and the increase is only partially explained by increased efficiency of detection.

leuko-, leuco-, combining form meaning 'white', or 'white blood cell'.

leukocyte ('lookə,siet) a white blood corpuscle. There are three types: (a) granular (polymorphonuclear cells) formed in bone marrow, consisting of neutrophils, eosinophils, and basophils; (b) lymphocytes (formed in the lymph glands); and (c) monocytes (*see* figure and table).

Type of leucocyte	*No. of cells per litre*
Neutrophils	$2.5–7.1 \times 10^9$
Eosinophils	$4–44 \times 10^9$
Basophils	$0–1 \times 10^9$
Lymphocytes	$1.5–3.5 \times 10^9$
Monocytes	$2–8 \times 10^9$

leukocytolysis (,lookohsie'toləsəs) destruction of white blood cells.

leukocytopoiesis (,lookoh,sietohpoy'eesəs) LEUCOPOIESIS.

leukocytosis (,lookohsie'tohsəs) an increase in the number of leukocytes in the blood. Often a response to infection.

leukoderma (,lookoh'dərmə) an absence of pigment in patches or bands, producing abnormal whiteness of the skin. VITILIGO.

leukodystrophy (,lookoh'distrəfee) a degenerative disorder of the brain which starts during the first few months of life and leads to mental, visual, and motor deterioration.

leukoma (loo'kohmə) a white spot on the cornea, usually the result of an injury to the eye.

leukonychia (,lookoh'niki·ə) white patches on the nails due to air underneath.

leukopaenia (,lookoh'peeni·ə) a decreased number of white cells, usually GRANULOCYTES, in the blood.

leukophoresis (,lookohfə'reesəs) withdrawal of blood for the selective removal of leukocytes. The remaining blood is retransfused.

leukoplakia (,lookoh'playki·ə) a chronic inflammation, characterised by white thickened patches on the mucous membranes, particularly on the tongue, gums, and inside of the cheeks. *L. vulvae* thickening of the mucous membrane of the labia with the appearance of scattered white patches.

leukopoiesis (,lookohpoy'eesəs) the formation of white blood cells. LEUKOCYTOPOIESIS.

leukorrhoea (,lookə'reeə) a viscid, whitish discharge from the vagina.

leukotomy (loo'kotəmee) a psychosurgical operation in which the white nerve fibres within the brain are severed. Prefrontal leukotomy has been largely replaced by a variety of stereotatic surgical techniques, whereby carefully controlled and very small lesions are made in one or more of the pathways of the limbic system. Now rarely used.

levator (lə'vaytə) a muscle that raises a structure or organ of the body.

levels of care ('levəlz) the six divisions of the HEALTH CARE SYSTEM: preventative care, primary care, secondary or acute care, tertiary care, restorative care, and continuing care.

Levin tube ('levən) a plastic catheter used in gastric intubation.

levodopa (,leevoh'dohpə) L-dopa; a synthetic drug used in the treatment of PARKINSONISM.

levonorgestrel (,leevohnaw'jestrel) a potent progestin used in com-

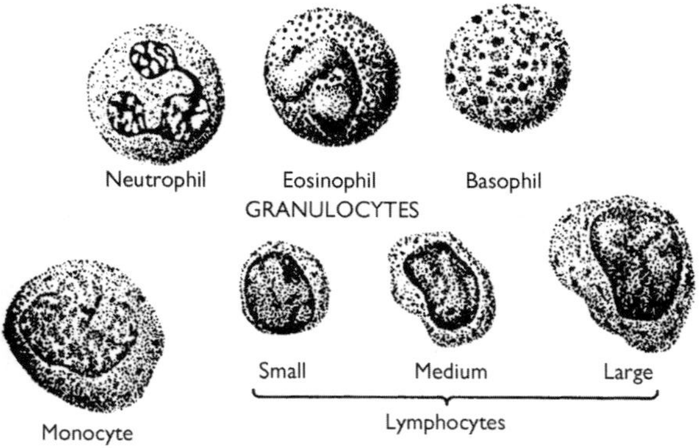

Types of Leukocyte

bination with an oestrogen as an oral contraceptive.

levorphanol (le'vawfənol) an analgesic somewhat resembling morphine in its action and addiction potentialities. It is used to relieve severe pain.

LFT liver function test.

Li symbol for *lithium*.

libido (lə'beedoh) 1. the vital force or impulse which brings about purposeful action. 2. sexual drive in Freudian psychoanalysis, the motive force of all human beings.

lichen ('liekən, 'lichən) a group of inflammatory affections of the skin in which the lesions consist of papular eruptions. *L. planus* raised flat patches of dull, reddish-purple colour, with smooth or scaly surface.

lichenification (lie,kenəfə'kayshən) the stage of an eruption when it resembles lichen.

lid (lid) eyelid. *Granular l.* trachoma. *L. lag* jerky movement of the upper lid when it is being lowered. A sign of exophthalmic GOITRE (thyrotoxicosis).

lidocaine ('liedoh,kayn) *see* LIGNOCAINE.

lie (lie) a position or direction. *L. of fetus* the position of the fetus in the uterus. The normal lie is longitudinal.

Lieberkühn's glands ('leebə,koonz) *J.N. Lieberkühn, German anatomist, 1711–56.* Tubular glands of the small intestine.

lien ('lie·en) the spleen.

lienculus (lie'engkyələs) an accessory spleen.

lienorenal (,lieənoh'reen'l) relating to the spleen and kidneys; splenorenal; splenonephric.

lientery ('lieəntə·ree) diarrhoea consisting mainly of undigested food.

life event (lief) a sociological term used to describe major events in a person's life, e.g. leaving home for the first time, getting married, moving house, changing a job.

life expectancy (lief ək'spektənsee) the average length of life based upon prevailing mortality trends.

life-support system (lief sə'pawt sis,təm) the equipment and technology used to maintain the life of a patient who is not otherwise able to survive.

lift assessment (lift ə'sesmənt) the choice of the most appropriate lift method to use when moving a patient, as from bed to a chair. Factors that need to be taken into account include: (i) whether the patient is conscious or unconscious; (ii) whether there is a visual, hearing, or cognitive impairment present; (iii) other equipment such as urinary drainage, IV lines, or monitors; and (iv) the body weight of the person. No particular method of lifting is suggested as correct or appropriate in all situations. Rather, safe lifting or manual handling practices should be used at all times, and lifting devices are the first option when implementing manual handling activities. *See* MANUAL HANDLING.

ligament ('ligəmənt) 1. a band of fibrous tissue connecting bones forming a joint. 2. a layer or layers of peritoneum connecting one abdominal organ to another or to the abdominal wall. *Annular l.* the ring-like band that fixes the head of the radius to the ulna. *Cruciate l.* crossed ligaments within the knee joint. *Inguinal l.* that between the pubic bone and anterior iliac crest. *Round l.* one of the two anterior ligaments of the uterus, passing through the inguinal canal and ending in the LABIA MAJORA. There are also round ligaments of the femur and of the liver.

ligation (lie'gayshən) the application of a ligature.

ligature ('ligəchə) a thread of silk, catgut, or other material used for tying around a blood vessel to stop it bleeding.

light (liet) electromagnetic waves which stimulate the retina of the eye. *L. adaptation* the changes that take place in the eye when the intensity of the light increases or decreases. *L. coagulation* a method of treating retinal detachment by directing a beam of strong light from a carbon arc through the pupil to the affected area.

lightening ('lietəning) the relief experienced in pregnancy, 2#3 weeks before labour, when the uterus sinks into the pelvis and ceases to press on the diaphragm.

lignocaine ('lignoh,kayn) a local anaesthetic administered by injection and by surface application. Also used intravenously in cases of cardiac ARRHYTHMIA, especially following MYOCARDIAL INFARCTION. Also lidocaine.

Likert-type scales ('likərt tiep skaylz, 'lie-) lists of statements on which respondents indicate whether they "strongly agree", agree", "disagree", or "strongly disagree".

limbus ('limbəs) an edge or border. *Corneal l.* the border where the cornea joins theSCLERA.

lime (liem) a citrus fruit with a high ascorbic acid content.

liminal ('limən'l) pertaining to the threshold of perception.

lincomycin (,linkoh'miesən) an antibiotic derived from the *Streptomyces* genus. Used in the treatment of streptococcal bone and joint infections, including OSTEOMYELITIS.

linctus ('lingktəs) a thick syrup, usually given to soothe and allay coughing.

linea ('lini·ə) [L.] *a line. L. alba* the tendinous area in the centre of the abdominal wall into which the transversalis and part of the oblique muscles are inserted. *L. albicantes* white streaks that appear on the abdomen when it is distended by pregnancy or a tumour. *L. aspera* the rough ridge on the back of the femur into which muscles are inserted. *L. nigra* the pigmented line that often appears in pregnancy on the abdomen between the umbilicus and the pubis.

linear ('lini·ə) pertaining to line. *L. accelerator* a megavoltage machine for accelerating electrons so that powerful X-rays are given off for use in the treatment of deep-seated tumours.

lingual ('ling·gwəl) pertaining to the tongue.

lingula ('ling·gyələ) a tongue-like structure, such as the projection of lung tissue from the left upper lobe.

liniment ('linəmənt) a liquid applied externally by rubbing on to the skin.

lip (lip) 1. the upper or lower fleshy margin of the mouth. 2. any lip-like part; labium. *Cleft l.* congenital fissure of the upper lip.

lip reading (lip 'reeding) understanding of speech through observation of the speaker's lip movements; called also 'speech reading'.

lipaemia (li'peemi·ə) the presence of excess fat in the blood. Sometimes a feature of diabetes. *L. retinalis* condition in which the retinal blood vessels appear to be filled with milk owing to the presence of an excess of fat in the blood.

lipase ('lipayz, -pays) fat-splitting enzyme; any enzyme that catalyses the splitting of fats into glycerol and fatty acids. Measurement of the serum lipase level is an important diagnostic test for acute and chronic PANCREATITIS.

lipid ('lipəd) one of a group of fatty substances that are insoluble in water but soluble in alcohol or chloroform. They form an important part of the diet and are normally present in the body tissues.

lipochondrodystrophy (ˌlipohˌkondroh'distrəfee) a congenital condition affecting the metabolism of fat and producing bone deformities, short stature, facial abnormalities, and learning difficulties. HURLER'S SYNDROME.

lipodystrophy (ˌlipoh'distrəfee) a disorder of fat metabolism. *Progressive l.* a rare condition occurring mainly in females in which there is progressive loss of fat over the upper half of the body.

lipoidosis (ˌlipoy'dohsəs) a group of diseases in which there is an error in lipoid metabolism producing RETICULOENDOTHELIAL hyperplasia. XANTHOMATA are common.

lipolysis (li'poləsəs) the breakdown of fats by the action of bile salts and enzymes to a fine emulsion and fatty acids.

lipoma (li'pohmə) a benign tumour composed of fatty tissue arising in any part of the body and developing in connective tissue. *Diffuse l.* a tumour of fat in an irregular mass, without a capsule, occurring above the pelvis.

lipoprotein (ˌlipoh'prohteen) one of a group of fatty proteins present in blood plasma.

liposarcoma (ˌlipohsah'kohmə) a malignant tumour of the fat cells.

lipuria (li'pyooə·ri·ə) the presence of fat in urine.

liquefaction (ˌlikwi'fakshən) reduction to liquid form.

liquid ('likwəd) 1. a substance that flows readily in its natural state. 2. flowing readily, neither solid nor gaseous. *L. diet* a diet limited to the intake of liquids or foods that can be changed to a liquid state. A liquid diet might be restricted to any liquids taken being clear liquids, or it might be a full liquid diet in which only liquids are taken.

liquor ('likə, 'liekwaw) a watery fluid; a solution. *L. amnii* the fluid in which the fetus floats; amniotic fluid.

Listeria (lis'tiə·ri·ə) *Baron J. Lister, British surgeon, 1827–1912*. A genus of Gram-negative bacteria which produce upper respiratory disease, septicaemia, and encephalitic disease in humans. They can be transmitted by the consumption of infected, unpasteurised dairy produce or infected leafy vegetables, or by direct contact with infected animals or contaminated soil. Newborn infants, pregnant women, the elderly, and the immunosuppressed are more susceptible to infection.

listeriosis (lisˌtiə·ree'ohsəs) infection with organisms of the genus *Listeria*.

lithagogue ('lithəˌgog) a drug that helps to expel calculi.

lithiasis (li'thieəsəs) the formation of calculi. *Conjunctival l.* the formation of small white chalky areas on the inner surface of the eyelids.

lithium ('lithi·əm) *symbol* Li. An alkaline metallic element. *L. carbonate* a drug used in the treatment of manic–depressive illness.

litholapaxy (li'tholəˌpaksee) the removal of fragments of a calculus from the bladder after LITHOTRIPSY.

lithonephrotomy (ˌlithohnə'frotəmee) incision into the kidney to remove a stone; NEPHROLITHOTOMY.

lithosis (li'thohsəs) PNEUMOCONIOSIS resulting from inhalation of particles of silica, etc., into the lungs.

lithotomy (li'thotəmee) incision into the bladder for the removal of calculi.

lithotripsy ('lithohˌtripsee) the crushing of calculi in the bladder; lithotrity.

lithotrite ('lithohˌtriet) an instrument used for LITHOTRIPSY.

lithuresis (ˌlithyə'reesəs) passage of small calculi or gravel in the urine.

litmus ('litməs) a blue pigment obtained from lichen and used for testing the reaction of fluids. *Blue l.* is turned red by an acid. *Red l.* is turned blue by an alkali.

litre ('leetə) *symbol* L. The SI unit of capacity. One cubic decimetre.

Little's disease ('lit'lz) *W.J. Little, British surgeon, 1810–94*. Spastic DIPLEGIA. A congenital muscle rigidity of the lower limbs causing 'scissor leg' deformity.

liver ('livə) the large gland situated in the right upper area of the abdominal cavity. Its chief functions are: (a) the secretion of bile; (b) the maintenance of the composition of the blood; and (c) the regulation of metabolic processes. *Cirrhotic l.* fibrotic changes which occur in the liver as the result of degeneration of the liver cells, often as a result of alcoholism. *L. transplant* the transplantation of a liver from a suitable donor who has recently died.

livid ('livəd) descriptive of the bluish-grey discolouration of the skin produced by congestion of blood.

LMP last monthly period.

LOA left occipito-anterior. Refers to a position that might be taken up by the fetus in the uterus.

lobar ('lohbə) relating to a lobe.

lobe (lohb) a section of an organ separated from neighbouring parts by fissures. The liver, lungs and brain are divided into lobes.

lobectomy (loh'bektəmee) removal of a lobe, e.g. of the lung.

lobular ('lobyələ) relating to a lobule.

lobule ('lobyool) a small lobe, particularly one making up a larger lobe.

localise ('lohkə,liez) 1. to limit the spread, e.g. of disease or infection, to a certain area. 2. to determine the site of a lesion.

lochia ('lohki·ə) the discharge of blood and tissue debris from the uterus after childbirth and lasting for 2–3 weeks. Initially, lochia is bright red and gradually becomes paler.

lochiometra (,lohkioh'meetrə) the retention of lochia in the uterus, causing its distension.

lockjaw ('lok,jor) tetanus.

locomotor (,lohkə'mohtə) pertaining to movement from one place to another. *L. ataxia* TABES dorsalis. *See* ATAXIA.

loculated ('lokyə,laytəd) divided into small locules or cavities.

loculus ('lokyələs) a small cystic cavity, one of a number.

log roll ('log ,rohl) a nursing technique used to turn a reclining patient from one side to the other. The patient lies on the back with arms folded across the chest, and legs extended. The nurses manipulate the underlying drawsheet so that the patient is rolled on to one side or the other.

logorrhoea (,logə'reeə) excessive and often unintelligible volubility.

loiasis (loh'ieəsəs) infestation of the conjunctiva and eyelids with a parasite worm. *Loa loa*. A tropical condition.

loin (loyn) the area of the back on each side between the thorax and the pelvis.

longitudinal study (,longətyoodən'l 'studee) a nonexperimental research design in which a researcher collects data from the sample group at different time points. Longitudinal studies are valuable as a means of studying human development or change and can also be used to observe change over time within an institution or organisation.

long sight (,long'siet) HYPERMETROPIA.

loosening ('loosəning) in psychiatry, a disorder of thinking in which associations of ideas become so shortened, fragmented and disturbed as to lack logical relationship.

LOP left occipito-posterior. Refers to a position that might be taken up by the fetus in the uterus.

lorazepam (lo'razipam, -ayzipam) a minor tranquilliser used to treat anxiety and insomnia.

lordosis (lor'dohsəs) a form of spinal curvature in which there is an abnormal forwards curve of the lumbar spine.

lotion ('lohshən) a medicinal solution for external application to the body.

Lotions usually have a soothing or antiseptic effect. *Calamine l.* a soothing mixture containing calamine and zinc oxide. *Evaporating l.* a dilute alcoholic solution applied to bruises.

loupe (loop) a magnifying lens, which can be used in eye examination.

louse (lows) a general term covering a number of small insects that are parasitic to humans and to other mammals and birds. Three varieties are parasitic to humans: (a) *Pediculus capitis*, the head louse; (b) *Pediculus corporis*, the body louse; and (c) *Phthirus pubis*, which infects the coarse hair on the body and also the eyebrows. Diseases known to be transmitted by lice are typhus fever, relapsing fever, and trench fever.

lozenge ('lozinj) a medicated tablet with a sugar basis, used to treat mouth and throat conditions.

LSD *see* LYSERGIDE.

lubb-dupp (lub'dup) representation of the sounds heard through the stethoscope when listening to the normal heart: *lubb* when the atrioventricular valves shut, and *dupp* when the semilunar valves meet each other.

lucid ('loosəd) clear, particularly of the mind. *L. interval* period of clear thinking that can occur in cerebral injury between two periods of unconsciousness or as a sane interval in a mental disorder.

Lugol's solution ('loogolz) *J.G.A. Lugol, French physician, 1786–1851.* A preparation of iodine and potassium iodide. It is best given in milk and is used in the treatment of toxic GOITRE.

lumbago (lum'baygoh) pain in the lower part of the back. It can be caused by muscular strain or by a prolapsed intervertebral disc ('slipped disc').

lumbar ('lumbə) pertaining to the loins. *L. puncture* insertion of a trocar and cannula into the spinal canal in the lower back and withdrawal of cerebrospinal fluid for diagnostic purposes.

lumbosacral (ˌlumboh'saykrəl) relating to both the lumbar vertebrae and the sacrum. *L. support* a corset aimed at both supporting and restricting movement in that region. *L. vertebra* one of the five vertebrae in the lower back lying between the thoracic vertebrae and the sacrum.

lumen ('loomən) the space inside a tube.

lumpectomy (ˌlump'ektəmee) the surgical excision of only the local lesion (benign or malignant) of the breast.

lunacy ('loonəsee) an obsolete term formerly applied to insanity.

Lund and Browder chart (luhnd ənd 'browdə) a chart that has been adopted by many burn centres for calculation of the surface area of a burn (*see* figures on pp 263–264). At birth, the size and area of the head is large compared with the adult, and the legs and thighs constitute a much smaller proportion of the total body surface. On admission to a burns unit or ward, the area of the body burned is mapped onto the Lund and Browder chart and the area of the burn affecting each portion of the body surface is calculated.

lung (lung) one of a pair of conical organs of the respiratory system,

Name ______________________ Age ______ Number ______________

Burn record Ages birth to $7\frac{1}{2}$ Date of observation ________

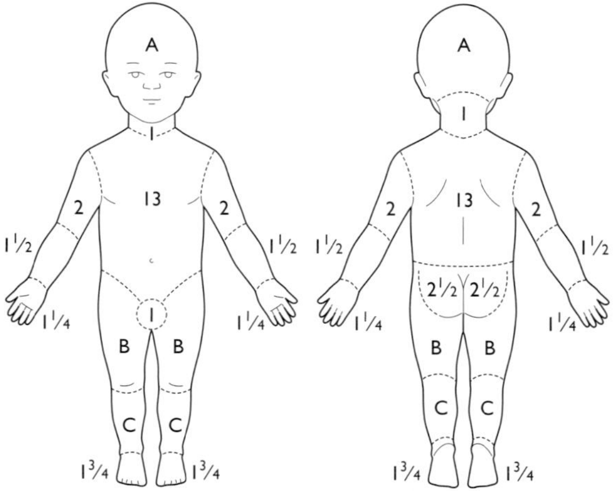

Relative percentages of areas affected by growth

Area	Age 0	1	5
A = $\frac{1}{2}$ of head	$9\frac{1}{2}$	$8\frac{1}{2}$	$6\frac{1}{2}$
B = $\frac{1}{2}$ of one thigh	$2\frac{3}{4}$	$3\frac{1}{4}$	4
C = $\frac{1}{2}$ of one leg	$2\frac{1}{2}$	$2\frac{1}{2}$	$2\frac{3}{4}$

% Burn by areas

Lund and Browder Chart
Estimation of extent of burn (birth–$7\frac{1}{2}$ yrs)

consisting of an arrangement of air tubes terminating in air vesicles (alveoli) and filling almost the whole of the thorax. The right lung has three lobes and the left lung two. They are connected with the air by means of the bronchi and trachea.

lunula ('loonyələ) the white semicircle near the root of each nail.

Name ______________________ Age ______ Number ______________

Burn record Ages $7\frac{1}{2}$ to adult Date of observation ________

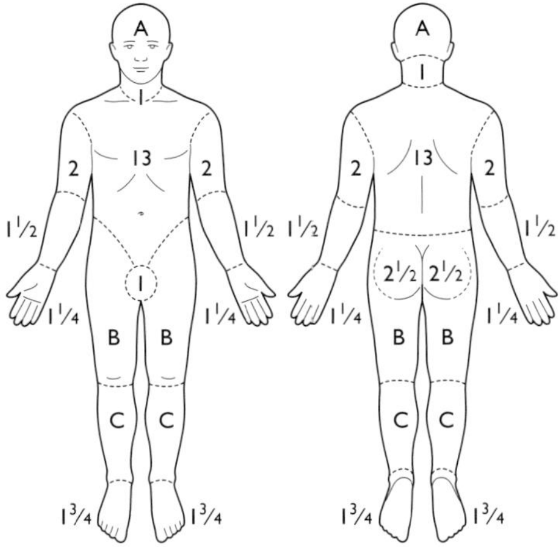

Relative percentages of areas affected by growth

Area	Age 10	15	Adult
A = $\frac{1}{2}$ of head	$5\frac{1}{2}$	$4\frac{1}{2}$	$3\frac{1}{2}$
B = $\frac{1}{2}$ of one thigh	$4\frac{1}{4}$	$4\frac{1}{2}$	$4\frac{3}{4}$
C = $\frac{1}{2}$ of one leg	3	$3\frac{1}{4}$	$3\frac{1}{2}$

% Burn by areas

Lund and Browder Chart
Estimation of extent of burn ($7\frac{1}{2}$ yrs–adult)

lupus ('loopəs) a chronic skin disease having many manifestations. *L. erythematosus* an inflammatory disease affecting both the internal organs and the skin which finally produces a round plaque-like area of HYPERKERATOSIS. It is thought to be due to an autoimmune reaction to sunlight, infection or other unknown cause. *L. vulgaris* a tuberculous disease of the skin producing brownish nodules, frequently on the nose or cheek, and severe scarring.

luteinising hormone ('lootee·ə-ˌniezing) abbreviated LH. One of three hormones produced by the anterior pituitary gland which control the activity of the gonads.

luteotrophin (ˌlooteeoh'trohfən) an anterior pituitary hormone which stimulates the formation of the corpus luteum and the production of milk. PROLACTIN.

luxation (luk'sayshən) the dislocation of a joint. *L. of the lens* displacement of the lens of the eye into the anterior chamber or posteriorly into the vitreous humour.

Lyme disease (liem) a ZOONOSIS transmitted by ticks and characterised by rash (erythema chronocium migrans), arthritis, and aseptic meningits, caused by the spirochaete *Borrelia burgdorferi*.

lymph (limf) the fluid from the blood which has transuded through capillary walls to supply nutriment to tissue cells. It is collected by lymph vessels which ultimately return it to the blood. *L. nodes* or *glands* structures placed along the course of lymph vessels, through which the lymph passes and is filtered of foreign substances, e.g. bacteria. These nodes also make lymphocytes. *Vaccine l.* a lymph preparation obtained from calves or other animals and used for vaccination.

lymphadenectomy (ˌlimfadə-'nektəmee) excision of a lymph gland or nodes.

lymphadenitis (ˌlimfadə'nietəs) inflammation of a lymph gland.

lymphadenoma (ˌlimfadə'nohmə) lymphoma. *Multiple l.* HODGKIN'S DISEASE.

lymphadenopathy (ˌlimfadə'nopəthee) any disease condition of the lymph nodes.

lymphangiectasis (ˌlimfanjee-'ektəsəs) dilatation of the lymph vessels due to some obstruction of the lymph flow. It can be congenital.

lymphangiography (ˌlimfanjee-'ogrəfee) radiographic examination of lymph vessels after the insertion of a radio-opaque contrast medium.

lymphangioma (ˌlimfanjee'ohmə) a swelling composed of dilated lymph vessels.

lymphangioplasty (lim'fanjeeoh-ˌplastee) any plastic operation the aim of which is to create artificial lymph drainage.

lymphangitis (ˌlimfan'jietəs) inflammation of lymph vessels manifested by red lines on the skin over them. It occurs in cases of severe infection through the skin.

lymphatic (lim'fatik) referring to lymph. *L. system* the system of vessels and glands through which the lymph is returned to the circulation. The vessels end in the thoracic duct and the right lymphatic duct.

lymphoblast ('limfəˌblast) an early developmental cell that will mature into a LYMPHOCYTE.

lymphocyte ('limfəˌsiet) a white blood cell formed in the lymphoid tissue. Lymphocytes produce immune bodies to overcome and protect against infection.

lymphocythaemia (ˌlimfohsie-'theemi·ə) an excessive number of lymphocytes in the blood. LYMPHOCYTOSIS.

lymphocytopaenia (ˌlimfohˌsietoh-'peeni·ə) absence or scarcity of lymphocytes in the blood. Lymphopaenia.

lymphocytosis (ˌlimfohsie'tohsəs) LYMPHOCYTHAEMIA.

lymphoedema (ˌlimfohə'deemə) a condition in which the intercellular spaces contain an abnormal amount of lymph due to obstruction of the lymph drainage.

lymphogranuloma (ˌlimfohˌgran-yə'lohmə) HODGKIN'S DISEASE. *L. venereum* a sexually transmitted disease, caused by a virus; primarily a tropical condition.

lymphoid ('limfoyd) relating to the lymph.

lymphoma (lim'fohmə) lymphadenoma. Used to denote any malignant condition of the lymphoid tissue. Generally these diseases are classified as either Hodgkin's or non-Hodgkin's lymphomata. *Burkitt's l.* a type of lymphoma found predominantly in Central Africa and affecting the jaws of children.

lymphopaenia (ˌlimfoh'peeni·ə) LYMPHOCYTOPAENIA.

lymphopoiesis (ˌlimfohpoy'eesəs) the production of lymphocytes. Occurs chiefly in the bone marrow, lymph nodes, thymus, spleen, and gut wall.

lymphorrhagia (ˌlimfə'rayji·ə) the escape of lymph from a ruptured lymphatic vessel. Lymphorrhoea.

lymphosarcoma (ˌlimfohsah-'kohmə) a term formerly used to denote a malignant lymphoma (with the exception of Hodgkin's disease).

lyophilisation (lieˌofəlie'zayshən) a method of preserving biological substances in a stable state by freeze drying. It can be used for plasma, sera, bacteria, viruses, and tissues.

lysergide (lie'sərjied) lysergic acid diethylamide (LSD). A hallucinogenic drug that can cause visual hallucinations and increased auditory acuity but can prove to be very disruptive to personality and can affect mental ability.

lysin ('liesən) a specific antibody present in the blood that can destroy cells. *See* BACTERIOLYSIN.

lysine ('lieseen) an essential amino acid formed by the digestion of dietary protein. It is vital for normal health.

lysis ('liesəs) 1. the gradual decline of a disease, especially of a fever. The temperature falls gradually, as in typhoid. *See* CRISIS. 2. the destruction of cells.

lysosome ('liesəˌsohm) a particle found in the cytoplasm of cells which causes the breakdown of metabolic substances and foreign particles (e.g., bacteria) within the cell.

lysozyme ('liesəˌziem) an enzyme present in tears, nasal mucus, and saliva that can kill most bacteria that come into contact with it.

lytic cocktail ('litik) a combination of chlorpromazine, promethazine, and pethidine used in the treatment of severe pre-eclampsia and ECLAMPSIA. It induces deep sleep, aids muscular relaxation, and lowers blood pressure. Used also during the induction and maintenance of HYPOTHERMIA.

Mm

M symbol for *molar*.
m symbol for *metre* and *misce* (mix).
McBurney's point (mək'bərneez) *C. McBurney, American surgeon, 1845–1913*. The spot two-thirds of the way along an imaginary line from the UMBILICUS to the right anterior superior iliac spine where tenderness is elicited if the appendix is inflamed.
McNaghten's Rules on Insanity at Law (mək'nawtənz) the rules that define the factors on which a defence to a charge of murder on grounds of insanity may be established.
maceration (ˌmasə'rayshən) softening of a solid by soaking it in liquid. *Neonatal m.* the natural softening of a dead fetus in the uterus.
Mackenrodt's ligaments ('makenˌrohts) *A.K. Mackenrodt, German gynaecologist, 1859–1925*. The transverse or cardinal ligaments that support the uterus in the pelvic cavity.
macrocheilia (ˌmakroh'kieli·ə) a congenital condition in which there is excessive development of the lips.
macrocyte ('makrohˌsiet) an abnormally large red cell found in the blood in some forms of anaemia.
macrocythaemia ('makrohsieˌtheemi·ə) the presence of abnormally large red cells in the blood. Macrocytosis.
macrodrip (ˌmacro'drip) intravenousgiving set which delivers an infusion at the rate of 15 drops per 1 mL.
macromastia (ˌmakroh'masti·ə) abnormal increase in the size of the breast.
macronutrient (ˌmakroh'nyootri·ənt) an essential nutrient that has a large minimal daily requirement (greater than 100 mg); calcium, phosphorus, magnesium, potassium, sodium and chloride are macronutrients.
macrophage ('makrohˌfayj) a large reticuloendothelial cell which has the power to ingest cell debris and bacteria. It is present in connective tissue, especially when there is inflammation.
macrophthalmia (ˌmakrof'thalmi·ə) a congenital condition of abnormally large eyes.
macroscopic (ˌmakroh'skopik) discernible with the naked eye. The opposite of microscopic.
macrostomia (ˌmakroh'stohmi·ə) an abnormal development of the mouth in which the mandibular and maxillary processes do not fuse and the mouth is excessively wide.
macula ('makyələ) a spot or

discoloured area of the skin, not raised above the surface; a macule. *M. corneae* a small area of opacity in the cornea, seen through an ophthalmoscope as a deeper red. *M. lutea* the yellow central area of the retina, where vision is clearest.

maculopapular (ˌmakyəloh'papyələ) displaying both maculae and papules. *M. eruption* a rash comprised of both, as in measles.

Madura foot (mə'dyoo·rə) MYCETOMA of the foot.

Madurella (ˌmadyə'relə) a genus of fungi causing MYCETOMA.

maduromycosis (məˌdyoo·rohmie'kohsəs) a chronic disease caused by *Madurella mycetoma*. The most common form is Madura foot.

Magendie's foramen (ˌmazhon'deez) *F. Magendie, French physiologist, 1783–1855*. Aperture in the roof of the fourth ventricle of the brain through which cerebrospinal fluid passes into the subarachnoid space.

magnesium (mag'neezi·əm) *symbol* Mg. A bluish-white metallic element. It occurs widely in mineral sources and is present in some of the body tissues. *M. carbonate* and *m. hydroxide* neutralising antacids used in hyperacidity. *M. sulphate* a saline purgative. Epsom salts. *M. trisilicate* an antacid powder taken after food for dyspepsia and peptic ulceration.

magnet ('magnət) in ophthalmology, an instrument used for removing metallic foreign bodies that have penetrated the eye.

magnetic resonance imaging (mag'netik) abbreviated MRI. An imaging technique based on the NUCLEAR MAGNETIC RESONANCE properties of the hydrogen nucleus. Cross-sectional images in any plane of the body for examination may be obtained. MRI is without hazard to the patient.

Makaton (ˌmak'əton) one of the sign languages.

mal (mal) [Fr.] *disease. M. de mer* seasickness. *Grand m., petit m.* forms of epilepsy.

malabsorption (ˌmaləb'sawpshən, -'zaw-) inability of the small intestine to absorb certain substances. It can be the cause of a deficiency disease due to the lack of an essential factor.

malacia (mə'layshi·ə) softening of tissues. *Kerato-m.* softening of the cornea. *Osteo-m.* softening of bone tissue.

maladjustment (ˌmalə'justmənt) in psychiatry, a failure to adjust to the environment.

malaise (ma'layz) a feeling of general discomfort and illness.

malalignment (ˌmalə'lienmənt) displacement, especially of the teeth from their normal relation to the line of the dental arch.

malaria (mə'lair·ri·ə) a serious, notifiable infectious illness characterised by periodic chills, fever, sweating, and SPLENOMEGALY. Serious and often fatal complications can arise in falciparum malaria. It is endemic in parts of Africa, Asia, and Central and South America, and is estimated to occur at the rate of 100 million cases each year throughout the world. Epidemics usually occur in areas in which mosquitoes persist in large numbers. The disease is caused by a parasite of the genus *Plasmodium* introduced into the blood by mosquitoes of the genus *Anopheles*. The attacks are periodic; every 48–72 hours according to the type of plasmodium. For *P. vivax,* it lasts 48 hours; *P. malariae,* 72 hours; and *P. falciparum,* 36–48 hours. *Airport* *m.* a term sometimes used to describe malaria occurring at or near an airport, in a country normally free of the disease, and spread by infected mosquitoes brought in on an aeroplane from an endemic area. Control measures include disinfection of aircraft if appropriate.

malformation (ˌmalfaw'mayshən) deformity; a structural defect.

malignant (mə'lignənt) tending to become progressively worse and to result in death; having the properties of ANAPLASIA, INVASIVENESS, and METASTASIS; said of tumours.

malingering (mə'ling·gə·ring) wilful, deliberate, and fraudulent feigning or exaggeration of the symptoms of illness or injury to attain a consciously desired end.

malleolus (mə'leeələs) one of the two protuberances on either side of the ankle joint. *Lateral m.* that on the outer surface at the lower end of the fibula. *Medial m.* that on the inner surface at the lower end of the tibia.

Mallory–Weiss syndrome (ˌmaləri-'vais) massive bleeding caused by a tear in the oesophagus, usually associated with protracted vomiting.

malleus ('mali·əs) the hammer-shaped bone in the middle ear.

malnutrition (ˌmalnyoo'trishən) the condition in which nutrition is defective in quantity or quality.

malocclusion (ˌmalə'kloozhən) an abnormality of dental development which causes overlapping of the bite.

Malpighian body (mal'pigi·ən) *M. Malpighi, Italian anatomist, physician and physiologist, 1628–94.* The GLOMERULUS and Bowman's capsule of the kidney.

malposition (ˌmalpə'zishən) an abnormal position of any part of the body.

malpractice (mal'praktəs) failure to maintain accepted ethical standards. Professional misconduct.

malpresentation (ˌmalprezən-'tayshən) any abnormal position of the fetus at birth that renders delivery difficult or impossible.

Malta fever ('mawltə) BRUCELLOSIS; undulant fever.

maltase ('mawltayz) a sugar-splitting enzyme which converts maltose to glucose. Present in pancreatic and intestinal juice.

maltose ('mawltohz, -tohs) the sugar formed by the action of digestive enzymes on starch.

malunion (mal'yooni·ən) faulty repair of a fracture.

mamilla (mə'milə) a nipple.

mamma ('mamə) a breast; a milk-secreting gland.

mammary ('mamə·ree) relating to the breasts.

mammography (mə'mografee) radiographic or infra-red examination of the breast to detect abnormalities.

mammoplasty ('mamohˌplastee) a plastic operation to reduce the size of abnormally large, pendulous breasts or augment the size of very small breasts.

mammothermography (ˌmamo-hthər'mografee) an examination of the breast that depends on the more active cells producing heat that can be shown on a thermograph and can indicate abnormalities of the breast tissue.

mandible ('mandəbəl) the lower jaw-bone.

manganese ('mang·gəneez) a common metallic element found in trace amounts in the body where it aids in the function of various enzymes.

mania ('mayni·ə) a disordered mental state of extreme excitement; specially, the manic type of manic–depressive psychosis. Also used as a word termination to denote obsessive preoccupation with something, as in TOMOMANIA.

maniac ('mayni͵ak) colloquial term for one suffering from a violent or extreme form of insanity.

manic ('manik) pertaining to mania. *M.–depressive psychosis* a mental illness characterised by mania and endogenous depression. The attacks can alternate between mania and depression or the patient can have recurrent attacks of mania or depression.

manipulation (mə͵nipyə'layshən) use of the hands to produce a desired movement, such as in reducing a fracture or a hernia or changing the position of a fetus. A skilfully applied forced movement upon a joint in order to relocate the joint or increase its range of movements by tearing adhesions round it.

mannitol ('manə͵tol) a sugar alcohol occurring widely in nature; an osmotic diuretic used for forced diuresis in drug overdose and in cerebral oedema.

manometer (mə'nomətə) an instrument for measuring the pressure of liquids or gases.

Mantoux test (man'too) *C. Mantoux, French physician, 1877–1947.* A tuberculin skin test in which a solution of PPD-tuberculin is injected intradermally into either the anterior or posterior surface of the forearm. The test is read 48–72 hours after injection. It is considered positive when the induration at the site of injection is more than 10 mm in diameter.

manual handling ('manyoo·əl) any activity needing the use of force by a healthcare professional to lift, move, or hold a person or object. *M. h risk* any hazard or action that has the potential to cause harm or illness to a person. *M. h equipment* any piece of equipment that facilitates the transfer of persons or objects. Examples include monkey bars, mechanical lifters/hoists, slide sheet, and Patslides.

manubrium (mə'nyoobri·əm) the upper part of the sternum to which the clavicle is attached.

MAOI *see* MONOAMINE OXIDASE.

map mean arterial pressure.

maple syrup urine disease ('maypəl 'sirəp 'yoo·rən) an inborn error of metabolism in which there is an excess in the urine of certain amino acids. The urine smells like maple syrup and there are learning difficulties, spasticity, and convulsions.

marasmus (mə'razməs) severe and chronic malnutrition producing a gradual wasting of the tissues, owing to insufficient or unassimilated food, occurring especially in infants. It is not always possible to discover the cause.

marble bone disease (͵mahbəl 'bohn) a condition in which there is increased density of bone, which is visible on radiographic examination. Albers–Schönberg's disease. OSTEOPETROSIS.

Marburg virus disease ('mahbərg) a Central African viral HAEMORRHAGIC FEVER with acute onset and characteristic MORBILLIFORM rash. The incubation period is 3–7 days. It was first reported in Europe in 1967, associated with the importation of green monkeys from Uganda. Since then, several isolated incidents have occurred in Africa. The reservoir of infection is not known. Person-to-person transmission (by inoculation of blood and tissue fluid and by sexual intercourse) has been reported.

Marfan's syndrome (mah'fanhz) *B.J.A. Marfan, French paediatrician, 1858–1942.* An hereditary disorder in which there is excessive height with very long digits, a high-arched palate, hypertonus, dislocation of the lens of the eyes, and cardiac lesions, the most common of which is atrial septal defect.

marijuana (ˌmarəyə'wahnə, ˌmarə'wahnə) *Cannabis indica*; Indian hemp or hashish. *See* CANNABIS.

marrow ('maroh) the substance contained in the middle of long bones and in the cancellous tissue of all bones. *M. puncture* investigatory procedure in which marrow cells are aspirated from the sternum or iliac crest. *Red m.* that found in all cancellous tissue at birth. Blood cells are made in it. *Yellow m.* the fatty substance contained in the centre of long bones in later life.

Marshall-Marchetti operation ('mahˌshəl mar'ketee) a surgical procedure performed to control stress incontinence.

masculinisation (ˌmaskyələnie'zayshən) the development in a woman of male secondary sexual characteristics.

Maslow's hierarchy of needs ('mazlohz ˌhie·rahkee əv 'needz) *A.H. Maslow, American psychologist, 1908–70.* A hierarchical ranking, in ascending order of importance, concerning human needs and the aim of realising one's full potential. Physiological needs (for oxygen, nutrition, shelter, sleep, etc.) are the most basic and need to be met first, before one is able to deal, in successive order, with the needs for safety, security, love and belonging, self-esteem and, ultimately, self-actualisation. (*See* figure.)

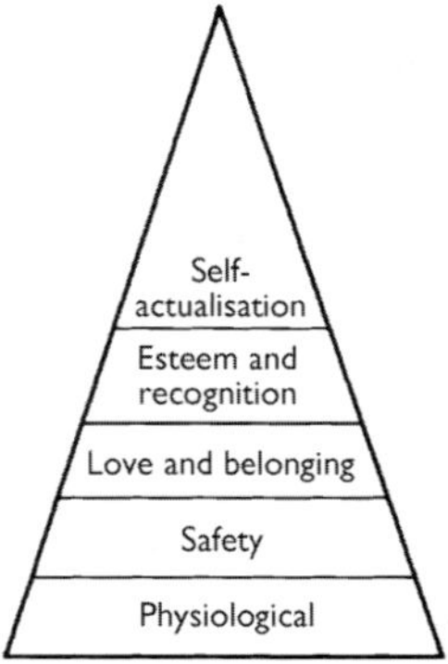

Maslow's Hierarchy of Needs

masochism ('masəˌkizəm) a sexual perversion in which pleasure is derived from suffering mental or physical pain.

massage ('masahzh, -sahj) a method of stroking, rubbing, kneading, and manipulating the body to stimulate circulation and to promote a sense of wellbeing. *External cardiac m.* the application of rhythmic pressure to the lower sternum to cause expulsion of blood from the ventricles and restart circulation in cases of cardiac arrest.

masseter (ma'seetə) the muscle of

the cheek chiefly concerned in mastication.

MAST medical anti-shock trouser.

mast cell (mahst) a large connective tissue cell found in many body tissues including the heart, liver, and lungs. Most cells contain granules which release heparin, serotinin, and histamine in response to inflammation or allergy.

mastalgia (ma'stalji·ə) pain in the breast.

mastatrophia (ˌmastə'trohfeeə) atrophy of the breast.

mastectomy (ma'stektəmee) amputation of the breast. *Radical m.* removal of the breast, axillary lymph glands, and the pectoral muscles.

mastication (ˌmastə'kayshən) the act of chewing food.

mastitis (ma'stietəs) inflammation of the breast, usually due to bacterial infection.

mastodynia (ˌmastoh'dini·ə) pain in the breast, which frequently occurs during the premenstrual phase.

mastoid ('mastoyd) breast- or nipple-shaped. *M. antrum* the cavity in the mastoid process which communicates with the middle ear and contains air. *M. cells* hollow spaces in the mastoid bone. *M. operation* drainage of mastoid cells when infection spreads from the middle ear. *M. process* the breast-shaped prominence on the temporal bone which projects downwards behind the ear and into which the sternocleidomastoid muscle is inserted.

mastoidectomy (ˌmastoy'dektəmee) removal of diseased bone and drainage of the mastoid antrum in severe purulent MASTOIDITIS.

mastoiditis (ˌmastoy'dietəs) inflammation of the mastoid antrum and cells.

masturbation (ˌmastə'bayshən) the production of sexual excitement by friction of the genitals.

materia medica (mə'tiə·ri·ə 'medikə) the science of the source and preparation of drugs used in medicine.

maternal (mə'tərn'l) pertaining to the mother. *M. mortality rate* the number of deaths in childbirth per 1000 births.

matrix ('maytriks) that tissue in which cells are embedded.

matter ('matə) substance. *Grey m.* a collection of nerve cells or non-medullated nerve fibres. *White m.* medullated nerve fibres massed together, as in the brain.

maturation (ˌmatyə'rayshən, ˌmachuh-) ripening or developing.

maxilla (mak'silə) one of the pair of bones forming the upper jaw and carrying the upper teeth.

maxillary (mak'silə·ree) pertaining to the upper jaw bones.

maxillofacial (ˌmaksiloh'fayshəl) pertaining to the maxilla and the face.

MCHC mean corpuscular haemoglobin concentration.

MCV mean corpuscular volume.

mean (meen) a measure of central tendency; the arithmetic average of all scores.

measles ('meezəlz) morbilli; rubeola. An acute, infectious, statutorily notifiable disease of childhood caused by a virus spread by droplets. Endemic and worldwide in distribution. Onset is catarrhal before the rash appears at the fourth day. KOPLIK'S SPOTS are diagnostic earlier. Secondary infection can give rise to the serious complication of OTITIS MEDIA or BRONCHOPNEUMONIA.

Vaccination provides a high degree of immunity. *German m.* *See* RUBELLA.

measures of central tendency ('mezhəz əv 'sentrəl 'tendənsee) descriptive statistical procedure that describes the average member of a sample (mean, median, and mode).

meatus (mee'aytəs) an opening or passage. *Auditory m.* the opening leading into the auditory canal. *Urethral m.* the opening of the urethra to the exterior.

mechanism of labour ('mekə,nizəm) the sequence of movements whereby the fetus adapts itself to pass through the maternal passages during the process of birth.

Meckel's diverticulum ('mekəlz) *J.F. Meckel, German anatomist and surgeon, 1781–1833.* The remains of a passage which, in the embryo, connected the yolk sac and intestine; evident as an enclosed sac or tube in the region of the ileum.

meconium (mə'kohni·əm) the first intestinal discharges of a newly born child. Dark green and consisting of epithelial cells, mucus, and bile. *M. ileus* intestinal obstruction due to blockage of the bowel by a plug of meconium in a neonate with CYSTIC FIBROSIS.

median ('meedi·ən) 1. placed in the centre. 2. in a series of values, the value middle in position.

mediastinum (,meedi·ə'stienəm) the space in the middle of the thorax, between the two pleurae; contains all the thoracic viscera other than the lungs.

medical ('medikəl) pertaining to medicine. *M. audit* an evaluative process applied to the quality of clinical practice, often by peer review of routine or specially collected records of individual cases. In the light of the outcome, judgments are frequently made on the appropriateness of the processes carried out during the management of the case.

medicalisation (,medikəlie'zayshən) 1. the extension of medical authority into areas previously regarded as being non-medical, in which the lay or a popular approach prevailed, e.g. pregnancy and childbirth. 2. the tendency to view undesirable conduct as illness and therefore requiring medical intervention.

medicament (mə'dikəmənt) any medicinal substance used in treatment.

medicated ('medə,kaytəd) impregnated with a medicinal substance.

medication (,medə'kayshən) 1. a substance administered to a patient for therapeutic purposes. 2. the treatment of a patient by means of drugs.

medicinal (mə'disən'l) 1. having therapeutic qualities. 2. pertaining to a medicine.

medicine ('medəsən, 'medsən) 1. any drug or remedy. 2. the art and science of the diagnosis and treatment of disease and the maintenance of health. 3. the non-surgical treatment of disease. *Community m.* that speciality which deals with all aspects of medical care in the community, including notification and control of infectious diseases, preschool and school health care, and factors affecting the health of the population as a whole. *Emergency m.* that speciality which deals with the acutely ill or injured who require immediate medical treatment. *Family m.* family practice; the medical speciality concerned with the provision of comprehensive primary health care. *Forensic m.* the application of medical knowledge to questions of law; medical jurisprudence. Called also legal medicine. *Group m.* the practice of medicine by a group of doctors, usually representing various specialities, who are associated together for the cooperative diagnosis, treatment, and prevention of disease. *Legal m.* forensic medicine. *Nuclear m.* that branch of medicine concerned with the use of radionuclides in the diagnosis and treatment of disease. *Physical m.* that branch of medicine using physical agents in the diagnosis and treatment of disease. It includes the use of heat, cold, light, water, electricity, manipulation, massage, exercise, and mechanical devices. *Preventive m.* science aimed at preventing disease. *Proprietary m.* any chemical, drug, or similar preparation used in the treatment of diseases, if such article is protected against free competition as to name, product, composition, or process of manufacture by secrecy, patent, trademark, copyright, or other means. *Psychosomatic m.* the study of the interrelations between bodily processes and emotional life. *Space m.* that branch of aviation medicine concerned with conditions to be encountered in space. *Sports m.* the field of medicine concerned with injuries sustained in athletic endeavours, including their prevention, diagnosis, and treatment.

medicosocial (ˌmedəkoh'sohshəl) applying to both medicine and the social factors involved.

meditation (ˌmedə'tayshən) the production of a state of relaxation by focusing the mind on a single thought and eliminating other stimuli.

medium ('meedi·əm) in bacteriology, a preparation for the culture of microorganisms. *Contrast m.* a substance used in radiography to make visible structures that could not otherwise be seen.

MEDLINE ('medˌlien) the print or computerised database of standard medical literature analysis and retrieval system on-line; it is also available on CD-Rom.

medroxyprogesterone (medˌroksee-proh'jestəˌrohn) a synthetic female sex hormone used to treat menstrual disorders, endometrial carcinoma, and ENDOMETRIOSIS, and as a short-term contraceptive.

medulla (mə'dulə) 1. bone marrow. 2. the innermost part of an organ, particularly the kidneys, lymph glands, and suprarenal glands. *M. oblongata* that portion of the spinal cord that is contained inside the cranium. In it are the nerve centres which govern respiration, the action of the heart, etc.

medullary (mə'dulə·ree) pertaining to the marrow or a medulla. *M. cavity* the hollow in the centre of long bones.

medullated ('medəˌlaytəd) having a myelin covering. *M. nerve fibre* one enclosed in a myelin sheath.

medulloblastoma (məˌdulohbla-'stohmə) a rapidly growing tumour of neuroepithelial origin occurring in childhood and appearing near the fourth ventricle of the brain. The tumour is very radiosensitive.

mefenamic acid (ˌmefə'namik) an analgesic and antipyretic drug used in the treatment of mild to moderate pain.

mega a combining form meaning large, enlarged, or of abnormally large size.

megacolon (ˌmegəˈkohlon) extreme dilatation and hypertrophy of the large intestine. When the condition is congenital, it is known as HIRSCHSPRUNG'S DISEASE.

megakaryocyte (ˌmegəˈkareeəˌsiet) a large cell of the bone marrow, responsible for blood platelet formation.

megaloblast (ˌmegəlohˈblast) an abnormally large nucleated cell from which mature red blood cells are derived.

megalocephaly (ˌmegəlohˈkefəlee, -ˈsef-) 1. abnormal largeness of the head. 2. LEONTIASIS OSSEA.

megalomania (ˌmegəlohˈmayni·ə) delusions of grandeur or self-importance characteristic of general paralysis of the insane.

megaureter (ˌmegəyəˈreeta) dilatation of the ureter.

Meibomian glands (mieˈbohmi·ən) *H. Meibom, German anatomist, 1638–1700*. Small sebaceous glands situated beneath the conjunctiva of the eyelid; tarsal glands. *M. cyst* a small swelling of the gland caused by obstruction of its duct. If untreated, it can become infected. ACHALAZION.

meibomianitis (mieˌbohmi·əˈnietəs) a bilateral chronic inflammation of the MEIBOMIAN glands.

meiosis (mieˈohsəs) 1. a stage of reduction cell division when the chromosomes of a GAMETE are halved in number ready for union at fertilisation. 2. contraction of the pupil of the eye; miosis.

melaena (məˈleenə) the passing of black, tarry faeces stained with blood pigments.

melancholia (ˌmelənˈkohleeə) a state of extreme depression. *See* DEPRESSION.

melanin (ˈmelənən) a dark pigment found in the hair, the choroid of the eye, the skin, and melanotic tumours.

melanism (ˈmeləˌnizəm) a condition marked by an abnormal deposit of dark pigment in the skin or other tissue. Melanosis.

melanocyte (ˈmelənohˌsiet) a cell of the skin pigment melanin. *M.-stimulating hormone* abbreviated MSH. Hormone produced in the pituitary gland which stimulates the formation of melanin.

melanoderma (ˌmelənohˈdərmə) a patchy pigmentation of the skin.

melanoma (ˌmeləˈnohmə) a malignant tumour arising in any pigment-containing tissues, especially the skin and the eye. *Amelanotic m.* an unpigmented malignant melanoma. *Juvenile m.* a benign lesion which usually occurs on the face before puberty. Can be mistaken for a malignant melanoma.

melanosis (ˌmeləˈnohsəs) *see* MELANISM.

melanotic (ˌmeləˈnotik) pertaining to melanosis. *M. sarcoma see* SARCOMA.

melanuria (ˌmeləˈnyoo·ri·ə) the presence of black pigment in the urine. Occurs in melanotic SARCOMA and PORPHYRIA.

melasma (meˈlazma) dark discolouration of the skin; CHLOASMA.

melphalan (ˈmelfəlan) a cytotoxic drug that is particularly useful in the treatment of multiple MYELOMA.

membrane (ˈmembrayn) a thin elastic tissue covering the surface of certain organs and lining the cavities of the body. *Basement m.*

the interface between epithelial cells and the underlying connective tissue. *Mucous m.* a membrane that secretes mucus and lines all cavities connected directly or indirectly with the skin. *Serous m.* membrane lining the abdominal cavity and thorax and covering most of the organs within.

memory ('meməree) the mental faculty that enables one to retain and recall previously experienced sensations, impressions, information, and ideas. The ability of the brain to retain and to use knowledge gained from past experience is essential to the process of learning. The exact way in which the brain remembers is not fully understood; it is believed that a portion of the temporal lobe of the brain acts as a memory centre, drawing on memories stored in other parts of the brain.

menarche ('menahk, 'menahkee) the first appearance of menstruation.

Mendel's theory ('mend'lz) *G.J. Mendel, Abbot of Brünn, 1822–84.* The theory that the characters of sexually reproducing organisms are handed on to the offspring in fixed ratios and without blending.

Mendelson's syndrome ('mend'l-ˌsənz) a condition in which there is severe oedema and spasm of the bronchioles due to the inhalation of acid gastric contents.

Menière's disease or **syndrome** ('meneeˌairz) *P. Menière, French physician, 1799–1862.* A disease of the inner ear causing attacks of vertigo and TINNITUS with progressive deafness.

meninges (mə'ninjeez, 'menin-) the membranes covering the brain and spinal cord. There are three: the dura mater (outer), arachnoid mater (middle), and pia mater (inner).

meningioma (mə'ninjeeˌohmə) a slow-growing, usually benign tumour developing from the arachnoid and pia mater.

meningism ('meninˌjizəm) a condition in which there are signs of cerebral irritation similar to meningitis, but in which no causative organism can be isolated.

meningitis (ˌmenən'jietəs) inflammation of the meninges; can be due to organisms (such as bacteria, viruses, and fungi), chemical toxins (such as lead and arsenic), contrast media (used in myelography), or metastatic malignant cells. Meningitis, and its causal organism (if known), is a notifiable disease. *Meningococcal m. See* MENINGOCOCCAL DISEASE. *Tuberculous m.* inflammation of tuberculous origin.

meningocele (mə'ning·gohˌseel) a protrusion of the meninges through the skull or spinal column, appearing as a cyst filled with cerebrospinal fluid. *See* SPINA bifida.

meningococcal disease (mə'ning-·gə'kokəl, məˌninjə'kokəl) a rare but potentially fatal bacterial infection. The disease manifests as either meningococcal meningitis (inflammation of the membranes surrounding the brain) or meningococcal septicaemia (bacteria in the blood). Caused by the bacterium *Neisseria meningitidis*. The most common groups are A, B, C (W135), and Y. In Australia, groups B and C are common. Transmitted either through the air by droplets of respiratory secretions or by direct contact with an infected person. Early signs and symptoms include

fever, severe headache, stiff neck, rash (tiny red or purple spots), nausea, and vomiting. Disease progression is rapid and urgent medical care is required if two or more of the signs and symptoms are experienced concurrently. Immunisation (except for group B) is available to reduce the risk of meningococcal menginitis.

meningococcus (məˌning·gə'kokəs) *Neisseria meningitidis*. A diplococcus, the microorganism of cerebrospinal meningitis.

meningoencephalitis (məˌning·goh-·enˌkefə'lietəs, -ˌsef-) inflammation of the brain and meninges.

meningomyelocele (məˌning·goh-'mieəlohˌseel) a protrusion of the spinal cord and meninges through a defect in the vertebral column. Myelomeningocele. *See* SPINA bifida.

meniscectomy (ˌmenə'sektəmee) surgical removal of a semilunar cartilage in a knee joint.

meniscus (mə'niskəs) 1. the convex or concave surface of a liquid as observed in its container. 2. a lens having one convex and one concave surface. 3. a semilunar cartilage of the knee joint.

menopause ('menəˌpawz) the span of time during which the menstrual cycle wanes and gradually stops; called also 'change of life' and 'climacteric'. It is the time when the ovaries stop functioning and, therefore, when menstruation and childbearing cease. Usually occurs between the 45th and 50th years of life. There can be an associated hormonal imbalance which causes symptoms including night sweats, hot flushes, diminished libido, and extreme lethargy. *Artificial m.* an induced cessation of menstruation by surgery or by irradiation.

menorrhagia (ˌmenə'rayji·ə) an excessive flow of the menses; menorrhoea.

menses ('menseez) the discharge from the uterus during menstruation.

menstrual ('menstrooəl) relating to the menses. *M. cycle* the monthly cycle commencing with the first day of menstruation, when the ENDOMETRIUM is shed, proceeding through a process of repair and hypertrophy until the next period. It is governed by the anterior pituitary gland and the ovarian hormones, oestrogen and progesterone (*see* figure).

menstruation (ˌmenstroo'ayshən) the monthly discharge of blood and ENDOMETRIUM from the uterus, starting at the age of puberty and lasting until the menopause. *Anovular m., anovulatory m.* peri-

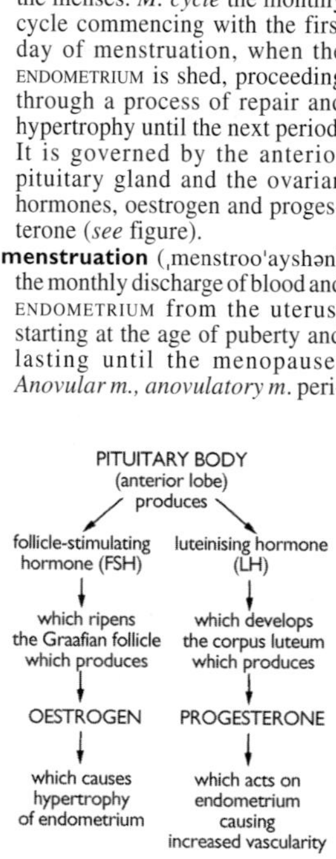

Hormone Influence on Menstruation

odic uterine bleeding without preceding ovulation. *Vicarious m.* discharge of blood at the time of menstruation from some organ other than the uterus, e.g. epistaxis, which is not uncommon.

mental ('ment'l) 1. pertaining to the mind. *M. age* the measurement of the intelligence level of an individual in terms of the average chronological age of children showing the same mental standard, as measured by a scale of mental tests. *M. illness* a term used to describe a number of disorders of the mind that affect the emotions, perceptions, reasoning, or memory of the individual, e.g. psychoses and neuroses. 2. pertaining to the chin.

menthol ('menthol) a crystalline substance derived from oil of peppermint and used in neuralgia and rhinitis, and as a local anodyne and antiseptic.

mentor ('mentaw) 1. a wise or trusted adviser or guide. 2. in nursing, a professional colleague who assists with the career development of a colleague and who facilitates and encourages that person's professional growth and awareness.

mepacrine ('mepə,krin) a synthetic drug used as an antimalarial agent and in the treatment of GIARDIASIS.

meprobamate (mə'prohbə,mayt) a tranquilliser used in the treatment of nervous anxiety.

meptazinol (mep'tazənol) a newer narcotic analgesic claimed to cause less repiratory depression than other narcotic analgesics. It has a relatively quick onset of action but a short duration of action of 2–4 hours. Nausea and vomiting are quite common and the drug does not appear to have any great advantage over more established agents.

mercaptopurine (mə,kaptoh'pyoo·reen) a drug which prevents nucleic acid synthesis and can be used in the treatment of some types of leukaemia.

mercury ('mərkyə·ree) *symbol* Hg. Quicksilver; a heavy liquid metallic element, the salts of which are used occasionally as antiseptics and disinfectants. Also used in the manufacture of various types of thermometers and manometers.

mesarteritis (,mesahtə'rietəs) inflammation of the middle coat of an artery.

mescaline ('meskə,leen) an alkaloid drug which produces intoxication and hallucinations. It is a drug of addiction.

mesencephalon (,mesən'kefə,lon, -'sef-) the middle brain.

mesenchyme ('mesəng,kiem) in the embryo, the connective tissue developed from the MESODERM.

mesentery ('mesəntə·ree, 'mez-) a fold of the peritoneum which connects the intestine to the posterior abdominal wall.

mesmerism ('mezmə,rizəm) *F.A. Mesmer, Austrian physician, 1734–1815.* HYPNOTISM.

mesoderm ('mesoh,dərm) the middle of the three primary layers of cells in the embryo from which the connective tissues develop.

mesometrium (,mesoh'meetri·əm) the broad ligament connecting the uterus with the abdominal wall.

mesomorph ('mesoh,mawf) a stocky individual of medium height with well-developed muscles.

mesothelioma (,mesoh,theelee'ohmə) a rapidly growing tumour of the pleura, peritoneum, or pericardium which might be seen in patients with ASBESTOSIS. However, this tumour can also occur in people who have no history of exposure to asbestos.

messenger RNA (ˌmesənjə ˌah'enˌay) abbreviated mRNA. The ribonucleic acid which acts as a template for the linking of amino acids during the formation of protein in the cells.

mestranol ('mestrəˌnol) a synthetic oestrogen commonly used in combination with a progesterone in contraceptive pills.

meta-analysis (ˌmetə·rə'naləsəs) a research method that takes the results of multiple studies in a specific area and synthesises the findings to make conclusions regarding the area of focus.

metabolic (ˌmetə'bolik) referring to metabolism.

metabolism (mə'tabəˌlizəm) the sum of the physical and chemical processes by which living organised substance is built up and maintained ANABOLISM, and by which large molecules are broken down into smaller molecules to make energy available to the organism (catabolism). Essentially, these processes are concerned with the disposition of the nutrients absorbed into the blood after digestion. *Basal m.* the minimal energy expended for the maintenance of respiration, circulation, peristalsis, muscle tonus, body temperature, glandular activity, and the other 'vegetative' functions of the body. *Inborn error of m.* a genetically determined biochemical disorder in which a specific enzyme defect produces a metabolic block that can have pathological consequences at birth, as in PHENYLKETONURIA, or in later life.

metabolite (mə'tabəˌliet) any product or substance taking part in metabolism. *Essential m.* a substance that is necessary for normal metabolism, e.g. a vitamin.

metacarpal (ˌmetə'kahpəl) one of the five bones of the hand which join the fingers to the wrist.

metacarpophalangeal (ˌmetəˌkahpohfə'lanji·əl) relating to the metacarpal bones and the phalanges.

metacarpus (ˌmetə'kahpəs) the five bones of the hand uniting the carpus with the phalanges of the fingers.

metamorphosis (ˌmetə'mawfəsəs) a structural change or transformation.

metaphase ('metəˌfayz) the second stage of mitosis or cell division.

metaphysis (mə'tafəsəs) the junction of the EPIPHYSIS with the DIAPHYSIS in a long bone.

metaplasia (ˌmetə'playzi·ə) abnormal change in the structure of a tissue. Can be indicative of malignant change.

metastasis (mə'tastəsəs) the transfer of a disease from one part of the body to another, through the blood vessels, via the lymph channels, or across the body cavities. (a) Secondary deposits can occur from a primary malignant growth. (b) Septic infection can arise in other organs from some original focus.

metatarsal (ˌmetə'tahsəl) one of the five bones of the foot which join the tarsus to the toes.

metatarsalgia (ˌmetətah'salji·ə) pain in the metatarsal bones.

metatarsus (ˌmetə'tahsəs) the five bones of the foot uniting the tarsus with the phalanges of the toes.

Metazoa (ˌmetə'zoh·ə) the division

of the animal kingdom that includes the multicellular animals, i.e. all animals except the PROTOZOA.

metformin (met'fawmən) a biguanide hypoglycaemic used in the treatment of DIABETES mellitus.

methadone ('methəˌdohn) a powerful analgesic with no sedative action. Similar in action to morphine, it is used to relieve pain in terminal illness and also in withdrawal programs for heroin addicts. Methadone is addictive, but less socially disabling than heroin. Amidone.

methaemalbumin (ˌmet·heem-'albyoomən) a compound of haem with plasma albumin found in the blood in some types of anaemia.

methaemoglobin ('met·heemə-'glohbən) an altered form of haemoglobin found in the blood and usually produced by the action of a drug on the red blood cells, causing a reduction in their oxygen-carrying ability. Can be associated with the use of phenacetin and other aniline derivatives.

methaemoglobinaemia (ˌmet·heeməˌglohbə'neemi·ə) CYANOSIS and inability of the red blood cells to transport oxygen because of the presence of methaemoglobin.

methane ('meethayn) marsh gas; an inflammable explosive gas produced by decomposition of organic matter.

methicillin (ˌmethi'silin) a form of penicillin that is resistant to staphylococcal penicillinase. *M-resistant staphyloccus aureus* (MRSA) is a nosocomial pathogen that is prevalent in most hospitals. MRSA is a virulent organism that can cause significant morbidity and mortality, and, although it does not seem to affect healthy individuals, it can be deadly to patients in hospital.

methionine (me'thieəˌneen) 1. a sulphur-containing essential amino acid occurring in proteins that is a vital component of the diet. 2. a drug used orally in the treatment of paracetamol poisoning.

methohexitone (ˌmethoh'heksə-tohn) a barbiturate anaesthetic agent; given intravenously it has a short recovery time.

methotrexate (ˌmethoh'treksayt) a cytotoxic drug that antagonises folic acid and prevents cell formation. It is used to treat various types of malignant disease.

methotrimeprazine (ˌmethohtrie-'meprəzeen) a phenothiazine with sedative and analgesic properties. Useful in SCHIZOPHRENIA and terminal illness.

methoxamine (me'thoksəˌmeen) a sympathomimetic amine used for its vasopressor effects in restoring blood pressure during anaesthesia.

methyl salicylate (ˌmethəl sə'lisəˌlayt, ˌmeethiel) a compound used externally for rheumatic pains, lumbago, etc. Oil of wintergreen.

methylated spirit (ˌmethəˌlaytəd 'spirət) a mixture of 95% ethyl alcohol and 5% methyl alcohol. An industrial spirit which, taken as a drink, is poisonous.

methylcellulose (ˌmethəl'selyəlohs, -lohz) a bulk-forming drug used as a laxative and to control diarrhoea.

methyldopa (ˌmethəl'dohpə) a hypotensive drug the action of which is increased if used with thiazide diuretics.

methylene blue ('methəˌleen) a synthetic organic compound, in dark-green crystals or lustrous crystalline powder, used in treatment of METHAEMOGLOBINAEMIA, as an antidote in cyanide poisoning, as a stain in pathology and bacteriology, and as an antiseptic.

methylphenobarbitone (ˌmethəlˌfenoh'bahbətohn) a white crystalline powder used as an anticonvulsant with a slight hypnotic action. Especially useful for senile tremor.

methylprednisolone (ˌmethəlpred'nisəˌlohn) a corticosteroid of the glucogenic type, having an anti-inflammatory action similar to that of prednisolone.

methysergide (ˌmethi'sərjied) a potent serotonin antagonist used in the prophylaxis of migraine.

metoclopramide (ˌmetoh'klohprəmied) a drug which speeds up gastric action and is used to treat nausea, heartburn, and vomiting.

metoprolol (me'tohprəˌlol) a cardioselective beta-blocker having a greater effect on β_1-adrenergic receptors of the heart than on the β_2-adrenergic receptors of the bronchi and blood vessels; used for treatment of hypertension. *See* BETA blockers.

metra ('meetrə) the uterus.

metre ('meetə) *symbol* m. The fundamental SI unit of length.

metritis (mə'trietəs) inflammation of the uterus.

metrocolpocele (ˌmeetroh'kolpəˌseel) the protrusion of the uterus into the vagina, the wall of the latter also being pushed forwards.

metronidazole (ˌmetroh'nidəˌzohl) a drug that is effective in overcoming *Trichomonas* infection of the genital tract of both sexes. Also used in the treatment of GIARDIASIS, acute amoebic dysentery, and infection by anaerobic bacteria.

metropathia (ˌmeetroh'pathi·ə) any disorder affecting the uterus; metropathy. *M. haemorrhagica* excessive loss of blood from the uterus due to disease; uterine haemorrhage.

metroptosis (ˌmeetrop'tohsəs) prolapse of the uterus.

metrorrhagia (ˌmeetrə'rayji·ə) irregular uterine bleeding not associated with menstruation.

metrostaxis (ˌmeetroh'staksəs) persistent slight haemorrhage from the uterus.

mexiletine (mek'silәteen) an antiarrhythmic agent used to treat ventricular ARRHYTHMIAS.

Michel's suture clips (mi'shelz) *G. Michel, French surgeon, 1875–1937.* Small metal clips used for suturing wounds.

miconazole (mie'konəˌzohl) an antifungal agent used topically for dermatophytic infections such as athlete's foot or vulvovaginal candidiasis, orally for CANDIDIASIS of the mouth and gastrointestinal tract, and systemically by intravenous infusion for systemic fungal infections.

microalbuminuria (ˌmiekrohˌalbyəmən'yoo·ri·a) the urinary excretion of small amounts of albumin, below the detection level of routine dipstick analysis. The condition is an early indicator of altered glomerular permeability in diabetes mellitus.

microbe ('miekrohb) a minute living organism, especially one causing disease. A microorganism.

microbiology (ˌmiekrohbie'oləjee) the study of microorganisms and their effect on living cells.

microcephalic (ˌmiekrohkə'falik, -sə-) having an abnormally small head.

Micrococcus (ˌmiekroh'kokəs) a genus of bacteria, each of which has a spherical shape. The bacteria occur in pairs or in groups and are Gram-positive. Found in soil and water.

microcornea (ˌmiekroh'kawni·ə) a condition in which the cornea is smaller than normal, producing HYPERMETROPIA and sometimes causing GLAUCOMA.

microcythaemia (ˌmiekrohsie'thee-mi·ə) the presence of abnormally small red cells in the blood; microcytosis.

microdrip (ˌmiekroh'drip) an intravenous-giving set that delivers an infusion rate of 60 drops per 1 mL.

micrognathia (ˌmiekroh'nathi·ə) failure of development of the lower jaw, causing a receding chin.

microgram ('miekrohˌgram) *symbol* μg. One millionth of a gram.

micrometre ('miekrohˌmeetə) *symbol* μm. One millionth of a metre. Formerly called micron.

micron ('miekron) *see* MICROMETRE.

micronutrient (ˌmiekroh'nyoo-tri·ənt) a dietary element essential only in small quantities.

microorganism (ˌmiekroh'awgə-ˌnizəm) a minute animal or vegetable, particularly a virus, a bacterium, a fungus, a rickettsia, or a protozoon.

microphage (ˌmiekroh'fayj) a minute PHAGOCYTE.

microphthalmos (ˌmiekrof'thalməs) a condition in which one or both eyes are smaller than normal. Their function might or might not be impaired.

microscope ('miekrəˌskohp) an instrument which produces a greatly enlarged image of objects that are normally invisible to the human eye. *Electron m.* a microscope in which a beam of electrons is used instead of a light beam, allowing magnification of as much as 500 000 diameters.

microscopic (ˌmiekrə'skopik) visible only by means of a microscope.

Microsporum (ˌmiekroh'spaw·rəm) a genus of fungi. The cause of some skin diseases, especially ringworm.

microsurgery (ˌmiekroh'sərjə·ree) the carrying out of surgical procedures using a microscope and miniature instruments.

micturition (ˌmiktyə'rishən) the act of passing urine.

midbrain ('midˌbrayn) that portion of the brain that connects the CEREBRUM with the pons and CEREBELLUM. The mesencephalon.

midlife crisis (ˌmidˌlief 'kriesəs) experienced by many people during the fifth decade of life, resulting in doubt, anxiety and, sometimes, depression. During this time, men and women might reflect on their lives, review the past, and be aware of physiological deterioration associated with ageing. Any children are growing up, moving away from home, and establishing their own adult relationships. 'Empty nest syndrome'.

midwifery (mid'wifə·ree, 'midˌwifə-·ree) dealing with childbirth. *See* OBSTETRICS. *M. process* the application of the nursing process to midwifery. It is a systematic, cyclical method of organising midwifery care, and is carried out by the assessment of actual and potential problems, and the planning, implementation, and evaluation of care.

migraine ('meegrayn, 'mie-)

paroxysmal attacks of severe headache, often with nausea, vomiting, and visual disturbance.

milestone ('miel,stohn) one of the 'norms' against which the motor, social, and psychological development of a child is measured.

miliaria (,milee'air·ri·ə) prickly heat, an itching skin eruption common among white people in tropical and subtropical areas.

miliary ('milyə·ree) resembling millet seed. *M. tuberculosis see* TUBERCULOSIS.

milium ('mili·əm) [L.] a whitish nodule in the skin, especially of the face, usually 1–4 mm in diameter. Milia are spheroidal, epithelial cysts of lamellated keratin lying just under the epidermis, often associated with vellus hair follicles. Popularly called 'whitehead'.

milk (milk) 1. a nutrient fluid produced by the mammary gland of many animals for nourishment of young mammals. 2. a liquid (emulsion or suspension) resembling the secretion of the mammary gland. *M. sugar* lactose, a disaccharide present in the milk of all mammals. *M. teeth* the first set of teeth. *Witch's m.* milk secreted from the breast of a newborn child.

Miller–Abbott tube (,milə'abət ,tyoob) *T.G. Miller, American physician, 1886–1981; W.O. Abbott, American physician, 1902–43.* A double-channel intestinal tube for treating obstruction, especially that due to paralytic ileus of the small intestine. It has an inflatable balloon at its distal end.

milliequivalent (,mileeə'kwivələnt) the amount of a substance that balances or is equivalent in combining power to 1 mg of hydrogen. A method of assessing the body's acid–base balance or needs during electrolyte upset.

milligram ('milə,gram) *symbol* mg. One thousandth of a gram.

millilitre ('milə,leetə) *symbol* mL. One thousandth of a litre (one cubic centimetre).

millimetre ('milə,meetə) *symbol* mm. One thousandth of a metre.

millimole ('milee,mohl) *symbol* mmol. The amount of a substance that balances or is equivalent in combining power to 1 mg of hydrogen. A method of assessing the body's acid–base balance or needs during electrolyte upset.

Millipore filter ('milee,paw) trade name for a device used to filter nutrient solutions as they are administered intravenously.

Milton ('miltən) trade name for an antiseptic consisting of a standardised 1% solution of electrolytic sodium hypochlorite. It is used especially for the sterilisation of babies' feeding bottles.

Milwaukee brace (mil'wawkee) a brace consisting of a leather girdle and neck ring connected by metal struts; used to brace the spine in the treatment of SCOLIOSIS.

mineralocorticoid (,minə·rəloh-'kawtə,koyd) a hormone produced by the adrenal cortex. Its function is to maintain the salt and water balance in the body.

Minims ('minəmz) trade name for eye drops packaged in single-use containers.

minocycline (,minoh'siekleen) a semisynthetic broad-spectrum antibiotic of the tetracycline group.

miosis (mie'ohsəs) contraction of the pupil of the eye, as in reaction to a bright light; MEIOSIS.

miotic (mie'otik) a drug which causes contraction of the pupil.

miscarriage ('mis,karij) abortion; the expulsion of the fetus before the 20th week of pregnancy, i.e. before it is legally viable.

mite (miet) a minute animal, frequently parasitic on humans and animals, which causes various forms of dermatitis.

mithramycin (,mithrə'miesən) an antitumour antibiotic which is particularly helpful in the treatment of HYPERCALCAEMIA.

mitochondrion (,mietoh'kondri·ən) a body which is found in the cytoplasm of cells and is concerned with energy production and the oxidation of food.

mitomycin (,mietoh'miesən) a group of highly toxic antineoplastics (mitomycin A, B, and C), produced by *Streptomyces caespitosus*; indicated for palliative treatment of certain neoplasms that do not respond to surgery, radiation, and other drugs.

mitosis (mie'tohsəs) a method of multiplication of cells by a specific process of division.

mitral ('mietrəl) shaped like a mitre. *M. incompetence* the result of a defective mitral valve, when there is a back flow, or regurgitation, after closure of the valve. *M. stenosis* the formation of fibrous tissue causing a narrowing of the valve; usually due to rheumatic heart disease and ENDOCARDITIS. *M. valve* the bicuspid valve between the left atrium and left ventricle of the heart. *M. valvotomy* an operation for overcoming stenosis by dividing the fibrous tissue to free the cusps.

mittelschmerz ('mit'l,shmərts) pain occurring between the menses, accompanying ovulation.

Mn symbol for *manganese*.

mobilisation (,mobəlie'zayshən) the bringing back into mobility of a limb, joint, or person following illness or injury.

modality (moh'dalətee) the number of peaks in a frequency distribution.

mode (mohd) a measure of central tendency; most frequent score or result.

molar ('mohlə) a back tooth used for grinding. There are three on either side of each jaw, making 12 in all (only eight in children).

mole (mohl) 1. the molecular weight of a substance expressed in grams. 2. a pigmented naevus or dark-coloured growth on the skin. Moles are of various sizes and are sometimes covered with hair. 3. a uterine tumour. *Carneous m.* an organised blood clot surrounding a shrivelled fetus in the uterus. *Hydatidiform m.* (vesicular m.) a condition in pregnancy in which the chorionic villi of the placenta degenerate into clusters of cysts like hydatids. Malignant growth is very likely to follow if any remnants are left in the uterus. *See* CHORIOCARCINOMA.

molecular (mə'lekyələ) pertaining to or composed of molecules. *M. weight* the weight of a molecule of a substance compared with that of an atom of carbon.

molecule ('molə,kyool) the chemical combination of two or more atoms which form a specific chemical substance, e.g. H_2O (water). The smallest amount of a substance that can exist independently.

molluscum (mo'luskəm) a skin disease characterised by the development of soft, round tumours. *M. contagiosum* a benign tumour arising in the epidermis caused by a virus, transmitted by direct contact or FOMITES.

monarticular (ˌmonah'tikyələ) referring to one joint only.

Mongolian spot (mong'gohli·ən) a smooth naevus consisting of an excess of melanocytes, situated in the sacral region, usually disappearing in childhood.

mongolism ('mong·gəˌlizəm) outdated term for Down's syndrome.

Monilia (mo'nili·ə) former name for the genus of fungi now known as *Candida*.

monitor ('monətə) 1. to check constantly on a given condition, state, or phenomenon, e.g. blood pressure, heart, respiration rate, or standards of care. 2. an apparatus by which such conditions or phenomena can be constantly observed and recorded. *Patient m.* the use of electrodes or transducers attached to the patient so that information such as temperature, pulse, respiration, and blood pressure can be seen on a screen or automatically recorded.

monoamine oxidase (ˌmonoh-ˌameen 'oksədayz) an enzyme that breaks down noradrenaline and serotonin in the body. *M. o. inhibitor* abbreviated MAOI. A drug that prevents the breakdown of serotonin and leads to an increase in mental and physical activity.

monochromatism (ˌmonoh'kromə-ˌtizəm) colour blindness. The patient sees all colours as black, grey, or white.

monoclonal (ˌmonoh'klohn'l) derived from a single cell. *M. antibodies* antibodies derived from a single clone of cells. All the antibody molecules are identical and will react with the same antigenic site.

monocular (mo'nokyələ) pertaining to or affecting one eye only.

monocyte ('monohˌsiet) a white blood cell having one nucleus, derived from the reticular cells, and having a phagocytic action.

mononucleosis (ˌmonohˌnyooklee-'ohsəs) an excessive number of monocytes in the blood; monocytosis. *Infectious m.* an infectious disease due to the Epstein–Barr virus; glandular fever.

monoplegia (ˌmonoh'pleeji·ə) paralysis of one limb or of a single muscle or a group of muscles.

monosaccharide (ˌmonoh'sakəˌried) a simple sugar. The end result of carbohydrate digestion. Examples are glucose, fructose, and galactose.

monosodium glutamate (ˌmonoh-ˌsohdi·əm 'glootəˌmayt) a chemical food flavour enhancer commonly added to Chinese dishes. Can result in nausea, faintness, facial flushing, and headache. (Sometimes called the 'Chinese restaurant syndrome'.)

monosomy (ˌmonoh'sohmee) a congenital defect in the number of human chromosomes. There is one fewer than the normal 46.

mons (monz) a prominence or mound. *M. pubis* or *m. veneris* the eminence, consisting of a pad of fat, that lies over the pubic symphysis in the female.

Montgomery's glands or **tubercles** (mənt'guməreez) *W.F. Montgomery, Irish obstetrician, 1797–1859.* Sebaceous glands around the nipple, which grow larger during pregnancy.

mood (mood) emotional reaction. Variations in mood are natural, but in certain psychiatric conditions there is severe depression in some cases and wild excitement in others, or alternations between each.

moon face ('moon,fays) one of the features occurring in Cushing's syndrome and as a result of prolonged treatment with steroid drugs.

morbid ('mawbəd) diseased, or relating to an abnormal or disordered condition.

morbidity (maw'bidətee) the state of being diseased. *M. rate* a figure that shows the susceptibility of a population to a certain disease. Usually shown statistically as the number of cases which occur annually per thousand or other unit of population.

morbilli (maw'bilie) measles.

morbilliform (maw'bilə,fawm) resembling measles.

moribund ('mo·rə,bund) in a dying condition.

morning sickness ('mawning) nausea and vomiting which sometimes occurs in early pregnancy.

Moro reflex ('mo·roh) *E. Moro, German paediatrician, 1874–1951.* The reaction to loud noise or sudden movement which should be present in the newborn. Startle reflex.

morphine ('mawfeen) the principal alkaloid obtained from opium and given mainly to relieve severe pain. It is a drug of addiction. Morphia.

mortality (maw'talətee) the state of being liable to die. *M. rate* the number of deaths, per 1000 or other unit of population, occurring annually from a certain disease or condition.

mortification (,mawtəfə'kayshən) gangrene or death of tissue; NECROSIS.

morula ('mo·ryələ) an early stage of development of the ovum when it is a solid mass of cells.

mosaic (moh'zayik) an individual who has cells of varying genetic composition.

motile ('mohtiel) capable of movement.

motion ('mohshən) 1. the process of moving. 2. evacuation of the bowels; defaecation. *M. sickness* sickness occurring as the result of travel by land, sea, or air. Appears to be caused by excessive stimulation of the vestibular apparatus within the inner ear.

motivation (,mohtə'vayshən) the reason or reasons, conscious or unconscious, behind a particular attitude or behaviour.

motive ('mohtiv) the incentive that determines a course of action or its direction.

motor ('mohtə) something that causes movement. *M. end-plate* the nuclei and cytoplasm of muscle fibres at the termination of motor nerves. *M. nerve* one of the nerves that convey an impulse from a nerve centre to a muscle or gland to promote activity. *M. neurone disease* a disease in which there is progressive degeneration of the anterior cells in the spinal cord, the motor nuclei of cranial nerves, and the corticospinal tracts. The cause is unknown.

mould (mohld) 1. a species of fungus. 2. the plastic shell used to immobilise a part of the body, usually the head, during radiotherapy.

moulding ('mohlding) the alteration

in shape of the infant's head as it is forced through the maternal passages during labour.

mountain sickness ('mowntən) DYSPNOEA, headache, rapid pulse, and vomiting, which occur on sudden change to the rarefied air of high altitudes.

mouth (mowth) an opening, particularly the external opening (in the face) of the alimentary canal. *M. ulcers* painful, greyish white sores occurring inside the mouth. Most are of unknown cause and disappear after a few days. Those that persist should be reported. Aphthous ulcers. *M.-wash* a solution for rinsing the mouth.

movement ('moovmənt) 1. an act of moving; motion. 2. an act of defaecation. *Active m.* movement produced by the person's own muscles. *Associated m.* movement of parts that act together, as the eyes. *Passive m.* a movement of the body or of the extremities of a patient performed by another person without voluntary motion on the part of the patient. *Vermicular m's* the wormlike movements of the intestines in peristalsis.

MRSA *See* METHICILLIN-RESISTANT *staphyloccus aureus*

mucinase ('myoosə͵nayz) an enzyme which acts upon mucin. Contained in some aerosols and useful in the treatment of CYSTIC FIBROSIS.

mucocele ('myookoh͵seel) a mucous tumour. *M. of the gallbladder* occurs if a stone obstructs the cystic duct. *Lacrimal m.* a distension of the lacrimal sac caused by a blockage of the nasolacrimal duct.

mucocutaneous (͵myookohkyoo'tayni·əs) pertaining to mucous membrane and skin.

mucoid ('myookoyd) resembling mucus.

mucolytic (͵myookoh'litik) a drug that has a mucous softening effect and so reduces the viscosity of the bronchial secretion in chest disorders.

mucopurulent (͵myookoh'pyoo·rələnt) containing mucus and pus.

mucosa (myoo'kohsə) mucous membrane.

mucous ('myookəs) pertaining to or secreting mucus. *M. membrane* a membrane that secretes mucus and lines many of the body cavities, particularly those of the respiratory and alimentary tract.

mucoviscidosis (͵myookoh͵visə'dohsəs) fibrocystic disease of the pancreas. *See* FIBROCYSTIC.

mucus ('myookəs) the viscous secretion of mucous membrane.

multicellular (͵multee'selyələ) consisting of many cells.

multidisciplinary (͵multee'disəplənree) involving two or more professional disciplines.

multigravida (͵multee'gravəda) a pregnant woman who has had two or more pregnancies.

mutilation (͵myootə'layshən) the act of depriving an individual of a limb or other body part; severe disfigurement.

multilocular (͵multee'lokyələ) having many locules. *M. cyst* a cyst, usually in the ovary, containing many compartments.

multinuclear (͵multee'nyookli·ə) possessing many nuclei.

multipara (mul'tipə·rə) a woman who has had two or more children.

multiple ('multəpəl) manifold, occurring in many parts of the body at once. *M. myeloma* malignant disease of the plasma cells which invade the bone marrow and suppress its functioning. *M. sclerosis* See SCLEROSIS. *M. regression* measure of the relationship between one interval level dependent variable and several independent variables.

multivariate analysis (ˌmultee-ˌvaireeət əˈnaləsəs) the analysis of data collected on several different variables but all having a relevance to the study; e.g. in a survey of the provision of community nursing services for a specific population, data might be collected on age, family size, and previous use of the services. In analysing the data, the effect of each of these variables and their interaction can be examined and considered.

multivitamin (ˌmulteeˈvietəmən, -vit-) a tablet containing a combination of different vitamins.

mumps (mumps) a communicable paramyxovirus disease which is statutorily notifiable and which attacks one or both of the parotid glands, the largest of the three pairs of salivary glands; called also epidemic PAROTITIS or epidemic parotiditis. Most common among children; characterised by inflammation and swelling of the parotid glands.Characterised by fever and a painful swelling in front of the ears that makes mastication difficult.

Munchausen's syndrome (ˈmuhn-ˌchowzənz) *Baron von Munchausen, 16th century German traveller noted for his exaggerated tales.* Habitual seeking of hospital treatment for apparent acute illness, the patient giving a plausible and dramatic history, all of which is false. *M. s. by proxy* an uncommon situation in which a parent (usually the mother) or both parents fabricate symptoms or signs in a child, who is then presented for hospital treatment; overlaps with other forms of child abuse, and fatal outcomes have been reported.

murmur (ˈmərmə) a sound, heard on auscultation, usually originating in the cardiovascular system. *Aortic m.* one indicating disease of the aortic valve. *Diastolic m.* one heard after the second heart sound. *Friction m.* one present when two inflamed surfaces of serous membrane rub on each other. *Mitral m.* a sign of incompetence of the mitral valve. *Systolic m.* one heard during systole.

Murphy's sign (ˈmərfeez) *J.B. Murphy, American surgeon, 1857–1916.* A sign denoting inflammation of the gallbladder. Continuous pressure over the organ causes the patient to 'catch' his or her breath at the zenith of inspiration.

muscae volitantes (ˈmuskə ˌvolətan-teez) black spots floating before the eyes. They do not obscure the sight.

muscarine (ˈmuskə·reen) a poisoning alkaloid that is found in certain fungi and causes muscle paralysis.

muscle (ˈmusəl) strong tissue composed of fibres which have the power of contraction, and thus produce movements of the body. *Cardiac m.* muscle composed of partially striped interlocking cells. Not under the control of the will. *M. relaxant* one of a group of drugs used to reduce muscular spasm and also to relax the muscles during surgery. *Smooth* or *non-striated m.* involuntary muscle of spindle-shaped cells, e.g. that of the intestinal wall. Contracts independently of the will. *Striped* or *striated m.* voluntary muscle. Transverse bands across the fibres give the characteristic appearance. It is under the control of the will.

muscular ('muskyələ) 1. pertaining to muscle. 2. well provided with strong muscles. *M. dystrophy* one of a number of inherited diseases in which there is progressive muscle wasting. *See* DUCHENNE DYSTROPHY.

musculocutaneous (ˌmuskyəloh-kyoo'tayni·əs) referring to the muscles and the skin. *M. nerve* one of the nerves which supply the muscles and the skin of the arms and legs.

musculoskeletal (ˌmuskyəloh-'skelət'l) referring to both the osseous and muscular systems.

mustine hydrochloride (ˌmusteen) nitrogen mustard. A cytotoxic drug which can be given intravenously for malignant disease of lymph glands and reticuloendothelial cells, such as HODGKIN'S DISEASE.

mutant ('myootənt) 1. in genetics, a variation that breeds true, owing to genetic changes. 2. produced by MUTATION.

mutation (myoo'tayshən) a chemical change in the genes of a cell causing it to show a new characteristic. Some produce evolutional changes, others produce disease.

mute (myoot) without the power of speech. *Deaf m.* one who cannot hear and therefore cannot speak.

mutism ('myootizəm) inability or refusal to speak. In almost all cases, mutes are unable to speak because deafness has prevented their hearing the spoken word. Speech is learnt by imitating the speech of others. Can also result from disease, the most common being a stroke. *Elective m.* psychological disorder of childhood.

myalgia (mie'alji·ə) pain in the muscles.

myasthenia (ˌmieəs'theeni·ə) muscle weakness. *M. gravis* an extreme form of muscle weakness which is progressive. There is a rapid onset of fatigue, thought to be due to the rapid destruction of acetylcholine at the neuromuscular junction. Commonly affected muscles are those of vision, speaking, chewing, and swallowing.

mycetoma (ˌmiesə'tohmə) a chronic fungus infection of the tissues, both external and internal, but most commonly affecting the hands and feet. There is swelling and the formation of sinuses. Madura foot.

Mycobacterium (ˌmiekohbak-'tiə·ri·əm) a genus of slender, rod-shaped, acid-fast, Gram-positive bacteria. *M. leprae* the causative organism of leprosy. *M. tuberculosis* the cause of tuberculosis.

mycology (mie'koləjee) the study of fungi.

mycosis (mie'kohsəs) any disease that is caused by a fungus. *M. fungoides* a rare malignant lymphoreticular neoplasm of the skin which later progresses to the lymph nodes and viscera.

mydriasis (mə'drieəsəs, mie-) abnormal dilatation of the pupil of the eye. Usually caused by injury to the pupil sphincter or by the use of MYDRIATIC drugs.

mydriatic (ˌmidree'atik) any drug that causes mydriasis. Used in examination of the eye and in the treatment of inflammatory conditions.

myelin ('mieələn) the fatty covering of medullated nerve fibres.

myelitis (ˌmieə'lietəs) 1. inflammation of the spinal cord, causing pain in the back and sometimes numbness and paralysis of the legs and the lower part of the trunk. 2. inflammation of the bone marrow; OSTEOMYELITIS.

myeloblast ('mieəlohˌblast) a primitive cell in the bone marrow, from which develop the granular leukocytes.

myelocyte ('mieəlohˌsiet) a cell of the bone marrow, derived from a myeloblast.

myelography (ˌmieə'logrəfee) radiographic examination of the spinal cord after the introduction of a radio-opaque substance into the subarachnoid space by means of lumbar puncture.

myeloid ('mieəˌloyd) 1. pertaining to, derived from or resembling bone marrow. 2. pertaining to the spinal cord. 3. having the appearance of MYELOCYTES, but not necessarily derived from bone marrow. *M. leukaemia* a malignant disease in which there is excessive production of LEUKOCYTES in the bone marrow. *M. tissue* red bone marrow.

myeloma (ˌmieə'lohmə) a tumour composed of plasma cells. *Multiple m.* a primary malignant tumour of plasma cells usually arising in bone marrow and usually associated with anaemia and with a paraprotein in the blood or Bence Jones protein in the urine.

myelomatosis (ˌmieəlohmə'tohsəs) a malignant disease of the bone marrow in which multiple myelomas are present.

myelomeningocele (ˌmieəlohmə'ning·gəˌseel) MENINGOMYELOCELE.

myocardial (ˌmieoh'kahdi·əl) pertaining to the MYOCARDIUM. *M. infarction* necrosis of a part of the myocardium, usually following a coronary thrombosis. Ventricular fibrillation can occur, followed by death.

myocarditis (ˌmieohkah'dietəs) inflammation of the MYOCARDIUM.

myocardium (ˌmieoh'kahdi·əm) the muscle tissue of the heart.

myocele ('mieohˌseel) protrusion of muscle through a rupture of its sheath.

myoclonus (ˌmieoh'klohnəs) spasmodic contraction of the muscles.

myoelectric (ˌmieoh·ə'lektrik) pertaining to the electric properties of muscle.

myofibrosis (ˌmieohfie'brohsəs) a degenerative condition in which there is some replacement of muscle tissue by fibrous tissue.

myogenic (ˌmieoh'jenik) originating in myocytes or muscle tissue.

myoglobin (ˌmieoh'glohbən) MYOHAEMOGLOBIN.

myohaemoglobin (ˌmieohˌheemə'glohbən) a substance, resembling haemoglobin, which is present in muscle cells. It is a pigment and is responsible for the colour of muscle. It acts as an oxygen store. Myoglobin.

myohaemoglobinuria (ˌmieohˌheeməˌglohbə'nyoo·ri·ə) the presence of myohaemoglobin in the urine.

myokymia (ˌmieoh'kimi·ə) a benign condition in which there is persistent quivering of the muscles.

myoma (mie'ohmə) a benign tumour of muscle tissue. *See* FIBROMYOMA.

myomectomy (ˌmieə'mektəmee) removal of a myoma; usually referring to a uterine FIBROMA.

myometrium (ˌmieoh'meetri·əm) the muscular tissue of the uterus.

myoneural (ˌmieoh'nyoo·rəl) relating to both muscle and nerve. *M. junction* the point at which nerve endings terminate in a muscle; neuromuscular junction.

myopathy (mie'opəthee) any disease of the muscles. MUSCULAR DYSTROPHY is one of a group of inherited myopathies in which there is wasting and weakness of the muscles.

myopia (mie'ohpi·ə) shortsightedness. The light rays focus in front of the retina and a biconcave lens is needed to focus them correctly.

myoplasty ('mieohˌplastee) any operation in which muscle is detached and utilised, as can be done to correct deformities.

myosarcoma (ˌmieohsah'kohmə) a sarcomatous tumour of muscle.

myosin ('mieəsən) muscle protein.

myositis (ˌmieoh'sietəs) inflammation of a muscle. *M. ossificans* a condition in which bone cells deposited in muscle continue to grow and cause hard lumps. It can occur after fractures.

myotomy (mie'otəmee) the division or dissection of a muscle.

myotonia (ˌmieə'tohni·ə) lack of muscle tone. *M. congenita* a hereditary disease in which the muscle action has a prolonged contraction phase and slow relaxation.

myringa (mi'ring·gə) the eardrum or tympanic membrane.

myringitis (ˌmirin'jietəs) inflammation of the tympanic membrane.

myringoplasty (mə'ring·gohˌplastee) a plastic operation to repair the tympanic membrane; TYMPANOPLASTY.

myringotome (mə'ring·gəˌtohm) an instrument for puncturing the tympanic membrane in MYRINGOTOMY.

myringotomy (ˌmiring'gotəmee) incision of the tympanic membrane to drain fluid from an infected middle ear.

myxoedema (ˌmiksə'deemə) a condition caused by HYPOTHYROIDISM which is marked by mucoid infiltration of the skin. There is oedematous swelling of the face, limbs, and hands, dry and rough skin, loss of hair, slow pulse, subnormal temperature, slowed metabolism, and mental dullness. *Congenital m.* CRETINISM.

myxoma (mik'sohmə) a benign mucous tumour of connective tissue.

myxosarcoma (ˌmiksohsah'kohmə) a SARCOMA containing mucoid tissue.

myxovirus (ˌmiksoh'vierəs) the group name of a number of related viruses, including the causal viruses of influenza, para-influenza, mumps, and Newcastle disease (of fowl).

Nn

N symbol for *nitrogen* and *newton*.

Na symbol for *sodium*.

Naboth's follicle or cyst ('nayboths) *M. Naboth, German anatomist, 1675–1721*. Cystic swelling of a cervical gland, the duct of which has become blocked by regenerating SQUAMOUS epithelium.

naevus ('neevəs) a birthmark; a circumscribed area of pigmentation of the skin due to dilated blood vessels. AHAEMANGIOMA. *N. flammeus* a flat bluish-red area, usually on the neck or face; popularly known as 'port wine stain'. *N. pilosus* a hairy naevus. *Spider n.* a small red area surrounded by dilated capillaries. *Strawberry n.* a raised tumour-like structure of connective tissue containing spaces filled with blood.

naftidrofuryl (naf,tidroh'fyoorəl) an agent used in the treatment of peripheral and cerebral vascular disorders.

Nägele's rule ('naygələz) rule for calculating the estimated date of labour; subtract 3 months from the first day of the last menstrual period and add 7 days.

nail (nayl) the keratinised portion of epidermis covering the dorsal extremity of the fingers and toes. *N. bed* the skin underlying a nail. *Hang n.* a strip of epidermis hanging at one side or at the root of a nail. *Ingrowing n.* a condition in which the flesh overhangs the edge of the nail, a sharp corner of which can pierce the tissues, causing a wound which can become septic. *Spoon n.* a nail with a depression in the centre and raised edges. KOILONYCHIA.

nalidixic acid (,nalə'diksik) an antibacterial agent used in the treatment of urinary infections.

nalorphine ('nalawfeen) an antidote for morphine, pethidine, and methadone overdose.

naloxone (na'loksohn) a narcotic antagonist used as an antidote to narcotic overdosage and as an antagonist for pentazocine overdosage.

NANDA North American Nursing Diagnosis Association.

nandrolone ('nandrə,lohn) an anabolic steroid that promotes protein metabolism and skeletal growth.

nape (nayp) the back of the neck.

napkin rash ('napkin) an erythematous rash which can occur in infants in the napkin area. The many causes include the passage of frequent loose stools, thrush, ammoniacal dermatitis, and allergy to washing powders and detergents.

narcissism ('nahsi,sizəm) the stage

of infant development during which children are mainly interested in themselves and their own bodily needs. In adults, it can be a sign of mental disorder. The term is derived from the Greek legend of Narcissus.

narcoanalysis (ˌnahkoh·ə'naləsəs) a form of psychotherapy in which an injection of a narcotic drug produces a drowsy, relaxed state during which a patient talks more freely; in this way much repressed material can be brought to consciousness.

narcolepsy ('nahkəˌlepsee) a condition in which there is an uncontrollable desire for sleep.

narcosis (nah'kohsəs) a state of unconsciousness produced by a narcotic drug. *Basal n.* a state of unconsciousness produced before surgical anaesthesia.

narcosynthesis (ˌnahkoh'sinthəsəs) the inducement of an hypnotic state by means of drugs. An aid to psychotherapy.

narcotic (nah'kotik) a drug that produces narcosis or unnatural sleep.

nares ('nair·reez) the nostrils. *Posterior n.* the opening of the nares into the nasopharynx.

nasal (nayzəl) pertaining to the nose.

nascent ('nas'nt, 'nay-) 1. at the time of birth. 2. incipient.

nasogastric (ˌnayzoh'gastrik) referring to the nose and stomach. *N. tube* one passed into the stomach via the nose.

nasojejunal feeding (ˌnayzoh-jə'joonəl ˌfeeding) a method of feeding whereby a silicone-coated catheter is passed through the nose into the JEJUNUM to provide sufficient nutrition to a sick baby on a ventilator or receiving continuous inflating pressure (CIP) by mask or nasal tube. It is used to prevent the dangers of aspiration with a nasogastric tube feed.

nasolacrimal (ˌnayzoh'lakrəməl) concerning both the nose and lacrimal apparatus. *N. duct* the duct draining the tears from the inner aspect of the eye to the inferior meatus of the nose.

nasopharynx (ˌnayzoh'faringks) the upper part of the pharynx; that above the soft palate.

nasosinusitis (ˌnayzohˌsienə'sietəs) inflammation of the nose and adjacent sinuses.

nasotracheal tube (ˌnayzohˌtrə'keel) a catheter inserted into the trachea via the nose and pharynx.

natriuresis (ˌnatreeyə'reesəs) the excretion of abnormally high amounts of sodium in the urine.

natural childbirth ('nachərəl) a term used to describe an approach to LABOUR and delivery in which the parents are prepared for the event so that the mother is awake and cooperative and the father is able to assume an active and supportive role during the birth of their child. The underlying concept for all methods of natural childbirth is avoidance of medical interference and analgesia in labour, and education of the parents so that they can actively participate in and share the experience of childbirth.

naturopathy (ˌnaychə'ropəthee) a drugless system of healing by a combination of diet, fasting, exercise, hydrotherapy, and positive thinking.

nausea ('nawzi·ə) a sensation of sickness with an inclination to vomit.

navel ('nayvəl) the UMBILICUS.

navicular (nə'vikyələ) boat shaped.

N. bone one of the tarsal bones of the foot.

near drowning (niə) survival, at least temporarily, from immersion in a liquid medium.

nebula ('nebyələ) a slight opacity or cloudiness of the cornea, caused by injury or by corneal ulceration.

nebuliser ('nebyə,liezə) an apparatus for reducing a liquid to a fine spray. An atomiser.

neck (nek) 1. the narrow part of an organ or bone. 2. the part of the body which connects the head and the trunk. *Derbyshire n.* simple GOITRE. *Wry n.*TORTICOLLIS.

necrobiosis (,nekrohbie'ohsəs) localised death of a part as a result of degeneration.

necropsy ('nekropsee) autopsy; a postmortem examination of a body.

necrosis (nə'krohsəs) death of a portion of tissue.

necrotising enterocolitis ('nekrə-,tiezing) abbreviated NEC. A condition of neonates in which there is severe diarrhoea and blood in the stools. It occurs in preterm or low birthweight neonates. Exact cause not known but often associated with infection.

needle-stick injury (need'lstik ,injə·ree) an accidental injury with a needle that is contaminated with blood or body fluids. The term is also used sometimes to include other sharps injuries. The injuries have been reported as a means of infecting nurse or healthcare professionals with hepatitis or HIV.

needling ('needling) discission; the operation for cataract of lacerating and splitting up the lens so that it can be absorbed.

negative ('negətiv) the opposite of positive. The absence of some quality or substance.

negativism ('negəti,vizəm) a symptom of mental illness in which the patient does the opposite of what is required and so presents an uncooperative attitude. Common in SCHIZOPHRENIA.

negligence ('neglijəns) in law, the failure to do something that a reasonable person of ordinary prudence would do in a certain situation or the doing of something that such a person would not do. Negligence can provide the basis for a lawsuit if there is a legal duty involved (for example, the duty of a doctor or nurse to provide reasonable care to patients) and if the negligence results in damage to the patient.

Neisseria (nie'siə·ri·ə) *A.L.S. Neisser, German bacteriologist, 1855–1916.* A genus of paired, spherical, Gram-negative bacteria. *N. gonorrhoeae* the causative organism of GONORRHOEA. *N. meningitidis* the cause of MENINGOCOCCAL MENINGITIS.

Nelson's syndrome ('nelsənz) *D.H.Nelson, American physician, b.1925*. The development of an ACTH-producing tumour after bilateral adrenalectomy in CUSHING'S SYNDROME; it is characterised by aggressive growth of the tumour and hyperpigmentation of the skin.

Nematoda (,nemə'tohdə) a phylum of worms, including the *Ascaris* or roundworm and the *Enterobius* or threadworm.

neocerebellum (,neeoh,serə'beləm) the middle lobe of the CEREBELLUM.

neocortex (,neeoh'kawteks) the cerebral cortex, excluding the hippocampal formation and PIRIFORM area.

neoglycogenesis (ˌneeohˌgliekə'jenəsəs) the formation of liver glycogen from non-carbohydrate sources. Glyconeogenesis.

neologism (nee'oləˌjizəm) the formation of new words, either completely new ones or ones formed by contraction of two separate words. This is done particularly by schizophrenic patients.

neomycin (ˌneeoh'miesən) an antibiotic drug used against a wide range of bacteria, frequently those affecting the skin or the eyes. Also given orally to sterilise the bowel before surgery.

neonatal (ˌneeə'nayt'l) referring to the first month of life. *N. mortality rate* the number of deaths of infants up to 4 weeks old per 1000 live births in any 1 year.

neonate ('neeəˌnayt) newborn; specifically pertaining to a baby under 1 month old.

neonatologist (ˌneeənay'toləjəst) a doctor specialising in the management, assessment, diseases, and intensive care of newborn babies, especially those of low birthweight and those with congenital abnormalities.

neonatology (ˌneeənay'toləjee) the branch of medicine dealing with disorders of the newborn infant.

neoplasm ('neeohˌplazəm) a morbid new growth; a tumour. It can be benign or malignant.

neostigmine (ˌneeoh'stigmeen) a synthetic preparation akin to physostigmine used in the treatment of MYASTHENIA GRAVIS and as an antidote to some muscle-relaxant drugs, and as eye drops in the treatment of GLAUCOMA.

nephralgic (nə'fraljik) relating to pain arising from the kidney. *N. crises* spasms of pain in the lumbar region in TABES dorsalis.

nephrectomy (nə'frektəmee) excision of a kidney.

nephritis (nə'frietəs) inflammation of the kidney; a focal or diffuse proliferative or destructive disease that can involve the GLOMERULUS, tubule, or interstitial renal tissue. Also called BRIGHT'S DISEASE. The most usual form is GLOMERULONEPHRITIS.

nephroblastoma (ˌnefrohbla'stohmə) a rapidly developing malignant mixed tumour of the kidneys, made up of embryonic cells and occurring chiefly in children before the fifth year; WILMS' TUMOUR.

nephrocalcinosis (ˌnefrohˌkalsə'nohsəs) a condition in which there is deposition of calcium in the renal tubules resulting in calculi formation and renal insufficiency.

nephrocele ('nefrohˌseel) hernia of the kidney.

nephrogram ('nefrohˌgram) a radiograph of the kidney with contrast medium in the renal tubules. Usually the immediate film in an excretion urogram.

nephrolith ('nefrohˌlith) stone in the kidney; renal calculus.

nephrolithiasis (ˌnefrohlə'thieəsəs) the presence of a calculus or of gravel in the kidney.

nephrolithotomy (ˌnefrohlə'thotəmee) removal of a renal calculus by incising the kidney or by extraporeal shock wave LITHOTRIPSY.

nephroma (ne'frohmə) tumour of the kidney.

nephron ('nefron) the functional unit of the kidney, comprised of Bowman's capsule, the proximal and distal tubules, the loop of Henle, and the collecting duct which conveys urine to the renal pelvis. (*See* figure.)

nephropexy ('nefroh,peksee) the fixation of a floating (mobile) kidney, usually by sutures to neighbouring muscle.

nephroptosis (,nefrop'tohsəs) downwards displacement or undue mobility of a kidney.

nephropyeloplasty (,nefroh'pieəloh,plastee) a plastic operation on the pelvis of the kidney performed in cases of HYDRONEPHROSIS.

nephropyosis (,nefrohpie'ohsəs) suppuration in the kidney.

nephrosclerosis (,nefrohsklə'rohsəs) constriction of the arterioles of the kidney. Seen in benign and malignant hypertension and in ARTERIOSCLEROSIS in old age.

nephrosis (ne'frohsəs) any disease of the kidney, especially that characterised by oedema, ALBUMINURIA, and a low plasma albumin. Caused by non-inflammatory degenerative lesions of the tubules.

nephrostomy (nə'frostəmee)

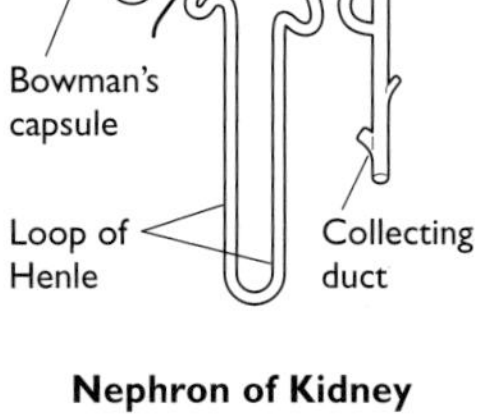

Nephron of Kidney

creation of a permanent opening into the renal pelvis.

nephrotic (nə'frotik) referring to or caused by nephrosis. *N. syndrome* a clinical syndrome in which there is ALBUMINURIA, low plasma protein, and gross oedema; the result of increased capillary permeability in the GLOMERULI. It can occur as a result of acute GLOMERULONEPHRITIS, in subacute NEPHRITIS, DIABETES mellitus, amyloid disease, systemic LUPUS ERYTHEMATOSUS, and renal vein thrombosis.

nephrotomogram (,nefroh'tohmə,gram) a tomogram of the kidney obtained by NEPHROTOMOGRAPHY.

nephrotomography (,nefrohtə'mogrəfee) radiological visualisation of the kidney by tomography after introduction of a contrast medium.

nephrotomy (nə'frotəmee) incision of the kidney.

nephrotoxic (,nehfroh'toksik) poisonous or destructive to the cells of the kidney.

nephroureterectomy (,nefroh·yə,reetə'rektəmee) surgical removal of the kidney and the ureter.

nerve (nərv) a bundle of conducting fibres enclosed in a sheath called the EPINEURIUM. Its function is to transmit impulses between any part of the body and a nerve centre. *N. block* a method of producing regional anaesthesia by injecting a local anaesthetic into the nerves supplying the area to be operated on. *N. fibre* the prolongation of the nerve cell, which conveys impulses. Each fibre has a sheath. Medullated nerve fibres have an insulating myelin sheath. *N. gas* a gas that interferes with the functioning of the nerves and muscles. Such gases can cause death from respiratory paralysis; some of them act through the skin and cannot be avoided by the use of gas masks. *Motor* (efferent) *n.* one that conveys impulses, causing activity from a nerve centre to a muscle or gland. *Sensory* (afferent) *n.* one that conveys sensation from an area to a nerve centre.

nervous ('nərvəs) 1. pertaining to or composed of nerves. 2. apprehensive. *N. breakdown* a popular and misleading term for any type of mental illness that interferes with a person's normal activities. A so-called 'nervous breakdown' can include any of the mental disorders, including NEUROSIS, PSYCHOSIS, or DEPRESSION, but is usually used to describe neurosis.

nervousness ('nərvəsnəs) excitability of the nervous system, characterised by a state of mental and physical unrest.

nettle rash ('net'l ˌrash) an allergic skin condition; URTICARIA.

network ('netˌwərk) 1. an interconnected group or system of voluntary organisations or of colleagues with similar interests. 2. a system of interconnected computer terminals in which the user has access to others using the system for sharing data, etc.

networking ('netˌwərking) 1. forming and maintaining professional connections and contacts through informal social meetings. 2. the interconnection of two or more computer networks in different places.

neural ('nyoo·rəl) pertaining to the nerves. *N. arch* the bony arch on each vertebra which encloses the spinal cord. *N. tube defect* any of a group of congenital malformations involving the neural tube, including ANENCEPHALY, hypocephalus, and SPINA BIFIDA.

neuralgia (nyə'raljə, -ji·ə) a sharp stabbing pain usually along the course of a nerve due to neuritis or functional disturbance.

neurapraxia (ˌnyoo·rə'praksi·ə) an injury to a nerve resulting in temporary loss of function and paralysis. It is usually caused by compression of the nerve and there is no lasting damage.

neurasthenia (ˌnyoo·rəs'theeni·ə) a neurosis in which there is much mental and physical fatigue, inability to concentrate, loss of appetite, and a failure of memory.

neurectomy (nyə'rektəmee) excision of part of a nerve.

neurilemma (ˌnyoo·rə'lemə) the membranous sheath surrounding a nerve fibre.

neurinoma (ˌnyoo·rə'nohma) a benign tumour arising in the NEURILEMMA of a nerve fibre.

neuritis (nyə'rietəs) inflammation of a nerve, with pain, tenderness, and loss of function. *Multiple n.* that involving several nerves; POLYNEURITIS. *Nutritional* (alcoholic) *n.* that which can be caused by alcoholism or lack of vitamin B complex. *Optic n.* that affecting the optic disc or nerve. *Peripheral n.* that involving the terminations of nerves. *Sciatic n.* SCIATICA. *Tabetic n.* a type occurring in TABES dorsalis. *Traumatic n.* that which results from an injury to a nerve.

neuroblast ('nyoo·rohˌblast) an embryonic nerve cell.

neuroblastoma (ˌnyoo·rohbla'stohmə) a malignant tumour of immature nerve cells, most often arising in the very young.

neurodermatitis (ˌnyoo·roh-ˌdərmə'tietəs) a localised PRURIGO of somatic and psychogenic origin. It irritates, and rubbing causes thickening and pigmentation of the skin.

neuroepithelioma (ˌnyoo·rohˌepee-ˌtheelee'ohmə) a malignant tumour of the retina of the eye which can spread into the brain.

neurofibroma (ˌnyoo·rohfie-'brohmə) a benign tumour of nerve and fibrous tissue.

neurofibromatosis (ˌnyoo·roh-ˌfiebrohmə'tosəs) von Recklinghausen's disease. A generalised hereditary disease in which there are numerous FIBROMATA of the skin and nervous system.

neurogenic (ˌnyoo·rə'jenik) derived from or caused by nerve stimulation. *N. bladder* a disorder of the urinary bladder caused by a lesion of the nervous system. *N. shock* shock originating in the nervous system.

neuroglia (nyə'rogli·ə) the special form of connective tissue supporting nerve tissues.

neurohypophysis (ˌnyoo·roh·hie-'pofəsəs) the posterior lobe of the pituitary gland.

neuroleptic (ˌnyoo·roh'leptik) a drug which acts on the nervous system.

neurological assessment (ˌnyoo·rə-'lojikəl) evaluation of the health status of a patient with a nervous system disorder or dysfunction. Purposes of the assessment include establishing nursing goals to guide the nurse in planning and implementing nursing measures to help the patient cope effectively with daily living activities. Nursing assessment of a patient's neurological status is concerned with identifying functional disabilities that interfere with the person's ability to provide self-care and lead an active life. A functionally oriented nursing assessment includes: (a) consciousness; (b) mental functions; (c) motor function; and (d) sensory function. Evaluation of these functions gives the nurse information about the patient's ability to perform everyday activities such as thinking, remembering, seeing, eating, speaking, moving, smelling, feeling, and hearing. A patient with an acute and life-threatening alteration in neurological function is evaluated and monitored in four general areas: (a) level of consciousness; (b) sensory and motor function; (c) pupillary changes; and (d) vital signs and pattern of respiration.

neurologist (nyə'roləjəst) a medical practitioner who specialises in neurology.

neurology (nyə'roləjee) 1. the scientific study of the nervous system. 2. the branch of medicine concerned with diseases of the nervous system.

neuroma (nyə'rohmə) a tumour consisting of nervous tissue.

neuromuscular (ˌnyoo·roh'mus-kyələ) appertaining to nerves and muscles. *N. junction* the small gap between the end of the motor nerve and the motor end-plate of the muscle fibre supplied. This gap is bridged by the release of acetylcholine whenever a nerve impulse arrives.

neuromyelitis (ˌnyoo·rohˌmieə-'lietəs) neuritis associated with MYELITIS. It is a condition akin to multiple sclerosis. *N. optica* a disease in which there is bilateral optic neuritis and PARAPLEGIA.

neurone (neuron) ('nyoo·rohn, 'nyoo·ron) a nerve cell. *Lower motor n.* the anterior horn cell and its neurone which conveys impulses to the appropriate muscles. *Upper motor n.* that in which the cell is in the cerebral cortex and the fibres conduct impulses to associated cells in the spinal cord.

neuroparalysis (ˌnyoo·rohpə'raləsəs) paralysis due to disease of a nerve or nerves.

neuropathy (nyə'ropəthee) a disease process of nerve degeneration and loss of function. *Alcoholic n.* neuropathy due to thiamine deficiency in chronic alcoholism. *Diabetic n.* that associated with diabetes. *Entrapment n.* any of a group of neuropathies, e.g. carpal tunnel syndrome, due to mechanical pressure on a peripheral nerve. *Ischaemic n.* that caused by a lack of blood supply.

neuroplasty ('nyoo·rohˌplastee) the surgical repair of a damaged nerve.

neurorrhaphy (nyə'ro·rəfee) the operation of suturing a divided nerve.

neurosis (nyə'rohsəs) a mental disorder which does not affect the whole personality, characterised by exaggerated anxiety and tension. *Anxiety n.* persistent anxiety and the accompanying symptoms of fear, rapid pulse, sweating, trembling, loss of appetite, and insomnia. *Obsessive-compulsive n.* one characterised by compulsions and obsessional rumination.

neurosurgery (ˌnyoo·roh'sərjə·ree) that branch of surgery dealing with the brain, spinal cord, and nerves.

neurosyphilis (ˌnyoo·roh'sifələs) a manifestation of third-stage syphilis in which the nervous system is involved. The three most common forms are: (a) meningovascular syphilis, affecting the blood vessels to the meninges; (b) tabes dorsalis (see ATAXIA); and (c) general paralysis of the insane.

neurotic (nyə'rotik) a loosely applied adjective denoting association with neurosis.

neurotmesis (ˌnyoo·rot'meesəs) degeneration of a nerve due to severance.

neurotoxic (ˌnyoo·roh'toksik) poisonous or destructive to nervous tissue.

neurotransmitter (ˌnyoo·rohtranz'mitə, -trahnz-) a substance (e.g. noradrenaline, acetylcholine, dopamine) that is released from the axon terminal to produce activity in other nerves.

neurotripsy ('nyoo·rohˌtripsee) the surgical bruising or crushing of a nerve.

neurotropic (ˌnyoo·roh'tropik) having an affinity for nerve tissue. *N. viruses* those that particularly attack the nervous system.

neutropaenia (ˌnyootrə'peeni·ə) a decrease in the number of neutrophils in the blood.

neutrophil ('nyootrəˌfil) a polymorphonuclear leukocyte which has a neutral reaction to acid and alkaline dyes.

nevus ('neevəs) *see* NAEVUS.

Newborn Screening Program ('nyooˌbawn) an extension of the Guthrie test. In Australia, all babies are screened for PKU and HYPOTHYROIDISM. Can also include screening for cystic fibrosis and GALACTOSAEMIA.

niacin ('nieəsən) NICOTINIC ACID.

niclosamide (ni'klohsəmied) an

anthelmintic used as a single dose in tapeworm infestations.

nicotine ('nikə,teen) a poisonous alkaloid in tobacco.

nicotinic acid (,nikə'tinik) niacin. A water-soluble vitamin in the B complex. A deficiency of this vitamin causes PELLAGRA.

nidation (nie'dayshən) implantation of the fertilised ovum in the uterus.

NIDDM non-insulin-dependent diabetes mellitus.

nidus ('niedəs) 1. a nest. 2. a place in which an organism finds conditions suitable for its growth and development. 3. the focus of an infection.

Niemann–Pick disease (,neemən-'pik) *A. Niemann, German paediatrician, 1880–1921; F. Pick, German physician, 1868–1935.* A rare inherited disease occurring primarily in Jewish children and resulting in learning difficulties. There is lipoid storage abnormality and widespread deposition of lecithin in the tissues.

nifedipine (nie'fedə,peen) a calcium channel blocker used as a coronary vasodilator in the treatment of ANGINA PECTORIS, and in the treatment of hypertension.

night blindness (niet) nyctalopia; difficulty in seeing in the dark. This can be a congenital defect or can be caused by a vitamin A deficiency. Also occurs as a result of retinal degeneration.

night sweat ('niet ,swet) profuse perspiration during sleep, especially typical of tuberculosis.

night terror ('niet ,terə) an unpleasant experience in which the subject, usually a young child, screams while asleep and seems terrified. On waking, the individual is unable to remember the cause of the fear.

nihilism ('nieə,lizəm) in psychiatry, a term used to describe feelings of not existing and hopelessness, that all is lost or destroyed.

nikethamide (ni'kethə,mied) a cardiac and respiratory stimulant given intravenously in cases of respiratory failure.

nipple ('nipəl) the small conical projection at the tip of the breast, through which, in the female, milk can be withdrawn. *Accessory n.* a rudimentary nipple anywhere in a line from the breast to the groin. *Depressed n.* one that does not protrude. *Retracted n.* one that is drawn inwards. It can be a sign of cancer of the breast. *N. shield* a shield fitted with a rubber teat which covers the AREOLA of a nursing mother when her nipple is sore or not sufficiently protractile for the baby to suck.

Nissl granules ('nisəl) *F. Nissl, German neuropathologist, 1860–1919.* RNA-containing units found in the cytoplasm of cells. Probably associated with protein synthesis.

nit (nit) the egg of the head louse, attached to the hair near the scalp.

nitrazepam (nie'trazə,pam) a hypnotic and sedative drug used to treat insomnia with early morning wakening.

nitrofurantoin (,nietrohfyoo'ran-toh·ən) a urinary antiseptic which is bactericidal and is effective against a range of organisms.

nitrogen ('nietrəjən) *symbol* N. A gaseous element. Air is largely composed of nitrogen, and it is one of the essential constituents of all protein foods. *N. balance* the state of the body with respect to the rate of protein intake and protein utilisation. A negative nitrogen balance occurs when more protein is utilised by the body than is taken in. A positive nitrogen balance implies a net gain of protein in the body. Negative nitrogen balance can be caused by such factors as malnutrition, debilitating disease, blood loss, and glucocorticoids. A positive balance can be caused by exercise, growth hormone, and testosterone. *N. mustards* a group of toxic, blistering alkylating agents, including nitrogen mustard itself (mechlorethamine hydrochloride) and related compounds; some have been used as antineoplastics in certain forms of cancer.

nitroglycerin (ˌnietroh'glisərən) glyceryl trinitrate. A drug which causes dilatation of the coronary arteries. In ANGINA PECTORIS, a tablet should be dissolved sublingually before exertion.

nitrous oxide ('nietrəs) N_2O; laughing gas. An inhalation anaesthetic ensuring a brief spell of unconsciousness.

nociassociation (ˌnohsee·əˌsohsee-'ayshən) the discharge of nervous energy which occurs unconsciously in trauma, as in surgical shock. *See* ANOCIASSOCIATION.

noctambulation (ˌnoktambyə'lay-shən) sleep walking; SOMNAMBULISM.

nocturia (nok'tyoo·ri·ə) the passing of urine at night, especially that associated with irritation of the bladder and urethra, or that associated with prostatic enlargement.

nocturnal (nok'tərn'l) referring to the night. *N. enuresis* bed wetting; incontinence of urine during sleep.

node (nohd) a swelling or protuberance. *Atrioventricular n.* the specialised tissue between the right atrium and the ventricle at the point where the coronary vein enters the atrium, from which is initiated the impulse of contraction down the atrioventricular bundle. *N. of Ranvier* a constriction occurring at intervals in a nerve fibre to enable the NEURILEMMA with its blood supply to reach and nourish the axon of the nerve. *Sinoatrial n.* the pacemaker of the heart. The specialised neuromuscular tissue at the junction of the superior vena cava and the right atrium which, stimulated by the right vagus nerve, controls the rhythm of contraction in the heart.

nodule ('nodyool) a small swelling or protuberance.

noma ('nohmə) a gangrenous condition of the mouth; CANCRUM ORIS.

nominal ('nomənəl) the level of measurement that simply assigns data into categories that are mutually exclusive.

nomogram ('noməˌgram, 'noh-) a graph with several scales arranged so that a ruler laid on the graph intersects the scales at related values of the variables; the values of any two variables can be used to find the values of the others. Increasingly used in the determination of drug therapy dosage, e.g. in paediatrics.

non compos mentis (non 'kompəs 'mentis) [L.] *not of sound mind*. Applied to people whose mental state is such that they are unable to manage their own affairs.

non-accidental injury (NAI) (ˌnonaksə'dent'l) injuries inflicted upon children or infants by those looking after them, usually the parents. The injuries are usually physical (beating, burning, biting) but the term includes the giving of poisons and dangerous drugs, sexual abuse, starvation, and any other form of physical assault..

non-compliance (ˌnonkəm'plieəns) describes the failure of a patient to comply with a drug or treatment regimen; this might be deliberate, or might be due to ignorance, forgetfulness, etc.

non-experimental research design (nonəkˌsperə'ment'l) research design in which an investigator observes a phenomenon without manipulating the independent variable(s).

non insulin-dependent diabetes mellitus (NIDDM) (ˌnon 'insyələn) a type of DIABETES mellitus (type II) in which the patient is not dependent on the use of insulin; usually occurs in later life.

nonparametric statistics (ˌnonˌparə'metrik) statistics that are usually utilised when variables are measured at the nominal or ordinal level because they do not estimate population parameters and involve less restrictive assumptions about the underlying distribution.

non-specific (ˌnonspə'sifik) 1. not due to any single known cause. 2. not directed against a particular agent, but rather having a general effect. *N. urethritis* a common, sexually transmitted disease which can be due to a variety of agents, e.g. *Chlamydia trachomatis* which causes 40% of cases. Also called non-gonococcal URETHRITIS.

non-steroidal anti-inflammatory drugs (nonˌstə'royd'l, ˌster-) abbreviated NSAIDs. A group of drugs with analgesic, antipyretic, and anti-inflammatory activity due to their ability to inhibit the synthesis of prostaglandins. It includes aspirin, phenylbutazone, indomethacin, tolmetic, ibuprofen, and related drugs.

non-union (non'yoonyən) in a fracture, failure of the two pieces of bone to unite.

noradrenaline (ˌnaw·rə'drenələn) a hormone present in extracts of the suprarenal medulla and at synapses in the peripheral sympathetic nervous system. It causes vasoconstriction and raises both the systolic and the diastolic blood pressures.

norepinephrine (ˌnawrˌepee'nefrən) *see* NORADRENALINE.

norethandrolone (ˌnaw·rə'thandrəˌlohn) an anabolic steroid that aids in the utlisation of protein. Can be used to treat severe wasting and osteoporosis.

norethisterone (ˌnaw·rə'thistəˌrohn) an anabolic steroid similar in action to progesterone. Used in the treatment of AMENORRHOEA. Also used in the combined contraceptive pill.

normal ('nawməl) conforming to a standard; regular or usual. *N. flora* bacteria which normally live on body tissues and have a beneficial effect. *N. saline* isotonic solution of sodium chloride. Physiological solution.

normoblast ('nawmohˌblast) a nucleated precursor red blood cell in bone marrow. *See* ERYTHROCYTE.

normochromic (ˌnawmoh'krohmik) normal in colour. Applied to the blood when the haemoglobin level is within normal limits.

normocyte ('nawmohˌsiet) a red blood cell that is normal in size, shape, and colour.

normoglycaemia (ˌnawmohglie'seemi·ə) normal blood sugar level.

normotension (ˌnawmoh'tenshən) normal tone, tension, or pressure. Usually used in relation to blood pressure.

North American Nursing Diagnosis Association (NANDA) ('nandə) formed as a professional organisation of registered nurses in 1982. The purpose of NANDA is 'to develop, refine and promote a taxonomy of nursing diagnostic terminology of general use to the professional'. Meets at regular intervals to review previously approved nursing diagnoses and to develop the classification systems.

Norton score ('nawtən) a pressure sore risk assessment scale devised by Norton, McLaren and Exton Smith and used primarily in the care of elderly patients. It is comprised of five health state components, each with a 4-point descending scale. Maximum points are 20 and the minimum 5; a 'score' of 14 and below indicates that the patient is at risk of developing pressure sores and needs 1–2 hourly changes of posture and the use of pressure-relieving aids. The system requires weekly application and whenever a change occurs in the patient's condition and/or circumstances of care.

nortriptyline (naw'triptəˌleen) a tricyclic antidepressant drug used for the relief of all types of depression.

nose (nohz) the organ of smell and the airway for respiration.

nosocomial (ˌnohzə'kohmieəl) pertaining to or acquired in hospital. *N. disease* for the patient a new disorder, not related to the original disease, that is caused or precipitated during hospitalisation. *N. infection* an infection acquired in hospital at least 72 hours after admission. Also called hospital-acquired infection (HAI).

nostril ('nostrəl) one of the anterior orifices of the nose.

notifiable ('nohtəˌfieəbəl) applied to such diseases as must by law be reported to the health authorities. These include measles, scarlet fever, typhus fever, typhoid fever, cholera, diphtheria, tuberculosis, dysentery, and various forms of food poisoning.

NSU non-specific URETHRITIS.

nuclear ('nyookli·ə) pertaining to a nucleus. *N. medicine* that branch of medicine concerned with the use of radionuclides in the diagnosis and treatment of disease.

nuclear magnetic resonance ('nyookli·ə mag'netik 'rezənəns) a phenomenon exhibited by atomic nuclei having a magnetic moment, i.e. those nuclei that behave as if they were tiny bar magnets. In the absence of a magnetic field these magnets are arranged randomly, but when a strong magnetic field is applied they align with the field. These signals can be analysed and used for chemical analysis (NMR spectroscopy) or for imaging (magnetic resonance imaging).

nuclease ('nyookleeˌayz) an enzyme which breaks down nucleic acids.

nucleic acids (nyoo'klee·ik, -'klay-) deoxyribonucleic acid (abbreviated DNA) and ribonucleic acid (abbreviated RNA), both of which are found in cell nuclei; RNA is also found in the cytoplasm. They are composed of series of nucleotides.

nucleolus (ˌnyooklee'ohləs, nyoo-'kleeələs) a small dense body in the cell nucleus which contains ribonucleic acid. It disappears during MITOSIS.

nucleoprotein (ˌnyookleeoh'proh-teen) a compound of nucleic acid and protein.

nucleotide ('nyookleeəˌtied) a compound formed from pentose sugar, phosphoric acid, and a nitrogen-containing base (a purine or a pyrimidine).

nucleotoxin (ˌnyookleeə'toksən) a toxin from cell nuclei, or one that affects cell nuclei.

nucleus ('nyookli·əs) 1. the essential part of a cell governing nutrition and reproduction, its division being essential for the formation of new cells. 2. the positively charged centre portion of an atom. 3. a group of nerve cells in the central nervous system. *Caudate n.* and *lenticular n.* part of the basal ganglia. *N. pulposus* the jelly-like centre of an intervertebral disc.

nullipara (nu'lipə·rə) a woman who has never given birth to a child.

nurse (nərs) 1. a person who is qualified in the art and science of nursing and meets certain prescribed standards of education and clinical competence (*see also* NURSING PRACTICE). 2. to provide services that are essential to or helpful in the promotion, maintenance, and restoration of health and wellbeing. 3. to nourish at the breast (see also breast feeding). *Wet n.* a woman who breastfeeds the infant of another.

nursing ('nərsing) the profession of performing the functions of a NURSE. *N. assessment* the systematic collection and analysis of patient data pertaining to an individual's health status, abilities, and preferences for care and treatment. The first step of the nursing process leading to a clinical nursing judgement. *See* ASSESSMENT. *N. audit* a systematic procedure for assessing the quality of nursing care rendered to a specific patient population. *N. care plan* devised by a nurse and based upon a nursing assessment and nursing diagnosis for an individual patient. The plan has four essential components: (a) identification of the nursing care problems; (b) an outline of the means and methods of solving these; (c) a statement of the anticipated benefit to the patient; and (4) an account of the specific actions used to achieve the goals specified. *N. diagnosis* a statement of a health problem or of a potential health problem in the patient's/client's health status that a nurse is professionally competent to treat. *N. goal* the objective that the nurse hopes to achieve through nursing interventions and activities related to the patient's health status, needs, and abilities, e.g. the development of self-care skills. *N. history* a written record providing data for assessing the nursing care needs of a patient. *N. models* a conceptual framework of nursing practice based on knowledge, ideas, and beliefs. A model or theory of nursing clarifies the meaning of nursing, provides criteria for policy, and gives direction to team nursing, thereby obviating conflicts in approach and giving the framework for continuity of care. It identifies the nurse's role, highlights areas of practice in which research is needed, and can be a basis for a nursing curriculum. *N. practice* the performance or compensation of any act in the observation, care, and counsel of the ill, injured, or infirm, or in the maintenance of health or prevention of illness of others, or in the supervision and teaching of other personnel, or in the administration of medications and treatments as prescribed by a doctor or dentist, requiring substantial specialised judgment and skill and based on knowledge and application of the principles of biological, physical, and social sciences. *N. process* a systematic approach to nursing care derived from many occupational groups. The system itself is not specific to nursing. It has been used as a framework for nursing care by American nurses and subsequently its principles have been adapted to the UK's culture and healthcare system by British and Australian nurses. It is an organised approach to the identification of a patient's nursing-care problems and the utilisation of nursing actions that effectively alleviate, minimise, or prevent the problems being presented or from developing. *Theories of n.* proposed explanations of the way in which nursing achieves its aims. They require a definition of the nurse's perception of the patient's needs, the nurse's own role, and the context in which nursing care is performed. An understanding of the relationship of these variables enables nursing care to be planned in such a way that the outcome can be predicted and set goals achieved.

nutation (nyoo'tayshən) uncontrollable nodding of the head.

nutrient ('nyootri·ənt) food; any substance that nourishes. The six classes of nutrients are fats, carbohydrates, proteins, vitamins, minerals, and water.

nutrition (nyoo'trishən) 1. the sum of the processes involved in taking in nutriments and assimilating and utilising them. 2. nutriment. *N. disease* one that is due to the continued absence of a necessary food factor. *Enteral n.* the provision of nutrients in fluid form to the alimentary tract by mouth, nasogastric tube, or an opening into the tract such as through a GASTROSTOMY. *Parenteral n.* a technique for meeting a patient's nutritional needs by means of intravenous feedings; sometimes called HYPERALIMENTATION.

nutritional status (nyoo'trishən'l ˌstaytəs) the condition of the body as a result of its receiving and using nutrients.

nyctalopia (ˌniktə'lohpi·ə) night blindness.

nymphomania (ˌnimfə'mayni·ə) excessive sexual desire in a woman.

nystagmus (ni'stagməs) an involuntary, rapid movement of the eyeball. It can be hereditary or result from disease of the semicircular canals or of the central nervous system. It can occur from visual defect or be associated with other muscle spasms.

nystatin (nie'statən, ni'-) an antibiotic drug effective against fungi. Used in the treatment of fungal infections of the ear.

Oo

O symbol for *oxygen*.

oat cell carcinoma (oht,sel ,kahsə'nohmə) malignant bronchogenic carcinoma.

obese (oh'bees) very fat; corpulent.

obesity (oh'beesətee) corpulence; excessive development of fat throughout the body. BMI of more than 30 kg/m^2.

objective (əb'jektiv) 1. in microscopy, the lens nearest the object being looked at. 2. a purpose; a desired end-result. 3. concerning matters outside oneself. *O. signs* signs that the observer notes as distinct from the subjective symptoms of which the patient complains. *O. data* data that are not influenced by the person who collects the information.

oblique (ə'bleek) slanting. *O. muscles* 1. a pair of muscles, the inferior (which turns the eye upwards and downwards) and the superior (which turns the eye inwards and outwards). 2. muscles found in the wall of the abdomen.

obsession (əb'seshən) an idea which persistently recurs to an individual although he or she resists it and regards it as being senseless. A compulsive thought. *See* COMPULSION.

obstetrician (,obstə'trishən) one who is trained and specialises in OBSTETRICS.

obstetrics (ob'stetriks) the branch of medicine and surgery dealing with pregnancy, labour, and the PUERPERIUM.

obstipation (obstə'payshən) intractable constipation.

obstruction (əb'strukshən) the act of blocking or clogging; state of being clogged. *Intestinal o.* any hindrance to the passage of faeces.

obturator (,obtyə,raytə) that which closes an opening. *O. foramen* the large hole in the hip bone closed by fascia and muscle.

obtusion (ob'tyoozhən) weakening or blunting of normal sensations, a condition produced by certain diseases.

occipital (ok'sipət'l) relating to the occiput. *O. bone* the bone forming the back and part of the base of the skull.

occipitoanterior (ok,sipətoh·an'tiə·ri·ə) referring to the position of the fetus's head when it is to the front of the pelvis as it comes through the birth canal. *Occipitoposterior* is the reverse position.

occiput ('oksi,puht) the back of the head.

occlusion (ə'kloozhən) closure, applied particularly to alignment of the teeth in the jaws. *Coronary o.* obstruction of the lumen of a coronary artery. *O. of the eye* covering a good eye to improve the visual acuity of the other, lazy, eye. *O. of the pupil* occlusion pupillae; obstruction of the pupil which can be congenital or can occur in IRIDOCYCLITIS or after injury.

occult ('okult) hidden, concealed. *O. blood* blood excreted in the stools in such a small quantity as to require chemical tests to detect it.

occupational (okyə'payshənəl) relating to work and working conditions. *O. disease* one likely to occur among workers in certain trades. An industrial disease. *O. health nursing* the branch of nursing that is concerned with the health of people in the workplace. *O. medicine* the branch of medicine concerned with people at work and the effects of work on health. Essentially, a branch of preventative or environmental medicine. It is concerned with ensuring that health and safety in the workplace are maintained and that legislation is complied with. *O. therapy* treatment by provision of interesting and congenial work within the limitations of the patient in cases of mental disability and in order to re-educate and coordinate muscles in physical defect.

ocular ('okyələ) relating to the eye. *O. myopathy* a gradual bilateral loss of mobility of the eyes. *O. myositis* inflammation of the orbital muscles.

oculentum (ˌokyə'lentəm) an eye ointment.

oculogyric (ˌokyəloh'jierik) causing movements of the eyeballs. *O. crisis* involuntary, violent movements of the eye, usually upwards.

oculomotor (ˌokyəloh'mohtə) relating to movements of the eye. *O. nerves* the third pair of cranial nerves, which control the eye muscles.

Oddi, sphincter of ('odee ˌsfingktə əv) *R. Oddi, Italian physician, 1864–1913.* The muscular sphincter situated at the junction of the duodenum with the conjoined common bile duct and pancreatic duct.

odontoid (oh'dontoyd) resembling a tooth. *O. process* a tooth-like projection from the axis vertebra upon which the head rotates.

odontolith (oh'dontohˌlith) tartar, the calcareous matter deposited upon teeth.

odontology (ˌohdon'toləjee) the science of treating teeth; dentistry.

odontoma (ˌodon'tohmə) a tumour of tooth structures.

oedema (ə'deemə) an excessive amount of fluid in the body tissues. If a finger is pressed upon an affected part, the surface pits and slowly regains its original contour. *Angioneurotic o.* temporary oedema suddenly appearing in areas of skin or mucous membrane and occasionally in the viscera. *Brain o.* an excessive accumulation of fluid in the brain substance (wet brain). *Cardiac o.* a manifestation of congestive heart failure due to increased venous and capillary pressures and often associated with renal sodium retention. *Dependent o.* oedema affecting most severely the lowermost parts of the body. *Famine o.* that due to protein deficiency. *Lymph o.* that due to blockage of the lymph vessels. *O. neonatorum* a disease of preterm and feeble infants resembling sclerema, marked by spreading oedema with cold, livid skin. *Pitting o.* oedema in which pressure leaves a persistent depression in the tissues. *Pulmonary o.* diffuse extravascular accumulation of fluid in the tissues and air spaces of the LUNG due to changes in hydrostatic forces in the capillaries or to increased capillary permeability.

Oedipus complex ('eedəpəs) the suppressed sexual desire of a son for his mother with hostility towards his father. It is a normal stage in the early development of the child but can become fixed if the child cannot solve the conflict during his early years or during adolescence. Named after a mythical Greek hero.

oesophageal (əˌsofə'jeeəl) pertaining to the oesophagus. *O. atresia* a congenital abnormality in which the oesophagus is not continuous between the pharynx and the stomach. Can be associated with a fistula into the trachea. *O. varices* varicose veins of the lower oesophagus secondary to portal hypertension.

oesophagitis (əˌsofə'jietəs) inflammation of the oesophagus. *Reflux o.* caused by regurgitation of acid stomach contents through the cardiac sphincter.

oesophagocele (ə'sofəgohˌseel) a protrusion of the mucous lining through a tear in the muscular wall of the oesophagus.

oesophagojejunostomy (əˌsofəgohˌjejə'nostəmee) the operation to create an anastomosis of the JEJUNUM with the oesophagus after a total gastrectomy.

oesophagoscope (ə'sofəgəˌskohp) an endoscope for viewing the inside of the oesophagus.

oesophagostomy (əˌsofə'gostəmee) the making of an artificial opening into the oesophagus.

oesophagotomy (əˌsofə'gotəmee) surgical incision of the oesophagus.

oesophagus (ə'sofəgəs) the canal that extends from the pharynx to the stomach. It is about 23 cm long. The gullet.

oestradiol (ˌeestrə'dieol) the chief naturally occurring female sex hormone produced by the ovary. Prepared synthetically, it is used to treat menopausal conditions and AMENORRHOEA.

oestrogen ('eestrəjən, -trəˌjen) one of several steroid hormones, including oestradiol, all of which have similar functions. Although they are largely produced in the ovary, they can also be extracted from the placenta, the adrenal cortex, and the testis. They control female sexual development.

ointment ('oyntmənt) an external application with a greasy base in which the remedy is incorporated.

olecranon (oh'lekrəˌnon, ˌohli'kraynən) the curved process of the ulna which forms the point of the elbow.

oleum ('ohli·əm) an oil.

olfactory (ol'faktə·ree) relating to the sense of smell. *O. nerves* the first pair of cranial nerves; those of smell.

oligaemia (ˌolə'geemi·ə) a deficiency in the volume of blood.

oligocythaemia (ˌoləgohsie'theemi·ə) a cell deficiency in the blood.

oligodendroglioma (ˌoləgohˌdendroglie'ohmə) a central nervous system tumour of the glial tissue.

oligohydramnios (ˌoləgoh·hie'dramneeəs) a deficiency in the amount of AMNIOTIC fluid.

oligomenorrhoea (ˌoləgohˌmenə'reeə) 1. a diminished flow at the menstrual period. 2. infrequent occurrence of menstruation.

oligospermia (ˌoləgoh'spərmi·ə) a diminished output of spermatozoa.

oliguria (ˌolə'gyoo·ri·ə) a deficient secretion of urine.

olivary ('olivə·ree) shaped like an olive. *O. body* a mass of grey matter situated behind the anterior pyramid of the MEDULLA oblongata.

omentectomy (ˌohmen'tektəmee) the surgical removal of all or part of the OMENTUM.

omentopexy (oh'mentəˌpeksee) the surgical fixation of the OMENTUM to some other tissue, usually the abdominal wall. *Cardio-o***.** attachment of the omentum to the heart to establish a collateral circulation following coronary occlusion.

omentum (oh'mentəm) a fold of peritoneum joining the stomach to other abdominal organs. *Greater o*. the fold reflected from the greater curvature of the stomach and lying in front of the intestines. *Lesser o*. the fold reflected from the lesser curvature and attaching the stomach to the undersurface of the liver.

omphalitis (ˌomfə'lietəs) inflammation of the UMBILICUS.

omphalocele ('omfəlohˌseel) an umbilical hernia.

Onchocerca ('ongkohˌsərkə) a genus of filarial worms found in tropical parts of Africa and America, which can give rise to skin and subcutaneous lesions and attack the eye.

onchocerciasis (ˌongkohsər'kieəsəs) a tropical skin disease caused by infestation with *Onchocerca*.

oncogenesis (ˌongkoh'jenəsəs) the causation and formation of tumours.

oncogenic (ˌongkoh'jenik) giving rise to tumour formation.

oncology (ong'koləjee) the scientific study of tumours.

onychia (o'niki·ə) inflammation of the matrix of a nail with suppuration which can cause the nail to fall off.

onychogryphosis (ˌoneekohgri'fohsəs) enlargement of the nails with excessive ridging and curvature, most commonly affecting the elderly.

onycholysis (ˌonee'koləsəs) loosening or separation of a nail from its bed.

onychomycosis (ˌoneekohmie'kohsəs) infection of the nails by a fungus.

onychosis (ˌonee'kohsəs) a disease or deformity of the nails or of a nail.

oöcyte ('oh·əˌsiet) the immature egg cell or ovum in the ovary.

oögenesis (ˌoh·ə'jenəsəs) the development and production of the ovum.

oöphorectomy (ˌoh·əfə'rektəmee) excision of an ovary; ovariectomy.

oöphoritis (ˌoh·əfə'rietəs) inflammation of an ovary.

oöphorocystectomy (ohˌofə·rohsə'stektəmee) surgical removal of an ovarian cyst.

oöphorocystosis (ohˌofə·rohsə'stohsəs) the development of one or more ovarian cysts.

oöphoron (oh'ofə·ron) an ovary.

oöphoropexy (oh'ofə·rohˌpeksee) the surgical fixation of a displaced ovary to the pelvic wall.

oöphorosalpingectomy (ohˌofə·rohˌsalpin'jektəmee) removal of an ovary and its associated uterine tube.

opacity (oh'pasitee) cloudiness, lack of transparency. Opacities occur in the lens of an eye when a cataract is forming. They also occur in the vitreous humour and appear as floating objects.

open-ended items (ˌohpən 'endəd) questions that the respondent can answer in his or her own words.

operant conditioning (ˌopə·rənt) a form of behaviour therapy in which a reward is given when the subject performs the action required. The reward serves to encourage repetition of the action.

operation (ˌopə'rayshən) a surgical procedure in which instruments or hands are used by the operator.

operational definition (ˌopə'ray-shənəl) the measurements used to observe or measure a variable; delineates the procedures or operations required to measure a concept.

ophthalmia (of'thalmi·ə) severe inflammation of the eye or of the conjunctiva or deeper structures of the eye. *O. neonatorum* any hyper-acute purulent conjunctivitis which can be caused by the gonococcus, *Escherichia coli*, staphylococci or *Chlamydia trachomatis*, occurring within the first 21 days of life, usually contracted during birth from infected vaginal discharge of the mother. *Sympathetic o.* granulomatous inflammation of the uveal tract of the uninjured eye following a wound involving the uveal tract of the other eye, resulting in bilateral granulomatous inflammation of the entire uveal tract. Called also sympathetic UVEITIS.

ophthalmitis (ˌofthal'mietəs) inflammation of the eyeball.

ophthalmologist (ˌofthal'moləjəst) a specialist in diseases of the eye.

ophthalmology (ˌofthal'moləjee) the study of the eye and its diseases.

ophthalmoplegia (ofˌthalmoh-'pleeji·ə) paralysis of the muscles of the eye.

ophthalmoscope (of'thalməˌskohp) an instrument fitted with a light and lenses by which the interior of the eye can be illuminated and examined.

ophthalmotomy (ˌofthal'motəmee) incision of the eyeball.

opiate ('ohpeeət, 'ohpeeˌayt) any medicine containing opium.

opisthotonos (ˌohpee'thotənəs) a muscle spasm causing the back to be arched and the head retracted, with rigidity of the muscles of the neck and back. This condition can be present in acute cases of meningitis, tetanus, and strychnine poisoning.

opium ('ohpi·əm) a drug derived from dried poppy juice and used as a narcotic. It produces deep sleep, slows the pulse and respiration, contracts the pupils, and decreases all secretions of the body except sweat. It is a highly addictive drug. Opium derivatives include apomorphine, codeine, morphine, and papaverine.

opponens (o'pohnənz) opposing. A term applied to certain muscles controlling the movements of the fingers. *O. pollicis* a muscle that adducts the thumb so that it and the little finger can be brought together.

opportunistic (ˌopətyoo'nistik) 1. denoting a microorganism which does not ordinarily cause disease but becomes pathogenic under certain circumstances. 2. denoting a disease or infection caused by such an organism.

opsonic index (opˌsonik 'indeks) a measurement of the bactericidal power of the phagocytes in the blood of an individual.

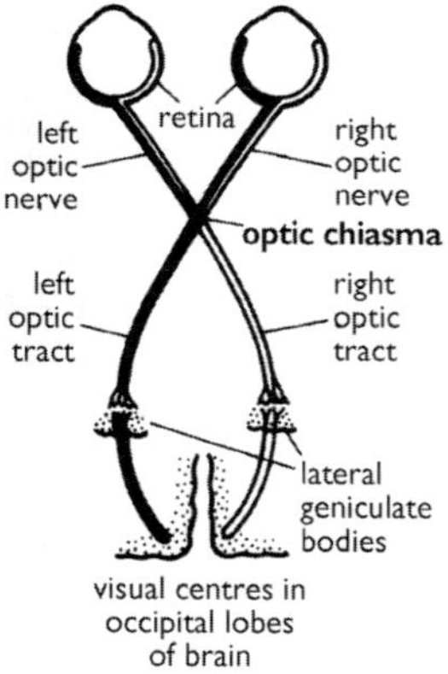

Optic Chiasma

opsonin (ˌopsənən) an antibody present in the blood which renders bacteria more easily destroyed by the phagocytes. Each kind of bacteria has its specific opsonin.

optic ('optik) relating to vision. *O. atrophy* degeneration of the optic nerve. *O chiasma* the crossing of the fibres of the optic nerves at the base of the brain (*see* figure). *O. disc* the point where the optic nerve enters the eyeball. *O. foramen* the opening in the posterior part of the orbit through which pass the optic nerve and the ophthalmic artery. *O. nerve* a bundle of nerve fibres running from the optic chiasma in the brain to the optic disc on the eyeball.

optical ('optikəl) pertaining to sight. *O. density* the refractive power of the transparent tissues through which light rays pass, changing the direction of the ray.

optician (op'tishən) a professional trained in the detection of refractive errors and the dispensing of appropriate spectacles or contact lenses.

optimum ('optəməm) the best and most favourable.

optometry (op'tomətree) the measuring of visual acuity and the fitting of glasses to correct visual defects.

ora ('ohra) [L.] *a margin. O. serrata* the jagged edge of the retina.

oral ('orəl) 1. pertaining to the mouth; taken through or applied in the mouth as an oral medication or an oral thermometer. 2. denoting that aspect of the teeth which faces the oral cavity or tongue.

orbit ('awbət) 1. the bony cavity containing the eyeball. 2. the path of an object moving around another object.

orchidectomy (ˌawkə'dektəmee) excision of a testicle. *Bilateral o.* the operation of castration.

orchidopexy (ˌawkədoh'peksee) an operation to free an undescended testicle and place it in the scrotum.

orchiepididymitis (ˌawkeeˌepeedidə'mietəs) inflammation of a testicle and its EPIDIDYMIS.

orchis ('awkəs) a testicle.

orchitis (aw'kietəs) inflammation of a testicle.

ordinal ('awdənəl) the level of measurement that systematically categorises data in an ordered or ranked manner. Ordinal measures do not permit a high level of differentiation among subjects.

orf (awf) a virus infection transmitted from sheep to humans. It can give rise to a boil-like lesion on the hands of meat handlers.

organ ('awgən) a part of the body designed to perform a particular function.

organ of Corti ('kawtee) terminal acoustic apparatus of the cochlea.

organelle (ˌawgə'nel) a structure within a cell which has specialised functions, e.g. nucleus, endoplasmic reticulum, mitochondrion, etc.

organic (aw'ganik) 1. pertaining to the organs. *O. disease* disease of an organ, accompanied by structural changes. 2. pertaining to chemicals containing carbon.

organism ('awgəˌnizəm) an individual living being, animal, or vegetable.

orgasm ('awgazəm) the climax of sexual excitement.

orientation (ˌawreeən'tayshən) a sense of direction. 1. The ability of a person to estimate his or her position in regard to time, place, and persons. 2. The imparting of relevant information at the onset of a course or conference so that its content and objects can be understood. *Reality O.* the way in which older people who are confused or mentally ill are assisted in keeping in touch with the world around them on a day-to-day basis. This can be achieved in a variety of ways, with large clocks, calendar boards, signs on doors, and daily newspapers.

orifice ('o·rəfəs) any opening in the body.

origin ('o·rəjən) in anatomy: 1. the point of attachment of a muscle; 2. the point at which a nerve or a blood vessel branches from the main stem.

ornithosis (ˌawnə'thohsəs) a virus disease of birds, usually pigeons, which can be transmitted to humans in a form resembling BRONCHOPNEUMONIA.

orogenital (ˌor·roh'jenət'l) pertaining to the mouth and external genitalia.

oropharynx (ˌor·roh'faringks) the lower portion of the pharynx behind the mouth and above the oesophagus and larynx.

orphenadrine (aw'fenəˌdrin) a drug used to treat PARKINSONISM, especially when accompanied by depression.

orthodontics (ˌawthoh'dontiks) dentistry that deals with the prevention and correction of malocclusion and irregularities of the teeth.

orthopaedics (ˌawthə'peediks) the science dealing with deformities, injuries, and diseases of the bones and joints.

orthopnoea (ˌawthop'neeə) difficulty in breathing unless in an upright position, e.g. sitting up in bed.

orthoptics (aw'thoptiks) the practice of treating by non-surgical methods (usually eye exercises) abnormalities of vision such as STRABISMUS (squint).

orthostatic (ˌawthoh'statik) pertaining to or caused by standing erect. *O. albuminuria see* ALBUMINURIA. *O. hypotension* low blood pressure occurring when a person stands up.

orthotic (aw'thotik) serving to protect or to restore or improve function; pertaining to the use or application of an orthosis (an appliance that can be applied to or around the body in the care/treatment of physical impairment or disability).

orthotist ('awthəˌtist) a person skilled in orthotics and practising its application in individual cases.

Ortolani's sign (ˌawtoh'lahneez) *M. Ortolani, 20th century Italian* *orthopaedic surgeon.* A test performed soon after birth to detect possible congenital dislocation of the hip. A 'click' is felt on reversing the movements of abduction and rotation of the hip while the child is lying with knees flexed.

os[1] (ohs) pl. ora [L.] 1. any body orifice. 2. the mouth.

os[2] (os) pl. ossa [L.] *a bone.*

oscillation (ˌosəˈlayshən) 1. a backwards and forwards motion. 2. vibration.

oscilloscope (əˈsiləˌskohp) an apparatus using a cathode-ray tube to depict visibly data fed into it electronically, e.g. the way in which the heart is performing.

Osler's nodes (ˈohsləz) *Sir W. Osler, Canadian physician, 1849–1919.* Small painful swellings which occur in or beneath the skin, especially of the extremities in subacute bacterial ENDOCARDITIS, caused by minute emboli. They usually disappear in 1–3 days.

osmolality (ˌozmohˈlalətee) the osmotic pressure of a solution expressed in osmols or milliosmols per kilogram of water.

osmolarity (ˌozmohˈlarətee) the osmotic pressure of a solution expressed in osmols or milliosmols per kilogram of the solution.

osmoreceptor (ˌozmohrəˈseptə) one of a group of specialised nerve cells which monitor the osmotic pressure of the blood and the extracellular fluid. Impulses from these receptors are relayed to the HYPOTHALAMUS.

osmosis (ozˈmohsəs, os-) the passage of fluid from a low concentration solution to one of a higher concentration through a semipermeable membrane.

osmotic (ozˈmotik) pertaining to osmosis. *O. pressure* the pressure exerted by large molecules in the blood, e.g. albumin and globulin proteins, which draws fluid into the bloodstream from the surrounding tissues.

osseous (ˈosi·əs) bony.

ossicle (ˈosikəl) a small bone. *Auditory o.* one of the three bones in the middle ear: the MALLEUS, INCUS and STAPES.

ossification (ˌosəfəˈkayshən) the process by which bone is developed; osteogenesis.

ostalgia (ˌostˈalji·ə) pain in a bone.

osteitis (ˌostˈietəs) inflammation of bone. *O. deformans see* PAGET'S DISEASE. *O. fibrosa cystica* or *parathyroid o.* defects of ossification with fibrous tissue production leading to weakening and deformity. It affects children chiefly, and is associated with parathyroid tumour, removal of which checks it. *See* RECKLINGHAUSEN'S DISEASE.

osteoarthritis (ˌosteeoh·ahˈthrietəs) *see* ARTHRITIS.

osteoarthrotomy (ˌosteeoh·ahˈthrotəmee) surgical excision of the jointed end of a bone.

osteoblast (ˈosteeohˌblast) a cell which develops into an osteocyte and turns into bone.

osteochondritis (ˌosteeohkonˈdrietəs) inflammation of bone and cartilage, particularly a degenerative disease of an EPIPHYSIS, causing pain and deformity. *O. of the hip* PERTHES' DISEASE. *O. of the tarsal scaphoid bone* Khler's disease. *O. of the tibial tuberosity* Osgood–Schlatter disease.

osteochondroma (ˌosteeohkonˈdrohmə) a tumour consisting of both bone and cartilage.

osteoclasis (ˌosteeˈokləsəs) 1. the

surgical fracture of bones to correct a deformity such as bowleg. 2. the restructuring of bone by osteoclasts during growth or the repair of damaged bone.

osteoclast ('osteeoh,klast) 1. a large cell that breaks down and absorbs bone and callus. 2. an instrument designed for surgical fracture of bone.

osteocyte ('osteeoh,siet) a bone cell.

osteodystrophy (,osteeoh'distrəfee) a metabolic disease of bone.

osteogenesis (,osteeoh'jenəsəs) the formation of bone. *O. imperfecta* a congenital disorder of the bones, which are very brittle and fracture easily. Fragilitas osseum.

osteoma (,ostee'ohmə) a benign tumour arising from bone.

osteomalacia (,osteeohmə'layshi·ə) a disease characterised by painful softening of bones. Due to vitamin D deficiency.

osteomyelitis (,osteeoh,mieə'lietəs) inflammation of bone, localised or generalised, due to a pyogenic infection. It can result in bone destruction, stiffening of joints and, in extreme cases occurring before the end of the growth period, in the shortening of a limb if the growth centre is destroyed. Acute osteomyelitis is caused by bacteria that enter the body through a wound, spread from an infection near the bone, or come from a skin or throat infection. The infection usually affects the long bones of the arms and legs and causes pain and fever. It most often occurs in children and adolescents, particularly boys.

osteopath ('osteeoh,path) one who practises OSTEOPATHY.

osteopathy (,ostee'opəthee) a system of treatment of disease by bone manipulation. Osteopathic treatment is manipulative and is aimed at freeing and loosening joints and re-establishing proper relationships of the spinal column and its component bones with the pelvis and limb bones.

osteoperiostitis (,osteeoh,pereeoh-'stietəs) inflammation of bone and PERIOSTEUM.

osteopetrosis (,osteeohpə'trohsəs) a rare congenital disease in which the bones become abnormally dense. Albers–Schönberg disease.

osteophyte ('osteeoh,fiet) a small outgrowth of bone.

osteoplasty ('osteeoh,plastee) a plastic operation on bone.

osteoporosis (,osteeohpaw'rohsəs) abnormal rarefaction of bone which can be idiopathic or secondary to other conditions. The disorder leads to thinning of the skeleton and decreased precipitation of lime salts. There can also be inadequate calcium absorption into the bone and excessive bone resorption. The principal causes are lack of physical activity, lack of oestrogens or androgens, and nutritional deficiency. There is almost always some degree of osteoporosis that occurs with ageing. Symptoms include pathological fractures and collapse of the vertebrae without compression of the spinal cord.

osteosarcoma (,osteeohsah'kohmə) an osteogenic sarcoma; a malignant bone tumour.

osteosclerosis (,osteeohsklə'rohsəs) an increase in density and a hardening of bone. *O. congenita* ACHONDROPLASIA. *O. fragilis* osteopetrosis.

osteotomy (,ostee'otəmee) the cutting into or through a bone, sometimes performed to correct deformity. *O. of the hip* a method of treating osteoarthritis by cutting the bone and altering the line of weight bearing.

ostium ('osti·əm) a mouth. *Abdominal o.* the opening at the end of the uterine tube into the peritoneal cavity.

otic ('ohtik) relating to the ear.

otitis (oh'tietəs) inflammation of the ear. *Aviation o.* a symptom complex resulting from fluctuations between atmospheric pressure and air pressure in the middle ear; also called barotitis media. *O. externa* inflammation of the external ear. *Furuncular o.* the formation of FURUNCLES in the external ear. *O. interna, o. labyrinthica* LABYRINTHITIS. *O. mastoidea* inflammation of the MASTOID spaces. *O. media* inflammation of the middle ear occurring most often in infants and young children and classified as serous, secretory, and suppurative.

otolaryngology (ˌohtohˌlaring'goləjee) the scientific study of the ear and the larynx and the diseases affecting them.

otolith ('otohˌlith) 1. a calculus in the middle ear. 2. one of a number of small calcareous concretions of the inner ear, at the base of semicircular canals.

otology (oh'toləjee) the scientific study of the ear and its diseases.

otomycosis (ˌohtohmie'kohsəs) a fungal infection of the auditory canal.

otorrhoea (ˌohtə'reeə) discharge from the ear, especially of pus.

otosclerosis (ˌohtohsklə'rohsəs) the formation of spongy bone in the labyrinth of the ear causing the auditory ossicles to become fixed and less able to pass on vibrations when sound enters the ear. The cause of otosclerosis is still unknown. It can be hereditary or related to vitamin deficiency or OTITIS media. An early symptom is ringing in the ears but the most noticeable symptom is progressive loss of hearing.

otoscope ('ohtohˌskohp) an auriscope; an instrument for examining the ear.

otoscopy (oh'toskəpee) an examination of the tympanic membrane and auditory canal by means of an OTOSCOPE.

Otosporin (ohtə'sporən) trade name for a combination preparation of ear drops containing hydrocortisone, neomycin, and polymyxin.

ototoxic (ˌohtoh'toksik) anything which has a deleterious effect on the 8th cranial nerve or on the organs of hearing.

ouabain (wah'bah·in, 'wahbayn) a cardiac glycoside; its effect is similar to that of digitalis, but digitalisation is achieved more rapidly.

ovarian (oh'vair·ri·ən) relating to an ovary. *O. cyst* a tumour of the ovary containing fluid.

ovariectomy (ˌohvə·ri'ektəmee) OÖPHORECTOMY; excision of an ovary.

ovariotomy (ohˌvair·ree'otəmee) 1. surgical removal of an ovary. 2. excision of an ovarian tumour.

ovaritis (ˌohvə'rietəs) OÖPHORITIS; inflammation of an ovary.

ovary ('ohvə·ree) one of a pair of glandular organs in the female pelvis. They produce ova which pass through the uterine tubes into the uterus, and steroid hormones which control the menstrual cycle.

overbite ('ohvəˌbiet) an overlapping

of the lower teeth by the upper teeth.

overcompensation (ˌohvaˌkompən'sayshən) a mental mechanism by which a person tries to assert himself or herself by aggressive behaviour or by talking or acting 'big' to compensate for a feeling of inadequacy.

oviduct ('ohviˌdukt, 'ovi-) a uterine tube.

ovulation (ˌovyə'layshən, ˌoh-) the process of rupture of the mature Graafian follicle when the ovum is shed from the ovary.

ovum ('ohvəm) [L.] an egg. The reproductive cell of the female.

oxidisation (ˌoksədie'zayshən) oxidation. The process by which combustion occurs and breaking up of matter takes place, e.g. oxidation of carbohydrates gives carbon dioxide and water: $C_6H_{12}O_6 + 6O_2 = 6CO_2 + 6H_2O$.

oximeter (ok'simətə) a photoelectric cell used to determine the oxygen saturation of blood. *Ear o.* one attached to the ear by which the oxygen content of blood flowing through the ear can be measured.

oxprenolol (oks'prenəˌlol) a beta-blocking drug used in the treatment of angina, hypertension, and cardiac ARRHYTHMIAS.

oxygen ('oksəjən) *symbol* O. A colourless, odourless gas constituting one-fifth of the atmosphere. It is stored in cylinders at high pressure or as liquid oxygen. It is used medicinally to enrich the air when either respiration or circulation is impaired. *O. saturation* the amount of oxygen bound to haemoglobin in the blood. *O. tent* a large plastic canopy that encloses the patient in a controlled environment; used for oxygen therapy, humidity therapy, or aerosol therapy. *O. therapy* supplementary oxygen administered for the purpose of relieving HYPOXAEMIA and preventing damage to the tissue cells as a result of lack of oxygen.

oxygenation (ˌoksəjə'nayshən) saturation with oxygen; a process (which occurs in the lungs) whereby the haemoglobin of blood is saturated with oxygen to form OXYHAEMOGLOBIN.

oxygenator ('oksəjəˌnaytə) a machine through which the blood is passed to oxygenate it during open heart surgery. *Pump o.* a machine which pumps oxygenated blood through the body during heart surgery.

oxyhaemoglobin (ˌokseeˌheemə'glohbən) haemoglobin that has been oxygenated, as in arterial blood.

oxyntic (ok'sintik) acid forming. *O. cell* a parietal cell of the gastric glands which secretes hydrochloric acid.

oxypertine (ˌoksee'pərteen) an antipsychotic tranquillising drug used in the treatment of SCHIZOPHRENIA and related psychoses, and of mania and HYPERACTIVITY.

oxytetracycline (ˌokseeˌtetrə'siekleen) a broad-spectrum antibiotic, chiefly used against infections caused by *Chlamydia*, *Rickettsia*, and *Brucella*.

oxytocic (ˌoksee'tohsik) any drug that stimulates uterine contractions; can be used to hasten delivery.

oxytocin (ˌoksee'tohsən) a pituitary hormone which stimulates uterine contractions and the ejection of milk. Synthetically prepared, it is used to induce labour and to control POSTPARTUM haemorrhage.

oxyuriasis (ˌokseeyəˈrieəsəs) infestation by threadworms of the genus *Enterobius*.

ozaena (ohˈzeenə) atrophic RHINITIS. A condition of the nose in which there is loss and shrinkage of the ciliated mucous membrane and of the turbinate bones. There can be an offensive nasal discharge.

ozone (ˈohzohn) an intensified form of oxygen containing three O atoms to the molecule (i.e. O_3), and often discharged by electrical machines, such as X-ray apparatus. In medicine, it is employed as an antiseptic and oxidising agent.

Pp

P symbol for *phosphorus*.

pacemaker ('pays,maykə) an object or substance that controls the rate at which a certain phenomenon occurs. The natural pacemaker of the heart is the sinoatrial NODE. *Electronic cardiac p.* an electrically operated mechanical device which stimulates the MYOCARDIUM to contract. It consists of an energy source, usually batteries, and electrical circuitry connected to an electrode which is in direct contact with the myocardium. Pacemakers can be temporary or permanent. Temporary ones usually have an external energy source, whereas permanent ones have a subcutaneously implanted one. The rate the pacemaker delivers pulses can be either fixed or on demand. *Fixed* pacing means that pulses are delivered to the heart at a predetermined rate irrespective of any cardiac activity. A *demand* pacemaker is programmed to deliver pulses only in the absence of spontaneous cardiac activity. The need for replacement batteries is usually indicated when the rate of the pulse slows by five beats or more.

pachydactyly (,pakee'daktəlee) abnormal thickening of the fingers or toes.

pachydermia (,pakee'dərmi·ə) an abnormal thickening of the skin. *P. laryngis* chronic HYPERTROPHY of the vocal cords.

pachyonychia (,pakeeo'niki·ə) abnormal thickening of the nails.

pachysomia (,pakee'sohmi·ə) abnormal thickening of parts of the body, as in ACROMEGALY.

Pacini's corpuscle (pa'cheeneez) *F. Pacini, Italian anatomist, 1812–83.* Specialised sensory end organ resembling a small white bulb. Each is attached to the end of a single nerve fibre in the subcutaneous tissue of many parts of the body (such as the palm of the hand, the sole of the foot, the genital organs, and joints) where they react to firm pressure.

paediatrician (,peedi·ə'trishən) a specialist in the diseases of children.

paediatrics (,peedi'atriks) the branch of medicine dealing with the care and development of children and with the treatment of diseases that affect them.

paedophilia (,peedə'fili·ə) a sexual attraction towards young children.

Paget's disease ('pajəts) *Sir J. Paget, British surgeon, 1814–99.* 1. a chronic disease of bone in which overactivity of the OSTEOBLASTS and OSTEOCLASTS leads to dense bone formation with areas of rarefaction. OSTEITIS deformans. 2. an inflammation of the nipple caused by cancer of the milk ducts of the breast.

pain (payn) a feeling of distress, suffering, or agony caused by stimulation of specialised nerve endings. Its purpose is chiefly protective; it acts as a warning that tissues are being damaged and induces the sufferer to remove or withdraw from the source of damage. Pain is a subjective experience and one person's pain cannot be compared to another's experience. *Bearing-down p.* pain accompanying uterine contractions during the second stage of LABOUR. *False p's* ineffective pains during pregnancy which resemble labour pains; not accompanied by cervical dilatation; called also false labour. *See also* BRAXTON HICKS CONTRACTIONS. *Gas p's* pains caused by distension of the stomach or intestine by accumulations of air or other gases. *Hunger p.* pain coming on at the time of feeling hunger for a meal; a symptom of gastric disorder. *Intermenstrual p.* pain accompanying ovulation occurring during the period between the menses, usually about midway. Also called MITTELSCHMERZ. *Labour p's* the rhythmic pains of increasing severity and frequency due to contraction of the uterus at childbirth. *See* also LABOUR. *Lancinating p.* sharp, darting pain. *Phantom p.* pain felt as if it were arising in an absent (amputated) limb. *See also* AMPUTATION. *Referred p.* pain in a part other than that in which the cause that produced it is situated. Referred pain usually originates in one of the visceral organs but is felt in the skin or sometimes in another area deep inside the body. Referred pain probably occurs because pain signals from the viscera travel along the same neural pathways used by pain signals from the skin. The person perceives the pain but interprets it as having originated in the skin rather than in a deep-seated visceral organ. *Rest p.* a continuous burning pain due to ISCHAEMIA of the lower leg, which begins or is aggravated after reclining and is relieved by sitting or standing.

palate ('palət) the roof of the mouth. *Artificial p.* a plate made to close a cleft palate. *Cleft p.* a congenital deformity where there is lack of fusion of the two bones forming the palate. *Hard p.* the bony part at the front. *Soft p.* a fold of mucous membrane that continues from the hard palate to the UVULA.

palatine bone ('palə,tien) one of a pair of bones which form a part of the nasal cavity and the hard palate.

palliative ('pali·ətiv) treatment that relieves symptoms but does not cure disease.

pallidectomy (,pali'dektəmee) an operation performed to decrease the activity of the globus pallidus, the medial part of the lentiform nucleus in the base of the cerebrum. It has brought about a marked improvement in severely agitated cases of PARKINSONISM.

pallor ('palə) abnormal paleness of the skin.

palmar ('palmə) relating to the palm of the hand. *Deep* and *superficial p. arches* the chief arterial blood supply to the hand formed by the junction of the ulnar and radial arteries. *P. fascia* the arrangement of tendons in the palm of the hand.

palpation (pal'payshən) the examination of the organs by touch or pressure of the hand over the part.
palpebral ('palpibrəl) referring to the eyelids. *P. ligaments* a band of ligaments which stretches from the junction of the upper and lower lid to the orbital bones, both medially and laterally.
palpitation (ˌpalpə'tayshən) rapid and forceful contraction of the heart of which the patient is conscious.
palsy ('pawlzee) paralysis. *Bell's p.* paralysis of the facial muscles on one side supplied by the seventh cranial nerve. *Crutch p.* paralysis due to pressure of a crutch on the radial nerve and a cause of 'dropped wrist'. *Erb's p.* paralysis of one arm due to a birth injury to the BRACHIAL plexus. *Shaking p.* PARKINSONISM; paralysis agitans.
panacea (ˌpanə'seeə) a remedy for all diseases.
panarthritis (ˌpanah'thrietəs) inflammation of all the joints or of all the structures of a joint.
pancarditis (ˌpankahdi'ietəs) inflammation of all the structures of the heart.
Pancoast's tumour ('pankohsts) *H.K. Pancoast, American radiologist, 1875–1939.* Pain, wasting and weakness of the arm which occur as secondary features of carcinoma of the bronchus as a result of neurological involvement. The tumour is at the apex of the lung.
pancreas ('pangkri·əs) an elongated, racemose gland about 15 cm long, lying behind the stomach with its head in the curve of the duodenum and its tail in contact with the spleen (*see* figure). It secretes a digestive fluid (pancreatic juice) containing ferments which act on all classes

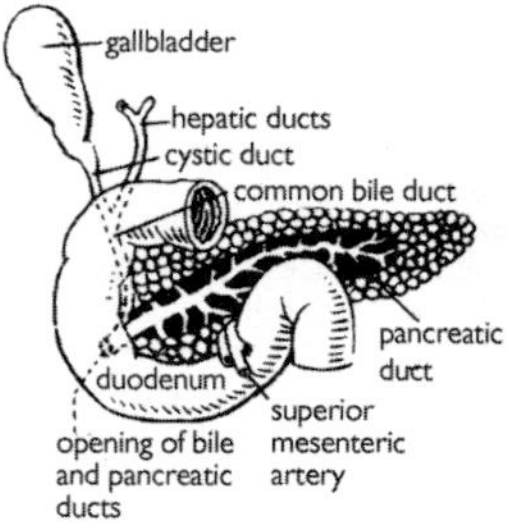

Pancreas

of foods. The fluid enters the duodenum by the pancreatic duct which usually joins the common bile duct. The pancreas also secretes the hormones insulin and glucagon.
pancreatectomy (ˌpangkri·ə'tektəmee) surgical excision of the whole or a part of the pancreas.
pancreatin ('pangkri·ətən, pan'kreeə-) an extract from the pancreas containing the digestive enzymes. Used to treat deficiency, as in cystic fibrosis, and after PANCREATECTOMY.
pancreatitis (ˌpangkri·ə'tietəs) inflammation of the pancreas. *Acute p.* a severe condition in which the patient experiences sudden pain in the upper abdomen and back. The patient often becomes severely shocked. *Chronic p.* chronic inflammation occurring after acute attacks. Pancreatic failure may lead to DIABETES mellitus.
pancreozymin (ˌpangkreeoh'ziemən) a hormone of the DUODENAL mucosa that stimulates the external secretory activity of the pancreas, especially its production of amylase.

pancuronium (ˌpangkyəˈrohni·əm) a neuromuscular blocking agent of the nerve depolarising type used as a muscle relaxant during surgery. It has a relatively long duration of action, a single intravenous dose lasting 45–60 min. It is often used in poor-risk patients.

pancytopenia (ˌpansietohˈpeeni·ə) a reduction in number of all types of blood cell due to failure of bone marrow formation.

pandemic (panˈdemik) an epidemic spreading over a wide area, sometimes all over the world.

panhysterectomy (ˌpanhistəˈrektəmee) surgical removal of the whole of the uterus.

panic (ˈpanik) an unreasoning and overwhelming fear or terror. It can occur in anxiety states and acute SCHIZOPHRENIA.

panleukopenia (ˌpanlookohˈpeeni·ə) a deficiency of all the white blood cells.

panmyelopathy (ˌpanmieəˈlopəthee) a disease affecting all the cells formed in the bone marrow.

panniculitis (peˌnikyəˈlietəs) inflammation of the subcutaneous fat causing tender nodules on the abdomen and thorax and on the thighs.

panniculus (pəˈnikyələs) a sheet of membrane. *P. adiposus* the fatty layer beneath the skin.

pannus (ˈpanəs) increased vascularity of the cornea leading to granulation tissue formation and impaired vision. It occurs after inflammation of the cornea.

panophthalmia (ˌpanofˈthalmi·ə) panophthalmitis; inflammation of all the tissues of the eyeball.

panosteitis (ˌpanostiˈietəs) inflammation of all the structures of a bone.

pansystolic murmur (ˌpansiˌstolik ˈmərmə) a heart murmur heard throughout the time the heart is in systole. *See* MURMUR.

pantothenic acid (ˌpantəˈthenik) one of the vitamins in the B complex.

PaO_2 partial pressure of oxygen (O_2) in arterial blood.

Papanicolaou test (Pap test) (ˌpapəˌnikəˈlayoo) *G.N. Papanicolaou, Greek physician, anatomist and cytologist, 1883–1962.* A smear test to detect diseases particularly cancer of the uterine cervix and ENDOMETRIUM.

papaveretum (pəˌpahvəˈreetəm) a preparation of the alkaloids of opium with an action similar to morphine. It is used to counteract severe pain.

papilla (pəˈpilə) a small nipple-shaped protuberance. *Circumvallate p.* one surrounded by a ridge. Several are found at the back of the tongue arranged in a V-shape and containing taste buds. *Filiform p.* one of the fine, slender filaments on the main part of the tongue which give it its velvety appearance. *Fungiform p.* a mushroom-shaped papilla of the tongue. *Optic p.* the optic disc where the optic nerve leaves the eyeball. *Tactile p.* a projection on the true skin which contains nerve endings responsible for relaying sensations of pressure to the brain. A touch corpuscle.

papillitis (ˌpapiˈlietəs) 1. inflammation of the optic disc. 2. inflammation of a papilla.

papilloedema (ˌpapiləˈdeemə) OEDEMA and HYPERAEMIA of the optic disc usually associated with increased intracranial pressure; also called choked disc.

papilloma (ˌpapəˈlohmə) a benign

growth of epithelial tissue, e.g. a wart.

papillomatosis (ˌpapəˌlohmə'tohsəs) the occurrence of multiple PAPILLOMATA.

papovavirus (pə'pohvəˌvierəs) a family of DNA-producing viruses which cause tumours, usually benign, such as warts.

papule ('papyool) a pimple or small solid elevation of the skin.

papulopustular (ˌpapyəloh'pustyəla) descriptive of skin eruptions of both PAPULES and pustules.

papulosquamous (ˌpapyəloh'skwayməs) descriptive of skin eruptions that are both papular and scaly. They include such conditions as LICHEN planus, PITYRIASIS and PSORIASIS.

para-aminobenzoic acid (ˌparəˌaminohben'zoh·ik) a member of the B group of vitamins. It is used in creams and lotions to prevent sunburn.

para-aminosalicylic acid (ˌparəˌaminohˌsalə'silik) abbreviated PAS. An acid, the salts of which are used together with other drugs, usually isoniazid (INH) or streptomycin, in the treatment of tuberculosis.

paracentesis (ˌparəsen'teesəs) puncture of the wall of a cavity with a hollow needle in order to draw off excess fluid or to obtain diagnostic material.

paracetamol (ˌparə'seetəˌmol, -'setə-) a mild analgesic drug used to treat headaches, toothache, rheumatic pains, and PYREXIA.

paracusis (ˌparə'kyoosəs) a perverted sense of hearing. *P. of Willis* an improvement in hearing when surrounded by noise.

paradigm ('parəˌdiem) any example or representative instance of a concept or theoretical approach.

paradoxical respiration (ˌparə'doksikəl) respiration in which part of the lung inflates on expiration and deflates on inspiration.

paradoxical sleep rapid eye movement sleep (REM). *See* SLEEP.

paraesthesia (ˌparəs'theezi·ə) an abnormal tingling sensation. 'Pins and needles'.

paraffin ('parəfən) any saturated hydrocarbon obtained from petroleum. *Liquid p.* a mineral oil which is used as a laxative. *Soft p.* petroleum jelly. Used as a barrier agent to protect the skin. *P. wax* a hard paraffin that can be used for wax treatment for chronic inflammation of joints.

Paragonimus (ˌparə'gonimǝs) a genus of trematode parasites. The flukes infest the lungs and are found mainly in tropical countries.

paraldehyde (pə'raldiˌhied) a sedative, hypnotic, and anticonvulsant drug that has an unpleasant taste and imparts an unpleasant odour to the breath. Its main use today is in the treatment of status epilepticus.

paralysis (pə'raləsəs) loss or impairment of motor function in a part owing to a lesion of the neural or muscular mechanism; also, by analogy, impairment of sensory function (sensory paralysis). Paralysis is a symptom of a wide variety of physical and emotional disorders rather than a disease in itself. Palsy. *P. agitans* Parkinsonism. *Bulbar p.* (labioglossopharyngeal p.) paralysis due to changes in the motor centre of the MEDULLA oblongata. It affects the muscles of the mouth, tongue and pharynx. *Facial p.* (Bell's palsy) paralysis that affects the muscles of the face and is due to injury to or inflammation of the facial nerve. *Flaccid p.* loss of tone and absence of reflexes in the paralysed muscles. *General p. of the insane* abbreviated GPI. Paralytic dementia occurring in the late stages of syphilis. *Infantile p.* the major form of poliomyelitis (*see* POLIOMYELITIS). *Spastic p.* paralysis characterised by rigidity of affected muscles.

paralytic (ˌparə'litik) affected by or relating to paralysis. *P. ileus* obstruction of the ileum due to absence of peristalsis in a portion of the intestine.

paramedian (ˌparə'meedi·ən) situated on the side of the median line.

paramedical (ˌparə'medikəl) associated with the medical profession and the delivery of health care. The paramedical services include occupational and speech therapy, physiotherapy, radiography, and social work.

parametric statistics (ˌparə'metrik) inferential statistics that involve the estimation of at least one parameter, require measurement at the interval level or above, and involve assumptions about the variables being studied. These assumptions usually include the fact that the variable is normally distributed.

parametritis (ˌparəmee'trietəs) inflammation of the parametrium; pelvic CELLULITIS.

parametrium (ˌparə'meetri·əm) the connective tissue surrounding the uterus.

paramnesia (ˌparam'neezi·ə) a defect of memory in which there is a false recollection. The patient might fill in the forgotten period with imaginary events which he or she describes in great detail.

paranoia (ˌparə'noyə) a mental disorder characterised by delusions of grandeur or persecution which can be fully systematised in logical form with the personality remaining fairly well preserved.

paranoid ('parəˌnoyd) resembling paranoia. Refers to a condition that can occur in many forms of mental disease. Delusions of persecution are a marked feature. *P. schizophrenia see* SCHIZOPHRENIA.

paraparesis (ˌparəpə'reesəs) an incomplete paralysis affecting the lower limbs.

paraphasia (ˌparə'fayzi·ə) a speech disorder involving the substitution of a similar sound or word for that intended, thereby producing a nonsensical utterance.

paraphimosis (ˌparəfie'mohsəs) retraction of the prepuce behind the glans penis with inability to replace it, resulting in a painful constriction.

paraphrenia (ˌparə'freeniə) schizophrenia occurring for the first time in later life and not accompanied by deterioration of the personality.

paraplegia (ˌparə'pleeji·ə) paralysis of the lower extremities and lower trunk. All parts below the point of lesion in the spinal cord are affected. It can be of sudden onset from injury to the cord or can develop slowly as the result of disease.

paraprofessional (ˌparəprə'feshənəl) 1. a person who is specially trained in a particular field or occupation to assist a professional. 2. allied health professional. 3. pertaining to a paraprofessional.

parapsychology (ˌparəsie'koləjee) the branch of psychology dealing with psychical effects and experiences that appear to fall outside the scope of physical law, e.g. telepathy and clairvoyance.

paraquat ('parə͵kwat) a poisonous compound used as a contact herbicide. Contact with concentrated solutions causes irritation of the skin, cracking and shedding of the nails, and delayed healing of cuts and wounds. After ingestion, renal and hepatic failure can develop followed by pulmonary insufficiency and death.

parasite ('parə͵siet) any animal or vegetable organism living upon or within another, from which it derives its nourishment.

parasiticide (͵parə'sitə͵sied) a drug that kills parasites.

parasympathetic system (͵parə͵simpə'thetik) the craniosacral part of the autonomic nervous system.

parasympatholytic (͵parə͵simpəthoh'litik) anticholinergic; an agent that opposes the effects of the parasympathetic nervous system.

parathormone (͵parə'thawmohn) the endocrine hormone secretion of the parathyroid glands.

parathyroid gland (͵parə'thieroyd) one of four small endocrine glands, two of which are associated with each lobe of the thyroid gland and sometimes embedded in it. The secretion from these has some control over calcium metabolism, and lack of it is a cause of TETANY.

parathyroidectomy (͵parə͵thieroy'dektəmee) the surgical removal of parathyroid glands.

paratyphoid (͵parə'tiefoyd) a notifiable infection caused by *Salmonella* of all groups except *S. typhi*. The disease is usually milder and has a shorter incubation period, more abrupt onset, and lower mortality rate than does typhoid. Clinically and pathologically, the two diseases cannot be distinguished. Called also paratyphoid fever.

parenchyma (pə'rengkima) the essential active cells of an organ, as distinguished from its vascular and connective tissue.

parenteral (pə'rentə·rəl) apart from the alimentary canal. Applied to the introduction into the body of drugs or fluids by routes other than the mouth or rectum, for instance, intravenously or subcutaneously.

paresis (pə'reesəs, 'parəsəs) partial paralysis.

parietal (pə'rieət'l) relating to the walls of any cavity. *P. bones* the two bones forming part of the roof and sides of the skull. *P. cells* the oxyntic cells in the gastric mucosa that secrete hydrochloric acid. *P. pleura* the pleura attached to the chest wall.

parity ('parətee) the classification of a woman with regard to the number of children that have been born live to her.

Parkinson's disease ('pahkənsənz) *J. Parkinson, British physician, 1755–1824*. Parkinsonism; paralysis agitans. A slowly progressive disease usually occurring in later life, characterised pathologically by degeneration within the nuclear masses of the extrapyramidal system, and clinically by mask-like facies (*see* FACIES Parkinson), a characteristic tremor of resting muscles, a slowing of voluntary movements, a festinating gait, peculiar posture, and muscular weakness. When this symptom complex occurs secondarily to another disorder, the condition is called Parkinsonism.

paronychia (ˌparəˈnikiə) an abscess near the fingernail; a whitlow or felon. *P. tendinosa* a pyogenic infection that involves the tendon sheath.

parosmia (paˈrozmi·ə) a disordered sense of smell.

parotid (pəˈrotid) situated near the ear. *P. glands* two salivary glands, one in front of each ear.

parotitis (ˌparəˈtietəs) inflammation of a parotid gland. Caused usually by ascending infection via its duct, when hygiene of the mouth is neglected or when the natural secretions are lessened, especially in severe illness or after operation. *Epidemic p.* mumps.

parous (ˈparəs) having borne one or more children.

paroxysm (ˈparokˌsizəm) 1. a sudden attack or recurrence of a symptom of a disease. 2. a convulsion.

paroxysmal (ˌparokˈsizməl) occurring in paroxysms. *P. cardiac dyspnoea* cardiac asthma. Recurrent attacks of DYSPNOEA associated with pulmonary oedema and left-sided heart failure. *P. tachycardia* recurrent attacks of rapid heart beats that can occur without apparent heart disease.

parrot disease (ˈparət) *see* PSITTACOSIS.

parthenogenesis (ˌpahthənohˈjenəsəs) asexual reproduction by means of an egg that has not been fertilised.

particle (ˈpahtikəl) a minute piece of substance.

parturient (pahˈtyoo·ri·ənt) giving birth; relating to childbirth.

parturition (ˌpahtyəˈrishən) the act of giving birth to a child.

PAS para-aminosalicylic acid.

pascal (paˈskal, ˈpaskəl) *symbol* Pa. The SI unit of pressure, which corresponds to a force of one newton per square metre.

passive (ˈpasiv) not active *P. immunity see* IMMUNITY. *P. movements* in massage, manipulation by a physiotherapist without the help of the patient.

passivity (paˈsivətee) in psychiatry, a delusional feeling that a person is under some outside control and must therefore be inactive.

Pasteurella (ˌpahstəˈrelə) *L. Pasteur, French chemist and bacteriologist 1833–95.* A genus of short Gram-negative bacilli. *P. pestis* the causative organism of plague transmitted by rat fleas to humans.

pasteurisation (ˌpastə·rieˈzayshən, ˌpahstyə-) the process of checking fermentation in milk and other fluids by heating them to a temperature of 72°C for 15–20 min or 63°C for 30 min, and then rapidly cooling. This kills most pathogenic bacteria.

patch test (pach) a test of skin sensitivity in which several possible allergens are applied to the skin under a plaster. The causal agent of the allergy will produce an area of inflammation.

patella (pəˈtelə) the small, circular, sesamoid bone forming the kneecap.

patellar (pəˈtelə) belonging to the patella. *P. reflex* a knee jerk obtained by tapping the tendon below the patella.

patellectomy (ˌpatəˈlektəmee) excision of the patella.

patent (ˈpaytənt) open. *P. ductus arteriosus* failure of the ductus arteriosus to close causing a shunt of blood from the aorta into the pulmonary artery and producing a

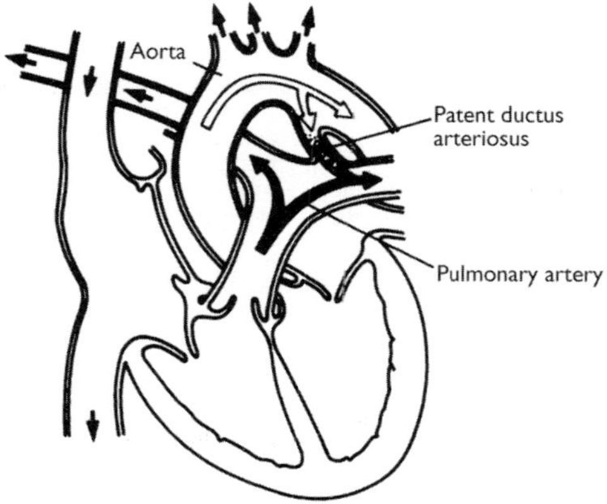

Patent Ductus Arteriosus

continuous heart murmur (*see* figure).

pathogen ('pathəjən) any disease-producing agent or microorganism.

pathogenicity (ˌpathəjə'nisətee) the ability of a microorganism to cause disease.

pathognomonic (ˌpathəgnə'monik) specifically characteristic of a disease. A sign or symptom by which a pathological condition can positively be identified.

pathological (ˌpathə'lojikəl) 1. pertaining to pathology. 2. causing or arising from disease. *P. fracture* a fracture occurring in diseased bone when there has been little or no external trauma.

pathology (pə'tholəjee) the branch of medicine that deals with the essential nature of disease, especially of the structural and functional changes in tissues and organs of the body which cause or are caused by disease.

pathophobia (ˌpathə'fohbi·ə) an exaggerated dread of disease.

patient ('payshənt) a person who is ill or is undergoing treatment for disease.

Paul–Bunnell test (ˌpawlbə'nel) *J.R. Paul, American physician 1893–1971; W.W. Bunnell, American physician, 1902–66.* An agglutination test which, if positive, confirms the diagnosis of glandular fever.

Pavlov's method ('pavlovz ˌmethəd) *I.P. Pavlov, Russian physiologist, 1849–1936.* A method for the study of the conditioned reflexes. Pavlov noticed that his experimental dogs salivated in anticipation of food when they heard a bell ring.

peak flowmeter (ˌpeek 'flohˌmeetə)

a hand-held device that is used to measure the highest flow during maximal expiration. The peak flow reading reflects changes in airway diameter.

peau d'orange (ˌpoh do'ronhzh) a dimpled appearance of the overlying skin. Blockage of the skin lymphatics causes dimpling of the hair follicle openings which resembles orange skin. Particularly associated with breast cancer.

pecten ('pektən) 1. the middle third of the anal canal. 2. a ridge on the pubic crest to which the inguinal ligament is attached.

pectoral ('pektə·rəl) relating to the chest. *P. muscles* two pairs of muscles, pectoralis major and pectoralis minor, which control the movements of the shoulder and upper arm.

pectus ('pektəs) the chest.

pedicle ('pedikəl) the stem or neck of a tumour. *P. graft* a tissue graft that is partially detached and inserted in its new position while temporarily still obtaining its blood supply from the original source.

pediculosis (pəˌdikyə'lohsəs) the condition of being infested with lice.

Pediculus (pə'dikyələs) genus of lice. *P. humanus* a species that feeds on human blood and is an important vector of relapsing fever, typhus, and trench fever; two subspecies are recognised; *P. humanus* var. *capitis* (head louse) found on the scalp hair, and *P. humanus* var. *corporis* (body or clothes louse) found elsewhere on the body.

peduncle (pə'dungkəl) a narrow part of a structure acting as a support. *Cerebellar p.* one of the collections of nerve fibres connecting the cerebellus with the MEDULLA oblongata.

PEEP positive end-expiratory pressure.

peer review (piə rə'vyoo) a basic component of a QUALITY ASSURANCE program in which the results of health and/or nursing care given to a specific patient population are evaluated according to defined criteria established by the peers of the professionals delivering the care. Peer review is focused on the patient and on the results of care given by a group of professionals rather than on individual professional practitioners.

Pel–Ebstein syndrome (pel'ebstien) *P.K. Pel, Dutch physician, 1852–1919; W. Ebstein, German physician, 1836–1912.* A recurrent pyrexia having a cycle of 15–21 days which occurs in cases of LYMPHADENOMA.

pellagra (pə'lagrə, -lay-) a syndrome caused by a diet seriously deficient in niacin (or by failure to convert tryptophan to niacin). Most persons with pellagra also suffer from deficiencies of vitamin B_2 (riboflavin) and other essential vitamins and minerals. The disease also occurs in persons suffering from alcoholism and drug addiction. Characterised by debility, digestive disorders, peripheral neuritis, ataxia, mental disturbance, and erythema with exfoliation of the skin.

pelvic ('pelvik) pertaining to the pelvis. *P. exenteration* removal of all the pelvic organs. *P. girdle* the ring of bone to which the lower limbs are jointed. It consists of the two hip bones and the sacrum and coccyx.

pelvimetry (pel'vimətree) measurement of the pelvis.

pelvirectal (ˌpelvi'rekt'l) pertaining to the flexure where the pelvic colon joins the rectum at an acute angle.

pelvis ('pelvəs) a basin-shaped cavity. *Bony p.* the pelvic girdle formed of the hip bones and the sacrum and coccyx. *Contracted p.* narrowing of the diameter of the pelvis. It can be of the true conjugate or the diagonal. Effective antenatal care recognises this condition and caesarean section might be necessary. *False p.* the part formed by the concavity of the iliac bones above the ileopectineal line. *Renal p.* the dilatation of the ureter which, by enclosing the hilus, surrounds the pyramids of the kidney substance. *True p.* the basin-like cavity below the false pelvis, its upper limit being the pelvic brim.

pemphigoid ('pemfəˌgoyd) 1. resembling pemphigus. 2. a bullous disease of the elderly with the blisters arising beneath the epidermis. The skin and the mucosa are affected, and, sometimes, the CONJUNCTIVA.

pemphigus ('pemfəgəs) a distinctive group of rare but serious diseases characterised by successive crops of large bullae ('water blisters'); the name is derived from the Greek word for blister, *pemphix*. Clusters of blisters usually appear first near the nose and mouth (sometimes inside them) and then gradually spread over the skin of the rest of the body. When the blisters burst, they leave round patches of raw and tender skin. Pemphigus is considered to be an autoimmune disorder.

pendulous ('pendyələs) hanging down. *P. abdomen* the hanging down of the abdomen over the pelvis, due to weakness and laxity of the abdominal muscles.

penicillamine (ˌpenə'siləˌmeen) a chelating agent that is used in heavy metal poisoning to aid excretion of the metal and in the treatment of HEPATOLENTICULAR degeneration (Wilson's disease). Also used in the treatment of severe rheumatoid arthritis.

penicillin (ˌpenə'silən) an antibiotic cultured from certain moulds of the genus *Penicillium*. The drug is used in various forms to treat a wide variety of bacterial infections. Discovered by Fleming in 1929, it was first used therapeutically in 1941. Varieties of the drug include: benethamine penicillin, benzylpenicillin, benzathine penicillin, procaine penicillin, cloxacillin, ampicillin, and amoxycillin.

penicillinase (ˌpenə'siləˌnayz) an enzyme that inactivates penicillin. Many bacteria, particularly staphylococci, produce this enzyme.

Penicillium (ˌpenə'sili·əm) a genus of mould-like fungi from some of which the penicillins are derived. Some species are pathogenic to humans.

penis ('peenəs) the male organ of copulation and urination.

pentagastrin (ˌpentə'gastrən) a synthetic hormone with a similar structure to gastrin. It has largely replaced histamine in gastric secretion tests because it has no apparent side-effects.

pentamidine (pen'tamədeen) an antiprotozoal drug used mainly in the treatment of *Pneumocystis carinii* infections.

pentazocine (pen'tazohˌseen) an

analgesic similar to morphine used in the treatment of moderate to severe pain.

pentose ('pentohz, -s) a monosaccharide containing five carbon atoms in a molecule.

pentosuria (ˌpentoh'syoo·ri·ə) a benign inborn error of metabolism due to a defect in the activity of the enzyme L-xylulose dehydrogenase resulting in pentose in the urine.

pepsin ('pepsən) an enzyme found in gastric juice. It partially digests proteins in an acid solution.

pepsinogen (pep'sinəjən) the precursor of pepsin, activated by hydrochloric acid.

peptic ('peptik) relating to pepsin or the action of the gastric juices in promoting digestion. *P. ulcer* an ulcer usually in the stomach or the duodenum caused by an excess of acid in the gastric juices.

peptide ('peptied) any of a class of compounds of low molecular weight which yield two or more amino acids on hydrolysis. Peptides form the constituent parts of proteins.

peptone ('peptohn) a substance produced by the action of pepsin on protein.

peptonuria (ˌpeptə'nyoo·ri·ə) presence of peptones in urine.

per os (pər os) [L.] *by the mouth.*

percept; perception ('pərsept; pə'sepshən) an awareness and understanding of an impression that has been presented to the senses. The mental process by which people perceive.

percussion (pə'kushən) a method of diagnosis by tapping with the fingers or with a light hammer upon any part of the body. Information can thus be gained as to the condition of underlying organs.

percutaneous (ˌpərkyoo'tayni·əs) through the skin, particularly in relation to ointments that are applied to unbroken skin.

perforation (ˌpərfə'rayshən) a hole or break in the containing walls or membranes of an organ or structure of the body. Perforation occurs when erosion, infection, or other factors create a weak spot in the organ and internal pressure causes a rupture. It can also result from a deep penetrating wound.

perfusion (pə'fyoozhən) the passage of liquid through a tissue or an organ, particularly the passage of blood through the lung tissue.

perianal (ˌperee'ayn'l) surrounding or located around the anus. *P. abscess* a small subcutaneous pocket of pus near the anal margin.

periarteritis (ˌpereeˌahtə'rietəs) inflammation of the outer coat and surrounding tissues of an artery.

periarthritis (ˌpereeah'thrietəs) inflammation of the tissues surrounding a joint.

pericardiectomy (ˌpereeˌkahdee'ektəmee) surgical removal of the pericardium; Used in the treatment of chronic constrictive pericarditis.

pericarditis (ˌpereekah'dietəs) inflammation of the pericardium. *Adhesive p.* the presence of adhesions between the two layers of pericardium owing to a thick fibrinous exudate. *Bacterial p.* inflammation of the pericardium due to bacterial infection. *Chronic constrictive p.* thickening and sometimes calcification of the pericardium which inhibits the action of the heart. *Rheumatic p.* pericarditis due to rheumatic fever.

pericardium (ˌperee'kahdi·əm) the

smooth membranous sac enveloping the heart, consisting of an outer fibrous and an inner serous coat. The sac contains a small amount of serous fluid.

perichondrium (ˌperee'kondri·əm) the membrane covering cartilaginous surfaces.

pericranium (ˌperee'krayni·əm) the periosteum of the cranial bones.

pericyazine (ˌperee'sieəˌzeen) a phenothiazine stronger than chlorpromazine; used in behavioural disturbances, schizophrenia, and related psychoses.

perilymph ('pereeˌlimf) the fluid that separates the bony and the membranous labyrinths of the ear.

perimeter (pə'rimətə) 1. the line marking the boundary of any area or geometrical figure; the circumference. 2. an instrument for measuring the field of vision.

perimetrium (ˌperee'meetri·əm) the peritoneal covering of the uterus.

perinatal (ˌperee'nayt'l) relating to the period shortly before and 7 days after birth. *P. mortality rate* the number of still births plus deaths of babies under 7 days old per 1000 total births in any one year.

perinatologist (ˌpereenay'toləjəst) a specialist in perinatology.

perinatology (ˌpereenay'toləjee) the branch of medicine (obstetrics and paediatrics) dealing with the fetus and infant during the perinatal period.

perineal (ˌperee'neeəl) relating to the perineum.

perineorrhaphy (ˌpereenee'o·rəfee) suture of the perineum to repair a laceration caused during childbirth.

perineum (ˌperee'neeəm) the tissues between the anus and external genitals. *Lacerated p.* a torn perineum (which can result from childbirth but is often forestalled by performing an episiotomy). Treatment is by perineorrhaphy.

periodic (ˌpiə·ree'odik) recurring at regular or irregular intervals. *P. apnoea of the newborn* occurring in the normal full-term infant, periodic episodes of rapid breathing followed by a brief period of apnoea which is associated with rapid eye movements. *P. syndrome* recurrent head, limb, or abdominal pains in children for which no organic cause can be found. It is often associated with migraine in adult life.

periodontitis (ˌperee·ədon'tietəs) inflammation of the periodontium.

periodontium (ˌperee·ə'donshi·əm) the connective tissue between the teeth and their bony sockets.

perioperative (ˌperee'opə·rətiv) pertaining or relating to the period immediately before or after an operation, as in perioperative care.

periosteal (ˌperee'osti·əl) pertaining to or composed of periosteum. *P. elevator* an instrument for separating the periosteum from the bone.

periosteum (ˌperee'osti·əm) the fibrous membrane covering the surface of bone. It consists of two layers, the inner or osteogenetic layer, which is closely adherent and forms new cells (by which the bone grows in girth), and, in close contact with it, the fibrous layer richly supplied with blood vessels.

periostitis (ˌpereeoh'stietəs) inflammation of the periosteum.

peripheral (pə'rifə·rəl) relating to the periphery. *P. iridectomy* excision of a small piece of iris from its peripheral edge. *P. nervous system* those parts of the nervous system lying outside the central nervous system. *P. neuritis* inflammation of terminal nerves. *P. resistance* the resistance in the walls of the arterioles, which is a major factor in the control of blood pressure. *P. vascular disease* an abnormal condition affecting blood vessels outside the heart causing pain or numbness, pallor, and elevated blood pressure

periphery (pə'rifə·ree) the outer surface or circumference.

peristalsis (ˌperee'stalsəs) a wavelike contraction preceded by a wave of dilatation which travels along the walls of a tubular organ, tending to press its contents onwards. It occurs in the muscle coat of the alimentary canal. *Reversed p.* a wave of contraction in the alimentary canal which passes *towards* the mouth. *Visible p.* a wave of contraction in the alimentary canal that is visible on the surface of the abdomen.

peritomy (pe'ritəmee) excision of a portion of the conjunctiva at the edge of the cornea, for the cure of PANNUS.

peritoneal (ˌperətə'neeəl) referring to the peritoneum. *P. cavity* the cavity between the parietal and the visceral peritoneum. *P. dialysis* a method of removing waste products from the blood by passing a cannula into the peritoneal cavity, running in a dialysing fluid, and after an interval, draining it off.

peritoneoscopy (ˌperətənee'oskəpee) visual examination of the peritoneum by means of a peritoneoscope.

peritoneum (ˌperətə'neeəm) the serous membrane lining the abdominal cavity and forming a covering for the abdominal organs. *Parietal p.* that which lines the abdominal cavity. *Visceral p.* the inner layer which closely covers the abdominal organs and includes the MESENTERIES.

peritonitis (ˌperətə'nietəs) inflammation of the peritoneum. *Acute p.* this can be produced by inflammation of abdominal organs, by irritating substances from a perforated gallbladder or gastric ulcer, by rupture of a cyst, or by irritation from blood, as in cases of internal bleeding. *Chronic p.* this is comparatively rare and is often associated with tuberculosis. Less frequently it can result from long-standing irritation caused by the presence in the abdomen of a foreign body, such as gunshot, or by chronic peritoneal dialysis.

peritonsillar (ˌperee'tonsələ) around the tonsil. *P. abscess* QUINSY.

perlèche (pər'lesh) inflammation with fissuring at the angles of the mouth; often due to vitamin B deficiency, poorly fitting dentures, or thrush infection.

permeability (ˌpərmi·ə'bilətee) the degree to which a fluid can pass from one structure through a wall or membrane to another.

pernicious (pə'nishəs) highly destructive; fatal. *P. anaemia* an anaemia due to lack of absorption of vitamin B_{12} that is required for the formation of red blood cells.

perniosis (ˌpərnee'ohsəs) a condition resulting from persistent exposure to cold which produces vascular spasm in the superficial arterioles of the hands and feet, causing thrombosis and necrosis. Perniosis includes chilblains and RAYNAUD'S PHENOMENON (disease).

per oral (pər'ro·rəl) by the mouth.

perphenazine (pərˈfenəˌzeen) an antiemetic and tranquillising drug similar to chlorpromazine. Used in the treatment of nausea and vomiting, and of SCHIZOPHRENIA and other psychoses.

perseveration (pərˌsevəˈrayshən) the constant recurrence of an idea or the tendency to keep repeating the same words or actions.

personality (ˌpərsəˈnalətee) the sum total of heredity and inborn tendencies with influences from environment and education which forms the mental make-up of a person and influences attitude to life. *Antisocial p.* a personality disorder in which repetitive antisocial behaviour is associated with ego eccentricity, lack of guilt or anxiety, and imperviousness to punishment. Called also sociopathic (psychopathic) personality. *Cyclothymic p.* a personality marked by alternate moods of elation and dejection. *Double p.*, *dual p.* multiple personality. *Multiple p.* a dissociative reaction in which an individual adopts two or more personalities alternatively, in none of which is there awareness of the experiences of the other(s). *Psychopathic p.* antisocial personality, sociopathic personality. *Schizoid p.* a personality disorder marked by timidness, self-consciousness, introversion, feelings of isolation and loneliness, and failure to form close interpersonal relationships; the individual is frequently ambitious, meticulous, and a perfectionist.

perspiration (ˌpərspəˈrayshən) sweat or the act of sweating. *Insensible p.* water evaporation from the moist surfaces of the body such as the respiratory tract and skin, that is not due to the activity of the sweat glands. It occurs at a constant rate of about 500 mL/day. When treating dehydration, this loss must be taken into account. *Sensible p.* sweat that is visible as droplets on the skin. Part of the mechanism for regulation of body temperature.

Perthes' disease (ˈpərtayz) *G.C. Perthes, German surgeon, 1869–1927.* Osteochondritis of the head of the femur. PSEUDOCOXALGIA (Legg–Calvé–Perthes disease).

pertussis (pəˈtusəs) whooping cough.

perversion (pəˈvərshən) morbid diversion from a normal course. *Sexual p.* abnormal sexual desires and behaviour. A deviation.

pes (payz, peez) the foot or any foot-like structure. *P. cavus* a foot with an abnormally high arch. Claw foot. *P. malleus valgus* hammer toe. *P. planus* flat foot.

pessary (ˈpesə·ree) 1. a plastic or metal ring-shaped device which is inserted in the vagina to support a prolapsed uterus. 2. a medicated suppository inserted into the vagina for antiseptic or contraceptive purposes.

petechia (pəˈteeki·ə) a small spot due to an effusion of blood under the skin, as in PURPURA.

pethidine (ˈpethəˌdeen, -in) a synthetic narcotic analgesic, less potent than morphine with quicker onset but shorter duration of action, used in obstetrics and preoperative and postoperative medication. Particularly useful, because it relaxes smooth muscle, in patients with ureteric and biliary colic and as an analgesic in patients with asthma.

petit mal (ˌpetee ˈmal) a mild form

of epilepsy common in children and characterised by a sudden and brief loss of consciousness.

pétrissage (paytri'sahzh) a kneading action used in massage.

petrositis (ˌpetroh'sietəs) inflammation of the petrous portion of the temporal bone, usually spread from a middle-ear infection.

petrous ('petrəs) resembling a stone. *P. bone* that part of the two temporal bones that forms the base of the skull and contains the middle and inner ear.

Peyer's glands or patches ('pieəz) *J.C. Peyer, Swiss anatomist, 1653–1712.* Small lymph nodules situated in the mucous membrane of the lower part of the small intestine.

Peyronie's disease ('payrəneez) induration of the corpora cavernosa of the penis, producing a fibrous CHORDEE leading to painful erection.

pH a measure of the hydrogen ion concentration, and so the acidity or alkalinity of a solution. Expressed numerically 1 to 14; 7 is neutral, below this is acid and above is alkaline. *See* HYDROGEN (ion concentration).

phacoemulsification (ˌfakoheeˌmulsəfə'kayshən) a technique of CATARACT extraction utilising high-frequency ultrasonic vibrations to fragment the lens nucleus combined with controlled irrigation to maintain normal pressure in the anterior chamber and suction to remove lens fragments and irrigating fluid.

phacoma (fə'kohmə) a congenital tumour of the lens of the eye.

phaeochromocytoma (ˌfeeohˌkrohmohsie'tohmə) a tumour of the adrenal medulla which gives rise to paroxysmal hypertension.

phage (fayj, fahzh) bacteriophage. A virus that lives on bacteria but is confined to a particular strain. *P.-typing* the identification of certain bacterial strains by determining the presence of strain-specific phages. Used in detecting the causative organisms of epidemics, especially food poisoning.

phagocyte ('fagəˌsiet) a blood cell that has the power of ingesting bacteria, protozoa, and foreign bodies in the blood.

phagocytosis (ˌfagəsie'tohsəs) the engulfing and destruction of microorganisms and foreign bodies by phagocytes in the blood.

phalanges (fə'lanjeez) the bones of the fingers or toes.

phallus ('faləs) the penis.

phantasy ('fantəsee) *see* FANTASY.

phantom ('fantəm) 1. an image or impression not evoked by actual stimuli. 2. a model of the body or of a specific part thereof. 3. a device for simulating the in vivo interaction of radiation with tissues. *P. pain* pain felt as if it were arising in an absent (amputated) limb. *P. pregnancy* see PSEUDOCYESIS. *P. tumour* a tumour-like swelling of the abdomen caused by contraction of the muscles or by localised gas.

pharmacogenetics (ˌfahməkohjə'netiks) the study of genetically determined variations in drug metabolism and the response of the individual.

pharmacology (ˌfahmə'koləjee) the science of the nature and preparation of drugs and particularly of their effects on the body.

pharmacopoeia (ˌfahməkə'pee·ə) an authoritative publication that gives the standard formulae and preparations of drugs used in a given country. *British P.* that authorised for use in the UK.

pharmacy ('fahməsee) 1. the art of preparing, compounding, and dispensing medicines. 2. the place where drugs are stored and dispensed.

pharyngeal (ˌfarən'jeeəl, fə'rinji·əl) relating to the pharynx. *P. pouch* dilatation of the lower part of the pharynx.

pharyngectomy (ˌfarən'jektəmee) excision of a section of the pharynx.

pharyngitis (ˌfarən'jietəs) inflammation of the pharynx.

pharyngolaryngeal (ˌfəˌring·goh-ˌlarən'jeeəl) referring to both the pharynx and larynx.

pharyngotympanic tube (fəˌring-·gohtim'panik) the tube that joins the middle ear to the pharynx; also called the Eustachian tube.

pharynx ('faringks) the muscular tube lined with mucous membrane situated at the back of the mouth. It leads into the oesophagus and also communicates with the nose through the posterior nares, with the ears through the pharyngotympanic (Eustachian) tubes, and with the larynx. *See* LARYNGOPHARYNX, NASOPHARYNX, and OROPHARYNX.

phenazocine (fe'nazohˌseen) an analgesic drug used to relieve severe pain. It is a drug of addiction.

phenelzine (fe'nelzeen) a monoamine oxidase inhibitor used in the treatment of depressive illness.

phenindione (ˌfenin'dieohn) an anticoagulant drug used in the treatment of deep vein thrombosis.

phenobarbitone (ˌfeenoh'bahbə-ˌtohn) a long-lasting barbiturate drug used to treat severe insomnia and also as an anticonvulsant drug in the treatment of epilepsy.

phenol ('feenol) carbolic acid. A disinfectant derived from coal tar.

phenolphthalein (ˌfeenəl'thaleen, -'thay-) a cathartic. Its use should be avoided because it can cause rashes, ALBUMINURIA, and HAEMOGLOBINURIA. Its laxative effects can continue for several days.

phenomenology (fəˌnomə'noləjee) a qualitative research approach that aims to describe experience as it is lived through, before it is conceptualised.

phenomenon (fə'nomənən) an objective sign or symptom. A noteworthy occurrence.

phenoperidine (ˌfeenoh'perədeen) synthetic narcotic analgesic used intraoperatively to supplement general anaesthesia. Also used in intensive care units to facilitate patients' acceptance of mechanical ventilation.

phenothiazine (ˌfeenoh'thieəzeen) one of a group of drugs used in the treatment of severe psychiatric disorders. The first to be used was chlorpromazine.

phenotype ('feenohˌtiep) the characteristics of an individual that are due to the environment and to genetic make-up.

phenoxybenzamine (feeˌnoksee-'benzəmeen) a vasodilator drug used in the treatment of peripheral conditions such as RAYNAUD'S DISEASE.

phenoxymethylpenicillin (feˌnoksee-ˌmethəlˌpenə'silən) a penicillinase-sensitive antibiotic similar in action to benzylpenicillin. Used mainly against streptococcal infections in children. It is taken orally. Pencillin V.

phentermine ('fentəˌmeen) an

appetite-suppressant drug used in the treatment of obesity.

phentolamine (fen'tolə,meen) a vasodilator used to reduce blood pressure in treating PHAEOCHROMOCYTOMA.

phenylalanine (,feenəl'aləneen) an essential amino acid which cannot be properly metabolised in persons suffering from PHENYLKETONURIA.

phenylbutazone (,feenəl'byootəzohn) an analgesic antipyretic drug used in the treatment of gout and rheumatic disorders.

phenylketonuria (,feenəl,keetə'nyoo·ri·ə) abbreviated PKU. A congenital disease due to a defect in the metabolism of the amino acid PHENYLALANINE. The condition is hereditary. It results from lack of an enyzme, phenylalanine hydroxylase, necessary for the conversion of phenylalanine into tyrosine. This causes an accumulation of phenylalanine in the blood with eventual excretion of phenylpyruvic acid in the urine. If untreated, the condition results in learning difficulties and other abnormalities. The condition can be detected soon after birth and screening of newborns for PKU entails a simple blood test. A sample of blood is taken from infants' heels at approximately 2 weeks and phenylalanine levels are assessed (Guthrie test). Treatment is with a diet low in phenylalanine.

phenylpyruvic acid (,feenəlpie'roovik) an abnormal constituent of the urine present in PHENYLKETONURIA.

phenytoin (,fenə'toh·ən) an anticonvulsant drug used in the treatment of major epileptic fits.

phimosis (fie'mohsəs) constriction of the prepuce so that it cannot be drawn back over the glans penis. The usual treatment is circumcision.

phlebectomy (flə'bektəmee) excision of a vein or a portion of a vein.

phlebitis (flə'bietəs) inflammation of a vein, usually in the leg, which tends to lead to the formation of a thrombus. The symptoms are pain, swelling, and redness along the course of the vein, which is later felt as a hard, tender cord.

phlebography (flə'bogrəfee) 1. Radiographic examination of a vein containing a contrast medium. 2. the graphic representation of the venous pulse.

phlebolith ('fleboh,lith) a stone formed in a vein by calcification of a blood clot.

phlebothrombosis (,flebohthrom'bohsəs) obstruction of a vein by a blood clot without local inflammation. It is usually in the deep veins of the calf of the leg causing tenderness and swelling. The clot can break away and cause an embolism.

Phlebotomus (flə'botəməs) a genus of sandflies, the various species of which transmit LEISHMANIASIS in its many forms and also SANDFLY fever.

phlebotomy (fli'botəmee) the puncture of a vein for the withdrawal of blood. Venesection.

phlegm (flem) mucus secreted by the lining of the air passages.

phlegmasia (fleg'mayzi·ə) an inflammation. *P. alba dolens* acute oedema in a leg due to lymphatic blockage. 'White leg'. Rarely occurs now but was seen most frequently in women after childbirth.

phlegmatic (fleg'matik) dull and apathetic.

phlycten ('fliktən) 1. a small blister caused by a burn. 2. a small vesicle containing lymph occurring in the conjunctiva or cornea of the eye. Often associated with tuberculosis.

phlyctenule ('fliktən,yool) a small vesicle on the conjunctiva or cornea.

phobia ('fohbi·ə) an irrational fear produced by a specific situation which the patient attempts to avoid.

phocomelia (,fohkə'meeli·ə) a rare congenital deformity in which the long bones of the limbs are minimal or absent and the individual has hands or feet resembling the flippers of seals, or stump-like limbs of various lengths. The drug thalidomide taken by the mother early in pregnancy has produced this deformity.

pholcodine ('folkoh,deen) a linctus for the suppression of a dry or painful cough.

phonation (foh'nayshən) the art of uttering meaningful vocal sounds.

phonocardiogram (,fohnoh'kahdeeə,gram) a record of the heart sounds made by a phonocardiograph.

phonocardiograph (,fohnoh'kahdeeə,grahf, -graf) an instrument that records graphically heart sounds and murmurs.

phonology (fə'noləjee) the study of speech sounds, their production and the relationship between sound as elements of language.

phosphatase ('fosfə,tayz) one of a group of enzymes involved in the metabolism of phosphate. *Alkaline p.* one formed by osteoblasts in the bones and by liver cells and excreted in the bile.

phosphate ('fosfayt) a salt or ester of phosphoric acid.

phosphaturia (,fosfə'tyoo·ri·ə) excess of phosphates in the urine.

phospholipid (,fosfə'lipəd) a lipid of glycerol fats found in cells, especially those of the nervous system.

phosphonecrosis (,fosfənə'krohsəs) necrosis, usually of the jaw bone, due to an excessive intake of phosphorus. An industrial disease occurring in workers engaged in the chemical industry.

phosphorus ('fosfə·rəs) *symbol* P. Phosphorus is an essential element in the diet. It is a major component of bone and is involved in almost all metabolic processes and also plays an important role in cell metabolism. It is obtained by the body from milk products, cereals, meat and fish. Its use by the body is controlled by vitamin D and calcium. Phosphorus is very inflammable and exceedingly poisonous. Inhalation of its vapour by workers in chemical industries can cause necrosis of the mandible (phosphonecrosis or phossy jaw). Free phosphorus causes fatty degeneration of the liver and other viscera.

phosphorylase (fos'fo·rə,layz) an enzyme found in the liver and kidneys which catalyses the breakdown of glycogen into glucose 1-phosphate.

photocoagulation (,fohtohkoh,agyə'layshən) the use of a powerful light source to induce inflammation of the retina and CHOROIDS to treat retinal detachment.

photophobia (,fohtoh'fohbi·ə) intolerance of light. It can occur in many eye conditions including conjunctivitis, corneal ulceration, IRITIS, and KERATITIS.

photophthalmia (,fohtof'thalmi·ə)

inflammation of the eye due to overexposure to bright light, especially to ultraviolet light.

photopic (foh'topik, -'toh-) pertaining to bright light. *P. vision* vision in bright light when the cones of the retina provide the visual appreciation of colour and shape.

photopsia (foh'topsi·ə) a sensation of flashes of light sometimes occurring in the early stages of retinal detachment.

photosensitivity (ˌfohtohˌsensə-'tivətee) an abnormal degree of sensitivity of the skin to sunlight.

phototherapy (ˌfohtoh'therəpee) treatment using fluorescent light containing a high output of blue light to reduce the amount of unconjugated BILIRUBIN in the skin of a mildly jaundiced neonate.

phrenemphraxis (ˌfrenem'fraksəs) an operation in which a phrenic nerve is crushed to paralyse one half of the diaphragm.

phrenic ('frenik) 1. relating to the mind. 2. pertaining to the diaphragm. *P. avulsion* the surgical extraction of a part of the phrenic nerve. *P. nerve* one of a pair of nerves controlling the muscles of the diaphragm.

phthalylsulphathiazole (ˌthaləl-ˌsulfə'thieəzohl) an insoluble sulphonamide, poorly absorbed in the intestine and so used to kill intestinal bacteria before surgery.

Phthirus pubis ('thirəs 'pyoobəs) the crab louse.

phthisis ('thisəs) pulmonary tuberculosis. *P. bulbi* a shrinking of the eyeball following inflammation or injury.

physical ('fisikəl) in medicine, relating to the body as opposed to the mental processes. *P. examination* examination of the bodily state of a patient by ordinary physical means, using inspection, palpation, percussion, and auscultation. *P. handicap* a term used when a physical disadvantage is due to impairment of physiological or anatomical structure of function. *P. medicine* the treatment and rehabilitation of patients with physical disabilities. It includes physiotherapy and manipulation. *P. signs* those observed by inspection, percussion, etc.

physician (fə'zishən) a medically qualified person who practises medicine as opposed to surgery.

physiological (ˌfizi·ə'lojikəl) relating to physiology. Normal, as opposed to pathological. *P. jaundice see* JAUNDICE. *P. solutions* those of the same salt composition and same osmotic pressure as blood plasma.

physiology (ˌfizee'oləjee) the science of the functioning of living organisms.

physiotherapy (ˌfizeeoh'therəpee) treatment and rehabilitation by natural forces, e.g. heat, light, electricity, massage, manipulation and remedial exercises.

physique (fə'zeek) the structure of the body.

physostigmine (ˌfiesoh'stigmeen) eserine, an alkaloid from the calabar bean. It is an antidote to curare; it constricts the pupils and is used with PILOCARPINE in the treatment of glaucoma.

phytomenadione (ˌfietohˌmenə-'dieohn) an intravenous preparation of vitamin K, effective in treating haemorrhage occurring during anticoagulant therapy.

pia mater (ˌpieə 'maytə) [L.] the innermost membrane enveloping the brain and spinal cord consisting of a network of small blood vessels connected by areolar tissue. This dips down into all the folds of the nerve substance.

pica ('piekə) an unnatural craving for strange foods and for things not fit to be eaten. It can occur in pregnancy and sometimes in children with learning disabilities.

Pick's disease (piks) *A. Pick, Czechoslovakian physician, 1851–1924.* A form of presenile brain failure (dementia) with an age of onset between 50 and 60 years. There is shrinkage of the brain and loss of cortical cells.

Pickwickian syndrome (pik'wiki·ən) (named after the fat boy 'Joe' in Pickwick Papers). A condition in which extreme obesity is associated with severe congestive cardiac failure.

picornavirus (pic'kawnə,vierəs) a family of small RNA-containing viruses including ECHOVIRUSES and RHINOVIRUSES.

PID pelvic inflammatory disease

pie chart ('pie ,chaht) a circular graph divided into sectors proportional to the magnitudes of the quantities represented.

pigeon breast ('pijən) a deformity in which the sternum is unduly prominent.

pigment ('pigmənt) colouring matter. *Bile p's* BILIRUBIN and BILIVERDIN. *Blood p.* haemoglobin. *Melanotic p.* MELANIN.

pigmentation (,pigmen'tayshən) the deposition in the tissues of an abnormal amount of pigment.

pile (piel) a HAEMORRHOID.

pill (pil) a rounded mass of one or more drugs, sometimes coated with sugar. Taken orally.

pilocarpine (,pieloh'kahpeen) an alkaloid prepared from jaborandi leaves. It is used to constrict the pupils in the treatment of GLAUCOMA.

pilomotor (,pieloh'mohtə) capable of moving the hair. *P. nerves* sympathetic nerves which control muscles in the skin connected with hair follicles. Stimulation causes the hair to be erected and also the condition of 'gooseflesh' of the skin.

pilonidal (,pielə'nied'l) having a growth of hair. *P. cyst* a congenital infolding of hair-bearing skin over the coccyx. It can become infected and lead to sinus formation.

pilot study ('pielət 'stuhdee) a small-scale version of a planned experiment or observation used to test the design of the larger study. A pilot study is helpful to see if any difficulties or problems arise in order that they can be clarified before embarking on the larger study, thus saving time and resources. A pilot study can also indicate possible extensions to the study or suggest restrictions of those aspects likely to be unhelpful.

pimple ('pimpəl) a small papule or pustule.

pineal ('pini·əl, 'pie-) shaped like a pine cone. *P. body* a small cone-shaped structure attached by a stalk to the posterior wall of the third ventricle of the brain and composed of glandular substance.

pinguecula (ping'gwekyələ) [L.] a small, benign, yellowish spot on the bulbar conjunctiva, seen usually in the elderly. Caused by degeneration of elastic tissue of conjunctiva.

pink disease (pink) ACRODYNIA.

pinkeye ('pingk,ie) acute contagious conjunctivitis.

pinna ('pinə) the projecting part of the external ear; the auricle.

pinta ('pintə) a non-venereal skin infection caused by *Treponema carateum* which is similar to the causative agent of syphilis. It is prevalent in the West Indies and Central America.

pinworm ('pin,wərm) a threadworm; *Enterobius vermiculasis*.

piperacillin (pie,perə'silən, pi-) a broad-spectrum semisynthetic penicillin active against a wide variety of Gram-negative, Gram-positive, and anaerobic bacteria.

piperazine (pie'perə,zeen, pi-) an anthelmintic drug used in the treatment of threadworms and roundworms.

pirenzepine (pi'renzə,peen) a drug which inhibits gastric acid secretion and promotes ulcer healing in the stomach.

piriform ('pirə,fawm) pear shaped. *P. fossa* one of a pair of depressions lying on either side of the opening into the larynx.

Piriton ('piriton) trade name for chlorpheniramine maleate; a preparation used for the relief of allergy and the emergency treatment of anaphylactic reactions.

piroxicam (pə'roksəkam) a non-steroidal anti-inflammatory drug used in the treatment of rheumatic diseases.

pituitary (pə'tyooətree) an endocrine gland suspended from the base of the brain and protected by the SELLA TURCICA in the sphenoid bone. It consists of two lobes: (a) the anterior, which secretes a number of different hormones including adrenocorticotrophic hormone (ACTH), GONADOTROPHIN, thyroid stimulating hormone (TSH), and prolactin; (b) the posterior, which secretes oxytocin and vasopressin.

pityriasis (,pitə'rieəsəs) a skin disease characterised by fine scaly desquamation. *P. alba* a condition common in children in which white scaly patches appear on the face. *P. capitis* dandruff. *P. rosea* an inflammatory form in which the affected areas are macular and ring shaped.

PKU phenylketonuria.

placebo (plə'seeboh) [L.] a substance given to a patient as medicine, or a procedure performed on a patient, that has no intrinsic therapeutic value and relieves symptoms or helps the patient in some way only because the patient believes or expects that it will. A placebo can be prescribed to satisfy a patient's psychological need for drug therapy and might also be given during controlled experiments. *P. effect* after the administration of a drug or treatment, a change (usually temporary) in a patient's physical or emotional condition following publicity or media interest in the drug or treatment. The placebo response is due more to the patient's expectations or to the expectations of the person giving the drug or treatment than to the result of any direct physiological or pharmacological substance response.

placenta (plə'sentə) the afterbirth. A vascular structure inside the pregnant uterus supplying the fetus with nourishment through the connecting umbilical cord. The placenta develops about the third month of pregnancy and is expelled after the birth of the child. *Battledore p.* one in which the cord is attached to the margin and not the centre. *P.*

praevia one attached to the lower part of the uterine wall. It can cause severe antepartum haemorrhage.

Placido's disc ('plasidohz) *A. Placido, Portuguese ophthalmologist 1848–1916.* A disc marked with black and white circles used in the diagnosis of corneal distortion.

plagiocephaly (ˌplayjeeoh'kefəlee, -'sef-) asymmetry of the head resulting from the irregular closing of the sutures.

plague (playg) an acute, febrile, infectious, highly fatal disease caused by the bacillus *Yersinia pestis*. It is a notifiable disease. Transmitted to humans by the bites of fleas that have derived the infection from diseased rats. *Bubonic p.* type in which the lymph glands are infected and buboes form in the groins and armpits. Known in mediaeval times as the 'Black Death'. *Pneumonic p.* type in which the infection attacks chiefly the lung tissues. A fatal form. *Septicaemic p.* a very severe and fatal form when the infection enters the bloodstream.

plantar (ˌplantə) relating to the sole of the foot. *P. arch* the arch made by anastomosis of the plantar arteries. *P. flexion* bending of the toes downwards and so arching the foot. *P. reflex* contraction of the toes on stroking the sole of the foot. *P. wart* a common WART located on the sole of the foot. Plantar warts are epidermal tumours caused by a virus which can be picked up by going barefoot. Called also VERRUCA plantaris.

plaque (plak; plahk) 1. a flat patch on the skin. 2. a deposit of food and bacteria on the enamel of teeth which can produce tartar and CARIES.

plasma ('plazmə) the fluid portion of the blood in which cells are suspended. Plasma is to be distinguished from serum which is plasma from which the FIBRINOGEN has been separated in the process of clotting. *P. proteins* those present in the blood plasma: albumin, globulin, and fibrinogen. *Reconstituted p.* dried plasma when again made liquid by addition of distilled water. *P. volume expander* a solution transfused instead of blood to increase the volume of fluid circulating in the blood vessels. Called also artificial plasma extender.

plasmapheresis (ˌplazməfə'reesəs) a method of removing a portion of the plasma from circulation. Venesection is performed, the blood is allowed to settle, the plasma is removed, and the red blood cells are returned to the circulation. Used in the treatment of those diseases caused by antibodies circulating in the patient's plasma.

plasmin ('plazmən) a FIBRINOLYSIS found in blood plasma which can dissolve fibrin clots.

plasminogen (plaz'minəjən) the inactive precursor of plasmin.

Plasmodium (plaz'mohdi·əm) a genus of protozoan parasites in the red blood cells of animals and humans. Four species, *P. falciparum*, *P. malariae*, *P. ovale*, and *P. vivax*, cause the four specific types of human malaria.

plaster ('plahstə, 'plasta) 1. a mixture of materials that hardens; used for immobilising or making impressions of body parts. 2. an adhesive substance spread on fabric or other suitable backing material for application to the skin. *Bohler's p.*

plaster for POTT'S FRACTURE. A leg splint of plaster of Paris in which is embedded an iron stirrup extending below the foot which enables the patient to walk without putting weight on the joint. *Corn p.* an adhesive strip or patch impregnated with salicyclic acid and applied to corns on the feet. *Frog p.* a plaster of Paris splint used to maintain the position after correction of the deformity due to congenital dislocation of the hip. *P. of Paris* calcium sulphate or gypsum which sets hard when water is added to it and is used to form a plaster cast to immobilise a part, and in dentistry for taking dental impressions.

plastic ('plastik) 1. constructive; tissue forming. 2. capable of being moulded; pliable. *P. lymph* the exudate which, in wounds and inflamed serous tissues, is organised into fibrous tissue and promotes healing. *P. surgery* the branch of surgery that deals with the repair and reconstruction of deformed or injured parts of the body, including their replacement, by tissue grafting or other means.

platelet ('playtlət) a disc-shaped structure present in the blood and concerned in the process of clotting. A THROMBOCYTE.

play (play) an occupation for either children or adults which is voluntary and can be a spontaneous or an organised activity providing enjoyment, entertainment, amusement, or diversion.

pleoptics (plee'optiks) an orthoptic method of improving the sight in cases of STRABISMUS by stimulating the use of the macular part of the retina.

plethora ('plethə·rə) a general term denoting a red, florid complexion or, specifically, an excessive amount of blood.

plethysmography (ˌplethiz'mografee) the measurement of changes in the volume of a limb due to alterations in blood pressure using an oncometer.

pleura ('ploo·rə) the serous membrane lining the thorax and enveloping each lung. *Parietal p.* the layer that lines the chest wall. *Visceral p.* the inner layer which is in close contact with the lung.

pleurisy; pleuritis ('ploo·rəsee; ploo'rietəs) inflammation of the pleura; it can be caused by infection, injury, or tumour. It can be a complication of lung diseases, particularly of pneumonia, or sometimes of tuberculosis, lung abscess, or influenza. The symptoms are cough, fever, chills, a sharp, sticking pain that is worse on inspiration, and rapid shallow breathing. *Dry* (fibrinous) *p.* pleurisy in which the membrane is inflamed and roughened, but no fluid is formed. *P. with effusion* (wet p). type that is characterised by inflammation and exudation of serous fluid into the pleural cavity. *Purulent p.* or *empyema* the formation of pus in the pleural cavity. An operation for drainage is usually necessary.

pleurocele ('ploo·rəˌseel) hernia of the lung or pleura.

peurodynia (ˌploo·rə'dini·ə) pain in the intercostal muscles, probably rheumatic in origin.

plexus ('pleksəs) a network of veins or nerves. *Auerbach's p.* the nerve ganglion situated between the longitudinal and circular muscle fibres of the intestine. They are motor nerves. *Brachial p.* the network of nerves of the neck and axilla. *Choroid p.* a capillary network situated in the ventricles of the brain which forms the cerebrospinal fluid. *Meissner's p.* the sensory nerve ganglion situated in the submucous layer of the intestinal wall. *Rectal p.* the network of veins which surrounds the rectum and forms a direct communication between the systemic and portal circulations. *Solar* or *coeliac p.* the network of nerves and ganglia at the back of the stomach which supply the abdominal viscera.

plication (plie'kayshən) the taking of tucks in a structure to shorten it; a folding to decrease the size of a structure or organ during a surgical procedure.

plumbism ('plumbizəm) lead poisoning.

Plummer–Vinson syndrome (ˌplum-ə'vinsən) difficulty in swallowing associated with GLOSSITIS and iron-deficiency anaemia.

pneumatocele (nyoo'matəˌseel) 1. a swelling containing a collection of gas. 2. hernia of the lung.

pneumaturia (ˌnyoomə'tyoo·ri·ə) the passing of flatus with the urine owing to a vesico-intestinal fistula and air from the bowel entering the bladder.

pneumocephalus (ˌnyoomoh-'kefələs, -'sef-) the presence of air in the ventricles of the brain caused usually by an anterior fracture of the base of the skull.

pneumococcus (ˌnyoomoh'kokəs) the causative agent of lobar and bronchopneumonia and of other bronchial diseases. A Gram-positive, ovoid diplococcus, *Streptococcus pneumoniae*.

pneumoconiosis (ˌnyoomoh-ˌkohnee'ohsəs) an industrial disease of the lung due to inhalation of dust particles over a period of time. *See* ANTHRACOSIS, ASBESTOSIS, and SILICOSIS.

Pneumocystis (ˌnyoomooh'sistəs) a genus of microorganisms of uncertain status but usually considered to be protozoans. *P. carinii* the causative organism of interstitial plasma cell pneumonia, particularly in immunosuppressed patients, people with HIV infection or small children.

pneumodynamics (ˌnyoomohdie-'namiks) the mechanics of respiration.

pneumoencephalography (ˌnyoo-moh·enˌkefə'logrəfee, ˌsef-) *see* ENCEPHALOGRAPHY.

pneumogastric (ˌnyoomoh'gastrik) pertaining to lungs and stomach. *P. nerve* the 10th cranial nerve to the lungs, stomach, etc. The VAGUS nerve.

pneumolysis (nyoo'moləsəs) the operation of detaching the pleura from the chest wall in order to collapse the lung when the two pleural layers are adherent. Pleurolysis.

pneumomycosis (ˌnyoomohmie-'kohsəs) infection of the lung by microfungi. *See* BRONCHOMYCOSIS.

pneumonectomy (ˌnyoomə'nek-təmee) partial or total removal of a lung.

pneumonia (nyoo'mohni·ə) inflammation of the lung with consolidation and exudation. *Aspiration p.* an acute condition caused by the aspiration of infected material into the lungs. *Broncho-p.* a descending infection starting around the bronchi and bronchioles. *Hypostatic p.* a form which occurs in weak, bedridden patients. *Lobar p.* an acute infectious disease caused by a pneumococcus and affecting whole lobes of either or both lungs. *Virus p.* inflammation of the lung occurring during some virus disease and secondary to it.

pneumonitis (ˌnyoomə'nietəs) an imprecise term denoting any inflammatory condition of the lung.

pneumoperitoneum (ˌnyoomoh-ˌperətə'neeəm) the presence of air or gas in the peritoneal cavity, occurring pathologically or introduced intentionally for diagnostic or therapeutic purposes.

pneumoradiography (ˌnyoomoh-ˌraydee'ogrəfee) radiographic examination of a cavity or part after air or a gas has been injected into it.

pneumotaxic (ˌnyoomoh'taksik) regulating the rate of respiration. *P. centre* the centre in the pons that influences inspiratory effort during respiration.

pneumothorax (ˌnyoomoh'thor-·raks) accumulation of air or gas in the pleural cavity, resulting in collapse of the lung on the affected side. The condition can occur spontaneously, as in the course of a pulmonary disease, or it can follow trauma to and perforation of the chest wall. *Artificial p.* a surgical procedure sometimes used in the treatment of tuberculosis or after PNEUMONECTOMY. *Spontaneous p.* sometimes occurs when there is an opening on the surface of the lung allowing leakage of air from the bronchi into the pleural cavity. *Tension p.* is a particularly dangerous form of pneumothorax that occurs when air escapes into the pleural cavity from a bronchus but cannot regain entry into the bronchus. As a result, continuously increasing air pressure in the pleural cavity causes progressive collapse of the lung tissue.

podagra (pə'dagrə) gout, particularly of the big toe.

podalic (pə'dalik) relating to the feet. *P. version* a method of changing the lie of a fetus so that its feet will present.

podarthritis (ˌpodah'thrietəs) inflammation of any of the joints of the foot.

pointillage (ˌpwanhti'lahzh) [Fr.] a method of massage using the tips of the fingers.

poison ('poyzən) any substance which, applied to the body externally or taken internally, can cause injury to any part or cause death.

poisoning ('poyzəning) the morbid condition produced by a poison. The poison might be swallowed, inhaled (*see* CARBON MONOXIDE), injected by a stinging insect as in a BEE STING, or spilled or otherwise brought into contact with the skin.

polioencephalitis (ˌpohleeoh·en-ˌkefə'lietəs, -ˌsef-) acute inflammation of the cortex of the brain.

poliomyelitis (ˌpohleeohˌmieə'lietəs) an acute, notifiable, infectious viral disease that attacks the central nervous system, injuring or destroying the nerve cells that control the muscles and sometimes causing paralysis; called also polio, infantile paralysis and HEINE–MEDIN DISEASE. Paralysis most often affects the limbs but can involve any muscles including those that control breathing and swallowing. Since the development and the use of vaccines against poliomyelitis, the disease has been virtually eliminated in developed, wealthy countries, where vaccination rates are high, but is still common in many other parts of the world.

poliovirus (ˌpohleeoh'vierəs) a small RNA-containing virus which causes poliomyelitis.

pollinosis (ˌpolə'nohsəs) hay fever; an allergy caused by various kinds of pollen. Pollenosis.

pollution (pə'looshən) the act of destroying the purity of or contaminating something.

polyarteritis (ˌpoleeˌahtə'rietəs) inflammatory changes in the walls of the small arteries.

polyarthralgia (ˌpoleeah'thralji·ə) pain in several joints.

polyarthritis (ˌpoleeah'thrietəs) inflammation of several joints at the same time, as seen in rheumatoid arthritis.

polycoria (ˌpolee'kor·ri·ə) a congenital abnormality in which there are one or more holes in the iris in addition to the pupil.

polycystic (ˌpolee'sistik) containing many cysts. *P. ovary disease* Stein–Leventhal syndrome. *P. renal disease* a hereditary disease in which there is massive enlargement of the kidney with the formation of many cysts. Severe bleeding into cysts can occur. End-stage renal disease can affect many members of one family.

polycythaemia (ˌpoleesie'theemi·ə) an abnormal increase in the number of red cells in the blood. Erythrocythaemia. *P. vera* a rare disease in which there is a greatly increased production of red blood cells and also of leukocytes and platelets. The skin becomes flushed, with cyanosis, thrombosis, and SPLENOMEGALY.

polydactylism (ˌpolee'daktəˌlizəm) the condition of having more than the normal number of fingers or toes.

polydipsia (ˌpoli'dipsi·ə) abnormal thirst. It can be a symptom of diabetes.

polymorphonuclear (ˌpoleeˌmawfoh'nyookli·ə) 1. having nuclei of many different shapes. 2. a polymorphonuclear leukocyte.

polymorphous (ˌpolee'mawfəs) occurring in several or many different forms.

polymyalgia rheumatica (ˌpoleemieˌalji·ə roo'matikə) persistent aching pain in the muscles, often involving the shoulder or the pelvic girdle.

polymyositis (ˌpoleeˌmieoh'sietəs) a generalised inflammation of the muscles with weakness and joint stiffness, particularly around the hips and shoulders.

polymyxin (ˌpolee'miksən) an antibiotic drug used in the treatment of Gram-negative bacteria, particularly *Pseudomonas*.

polyneuritis (ˌpoleenyə'rietəs) inflammation of many nerves at the same time.

polyneuropathy (ˌpoleenyə'ropəthee) a number of disease conditions of the nervous system.

polyopia (ˌpolee'ohpi·ə) the perception of two or more images of the same object. Multiple vision.

polyp ('polip) a pedunculated tumour of mucous membrane. A polypus.

polypharmacy (ˌpolee'fahməsee) 1. the administration of many drugs together. This increases the likelihood of side-effects from drug interactions and of noncompliance by the patient. 2. the administration of excessive medication.

polyposis (ˌpolə'pohsəs) the presence of many polyps in an organ. *Familial p.* an hereditary condition in which large numbers of polyps develop in the colon which can become malignant.

polyuria (ˌpolee'yoo·ri·ə) an abnormally large output of urine due either to an excessive intake of liquid or to disease, often diabetes.

pompholyx ('pomfəliks) an intensely pruritic skin condition in which vesicles appear on the hands and feet, particularly on the palms and soles. Typically occurring in repeated, self-limiting attacks.

pons (ponz) a bridge of tissue connecting two parts of an organ. *P. varolii* the part of the brain that connects the cerebrum, cerebellum, and MEDULLA oblongata.

Pontiac fever ('pontee͵ak) an influenza-like illness with little or no pulmonary involvement, caused by *Legionella pneumophila*. It is not life-threatening (unlike the pulmonary form known as legionnaires' disease). The name Pontiac fever comes from an outbreak of the disease in Pontiac, Michigan, USA.

popliteal (ˌpoplə'teeəl, pop'liti·əl) relating to the posterior part of the knee joint.

popliteus (ˌpoplə'teeəs, pop'liti·əs) the flat triangular muscle at the back of the knee joint.

population (ˌpopyə'layshən) 1. the total number of persons inhabiting a given geographical area or location. 2. in statistics, the aggregate of individuals or items from which a sample for a study is drawn. 3. any group that is distinguished by a particular trait or situation.

pore (por) a minute circular opening on a surface. *Sweat p.* an opening of a sweat gland on the skin surface.

porphyria (paw'firi·ə) an inborn error in the metabolism of porphyrins, resulting in PORPHYRINURIA. Two general types of porphyria are known: erythropoietic porphyrias which are concerned with the formation of erythrocytes in the bone marrow, and hepatic porphyrias which are responsible for liver dysfunction. The manifestations of porphyria include gastrointestinal, neurological, and psychological symptoms, cutaneous photosensitivity, pigmentation of the face (and later of the bones), and anaemia. with enlargement of the spleen.

porphyrin ('pawfərən) one of a number of pigments used in the production of the haem portion of haemoglobin.

porphyrinuria (ˌpawfərə'nyoo·ri·ə) the presence of an excess of porphyrin in the urine.

porta ('pawtə) an opening in an organ through which pass the main vessels.

Portacath ('pawtə͵kath) a catheter to provide a central venous line; attached to it is an injectable depot which is placed under the skin.

portacaval (ˌpawtə'kayvəl) pertaining to the portal vein and the inferior vena cava. *P. anastomosis* the joining of the portal vein to the inferior VENA CAVA so that much of the blood bypasses the liver. It is used in the treatment of portal hypertension.

Portage system ('pawtij ͵sistəm) a method of behaviour modification taught to family members to enable them to assist their handicapped child in development and acquiring skills for everyday living.

portal hypertension ('pawt'l ˌhiepə'tenshən) increased venous pressure in the portal system caused by compression of the portal or hepatic vascular system.

portal of entry the route by which infection enters the body.

position (pə'zishən) attitude of posture. *Dorsal p.* lying flat on the back. *Genupectoral* or *knee-chest p.* resting on the knees and chest with arms crossed above the head. *Lithotomy p.* lying on the back with thighs raised and knees supported and held widely apart. *Prone p.* face down. *Sims' p.* or *semiprone p.* lying on the left side with the right knee well flexed and the left arm drawn back over the edge of the bed. *Trendelenburg p.* lying down on a tilted plane (usually an operating table at an angle of 30–45 degrees to the floor), with the head lowermost, the shoulders supported and the legs hanging over the raised end of the table. (*See* figure).

positive ('pozətiv) having a value greater than zero; indicating existence or presence, as chromatin positive or Wassermann positive; characterised by affirmation or cooperation.

positive end-expiratory pressure abbreviated PEEP. In mechanical ventilation, a positive airway pressure maintained until the end of expiration. A PEEP higher than the critical closing pressure holds alveoli open until the end of expiration and can markedly improve the arterial $P0_2$ in patients with a lowered functional residual capacity (FRC), as in acute respiratory failure.

posseting ('posəting) regurgitation of a small amount of milk by an infant immediately after a feed.

Possum ('posəm) Patient-Operated Selector Mechanism; a machine that can be operated with a very slight degree of pressure or suction, using the mouth if no other muscle movement is possible. It can transmit messages from a light panel or be adapted for typing, telephoning, or working certain machinery.

postconcussional syndrome (ˌpohstkən'kushən'l) constant headaches with mental fatigue, difficulty in concentration, and insomnia that can persist after head injury.

posterior (po'stiə·ri·ə) behind a part. Dorsal. *P. chamber* that part of the aqueous chamber that lies behind the iris but in front of the lens.

posteroanterior (ˌpostə·roh·an'tie·ri·ə) from the back to the front.

postganglionic (ˌpohstgang·glee'onik) situated posterior or distal to a ganglion. *P. fibre* a nerve fibre posterior to a ganglion of the autonomic nervous system.

postgastrectomy syndrome (ˌpohstga'strektəmee) *see* DUMPING.

posthitis (pos'thietəs) inflammation of the prepuce.

posthumous ('postyəməs) occurring after death. *P. birth* one occurring after the death of the father, or by caesarean section after the death of the mother.

postmature (pohstmə'tyooə) a state in which the pregnancy is prolonged after the expected date of delivery. Because of the many variables, it is difficult to estimate, but might be said to exist when a pregnancy has lasted 41–42 weeks from the last menstrual period. There is

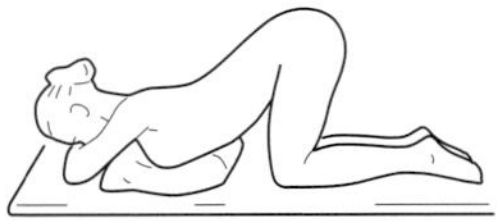

Genupectoral

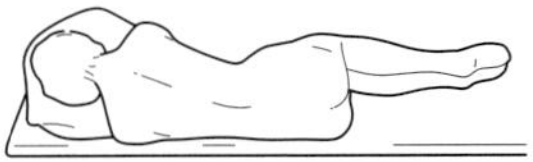

Left lateral

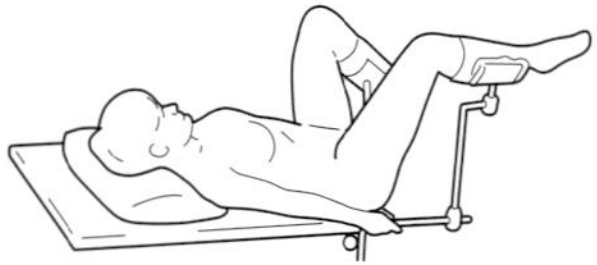

Lithotomy

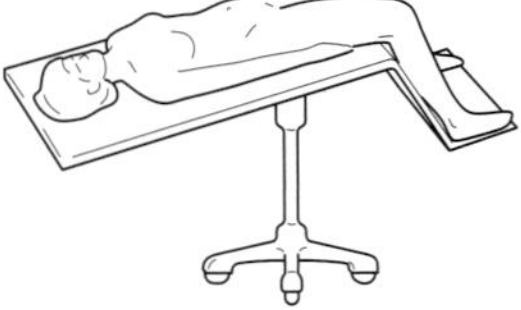

Trendelenburg

Gynaecological Positions

a danger of hypoxia to the fetus.

postmortem (pohst'mawtəm) after death. *P. examination* autopsy.

postnatal (pohst'nayt'l) after childbirth. *P. care* includes the care of the mother for at least 6 weeks after delivery. *P. clinic* an examination centre where the patient can be examined (postnatally), preferably 6 weeks after childbirth regarding: (a) her general health; and (b) the state of the uterus, pelvic floor, and vagina. *P. depression* a low mood after the birth of a baby; can be severe and incapacitating.

postpartum (pohst'pahtəm) occurring after labour.

postprandial (pohst'prandi·əl) occurring after a meal.

post-traumatic stress disorder (pohst traw'matik stres dis'awdə) psychiatric disorder following the experience of, or witnessing of, life-threatening events. The condition is characterised by sleep disturbances and flashbacks.

postural ('postyərəl) relating to a position or posture. *P. drainage* drainage of secretions from specific lobes or segments of the lung, aided by careful positioning of the patient.

potassium (pə'tasi·əm) *symbol* K. A metallic alkaline element which is a constituent of all plants and animals. Its salts are widely used in medicine. *P. chloride* a compound used orally or intravenously as an electrolyte replenisher. *P. citrate* a diuretic, expectorant, and systemic alkaliser. *P. gluconate* an electrolyte replenisher used in the prophylaxis and treatment of HYPOKALAEMIA. *P. iodide* an expectorant and antithyroid agent. *P. permanganate* a topical anti-infective, oxidising agent, and antidote for many poisons. *P. sodium tartrate* a compound used as a saline cathartic and also in combination with sodium bicarbonate and tartaric acid.

Pott's disease (pots) *P. Pott, British surgeon, 1714–88.* Tuberculosis of the spine.

Pott's fracture a fracture-dislocation of the ankle, involving fracture of the lower end of the tibia, displacement of the talus and, sometimes, fracture of the medial MALLEOLUS.

pouch (powch) a pocket-like space or cavity. *P. of Douglas*, the lowest fold of the peritoneum between the uterus and rectum. *Morison's p.* a fold of peritoneum below the liver.

poultice ('pohltəs) a soft, moist mass about the consistency of cooked cereal, spread between layers of muslin, linen, gauze, or towels and applied hot to a given area in order to create moist local heat or counter irritation.

Poupart's ligament ('poopahts) *F. Poupart, French anatomist, 1616–1708.* The inguinal ligament. The tendinous lower border of the external oblique muscle of the abdominal wall which passes from the anterior spine of the ilium to the os pubis.

Povidone-iodine (ˌpohvədohn-'ieəˌdeen) a complex of iodine with the polymer povidone; used as a topical anti-infective and in pre-operative skin preparation.

PPS pelvic pain syndrome.

practolol ('praktəˌlol) a drug used in the treatment of TACHYCARDIA and irregular heart rhythms. It is a beta-blocker and can be given only by injection.

precancerous (pree'kansə·rəs) applied to conditions or histological changes that can precede cancer.

preceptor (prə'septə) 1. a teacher, an instructor. 2. a registered nurse who provides newly registered practitioners with support and guidance in making the transition from student to registered practitioner.

precipitate (prə'sipəˌtayt) a deposit of solid matter which was previously in solution.

precipitate labour unusually rapid labour with extremely quick delivery. There is danger to the mother of severe perineal lacerations, and to the child of intracranial trauma as a result of the rapid passage through the birth canal.

precipitin (prə'sipətən) an antibody present in the blood which when mixed in solution with its antigen forms a precipitate.

precocious (prə'kohshəs) developed in advance of the norm, either mentally or physically or both.

precognition (ˌpreekog'nishən) a direct perception of a future event which is beyond the reach of inference.

precordium (pree'kawdi·əm) the area lying over the heart.

prediabetes (preeˌdie·ə'beetis, -teez) a state which precedes DIABETES mellitus in which the disease is not yet clinically manifest. In pregnancy, the diabetes might become evident or the patient might remain well but give birth to an unusually large child. Screening by urine testing can detect the condition.

predigestion (ˌpreedie'jeschən, -di-) partial digestion of food by artificial means before it is taken into the body.

predisposition (ˌpreedispəˈzishən) susceptibility to a specific disease.

prednisolone (predˈnisəlohn) a synthetic corticosteroid used in the treatment of inflammatory and rheumatic conditions, and of asthma and allergic skin diseases.

prednisone (ˈprednəˌsohn) a synthetic drug with an action and usage similar to prednisolone.

pre-eclampsia (ˌpree·əˈklampsi·ə) a condition occurring in late pregnancy. The signs include PROTEINURIA, hypertension, and oedema.

pregnancy (ˈpregnənsee) being with child; the condition from conception to the expulsion of the fetus. The normal period is 280 days or 40 weeks. *Ectopic* or *extrauterine p.* pregnancy occurring outside the uterus, in the uterine tube (tubal p.) or, very rarely, in the abdominal cavity. *P. tests* tests used to demonstrate whether conception has occurred. These detect the human chorionic gonadotrophin (HCG) produced by the embryo 8 days after the first missed period. Immunological laboratory tests are more accurate and less likely to give a false positive result than an over-the-counter kit.

premature (ˌpreməˈtyooə) occurring before the anticipated time. *P. contraction* a form of cardiac irregularity in which the ventricle contracts before its anticipated time. *See* SYSTOLE. *P. ejaculation* emission of semen before or at the beginning of sexual intercourse. *P. infant* a child weighing 2500 g or less at birth. *See also* PRETERM INFANT.

premedication (ˌpreemedəˈkayshən) drugs given preoperatively in order to reduce fear and anxiety and to facilitate the induction and maintenance of and recovery from anaesthesia.

premenstrual (preeˈmenstrooəl) preceding menstruation. *P. endometrium* the hypertrophied and vascular mucous lining of the uterus immediately before the menstrual flow starts. *P. tension* feelings of nervousness, depression, and irritability experienced by some women in the days before their menstrual periods. Emotional and physical symptoms usually disappear with the onset of menstruation.

premolar (preeˈmohlə) a bicuspid tooth in front of the molars on each side of the upper and lower jaws.

prenatal (preeˈnayt'l) preceding birth; antenatal. *P. care* care of the pregnant woman before delivery of the infant.

prepuce (ˈpreepyoos) foreskin; the loose fold of skin covering the GLANS PENIS.

presbycusis (ˌpresbəˈkyoosəs) progressive bilateral deafness in old age.

presbyopia (ˌpresbeeˈohpi·ə) diminution of accommodation of the lens of the eye due to a loss of elasticity, occurring normally with ageing and usually resulting in hyperopia, or farsightedness.

prescription (prəˈskripshən) a formula written by a medically qualified doctor, directing the pharmacist to supply the medication.

presenile (preeˈseeniel) prematurely aged in mind and body. *See* DEMENTIA.

presentation (ˌprezənˈtayshən) in obstetrics, that portion of the fetus that appears in the centre of the neck of the uterus (*see* figure on p. 350).

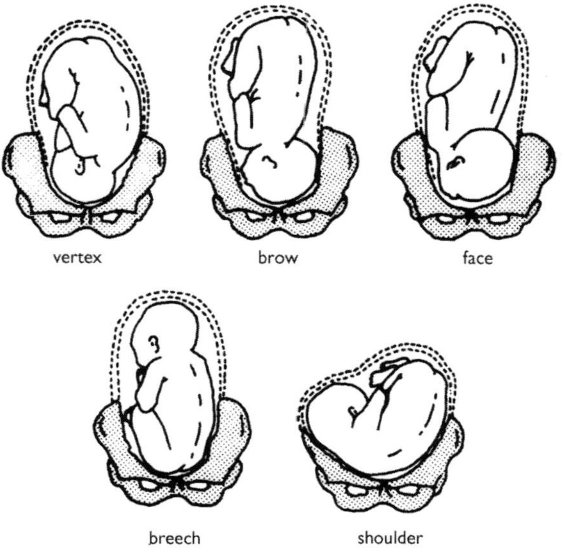

Fetal Presentation

pressor ('presə) a substance that can cause a rise in the blood pressure.

pressure ('preshə) stress or strain. The force exerted by one object upon another. *P. areas* areas of the body where the tissues might be compressed between the bed and the underlying bone, especially the sacrum, greater trochanters, and heels (*see* figure); the tissues become ischaemic. *P. point* the point at which an artery can be compressed against a bone in order to stop bleeding (*see* figure on page 352). *P. sore* a decubitus ulcer; a bedsore. Ulceration of the skin due to pressure which causes interference with the blood supply to the area.

presystole (pree'sistəlee) the period in the cardiac cycle just before systole.

preterm infant ('preetərm) one with a gestational age of less than 37 weeks.

priapism ('prieə,pizəm) persistent erection of the penis, usually without sexual desire. It can be caused by local or spinal cord injury.

prickle cell ('prikəl) a cell from the

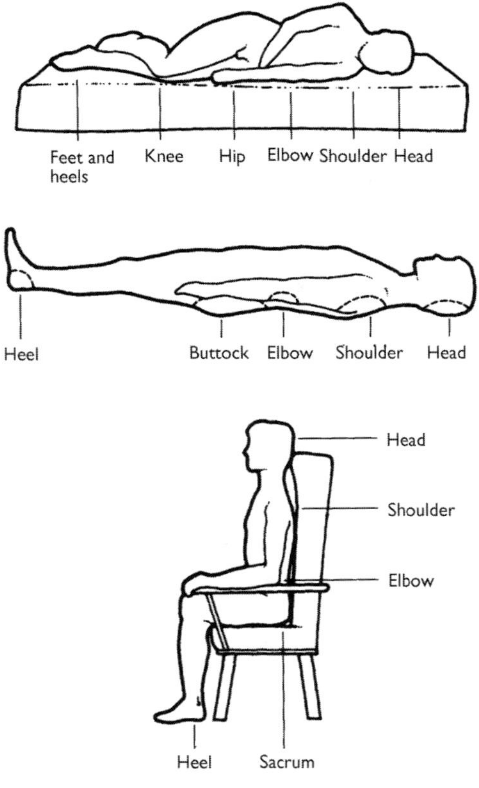

Pressure Areas

inner layer of the epidermis possessing delicate rod-shaped processes by which it is connected to other cells. *P. c. layer* the layer of the epidermis immediately above the basal cell layer.

prickly heat ('priklee) MILIARIA; heat rash. A skin eruption characterised

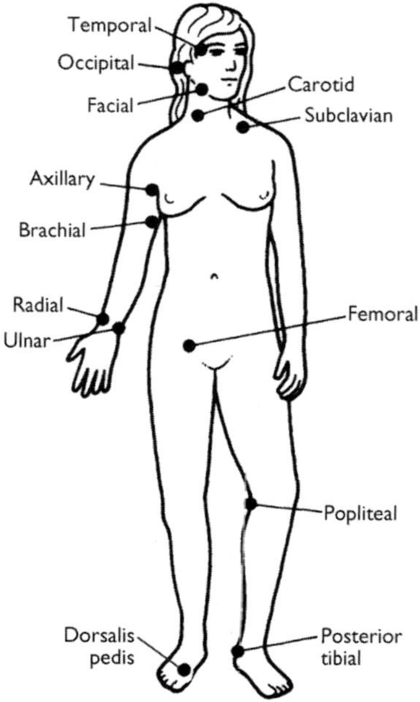

Arterial Pressure Points

by minute red spots with central vesicles.

primaquine ('primə,kween) a drug used in the treatment of benign tertian malaria after initial treatment with other antimalarial drugs.

primary care (,priemәree 'kair) the level of care in the HEALTHCARE SYSTEM that consists of initial care outside institutions. *P. health care* the care given to individuals in the community at the first point of contact with the primary healthcare team. First contact might be the general practitioner, a health visitor, or a community nurse. *P. healthcare team* usually made up of a general practitioner, community nurse, health visitors and, possibly, paramedical staff such as a physiotherapist. They might serve a geographical area and be based in a health centre or a general practice area.

primary nurse (ˌpriemәree 'nәrs) a nurse who is responsible for the planning, implementation, and evaluation of nursing care for assigned patients and their families for the duration of the patients' stays in hospital. The primary nurse delegates to an associate nurse when off duty but the primary nurse remains responsible and accountable for the patient's nursing care.

primary nursing (ˌpriemәree 'nәrsing) Manthey (1980) described a system for delivering nursing care that consists of four design elements: (a) allocation and acceptance of individual responsibility for decision-making to one individual; (b) individual assignment of daily care; (c) direct communication channels; and (d) one person responsible for the quality of care administered to patients on a unit 24 hours a day, 7 days a week.

primidone ('primәˌdohn) an anticonvulsant drug used in the treatment of major epilepsy.

primigravida (ˌpriemә'gravidә) a woman who is pregnant for the first time.

primipara (ˌpriemi'parә, prie'mipәrә) a woman who has given birth to her first child.

probability (ˌprobә'bilәtee) a statistical term assessing the likelihood of an association between variables being due to chance.

probenecid (proh'benәsid) a drug which increases the excretion of uric acid and is used between attacks of gout to prevent their occurrence.

problem-oriented record (ˌproblәm ˌorientәd 'reˌkord) a multiprofessional approach to patient care recordkeeping that focuses on the patient's specific health problems requiring immediate attention and the structuring of a healthcare plan designed to cope with the identified problems.

procainamide (proh'kaynәˌmied) a cardiac depressant drug used in the treatment of abnormal heart rhythms.

procaine ('prohkayn) a local anaesthetic used by infiltration. *P. penicillin* a long-acting antibiotic drug chiefly used in the treatment of venereal diseases.

procarbazine (proh'kahbәˌzen) a monoamine oxidase inhibitor used in the treatment of some malignant conditions such as LYMPHADENOMA.

process ('prohses) in anatomy, a prominence or outgrowth of any part. *P. of nursing see* NURSING (process).

prochlorperazine (ˌprohklor'perәˌzeen) a tranquillising drug used in the treatment of schizophrenia and other psychoses and also of vertigo, nausea, and vomiting.

procidentia (ˌprohsә'denshi·ә) complete prolapse of an organ, particularly the uterus so that the cervix extrudes through the vagina.

proctalgia (prok'talji·ә) pain in the rectum and anus; proctodynia.

proctectomy (prok'tektәmee) surgical removal of the rectum.

proctitis (prok'tietәs) inflammation of the rectum.

proctodynia (ˌproktoh'dini·ә) pain in the rectum and anus; proctalgia.

proctorrhaphy (prok'to·rәfee) suture of a wound in the rectum or anus.

proctoscope ('proktәˌskohp) an instrument for examination of the rectum. *Tuttle's p.* a speculum illuminated by an electric bulb combined with an arrangement by which the rectum can be dilated with air.

proctosigmoiditis (ˌproktohˌsigmoy'dietəs) inflammation of the rectum and sigmoid colon.

procyclidine (proh'siekləˌdeen) a drug used in the treatment of PARKINSONISM because it reduces muscle tremor and rigidity.

prodrome ('prohdrohm) a symptom which appears before the true diagnostic signs of a disease.

prodrug ('prohˌdrug) a compound that on administration must undergo chemical conversion by metabolic processes before becoming an active pharmacological agent, thus avoiding gastrointestinal side-effects.

profession (prə'feshən) 1. an avowed, public declaration or statement of intention or purpose. 2. a calling or vocation requiring specialised knowledge, methods, and skills, as well as preparation in an institution of higher learning in the scholarly, scientific, and historical principles underlying such methods and skills. Members of a profession are committed to continuing study, to enlarging their body of knowledge, to placing service above personal gain, and to providing practical services vital to human and social welfare. A profession functions autonomously and is committed to higher standards of achievement and conduct.

professional (prə'feshən'l) 1. pertaining to one's profession or occupation. 2. one who is a specialist in a particular field or occupation. *Allied health p.* a person with special training, and licensed when necessary, who works under the supervision of a health professional, with responsibilities bearing on patient care.

profile ('prohˌfiel) 1. a simple outline, as of the side view of the head or face; by extension, a graph representing quantitatively a set of characteristics determined by tests. 2. A record of achievements developed during a course of study, or subsequently.

progeny ('projənee) issue. Descendants.

progeria (proh'jeeri·ə) premature ageing, the signs of which appear in childhood.

progesterone (proh'jestəˌrohn) a hormone of the corpus luteum which plays an important part in the regulation of the menstrual cycle and in pregnancy.

progestogen (proh'jestəjən) one of a group of steroid hormones having an action similar to that of progesterone.

prognathism ('prognəˌthizəm) enlargement and protrusion of one or both jaws.

prognosis (prog'nohsəs) a forecast of the probable course and outcome of an attack of disease and the prospects of recovery, as indicated by the nature of the disease and the signs and symptoms of the case. *Nursing p.* the application of information obtained during a nursing assessment in order to determine the prospect for altering, through nursing intervention, a client's/patient's response to illness or injury. The prognosis provides a rationale for setting priorities for meeting a particular client's/patient's nursing care needs and enhances continuity of nursing care by clearly indicating agreed priorities.

proguanil (proh'gwahnəl) a widely used drug taken daily to prevent malarial infection.

projection (prə'jekshən) in psychology, an unconscious process by which painful thoughts or impulses are made acceptable by transferring them on to another person or object in the environment.

prolactin (proh'laktən) a milk-producing hormone of the anterior lobe of the pituitary body which stimulates the mammary gland.

prolapse ('prohlaps) the downwards displacement of an organ or part of one. *P. of the cord* expulsion of the umbilical cord before the fetus presents. *P. of an intervertebral disc.* Displacement of part of an intervertebral disc; 'slipped disc'. *P. of the iris* protrusion of a part of the iris through a wound in the cornea. *P. of the rectum* protusion of the mucous membrane through the anal canal to the exterior. *P. of the uterus* descent of the cervix or of the whole uterus into the vagina owing to a weakening of its supporting ligaments.

proliferation (prə,lifə'rayshən) rapid multiplication of cells as can occur in a malignant growth and during wound healing.

promazine ('prohmə,zeen) a tranquillising drug used to treat confusion and anxiety in elderly patients.

promethazine (proh'methə,zeen) a powerful long-acting antihistamine drug used in conditions of hypersensitivity, e.g. hay fever, contact dermatitis, drug rashes, etc.

prominence ('prominəns) in anatomy, a projection, usually on a bone.

pronation (proh'nayshən) turning the palm of the hand downwards.

prone (prohn) lying face downwards.

propantheline (proh'panthə,leen) an antispasmodic drug that blocks the impulses from the VAGUS nerve to the stomach and is used in the treatment of peptic ulcer and spastic colon.

prophylactic (,profə'laktik) 1. relating to prophylaxis. 2. a drug used to prevent a disease developing.

prophylaxis (,profə'laksəs) measures taken to prevent a disease.

propanolol (proh'pranə,lol) a beta-blocking drug used in the treatment of cardiac ARRHYTHMIAS, angina, THYROTOXICOSIS, and anxiety states.

proprietary name (prə'prieətree) the name assigned to a drug by the firm that first made it. A drug can have several different proprietary names.

proprioceptor (,prohpreeoh'septə) one of the sensory nerves that provide information about movements and position of the body. They occur chiefly in the muscles, tendons, joint capsules, and labyrinth.

proptosis (prop'tohsəs) forwards displacement of the eyeball; EXOPHTHALMUS.

propylthiouracil (,prohpəl,thieoh-'yoo·rəsil) a thyroid inhibitor used in the treatment of THYROTOXICOSIS.

prospective study (prə'spektiv) non-experimental study that begins with an exploration of assumed causes and then moves forwards in time to the presumed effect.

prostacyclin (,prostə'sieklən) an intermediate in the metabolic pathway of arachidonic acid formed from prostaglandin endoperoxides in the walls of arteries and veins; it is a potent vasodilator and a potent inhibitor of platelet aggregation.

prostaglandin (ˌprostəˈglandən) one of several hormone substances produced in many body tissues including the brain, lungs, uterus, and semen. They are active in many ways, having cardiac, gastric, and respiratory effects, and causing uterine contractions. They are sometimes used for the induction of abortion. Chemically they are fatty acids.

prostate (ˈprostayt) the gland surrounding the male urethra at its junction with the bladder; during ejaculation, it produces a fluid which forms part of the semen. It often becomes enlarged after middle age and might require removal if it causes obstruction to the outflow of urine.

prostatectomy (ˌprostəˈtektəmee) surgical removal of the whole or a part of the prostate gland. *Retropubic p.* removal of the gland by incising the capsule of the prostate after making a suprapubic abdominal incision. *Transurethral p.* resection of the gland through the urethra using a resectoscope. *Transvesical p.* removal of the gland by incising the bladder after making a low abdominal incision.

prostatitis (ˌprostəˈtietəs) inflammation of the prostate gland.

prostatorrhoea (ˌprostatəˈreeə) a thin urethal discharge from the prostate gland occurring in PROSTATITIS.

prosthesis (prosˈtheesəs) [Gr.] 1. the replacement of an absent part by an artificial substitute. 2. an artificial substitute for a missing part.

prostration (proˈstrayshən) a condition of extreme exhaustion.

protamine (ˈprohtəˌmeen) one of a number of proteins occurring only in fish sperm. *P. sulphate* a drug used to neutralise circulating heparin should haemorrhage arise during anticoagulant therapy.

protease (ˈprohteeˌayz) a proteolytic enzyme in the digestive juices that causes the breakdown of protein.

protective isolation (prətektiv ˌiesəˈlayshən) a type of ISOLATION designed to prevent contact between potentially pathogenic microorganisms and uninfected persons who have seriously impaired resistance. Called also reverse isolation.

protein (ˈprohteen) one of a group of complex organic nitrogenous compounds formed from amino acids and occurring in every living cell of animal and vegetable tissue. *Bence Jones p.* an abnormal protein found in the urine of patients suffering from MULTIPLE MYELOMA. *First class p.* one that provides the essential amino acids. Sources are meat, poultry, fish, cheese, eggs, and milk. *Second class p.* one that comes from a vegetable source (e.g. peas, beans, and whole cereal) that cannot supply all the body's needs. *P.-bound iodine* the iodine in the plasma which is combined with protein. Measurement of this is made when assessing thyroid function. *P.-losing enteropathy* a condition in which protein is lost from the lumen of the intestine. This causes HYPOPROTEINAEMIA and OEDEMA.

proteinuria (ˌprohtəˈnyoo·ri·ə) an excess of serum proteins in the urine.

proteolysis (ˌprohteeˈoləsəs) the processes by which proteins are reduced to an absorbable form by digestive enzymes in the stomach and intestines.

proteolytic (ˌprohteeoh'litik) 1. pertaining to, characterised by, or promoting proteolysis. 2. a proteolytic enzyme.

proteose ('prohteeˌohz) one of the first products in the breakdown of proteins.

Proteus ('prohtee·əs) a genus of Gram-negative bacteria common in the intestines of humans and animals and in decaying matter. They are frequently to be found in secondary infections of wounds and in the urinary tract.

prothrombin (proh'thrombən) a constituent of blood plasma, the precursor of THROMBIN, which is formed in the presence of calcium salts and THROMBOKINASE when blood is shed. *P. time* a test to measure the activity of clotting factors. Deficiency of any of these factors leads to a prolongation of clotting time. This test is widely used for the establishment and maintenance of anticoagulant therapy.

protoplasm ('prohtəˌplazəm) the essential chemical compound of which living cells are made.

prototype ('prohtəˌtiep) the original form from which all other forms are derived.

Protozoa (ˌprohtə'zoh·ə) a phylum comprising the unicellular eukaryotic organisms; most are free living but some lead commensalistic, mutualistic, or parasitic existences. Pathogenic protozoa include *Entamoeba histolytica* (cause of amoebic dysentery) and *Plasmodium vivax* (cause of malaria). *See* METAZOA.

protriptylene (proh'triptəˌleen) an antidepressant drug used in the treatment of extreme apathy and withdrawal.

protuberance (prə'tyoobə·rəns) in anatomy, a rounded projecting part.

provider (prə'viedə) of health services, a person, group of people or organisation supplying a service.

provitamin (proh'vitəmən, -'viet-) a precursor of a vitamin. *P. 'A'* carotene. *P. 'D'* ergosterol.

proximal ('proksəməl) in anatomy, nearest that point which is considered the centre of a system; the opposite to distal.

prurigo (proo'riegoh) a chronic skin disease with an irritating papular eruption.

pruritus (proo'rietəs) irritation of the skin. It can affect the whole surface of the body, as in certain skin diseases and nervous dis-orders, or it can be limited in area, especially involving the anus and vulva.

pseudarthrosis (ˌsyoodah'throhsəs) a false joint formed when the two parts of a fractured bone have failed to unite.

pseudoangina (ˌsyoodoh·an'jienə) false angina. Precordial pain occurring in anxious individuals without evidence of organic heart disease.

pseudocoxalgia (ˌsyoodohkok-'salji·ə) osteochondritis of the head of the femur. PERTHES' DISEASE.

pseudocyesis (ˌsyoodohsie'eesəs) false pregnancy; development of all the signs of pregnancy without the presence of an embryo.

pseudogynaecomastia (ˌsyoodohˌgienəkoh'masti·ə) the deposition of adipose tissue in the male breast which can give the appearance of enlarged mammary glands.

pseudohermaphroditism (ˌsyoodoh·hər'mafrədəˌtizəm) a congenital abnormality in which the external genitalia are characteristic of the opposite sex and confusion can arise as to the true sex of the individual.

pseudoisochromatic chart (ˌsyoo-dohˌiesohkrə'matik) a chart of coloured dots for testing colour blindness. ISHIHARA COLOUR CHART.

Pseudomonas (ˌsyoodoh'mohnəs) a genus of Gram-negative motile bacilli commonly found in decaying organic matter. *P. pyocyanea* (P. aeruginosa) one found in pus from wounds ('blue pus') and in urinary tract infections.

pseudomyopia (ˌsyoodohmie'ohpi·ə) spasm of the cilary muscle causing the same focusing defect as in myopia.

pseudoparalysis (ˌsyoodohpə'raləsəs) apparent loss of muscular power without real paralysis. *Arthritic general p.* a condition resembling dementia paralytica, dependent on intracranial ATHEROMA in arthritic patients. Called also Klippel's disease. *Parrot's p., syphilitic p.* pseudoparalysis of one or more extremities in infants due to syphilitic OSTEOCHRONDRITIS of an epiphysis.

psittacosis (ˌsitə'kohsəs) a disease of parrots and budgerigars due to *Chlamydia psittaci*. Communicable to humans, the symptoms resemble paratyphoid fever with bronchopneumonia.

psoas ('soh·əs) a long muscle originating from the lumbar spine and inserting into the lesser trochanter of the femur. It flexes the hip joint. *P. abscess* one that arises in the lumbar region and is due to spinal caries as a result of tuberculous infection.

psoriasis (sə'rieəsəs) a chronic, recurrent skin disease characterised by reddish marginated patches with profuse silvery scaling on extensor surfaces such as the knees and elbow but which can be more widespread. It is non-infectious and the cause is unknown. It tends to occur in families; about one-third of the cases are believed to be related to a hereditary factor.

psyche ('siekee) the mind, both conscious and unconscious.

psychedelic (ˌsiekə'delik) mind-altering; a term applied to hallucinatory or psychotomimetic drugs capable of profound effects upon the nature of the perception and conscious experience. *See also* HALLUCINOGEN.

psychiatrist (sie'kieətrəst) a doctor who specialises in psychiatry.

psychiatry (sie'kieətree) the branch of medicine that deals with the study, treatment, and prevention of mental illness.

psychoanalysis (ˌsiekoh·ə'naləsəs) 1. a method of investigating mental processes developed by Sigmund Freud which uses the techniques of free association, interpretation, and dream analysis. 2. a system of theoretical psychology formulated by Freud, based on the recognition of unconscious mental processes such as resistance, repression, and transference, and of the importance of infantile experience as a determinant of adult behaviour. 3. a method of psychotherapy based on the psychoanalytical method and psychoanalytical psychology.

psychoanalyst (ˌsiekoh'anələst) one who specialises in psychoanalysis.

psychodrama (ˌsiekoh'drahmə) group PSYCHOTHERAPY in which patients dramatise their individual conflicting situations of daily life.

psychodynamics (ˌsiekohdie-

'namiks) the understanding and interpretation of psychiatric symptoms or abnormal behaviour in terms of unconscious mental mechanisms.

psychogenic (ˌsiekoh'jenik) originating in the mind. *P. illness* a disorder that has a psychological as opposed to an organic origin.

psychogeriatrics (ˌsiekohˌjeri'atriks) the study and treatment of the psychological and psychiatric problems of the aged.

psychologist (sie'koləjəst) one who studies normal and abnormal mental processes, development and behaviour.

psychology (sie'koləjee) the study of the mind and mental processes.

psychometrics (ˌsiekoh'metriks) the measurement of mental characteristics by means of a series of tests.

psychomotor (ˌsiekoh'mohtə) related to the motor effects of mental activity. The term is applied to those mental disorders that affect muscular activity.

psychoneurosis (ˌsiekohnyə'rohsəs) a mental disorder characterised by an abnormal mental response to a normal stimulus. The psychoneuroses include anxiety states, depression, hysteria, and obsessive-compulsive neurosis.

psychopath ('siekəˌpath) *see* SOCIOPATH.

psychopathic disorder (ˌsiekə'pathik) a persistent disorder or disability of the mind (whether or not including significant impairment of intelligence) which results in abnormally aggressive or seriously irresponsible conduct on the part of the patient.

psychopathology (ˌsiekohpə'tholəjee) the study of the causes and processes of mental disorders.

psychopharmacology (ˌsiekohˌfahmə'koləjee) the study of drugs that have an action on the mind and how such action is produced.

psychoprophylaxis (ˌsiekohˌprofə'laksəs) 1. a psychological technique used to prevent emotional disturbances. 2. a technique involving breathing control and exercises used to relieve pain during childbirth.

psychosexual (ˌsiekoh'sekshooəl) relating to the mental aspects of sex. *P. development* the stages through which an individual passes from birth to full maturity, especially with respect to sexual urges, in the total development of the person.

psychosis (sie'kohsəs) any major mental disorder of organic or emotional origin marked by derangement of the personality and loss of contact with reality, often with delusions, hallucinations, or illusions. Psychoses are usually classified as functional psychoses, those for which no physical cause has been discovered, and organic psychoses, which are the result of organic damage to the brain.

psychosomatic (ˌsiekohsə'matik) relating to the mind and the body. *P. disorders* those illnesses in some individuals in which emotional factors (either causative or aggravating) have a profound influence, including ANOREXIA NERVOSA and asthma respectively.

psychotherapy (ˌsiekoh'therəpee) any of a number of related techniques for treating mental illness by psychological methods. These techniques are similar in that they all mainly rely on establishing communication between the therapist and the patient as a means of understanding and modifying the patient's behaviour. On occasion, drugs can be used, but only in order to make this communication easier.

psychotomimetic (sieˌkotohmi'metik) a drug that produces symptoms similar to those of a psychosis, with an abnormal mental state, mood changes, and delusions.

psychotrophic (ˌsiekoh'trohfik) pertaining to drugs that have an effect on the psyche. These include antidepressants, stimulants, sedatives, and tranquillisers.

pterygium (tə'riji·əm) a wing-like structure, especially an abnormal triangular fold of membrane from the conjunctiva to the cornea.

ptosis ('tohsəs) 1. dropping of the upper eyelid due to paralysis of the third cranial nerve. It can be congenital or acquired. 2. prolapse of an organ, e.g. gastroptosis.

ptyalin ('tieələn) an enzyme (amylase) in saliva which metabolises starches.

ptyalism ('tieəˌlizəm) an abnormally large secretion of saliva; sialorrhoea.

puberty ('pyoobətee) the period during which secondary sexual characteristics develop and the reproductive organs become functional. Generally between the 12th and 17th years.

pubes ('pyoobeez) pubic hair or the area on which it grows.

pubic ('pyoobik) pertaining to the pubis.

pubiotomy (ˌpyoobee'otəmee) surgical division of a pubic bone during labour to increase the pelvic diameter.

pubis ('pyoobəs) the anterior part of a hip bone. The left and right pubic bones meet at the front of the pelvis at the pubic symphysis.

public health ('publik) the field of medicine that is concerned with safeguarding and improving the physical, mental and social wellbeing of the community as a whole.

pudendal block (pyoo'dend'l blok) a form of local analgesia induced by injecting a solution of 0.5 or 1% lignocaine around the pudendal nerve. Used mainly for EPISIOTOMY and forceps delivery.

pudendum (pyoo'dendəm) the external genitalia, especially those of a woman.

puerperal (pyoo'ərpə·rəl) pertaining to childbirth. *P. fever* or *sepsis* infection of the genital tract following childbirth.

puerperium (ˌpyooə'piə·ri·əm) a period of about 6 weeks following childbirth when the reproductive organs are returning to their normal state.

Pulex ('pyooleks) a genus of fleas. *P. irritans* are parasitic on humans. The type that infests rats can transmit plague to humans.

pulmonary ('pulməˌnə·ree, 'puhl-) pertaining to or affecting the lungs. *P. embolism* obstruction of the pulmonary artery or one of its branches by an EMBOLUS. *P. hypertension* an increase of blood pressure in the lungs usually as a result of disease of the lung. *P. oedema* an excess of fluid in the lungs. *P. stenosis* a narrowing of the passage between the right ventricle of the heart and the pulmonary artery. The condition is frequently congenital. *P. tuberculosis see* TUBERCULOSIS. *P. valve* the valve at the point where the pulmonary artery leaves the heart.

pulp (pulp) any soft, juicy animal or vegetable tissue. *P. cavity* the centre of a tooth containing blood tissue and nerves. *Digital p.* the soft pads at the ends of the fingers and toes. *Splenic p.* the reddish-brown tissue of the spleen.

pulsation (pul'sayshən) a beating or throbbing.

pulse (puls) the local rhythmic expansion of an artery which can be felt with the finger, corresponding to each contraction of the left ventricle of the heart. It can be felt in any artery sufficiently near the surface of the body. The normal adult rate is about 72/min. In childhood it is more rapid, varying from 130/min in infants to 80/min in older children. *Alternating p.* alternate strong and weak beats; pulsus alternans. *P. deficit* a sign of atrial fibrillation; the pulse rate is slower than the apex beat. *High-tension p.* cordy pulse. The duration of the impulse in the artery is long and the artery feels firm and like a cord between the beats. *Low-tension p.* one easily obliterated by pressure. *Paradoxical p.* pulsus paradoxus; the pulse rate slows on inspiration and quickens on expiration. It can occur in constrictive PERICARDITIS. *Running p.* little distinction between the beats. It occurs in haemorrhage. *Thready p.* thin and almost imperceptible pressure. *Venous p.* that felt in a vein; it is usually taken in the right jugular vein.

pulseless disease ('pulsləs) progressive obliteration of the vessels arising from the aortic arch leading to loss of the pulse in both arms and carotids and to symptoms associated with ischaemia of the brain, eyes, face, and arms.

punctate ('pungktayt) dotted. *P. erythema* a rash of very fine spots.

punctum ('pungktəm) a point or small spot. *P. lacrimalis* one of the two openings of the lacrimal ducts at the inner CANTHUS of the eye.

puncture ('pungkchə) 1. the act of piercing with a sharp object. 2. the wound so produced. *Cisternal p.* the withdrawal of fluid from the CISTERNA magna. *Lumbar p.* the removal of cerebrospinal fluid by puncture between the 3rd and 4th lumbar vertebrae. *Sternal p.* the withdrawal of bone marrow from the MANUBRIUM of the sternum. *Ventricular p.* the withdrawal of cerebrospinal fluid from a cerebral ventricle.

pupil ('pyoopəl) the circular aperture in the centre of the iris through which light passes into the eye. *Argyll Robertson p.* absence of response to light but not to accommodation; characteristic of syphilis of the central nervous system. *Artificial p.* one made by cutting a piece out of the iris when the centre part of the cornea or the lens is opaque. *Fixed p.* one that fails to respond to light or convergence. *Multiple p.* two or more openings of the iris. *Tonic p.* one that reacts slowly to light or to convergence or both.

pupillary (pyoo'pilə·ree) referring to the pupil.

purgative ('pərgətiv) a laxative; an aperient drug. Purgatives can be: (a) irritants such as cascara, senna, rhubarb, and castor oil; (b) lubricants such as liquid paraffin; or (c) mechanical agents that increase bulk, such as bran and agar preparations.

purine ('pyoo·reen) a heterocyclic compound that is the nucleus of the purine bases (or purines) such as adenine and guanine, which occur in DNA and RNA. *See* PYRIMIDINE.

purpura ('pərpyərə) a condition characterised by extravasation of blood in the skin and mucous membranes causing purple spots and patches. There are two general types of purpura: (a) primary or idiopathic (usually autoimmune) thrombocytopenic purpura, in which the cause is unknown; and (b) secondary or symptomatic thrombocytopaenic pupura, which can be associated with exposure to drugs or other chemical agents, systemic diseases such as systemic LUPUS ERYTHEMATOSUS, diseases affecting the bone marrow such as leukaemia, and infections such as septicaemia and viral infections. *Allergic p.*, *anaphylactic p.* Schönlein–Henoch purpura; also called Henoch–Schônlein. *Idiopathic thrombocytopaenic p.* abbreviated ITP. An acquired THROMBOCYTOPAENIA which can be acute or chronic in its course. Acute ITP is common in young children. The disorder is usually self-limiting and rarely fatal. Chronic ITP is more insidious in onset, and is more common in young adult women. *Schönlein–Henoch p.* non-thrombocytopaenic purpura of unknown cause, most often seen in children, associated with various clinical symptoms such as urticaria and erythema, arthropathy and arthritis, gastrointestinal symptoms, and renal involvement. *P. senilis* dark purplish-red ECCHYMOSES occurring on the forearms and backs of the hands in the elderly; the platelet count is normal. *Steroid p.* purpura secondary to prolonged use of steroids. The platelet count is normal, the basic defect being the loss of supporting connective tissue. *Thrombocytopaenic p.* purpura associated with a decrease in the number of platelets in the blood.

purulent ('pyoo·rələnt) containing or resembling pus.

pus (pus) a thick, yellow semiliquid substance consisting of dead leukocytes and bacteria, debris of cells, and tissue fluids. It results from inflammation caused by invading bacteria, mainly *Staphylococcus aureus* and *Streptococcus haemolyticus*, which have destroyed the phagocytes and set up local suppuration. *Blue p.* that produced by infection with *Pseudomonas pyocyanea*.

pustule ('pustyool) a small pimple or elevation of the skin containing pus. *Malignant p. see* ANTHRAX.

putative ('pyootətiv) supposed, reputed. *P. father* the man believed to be the father of an illegitimate child.

putrefaction (ˌpyootrə'fakshən) decomposition of animal or vegetable matter under the influence of microorganisms, usually accompanied by an offensive odour due to gas formation.

pyaemia (pie'eemi·ə) a condition resulting from the circulation of pyogenic microorganisms from some focus of infection. Multiple abscesses occur, the development of which causes rigor and high fever. *Portal p.* PYLEPHLEBITIS.

pyarthrosis (ˌpieah'throhsəs) suppuration in a joint.

pyelitis (ˌpieə'lietəs) inflammation of the renal pelvis. Pyelitis is a fairly common disease particularly among young children, affecting girls more often than boys. The most common presentation includes urgency of micturition, frequency, and DYSURIA. PYURIA is present.

pyelography (ˌpieə'lografee) *see* UROGRAPHY.

pyelolithotomy (ˌpieəlohli'thotəmee) the surgical removal of a stone from the renal pelvis.

pyelonephritis (ˌpieəlohnə'frietəs) inflammation of the renal pelvis and renal substance characterised by fever, acute loin pain, and increased frequency of micturition, with the presence of pus and albumin in the urine.

pyeloplasty ('pieəlohˌplastee) plastic repair of the renal pelvis.

pylephlebitis (ˌpieləflə'bietəs) inflammation of the portal vein which gives rise to severe symptoms of septicaemia or PYAEMIA.

pylethrombosis (ˌpieləthrom'bohsəs) thrombosis of the portal vein.

pyloric (pie'lo·rik) relating to the PYLORUS. *P. stenosis* stricture of the pyloric orifice. It can be: (a) hypertrophic when there is thickening of normal tissue; this is congenital and occurs in infants from 4–7 weeks old, usually males and first babies; (b) cicatricial when there is ulceration or a malignant growth near the pylorus.

pyloromyotomy (pieˌlo·rohmie'otəmee) Ramstedt's operation; an incision of the pylorus performed to relieve congenital pyloric stenosis.

pyloroplasty (pie'lo·rohˌplastee) plastic operation on the PYLORUS to enlarge the outlet. A longitudinal incision is made and it is resutured tranversely.

pylorospasm (pieˌlo·roh'spazəm) forceful muscle contraction of the pylorus which delays emptying of the stomach and causes vomiting.

pylorus (pie'law·rəs) the opening into the duodenum at the lower end of the stomach. It is surrounded by a circular muscle, the *pyloric sphincter*, which contracts to close the opening.

pyoderma (ˌpieoh'dərmə) any purulent skin disease. *P. gangrenosum* a rapidly evolving cutaneous ulcer or ulcers with undermining of the border. Once regarded as a complication peculiar to ulcerative colitis, it is now known to occur in other wasting diseases.

pyogenic (ˌpieoh'jenik) producing pus.

pyometra (ˌpieoh'meetrə) the presence of pus in the uterus.

pyonephrosis (ˌpieohnə'frohsəs) obstruction and infection of the pelvis of the kidney. The calyces and pelvis are dilated and contain pus.

pyopericarditis (ˌpieohˌpereekah'dietəs) suppurative infection of the PERICARDIUM.

pyopneumothorax (ˌpieohˌnyoomoh'thor·raks) pus and gas or air in the pleural cavity, usually associated with the partial or total collapse of the lung.

pyorrhoea (pieə'reeə) a discharge of pus. *P. alveolaris* pus in the sockets of the teeth; suppurative PERIODONTITIS.

pyosalpinx (ˌpieoh'salpingks) the presence of pus in a uterine tube.

pyothorax (ˌpieoh'thor·raks) the presence of pus in the pleural cavity; EMPYEMA.

pyramidal (pə'ramid'l) of pyramid shape. *P. cells* cortical cells shaped like a pyramid from which originate nerve impulses to voluntary muscle. *P. tract* the nerve fibres that transmit impulses from pyramidal cells through the cerebral cortex to the spinal cord.

pyrazinamide (ˌpirə'zinəmied) a drug used in the treatment of tuberculosis, especially tuberculous meningitis.

pyrexia (pie'reksi·ə) fever; a rise of body temperature to any point between 37 and 40°C; above this is hyperpyrexia.

pyridostigmine (ˌpirədoh'stigmeen) a drug that prevents destruction of acetylcholine at the neuromuscular junctions; used in treatment of MYASTHENIA gravis. It is less powerful than neostigmine but has a more prolonged action.

pyrixodine (ˌpirə'dokseen) vitamin B_6. This vitamin is concerned with protein metabolism and blood formation. It is found in many types of food, and deficiency is rare.

pyrimethamine (ˌpieri'methəmeen) a folic acid antagonist used as an antimalarial, especially for suppressive prophylaxis, and also used concomitantly with a sulphonamide in the treatment of TOXOPLASMOSIS.

pyrimidine (pie'rimiˌdeen) nitrogen-containing organic compound. Thymine and cytosine are essential constituents of DNA, and uracil and cytosine of RNA. *See* PURINE.

pyrogen ('pierohˌjen) a substance that can produce fever.

pyromania (ˌpieroh'mayni·ə) an irresistible desire to set things on fire.

pyrosis (pie'rohsəs) heartburn; a symptom of indigestion marked by a burning sensation in the stomach and oesophagus with eructation of acid fluid.

pyuria (pie'yoo·ri·ə) the presence of pus in the urine; more than three leukocytes per high-power field on microscopic examination.

Qq

Q fever ('kyoo ˌfeeva) an acute infectious disease of cattle which is transmitted to humans, usually by infected milk. It is caused by a RICKETTSIA, *Coxiella burnetii*, and has symptoms resembling pneumonia.

QRS complex (kyoo ah·r es 'kompleks) a group of waves depicted on an electrocardiogram; called also the QRS wave. It actually consists of three distinct waves created by the passage of the cardiac electrical impulse through the ventricles and occurs at the beginning of each contraction of the ventricles. In a normal ELECTROCARDIOGRAM the R wave is the most prominent of the three; the Q and S waves can be weak, and are sometimes absent.

quadratus (kwod'raytəs) four-sided. The term is used to describe a number of four-sided muscles.

quadriceps ('kwodrəˌseps) four-headed. *Q. femoris muscle* the principal extensor muscle of the thigh.

quadriplegia (ˌkwodrə'pleeji·ə) paralysis in which all four limbs are affected; tetraplegia.

quality ('kwolətee) 1. a distinguishing characteristic, property, or attribute. 2. a degree or standard of excellence. *Q. assurance* in the healthcare field, a pledge to the public by those within the various health disciplines that they will work towards the goal of an optimal achievable degree of excellence in the services rendered to every patient.

quarantine ('kwo·rənˌteen) the period of isolation of an infectious or suspected case to prevent the spread of disease. For contacts, this is the longest incubation period known for the specific disease.

quartan ('kwawtan) 1. recurring in 4-day cycles (that is, by inclusive reckoning, every third day). 2. a variety of intermittent fever of which the paroxysms recur on every third day (see MALARIA).

quasiexperiment (ˌkwahzee ək'sperəmənt) research design in which the researcher initiates an experimental treatment but some character of a true experiment is lacking.

Queckenstedt's test ('kwekənˌstets) *H.H.G. Queckenstedt, German physician, 1876–1918.* A test carried out during lumbar puncture by compression of the jugular veins. When normal, there is a sharp rise in pressure followed by a fall as the compression is released. Blockage of the spinal canal or thrombosis of the jugular vein will result in an absence of rise, or only a sluggish rise and fall.

Queensland tick tyhphus ('kweens,land) an infection transmitted by tick bites resembling mild Rocky Mountain spotted fever.

'quickening' ('kwikəning) the first perceptible fetal movement felt by the mother, usually between the 4th and 5th months of pregnancy.

quiescent (kwee'esənt) inactive or at rest. Descriptive of a time when the symptoms of a disease are not evident.

quinalbarbitone (,kwinal'bahbə,tohn) an intermediate-acting barbiturate drug used in the treatment of severe insomnia.

quinestrol (kwi'neestrol) a synthetic oestrogen.

quinidine ('kwinə,deen) an alkaloid obtained from cinchona. It is used in the treatment of cardiac ARRHYTHMIAS.

quinine ('kwineen, kwi'neen) an alkaloid obtained from cinchona. Formerly used in the prevention and treatment of malaria. Still used to treat malignant tertian malaria.

quinsy ('kwinzee) a peritonsillar abscess; acute inflammation of the tonsil and surrounding cellular tissue with suppuration. This can cause obstruction to the airway and can be life-threatening, especially in young children.

quotidian (kwo'tidi·ən) recurring every day. *Q. fever* a variety of malaria in which the fever recurs daily.

quotient ('kwohshənt) a number obtained by dividing one number by another. *Intelligence q.* abbreviated IQ. The degree of intelligence, estimated by dividing the mental age, reckoned from standard tests, by the age in years. *Respiratory q.* the ratio between the carbon dioxide expired and the oxygen inspired during a specified time.

Rr

R symbol for the *roentgen* unit.
R wave *see* QRS complex.
rabid ('rabid) infected with rabies.
rabies ('raybeez) HYDROPHOBIA; a notifiable infectious disease of the central nervous system of animals, especially dogs, foxes, wolves, and bats. The virus is found in the saliva of infected animals and is usually transmitted by a bite. Symptoms include fever, muscle spasms, and intense excitement, followed by convulsions and paralysis; death usually occurs. Vaccines are available.
racemose ('rasə,mohz) grape-like *R. gland* a compound gland composed of a number of small sacs, e.g. the salivary gland.
radiant ('raydi·ənt) emitting rays.
radiation (,raydee'ayshən) the emanation of energy in the form of electromagnetic waves, including gamma rays, X-rays, infra-red rays, ultraviolet rays, and visible light rays. Radiation can cause damage to living tissues. *R. pneumonitis* inflammatory changes in the alveoli and interstitial tissue caused by radiation and which can lead to fibrosis. *R. sickness* a toxic reaction of the body to radiation. Any or all of the following can be present: anorexia, nausea, vomiting, and diarrhoea.
radical ('radikəl) dealing with the root or cause of a disease. *R. cure* one which cures by complete removal of the cause.
radioactivity (,raydeeoh·ak'tivətee) disintegration of certain elements to ones of lower atomic weight with the emission of alpha and beta particles and gamma rays. *Induced r.* that brought about by bombarding the nuclei of certain elements with neutrons.
radiobiology (,raydeeohbie'oləjee) the branch of medical science that studies the effect of radiation on live animal and human tissues.
radiocolloid (,raydeeoh'koloyd) a radioactive isotope in the form of a large molecule solution that can be instilled into the body cavities to treat malignant ASCITES.
radiodermatitis (,raydeeoh,dərmə'tietəs) a late skin complication of radiotherapy in which there is atrophy, scarring, pigmentation, and TELANGIECTASES of the skin.
radiograph ('raydeeoh,grahf, -,graf) skiagram; the picture obtained on specially sensitised film by passing X-rays through the body.
radiographer (,raydee'ogrəfə) a professional health care worker in a diagnostic X-ray department (diagnostic radiographer) or in a

radiotherapy department (therapy radiographer).

radiography (ˌraydee'ogrəfee) the making of film records (radiographs) of internal structures of the body by exposure of film especially sensitised to X-rays or gamma rays. *Body-section r.* a special technique to show in detail images and structures lying in a predetermined plane of tissue, while blurring or eliminating detail in images in other planes; various mechanisms and methods for such radiography have been given various names, e.g. laminagraphy, tomography, etc. *Double-contrast r.* a technique for revealing an abnormality of the intestinal mucosa; it involves injection and evacuation of a barium enema followed by inflation of the intestine with air under light pressure. *Neutron r.* that in which a narrow beam of neutrons from a nuclear reactor is passed through tissues; especially useful in visualising bony tissue. *Serial r.* the making of several exposures of a particular area at arbitrary intervals.

radioisotope (ˌraydeeoh'iesəˌtohp) an isotope of an element that emits radioactivity. These isotopes can occur naturally or be produced artificially by bombardment with neutrons.

radiologist (ˌraydee'oləjəst) a doctor who specialises in the science of radiology.

radiology (ˌraydee'oləjee) the science of radiation. In medicine, the term refers to its use in the diagnosis and treatment of disease.

radiomimetic (ˌraydeeohmi'metik) producing effects similar to those of ionising radiations.

radionuclide (ˌraydeeoh'nyooklied) a radioactive substance that is inherently unstable. It is used in both radiodiagnosis and in radiotherapy.

radioscopy (ˌraydee'oskəpee) the examination of X-ray images on a fluorescent screen.

radiosensitive (ˌraydeeoh'sensətiv) pertaining to those structures that respond readily to radiotherapy.

radiotherapist (ˌraydeeoh'therəpəst) a doctor or technician specialising in radiotherapy.

radiotherapy (ˌradeeoh'therəpee) treatment of disease by X-rays or radioactive isotopes.

radium ('raydi·əm) *symbol* Ra. A radioactive element obtained from uranium ores which gives off emanations of great radioactive power. Used in the treatment of some malignant diseases.

râle (rahl) an abnormal rattling sound, heard on auscultation of the chest during respiration when there is fluid in the bronchi.

Ramstedt's operation ('ramshtets) *W.C. Ramstedt, German surgeon, 1867–1963.* Operation for congenital stricture of the PYLORUS in which the fibres of the sphincter muscle are divided leaving the mucous lining intact.

random sample ('randəm 'sahmpəl, -'sampəl) sample from a population obtained by ensuring that each member of that population has an equal chance of being selected. The sample selected should then demonstrate the same profile as the parent population.

range (raynj) a measure of variability; difference between the highest and lowest scores in a set of sample data.

ranula ('ranyələ) a retention cyst usually under the tongue when blockage occurs in a submaxillary or sublingual duct, or in a mucous gland.

rape (rayp) sexual assault or abuse; criminal forcible sexual intercourse (i.e. penetration) without the consent of the adult or child.

raphe ('rayfee) a seam or ridge of tissue indicating the junction of two parts.

rapport (ra'paw) in psychiatry, a satisfactory relationship between two persons, either the doctor and patient or nurse and patient, or the patient with any significant other.

rarefaction (ˌrair·rə'fakshən) the process of becoming less dense.

rash (rash) a superficial eruption on the skin, frequently characteristic of some specific fever.

Rashkind catheter ('rashkint) A balloon catheter used to increase the size of the atrial septal defect in children who have transposition of the great vessels.

rate (rayt) the speed or frequency with which an event or circumstance occurs per unit of time, population, or other standard of comparison. *Basal metabolic r.* (BMR) an expression of the rate at which oxygen is utilised in a fasting subject at complete rest as a percentage of a value established as normal for such a subject. *Birth r.* the number of live births in a population in a specified period of time (crude birth rate), for the female population (refined birth rate), or for the female population of childbearing age (true birth rate), usually expressed per year per 1000 of the estimated mid-year population. *Death r.* the number of deaths per stated number of persons (1000, 10 000, or 100 000) in a certain region in a certain time (crude death rate). The death rate calculated with allowances made for age and sex distribution in the population is termed the standardised death rate. Called also *mortality rate. Glomerular filtration r.* an expression of the quantity of GLOMERULAR filtrate formed each minute in the nephrons of both kidneys, calculated by measuring the clearance of specific substances, e.g. insulin or creatinine.

ratio ('rayˌsheeoh) an expression of the quantity of one substance or entity in relation to that of another; the relationship between two quantities expressed as the quotient of one divided by the other or the highest level of measurement that possesses the characteristics of categorising, ordering, and ranking and also has an absolute or natural zero that has empirical meaning. *Lecithin–sphingomyelin r.* the ratio of lecithin to SPHINGOMYELIN in AMNIOTIC fluid.

rationalisation (ˌrashənəlie'zayshən) in psychiatry, the mental process by which individuals explain their behaviour, giving reasons that are advantageous to themselves or are socially acceptable. It can be a conscious or an unconscious act.

Rauwolfia (raw'wuhlfi·ə, row-) a genus of tropical trees and shrubs. The dried root of *R. serpentina* is sometimes used as an antihypertensive and sedative, e.g. reserpine.

Raynaud's phenomenon (disease) ('raynohz) *M. Raynaud, French physician, 1834–81.* Raynaud's phenomenon is characterised by episodic digital ischaemia provoked by stimuli such as emotion, cold, trauma, hormones, and drugs. It includes both Raynaud's disease (in which no underlying cause can be found) and Raynaud's syndrome (in which there is an associated underlying disorder). These disorders include SCLERODERMA, mixed connective tissue disease, systemic LUPUS ERYTHEMATOSUS (SLE), POLYMYOSITIS, rheumatoid arthritis, neurovascular entrapment syndromes and occlusive arterial disease.

RBC red blood cell (erythrocyte).

RDS respiratory distress syndrome (infants).

reaction (ree'akshən) counteraction; a response to the application of a stimulus.

reactive (ree'aktiv) in psychiatry, used to describe a mental condition brought about by adverse external circumstances. *R. depression* one that arises in this way and is not endogenous.

reagent (ree'ayjənt) employed to produce a chemical reaction.

reality (ree'alətee) agreed as an absolute by members of the same culture as the total of all things related to perception, meaning, and behaviour. Not imaginary, fictitious, or pretended. *R. orientation see* ORIENTATION.

rebound (rə'bownd) sudden contraction of a muscle after a period of relaxation.

rebreathing bag (ree'breedhing) a flexible bag (attached to a mask) which is squeezed to pump gas or air into the lungs.

recall (rə'kawl, 'reekawl) to bring back to consciousness.

receptor (rə'septə) 1. a sensory nerve ending that receives stimuli for transmission through the sensory nervous system. 2. a molecule on the surface or within a cell that recognises and binds with specific molecules, producing some effect in the cell.

recessive (rə'sesiv) tending to recede. The opposite to dominant. *R. gene* a gene that will produce its characteristics only when present in a HOMOZYGOUS state; both parents need to possess the particular gene, and there is a 1 in 4 chance of a child inheriting it homozygously.

recipient (rə'sipi·ənt) one who receives, as a blood transfusion, or a tissue or organ graft. *Universal r.* a person thought to be able to receive blood of any 'type' without agglutination of the donor cells.

recrudescence (ˌreekroo'desəns) renewed aggravation of symptoms after an interval of abatement.

rectal ('rekt'l) relating to the rectum. *R. examination* inspection by insertion of a glove-covered finger or with the aid of a PROCTOSCOPE.

rectocele ('rektohˌseel) hernia or prolapse of the rectum, usually caused by overstretching of the vaginal wall at childbirth. Proctocele.

rectopexy ('rektohˌpeksee) the operation for fixation of a prolapsed rectum.

rectosigmoid (ˌrektoh'sigmoyd) the junction of the pelvic colon with the rectum.

rectovaginal (ˌrektohvə'jienəl) concerning the rectum and vagina.

rectovesical (ˌrektoh'vesikəl) concerning the rectum and bladder.

rectum ('rektəm) the lower end of the large intestine from the sigmoid flexure to the anus.

recumbent (ree'kumbənt) lying down in the dorsal position.

recuperation (reeˌkoopə'rayshən) convalescence; recovery of health and strength.

recurrent (ree'kurənt) liable to recur. *R. fever* relapsing fever.

Redivac drainage tube ('redi,vak) a proprietary closed suction drainage system used mainly post-operatively for abdominal wounds.

reduction (ree'dukshən, rə-) 1. the correction of a fracture, dislocation or hernia. 2. the addition of hydrogen to a substance or, more generally, the gain of electrons; the opposite of oxidation. *Closed r.* the manipulative reduction of a fracture without incision. *Open r.* reduction of a fracture after incision into the fracture site.

re-education (,ree·edyə'kayshən) the education and training of the physically handicapped or those with learning difficulties to enable them to develop their potential.

referred pain (rə,fərd 'payn) that which occurs at a distance from the place of origin due to the sensory nerves entering the cord at the same level, e.g. the phrenic nerve supplying the diaphragm enters the cord in the cervical region, as do the nerves from the shoulder, and so an abscess on the diaphragm can cause pain in the shoulder. SYNALGIA.

reflection (rə'flekshən) a turning or bending back; for example, the folds produced when a membrane passes over the surface of an organ and then passes back to the body wall that it lines.

reflex ('reefleks) reflected or thrown back. *Accommodation r.* the alteration in the shape of the lens according to the distance of the image viewed. *R. action* an involuntary action following immediately upon some stimulus, e.g. the knee jerk or the withdrawal of a limb from a pin-prick. *R. arc* the sensory and motor neurones, together with the connector neurone, which carry out a reflex action (*see* figure). *Conditioned r.* that which is not natural but is developed by association and frequent repetition until it appears natural. *Corneal r.* the automatic reaction of closing the eyelids after exertion of light pressure on the cornea. This is a test for unconsciousness which is absolute when there is no response. *Deep r.* a muscle reflex elicited by tapping the tendon or bone of attachment. *Light r.* alteration of the size of the pupil in response to exposure to light. *R. zone therapy* palpation of the feet in order to alleviate pain and/or to treat symptoms by stimulating the self-healing capacity of the body.

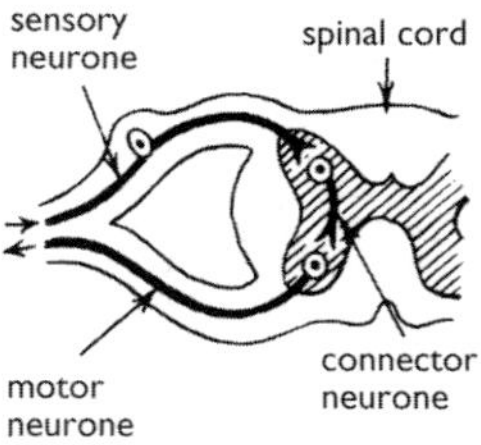

Reflex Arc

reflexology (,reefleks'oləjee) technique of deep massage to the soles of the feet and occasionally the palms of the hands to relieve somatic symptoms.

reflux ('reefluks) a backwards flow; regurgitation.

refraction (rə'frakshən) 1. the bending or deviation of rays of light as they pass obliquely through one transparent medium and penetrate another of different density. 2. in ophthalmology, the testing of the eyes to ascertain the amount and variety of refractive error that is present in each of them.

refractory (rə'fraktə·ree) not yielding to or resistant to treatment. *R. period* the period immediately after some activity during which a nerve or muscle is unable to react to a fresh impulse.

regeneration (rəˌjenə'rayshən, ree-) renewal, as in new growth of tissue in its specific form after injury.

register ('rejəstə) an epidemiological term meaning an index on file of all cases with a particular disease or condition in a defined population.

registrar ('rejəˌstrah) 1. an official keeper of records. 2. a doctor training to be a specialist.

regression (rə'greshən) 1. a return to a previous state of health. 2. in psychiatry, a tendency to return to primitive or child-like modes of behaviour. Some degree of regression frequently accompanies physical illness and hospitalisation. Patients who are mentally ill can exhibit regression to an extreme degree, reverting to infantile behaviour (atavistic regression).

regurgitation (rəˌgurjə'tayshən) backwards flow, e.g. of food from the stomach into the mouth. Fluids regurgitate through the nose in paralysis affecting the soft palate. *Aortic r.* backwards flow of blood into the left ventricle when the aortic valve is incompetent. *Mitral r.* mitral incompetence. *See* MITRAL.

rehabilitation (ˌreehəˌbilə'tayshən) re-education, particularly of one who has been ill or injured, so that he or she can again become capable of useful activity. *R. centre* one which provides for organised employment within the capacity of the patient and with special regard to the physical influence of the work.

reinforcement (ˌree·ən'fawsmənt) the increasing of force or strength. In behavioural science, the process of presenting a reinforcing stimulus to strengthen a response. *See* CONDITIONING. A positive reinforcer is a stimulus that is added to the environment immediately after the desired response. It serves to strengthen the response; that is, to increase the likelihood of its occurring again. Examples of a positive reinforcer are food, money, a special privilege, or some other reward that is satisfying to the subject.

Reiter's protein complement fixation ('rietəz) *H. Reiter, German bacteriologist, 1881–1969.* Abbreviated RPCF. A serological test used to aid the diagnosis of syphilis.

Reiter's syndrome a non-specific URETHRITIS affecting males, in which there is also arthritis and conjunctivitis.

rejection (rə'jekshən) in immunology, the formation of antibodies by the host against transplanted tissue, with eventual destruction of the transplanted tissue.

relapse (rə'laps, 'reeˌlaps) the return of a disease after an interval of convalescence.

relapsing fever (rə'lapsing) one of a group of similar notifiable infectious diseases transmitted to humans by the bites of ticks. Marked by alternating periods of normal temperature and periods of fever relapse. The diseases in the group are caused by several different species of SPIROCHAETES belonging to the genus *Borrelia*. Called also recurrent fever.

relaxant (rə'laksənt) a drug or other agent that brings about muscle relaxation or relieves tension.

relaxation (ree,lak'sayshən) a lessening of tension, which can be observed when muscles slacken after they have contracted. *R. therapy* classes in which patients are taught breathing and other exercises to use for the relief of pain, stress, and tension. Used as part of the preparation for childbirth.

relaxin (rə'laksən) a hormone that is produced by the CORPUS LUTEUM of the ovary; it softens the cervix and loosens the pelvic ligaments to aid the birth of the baby.

releasing factor (rə'leesing) a substance produced in the HYPOTHALAMUS which causes the anterior pituitary gland to release hormones.

REM (rem) rapid eye movement, a phase of SLEEP associated with dreaming and characterised by rapid movements of the eyes. Paradoxical sleep.

reliability (rə,lieə'bilətee) the consistency or constancy of a measuring instrument. *Interrater r.* the consistency of observations between two or more observers; often expressed as a percentage of agreement between observers or a coefficient of agreement that takes into account the element of chance. This usually is used with the direct observation method. *R. coefficient* a number between 0 and 1 that expresses the relationship between the error variance, true variance, and the observed score. A 0 correlation indicates no relationship. The closer to 1 the coefficient is, the more reliable the tool. *Test-retest r.* administration of the same instrument twice to the same subjects under the same conditions within a prescribed time interval, with a comparison of the paired scores to determine the stability of the measure.

reminiscence therapy (remə'nisəns) measures to stimulate long-term elderly patients with memorabilia, films, and songs meaningful to their generation. Used in conjunction with or as a prelude to reality orientation therapy. *See* ORIENTATION.

remission (rə'mishən) subsidence of the signs and symptoms of a disease for a long time.

remittent (rə'mitənt) decreasing at intervals. *R. fever* one in which a partial fall in the temperature occurs daily.

renal ('reenəl) relating to the kidney. *R. calculus* stone in the kidney. *R. clearance tests* laboratory tests that determine the ability of the kidney to remove certain substances from the blood. *R. dialysis* the application of the principles of dialysis for treatment of renal failure (see below). *See also* HAEMODIALYSIS and PERITONEAL dialysis. *R. failure* inability of the kidney to maintain normal function. It can be *acute* or *chronic*. Acute renal failure is a sudden, severe interruption of kidney function. It is normally the complication of another disorder and is reversible. Chronic renal failure is a progressive loss of kidney function. In its early stage, renal function can remain adequate but the GLOMERULAR filtration rate (GFR) is depressed and plasma chemistry begins to show abnormalities as waste products accumulate. In the later stage, known as end-stage renal disease (ESRD), the GFR deteriorates. When URAEMIA becomes evident and the patient becomes symptomatic, dialysis is started or the patient receives a transplant. *R. threshold* the level of the blood sugar beyond which it is excreted in the urine; normally 10 mmol/L (180 mg/100 mL). *R. tubule* the thin tubular part of a nephron. A uriniferous tubule.

renin ('reenən) a proteolytic enzyme released into the bloodstream when the kidneys are ischaemic. It causes vasoconstriction and increases the blood pressure.

rennin ('renən) an enzyme present in gastric juice that curdles milk.

reorganisation (ˌree·awgənie'zayshən) healing by formation of new tissue identical to that which was injured or destroyed.

reovirus (ˌreeoh'vierəs) any of a group of RNA viruses isolated from healthy children, children with some upper respiratory diseases, or children with some forms of diarrhoea.

repetitive strain injury (rə'petətiv) a soft-tissue disorder produced by repetitive use of muscle, especially if the muscle activity involves an awkward or uncomfortable position of the body. Particularly affects keyboard operators, musicians, packers, and machine operators.

replication (ˌreplə'kayshən) 1. the turning back of a tissue on itself. 2. the process by which DNA duplicates itself when the cell divides.

replogle tube (ri'plohgəl) a double-lumen aspiration catheter attached to low-pressure suction apparatus.

repolarisation (ˌreepohlə·rie'zayshən) the process by which the cell is restored to its resting potential.

representative sample (ˌreprə'zentətiv) a sample whose key characteristics closely approximate those of the population.

repression (rə'preshən) 1. the act of restraining, inhibiting, or suppressing. 2. in psychiatry, a defence mechanism whereby a person unconsciously banishes unacceptable ideas, feelings, or impulses from consciousness. A person using repression to obtain relief from mental conflict is unaware that he or she is 'forgetting' unpleasant situations as a way or avoiding them (motivated forgetting).

reproductive system (ˌreeprə'duktiv) all those parts of the male and female body associated with the production of children.

research (ˌreesərch) the systematic, logical and empirical inquiry into the possible relationships among particular phenomena to produce verifiable knowledge. *Applied r.* tests the practical limits of descriptive theories but does not examine the efficacy of actions taken by practitioners. *Basic r.* theoretical or pure research that generates, tests, and expands theories that explain or predict phenomenon. *R. design* the plan or blueprint for conduct of a study. *Qualitative r.* the study of research questions about human experiences. It is often conducted in natural settings, and uses data that are words or text rather than numerical in order to describe the experiences that are being studied. *Quantitative r.* the process of testing relationships, differences, and cause-and-effect interactions among and between variables. These processes are tested against hypotheses and/or research questions. *R. question* a key preliminary step wherein the foundation for a study is developed from the research problem, thus resulting in the research hypothesis.

resection (ree'sekshən) surgical removal of a part. *Submucous r.* removal of part of a deflected nasal septum from beneath a flap of mucous membrane which is then replaced. *Transurethral r.* a method of removing portions of an enlarged prostate gland via the urethra.

resectoscope (ree'sektə,skohp) a telescopic instrument by which pieces of tissue can also be removed. Used for transurethral PROSTATECTOMY.

reserpine ('rezə,peen) an alkaloid from *Rauwolfia*, a drug used to reduce the blood pressure in hypertension.

reservoir ('rezə,vwah) 1. a storage place or cavity. 2. the host or environment in which an organism lives and from which it is able to infect susceptible individuals, e.g. hands, skin, nose, bowel.

residential care (,rezə'denshəl) the provision of care for frail, elderly people in a variety of settings, e.g. local authority residential homes for the elderly or private residential homes.

residual (rə'zidyooəl) remaining. *R. air, r. volume* the amount of air remaining in the lungs after breathing out fully. *R. urine* urine remaining in the bladder after voiding; seen with bladder outlet obstruction and disorders affecting nerves controlling bladder function.

resistance (rə'zistəns) the degree of opposition to a force. 1. in electricity, the opposition made by a non-conducting substance to the passage of a current. 2. in psychology, the opposition, stemming from the unconscious, to repressed ideas being brought to consciousness. *Drug. r.* the ability of a micro-organism to withstand the effects of a drug that is lethal to most members of its species. *R. to infection* the natural power of the body to withstand the toxins of disease. *Peripheral r.* that offered to the passage of blood through small vessels and capillaries.

resolution (,rezə'looshən) 1. in medicine, the process of returning to normal. 2. the disappearance of inflammation without the formation of pus.

resonance ('rezənəns) in medicine, the reverberating sound obtained on percussion over a cavity or hollow organ, such as the lung.

respiration (,respə'rayshən) the gaseous interchange between the tissue cells and the atmosphere. *Artificial r.* the production of respiratory movements by external effort. *External r.* breathing, which is comprised of inspiration (when the external intercostal muscles and the diaphragm contract and air is drawn into the lungs) and expiration (when the air is breathed out). *Intermittent positive pressure r.* abbreviated IPPR. Respiration produced by a ventilator. *Internal* or *tissue r.* the interchange of gases that occurs between tissues and blood through the walls of capillaries. *Laboured r.* that which is difficult and distressed. *Stertorous r.* snorting; a noisy breathing. *See* CHEYNE–STOKES RESPIRATION.

respirator ('respə,raytə) an apparatus to qualify the air breathed through it, or a device for giving artificial respiration or to assist pulmonary ventilation (see also ventilator).

respiratory (rə'spirətree) pertaining to respiration. *Adult r. distress syndrome* abbreviated to ARDS. A group of signs and symptoms resulting in acute respiratory failure; characterised clinically by TACHYPNOEA, DYSPNOEA, TACHYCARDIA, CYANOSIS, and low PaO_2 that persists even with oxygen therapy. *R. acidosis* reduced alveolar ventilation resulting in raised arterial PCO_2 and carbonic acid. *R. alkalosis* an abnormal condition characterised by raised blood pH and decreased arterial PCO_2. *R. arrest* cessation of breathing. *R. distress syndrome of newborn* (abbreviated RDS), *idiopathic r. distress syndrome*, *infant r. distress syndrome* (abbreviated IRDS) a condition occurring in preterm infants, full-term infants of diabetic mothers, and infants delivered by caesarean section, and associated with pulmonary maturity and inability to produce sufficient lung surfactant. Also called hyaline membrane disease. *R. failure* a life-threatening condition in which respiratory function is inadequate to maintain the body's need for oxygen supply and carbon dioxide removal while at rest; called also acute ventilatory failure. *R. insufficiency* a condition in which respiratory function is inadequate to meet the body's needs when increased physical activity places extra demands on it. *R. quotient* the ratio of the volume of expired carbon dioxide to the volume of oxygen absorbed by the lungs per unit of time. *R. syncytial virus* a virus isolated from children with bronchopneumonia and bronchitis, characteristically causing severe respiratory infection in very young children but less severe infections as the children grow older. *R. therapy* the technical speciality concerned with the treatment, management and care of patients with respiratory problems including administration of medical gases.

resuscitation (rə,susə'tayshən) restoration to life or consciousness of one apparently dead, or whose respirations have ceased. *See also* ARTIFICIAL (respiration). *Cardiopulmonary r.* an emergency technique used in cardiac arrest to re-establish heart and lung function until more advanced life support is available.

retardation (,reetah'dayshən) delay; hindrance; delayed development. *Mental r.* low general intellectual development, associated with impairment either of learning and social adjustment or of maturation, or of both.

retching ('reching) strong, involuntary effort to vomit.

retention (rə'tenshən) holding back. R. cyst *see* CYST. *R. defect* a defect of memory. Inability to retain material in the mind so that it can be recalled when required. *R. of urine* inability to pass urine from the bladder which can be due to obstruction or can be of neurological origin.

reticular (rə'tikyələ) resembling a network. *R. formation* areas in the brain stem from which nerve fibres extend to the cerebral cortex.

reticulocyte (rə'tikyəloh,siet) a

red blood cell that is not fully mature; it retains strands of nuclear material.

reticulocytosis (rəˌtikyəlohsie'tohsis) the presence of an increased number of immature red cells in the blood, indicating overactivity of the bone marrow.

reticuloendothelial system (rəˌtikyəlohˌendə'theeli·əl) a collection of endothelial cells in the liver, spleen, bone marrow, and lymph glands that produce large mononuclear cells or MACROPHAGES. They are phagocytic, destroy red blood cells, and are able to make some antibodies.

retina ('retənə) the innermost coat of the eyeball formed of nerve cells and fibres from which the optic nerve leaves the eyeball and passes to the visual area of the cerebrum. The impression of the image is focused upon it.

retinal ('retənəl) relating to the retina. *R. detachment* partial detachment of the retina from the underlying choroid layer, resulting in loss of vision. It can result from several causes, including trauma or the presence of a tumour.

retinitis (ˌretə'nietəs) inflammation of the retina. *R. pigmentosa* a group of diseases frequently hereditary marked by progressive loss of retinal function, especially associated with contraction of the visual field and impairment of vision. The disorder often follows a slow course over a period of many years, but there is considerable variation in the progression of the disease.

retinoblastoma (ˌretənohbla'stohmə) a malignant tumour arising from retinal cells. Occurs in infancy and can be hereditary. Treatment includes cryosurgery, irradiation, and photocoagulation, but ENUCLEATION can be required.

retinopathy (ˌretə'nopəthee) any non-inflammatory disease of the retina. *Diabetic r.* a disorder of retinal blood vessels. It is characterised by capillary microaneurysms, haemorrhages, exudates, and the formation of new vessels and connective tissue. The disorder occurs most frequently in patients with poorly controlled diabetes mellitus. Repeated haemorrhages can cause permanent opacity of the vitreous humor, and, eventually, blindness. Photocoagulation of damaged retinal blood vessels by a laser beam can be performed to prevent haemorrhage from the vessels. *Hypertensive r.* retinal change occurring as a result of high blood pressure.

retinoscope ('retinəˌskohp) an instrument which illuminates the retina and is used to detect and measure refractive errors. Retinoscopy.

retrobulbar (ˌretroh'bulbə) pertaining to the back of the eyeball. *R. neuritis* dimness of vision due to inflammation of the optic nerve.

retroflexion (ˌretroh'flekshən) a bending back, particularly the bending posteriorly of the body of the uterus towards the cervix, resulting in a sharp angle at the point of bending. *See* RETROVERSION.

retrograde ('retrəˌgrayd) going backwards. *R. amnesia* forgetfulness of events occurring immediately before an illness or injury. *R. urography* radiographic examination of the kidney after the introduction of a radio-opaque substance into the renal pelvis through the urethra.

retrolental fibroplasia (ˌretroh-ˈlent'l) a fibrous condition of the anterior vitreous body which develops when a premature infant is exposed to high concentrations of oxygen. Both eyes are affected, seriously interfering with vision and leading to retinal detachment.

retroperitoneal (ˌretrohˌperətə-ˈneeəl) behind the peritoneum.

retropharyngeal (ˌretrohfəˈrinji·əl, -ˌfarənˈjeeəl) behind the pharynx.

retropubic (ˌretrohˈpyoobik) behind the pubic bone.

retrospection (ˌretrohˈspekshən) looking back, especially into the past.

retrospective study (ˌretrohˈspektiv) a nonexperimental research design that begins with the phenomenon of interest (dependent variable) in the present and examines the relationship to another variable (independent variable) in the past.

retrosternal (ˌretrohˈstərnəl) behind the sternum.

retroversion (ˌretrohˈvərshən) a lifting backwards, particularly of the uterus when the whole organ is tilted backwards (*see* figure). *See* RETROFLEXION.

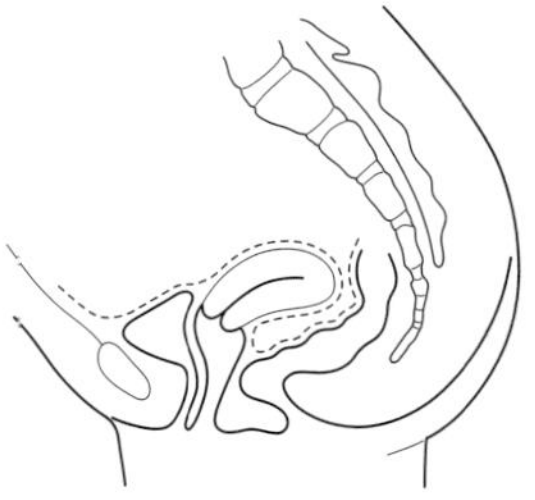

Retroversion of Uterus

Reverdin's graft (ˈrevərdahnz) *J.L. Reverdin, Swiss surgeon, 1842–1929.* A form of skin graft in which pieces of skin are placed as islands over the area.

Reye's syndrome (riez) *R.D.K. Reye, 20th century Australian pathologist.* An acute, potentially fatal illness occurring in children, in which there is fatty degeneration of the liver and the brain and raised intracranial pressure, accompanied by vomiting, convulsions, and coma. The cause of Reye's syndrome is unknown but administration of salicylates in children under the age of 12 years is not recommended. This follows evidence that aspirin might be a contributory factor in the development of Reye's syndrome.

rhabdomyosarcoma (ˌrabdohˌmieohsahˈkohmə) a rare malignant growth of striated muscle. It grows rapidly and metastasises early.

rhagades (ˈragəˌdeez) cracks or fissures in the skin, especially those round the mouth.

rhesus factor (ˈreesəs) abbreviated Rh factor. The red blood cells of most humans carry a group of genetically determined antigens and are said to be rhesus positive (Rh+). Those that do not are said to be rhesus negative (Rh–). This is of importance as a cause of anaemia and jaundice in the newly born when the infant is Rh+ and the mother Rh–. The result of this incompatibility (isoimmunisation) is the formation of an antibody which causes excessive HAEMOLYSIS in the child's blood. *See* ANTI-RHESUS SERUM.

rheumatism ('rooma,tizəm) any of a variety of disorders marked by inflammation, degeneration or metabolic derangement of the connective tissue structures, especially the joints and related structures, and attended by pain, stiffness, or limitation of motion. *Acute r.* or *rheumatic fever* an acute fever associated with previous streptococcal infection and occurring most commonly in children. The onset is usually sudden, with pain, swelling, and stiffness in one or more joints. There is fever, sweating, and TACHYCARDIA, and CARDITIS is present in most cases. Sometimes the symptoms are minor and ignored. This disease is the most common cause of MITRAL STENOSIS because scar tissue results from the inflammation.

rheumatoid ('rooma,toyd) resembling rheumatism. *R. arthritis see* ARTHRITIS.

rheumatology (,roomə'toləjee) the branch of medicine dealing with disorders of the joints, muscles, tendons, and ligaments.

rhinitis (rie'nietəs) inflammation of the mucous membrane of the nose.

rhinoplasty ('rienoh,plastee) a plastic operation on the nose; repairing a part of or forming an entirely new nose.

rhinorrhoea (,rienə'reeə) an abnormal discharge of mucus from the nose.

rhinoscopy (rie'noskəpee) examination of the interior of the nose. *Anterior r.* examination through the nostrils with the aid of a speculum. *Posterior r.* examination through the nasopharynx by means of a rhinoscope.

rhinovirus (,rienoh'vierəs) one of a genus of small RNA-containing viruses that cause respiratory diseases including the common cold.

Rhipicephalus (,riepi'kefələs, -'sef-) a genus of ticks that can transmit the RICKETTSIAE which cause typhus and relapsing fever.

rhodopsin (roh'dopsən) the visual purple of the retina, the formation of which is dependent upon vitamin A in the diet.

rhomboid ('romboyd) any one of two pairs of muscles in the upper back which control the shoulder blades.

rhonchus ('rongkəs) a wheezing sound produced in the bronchial tubes which is caused by partial obstruction and can be heard on auscultation.

rhythm ('ridhəm) a regular recurring action. *Cardiac r.* the smooth action of the heart when systole is followed by diastole. *R. method* a contraceptive technique in which intercourse is limited to the 'safe period' (avoiding the 2–3 days immediately before and after ovulation).

rib (rib) any one of the 12 pairs of long, flat curved bones of the thorax, each united by cartilage to the spinal vertebrae at the back. *Cervical r.* a short extra rib, often bilateral. Pressure on this can cause impairment of nerve or vascular function. *See* SCALENUS (syndrome). *False r's* the last 5 pairs, the upper 3 of which are attached by cartilage to each other. *Floating r's* the last two pairs connected only to the vertebrae. *True r's* the 7 pairs attached directly to the sternum.

riboflavin (,rieboh'flayvən) a chemical factor in the vitamin B complex.

ribonuclease (,rieboh'nyooklee,ayz) an enzyme from the pancreas which is responsible for the breakdown of nucleic acid.

ribonucleic acid (ˌriebohnyoo-ˈklee·ik, -ˈklay-) abbreviated RNA. A complex chemical found in the cytoplasm of animal cells and concerned with protein synthesis. Certain viruses contain RNA.

ribosome (ˌriebəˈsohm) an RNA and protein-containing particle which is the site of protein synthesis in the cell.

rickets (ˈrikəts) a condition of infancy and childhood caused by deficiency of vitamin D which leads to altered calcium and phosphorus metabolism and consequent disturbance of ossification of bone, resulting in deformity such as bowing of the legs. Because the action of sunlight on the skin produces vitamin D in the human body, rickets often occurs in parts of the world where the winter is especially long, and where smoke and fog constantly intercept the sun. *Adult r.* osteomalacia; a rickets-like disease affecting adults. *Fetal r.* ACHONDROPLASIA. *Late r.* OSTEOMALACIA, that occurring in older children. *Vitamin D-resistant r.* a condition almost indistinguishable from ordinary rickets clinically but resistant to unusually large doses of vitamin D; it is often familial.

Rickettsia (riˈketsi·ə) a genus of microorganisms which are parasitic in lice and similar insects. The bite of the host is thus the means of transmitting the organisms, some of which are responsible for the typhus group of fevers.

rifampicin (riˈfampəsən) an antibiotic drug used in leprosy and, with other drugs, in the treatment of tuberculosis.

rigor (ˈrigə) an attack of intense shivering occurring when heat regulation is disturbed. The temperature rises rapidly and can stay elevated or fall rapidly as profuse sweating occurs. *R. mortis* stiffening of the body which occurs soon after death.

Ringer's solution (ˈringəz) *S. Ringer, British physiologist, 1835–1910.* A physiological solution of saline to which small amounts of calcium and potassium salts have been added. Used to replace fluids and electrolytes intravenously.

ringworm (ˈringˌwərm) tinea. A contagious skin disease characterised by circular patches, pinkish in colour, with a desquamating surface, and due to a parasitic fungus.

Rinne's test (ˈrinəz) *H.A. Rinne, German biologist, 1819–68.* A test for deafness in which the degree of conductivity through bone is tested by holding a vibrating tuning fork alternately in front of the ear and over the mastoid bone.

risk (risk) hazard, or chance of developing a disease or of complications during or after treatment. This can arise because of inherent problems with the treatment itself (e.g. drug side-effects) or because of the frailty of the patient. *R. factor* a factor which, when added to others, increases the likelihood of a disease or complication (e.g. smoking and obesity are risk factors for the development of coronary artery disease). *Relative r.* the likelihood of developing a disease after a given exposure; in epidemiological terms, calculated as incidence rate of disease in an exposed group divided by incidence rate in the non-exposed group.

risus ('riesəs) laughter. *R. sardonicus* a peculiar grin caused by muscle spasm around the mouth; seen in tetanus and in strychnine poisoning.

RNA ribonucleic acid. *rna viruses* viruses which contain ribonucleic acid as their genetic material.

Rocky Mountain spotted fever ('rokee ˌmowntən, -tayn) a tick-borne infection caused by a *Rickettsia*, common in the USA, with rash, fever, muscle pain and, often, an enlarged liver. The disease lasts about three weeks.

rod (rod) a straight thin structure. *Retinal r.* one of the two types of light-sensitive end-organs of the retina, which contain RHODOPSIN and are responsible for night vision.

role (rohl) a pattern of behaviour developed in response to the demands or expectations of others; the pattern of responses to the persons with whom an individual interacts in a particular situation. *Sick r.* the role played by people who have defined themselves as ill. Adoption of the sick role changes the behavioural expectations of others towards the sick person, who is exempted from normal social responsibilities and is not held responsible for the condition. The patient is obliged to 'want to get well' and to seek competent medical help.

Romberg's sign ('rombərgz) *M.H. Romberg, German physician, 1795–1873.* Inability to stand erect with the feet close together without swaying if the eyes are closed. A sign of TABES dorsalis and other diseases of the posterior columns.

Rorschach test ('rorshahk) *H. Rorschach, Swiss psychiatrist, 1884–1922.* A personality trait test that consists of 10 ink-blot designs, some in colour and some in black and white.

rosacea (roh'zayshi·ə) *see* ACNE (rosacea).

roseola (roh'zeeələ) 1. a rose-coloured rash. 2. roseola infantum. *R. infantum* a common acute viral disease that usually occurs in children under 24 months old; it attacks suddenly but disappears in a few days, leaving no permanent marks. *Syphilitic r.* an eruption of rose-coloured spots in early secondary syphilis.

Ross River virus ('ros ˌrivə) Australian epidemic polyarthritis virus. An acute febrile illness characterised by fever and arthritic pain in the joints, often accompanied by a rash. Caused by a virus infection spread by mosquitoes.

Roth's spots (rohts) *M. Roth, Swiss physician, 1839–1915.* Small white spots seen in the retina early in the course of subacute bacterial ENDOCARDITIS.

roughage ('rufij) coarse vegetable fibres and cellulose that give bulk to the diet and stimulate peristalsis.

rouleau ('rooloh) a rounded formation found in blood, caused by red cells piling on each other.

roundworm ('rownd,wərm) any of various types of parasitic nematode worms, somewhat resembling the common earthworm, which sometimes invade the human intestinal tract and multiply there. Includes the pinworm, or threadworm.

Rovsing's sign ('rohvsingz) *N.T. Rovsing, Danish surgeon, 1868–1927.* A test for acute appendicitis in which pressure in the left iliac fossa causes pain in the right iliac fossa.

rubefacient (ˌroobə'fayshənt) an

agent causing redness of the skin.

rubella (roo'belə) German measles. An acute, notifiable virus infection of short duration, characterised by PYREXIA, enlarged cervical lymph glands, and a transient rash. The greatest risk from this disease is to the offspring of mothers who contract it during the early weeks of pregnancy. The child can be born with cataract or deformities, be a deaf mute, or have other congenital defects.

rumination (ˌroomə'nayshən) recurring thoughts. *Obsessional r.* thoughts which persistently recur against the patient's will and from which he or she cannot be rid.

rupture ('rupchə) 1. tearing or bursting of a part, as in rupture of an aneurysm; of the membranes during labour; or of a tubal pregnancy. 2. a term commonly applied to refer to a hernia.

Ryle's tube ('rieəlz) *G.A. Ryle, British physician, 1889–1950.* A thin tube with a weighted end, introduced via the nose into the stomach. It can be used for the withdrawal of gastric contents or for the administration of fluids.

Ss

Sabin vaccine ('saybin) *A.B. Sabin, American biologist, 1906–93.* A live oral attenuated poliovirus vaccine active against poliomyelitis.

saccharide ('sakə,ried) one of a series of carbohydrates, including the sugars.

saccule ('sakyool) a small sac, particularly the smaller of the two sacs within the membranous labyrinth of the ear.

sacral ('saykrəl) relating to the sacrum.

sacroiliac (,saykroh'ili·ak) relating to the sacrum and the ilium.

sacrum ('saykrəm) a triangular bone composed of five united vertebrae situated between the lowest lumbar vertebra and the coccyx. It forms the back of the pelvis.

sadism ('saydizem) a form of sexual perversion in which the individual takes pleasure in inflicting mental and physical pain on others.

sagittal ('sajət'l) arrow-shaped. *S. suture* the junction of the PARIETAL bones.

salbutamol (sal'byootəmol) a sympathomimetic drug used in the treatment of bronchospasm.

salicylate (sə'lisə,layt) a salt of salicylic acid. *Methyl s.* the active ingredient in ointments and lotions for joint pains and sprains. *Sodium s.* the specific drug used for rheumatic fever. It reduces the PYREXIA and relieves the pain but does not prevent cardiac complications.

salicylic acid (,salə'silik) a drug with bacteriostatic and fungicidal properties used in the treatment of skin diseases and, in concentrated form, to remove warts and corns.

saline ('saylien, -een) a solution of sodium chloride and water. *Hypertonic s.* a stronger than normal strength. *Hypotonic s.* a weaker than normal strength. *Normal* or *physiological s.* a 0.9% solution which is isotonic with blood.

saliva (sə'lievə) the secretion of the salivary glands. When food is taken, it moistens and partially digests carbohydrates by the action of its enzyme, PTYALIN amylase.

salivary (sə'lievə·ree, 'saləvə·ree) relating to saliva. *S. calculus* a duct. *S. fistula* an abnormal opening on the skin of the face leading into a salivary duct or gland. *S. glands* the parotid, submaxillary, and sublingual glands.

salivation (,salə'vayshən) 1. the process of salivating. 2. excessive salivation which can lead to soreness of mouth and gums. Ptyalism.

Salk vaccine (sawlk) *J.E. Salk,*

American virologist, 1914–95. The first poliomyelitis vaccine of killed viruses, given by injection. *See* VACCINE.

Salmonella (ˌsalməˈnelə) any of the genus of Gram-negative, non-sporing, rod-like bacteria that are parasites of the intestinal tract of man and animals. *S. typhi* and *S. paratyphi* are exclusively human pathogens which cause typhoid and paratyphoid fevers.

salmonellosis (ˌsalmənəˈlohsəs) infection with the genus *Salmonella*, usually caused by the ingestion of food containing salmonellae or their products. The organisms can be found in raw meats, raw poultry, eggs, and dairy products; they multiply rapidly at temperatures between 7 and 46°C. Symptoms of salmonellosis include violent diarrhoea attended by abdominal cramps, nausea and vomiting, and fever. It is rarely fatal and can be prevented by adequate cooking.

salpingectomy (ˌsalpinˈjektəmee) excision of one or both of the uterine tubes.

salpingitis (ˌsalpinˈjietəs) 1. inflammation of the uterine tubes. *Acute s.* most often a bilateral ascending infection due to a streptococcus or a gonococcus. *Chronic s.* a less acute form that can be blood borne. 2. inflammation of the PHARYNGOTYMPANIC (Eustachian) tubes.

salpingography (ˌsalpingˈgogrəfee) radiographic examination of the uterine tubes after injection of a radio-opaque substance to determine their patency.

salpingo-oöphorectomy (salˌping-·gohoh·əfəˈrektəmee) removal of a uterine tube and its ovary.

salpingostomy (ˌsalpingˈgostəmee) the making of a surgical opening in a uterine tube near the uterus to restore patency.

salpinx (ˈsalpingks) a tube. Applied to the uterine or PHARYNGOTYMPANIC (Eustachian) tubes.

salt (solt, sawlt) 1. sodium chloride, common salt, used in solution as a cleansing lotion, a stimulating bath, or for infusion into the blood, etc. 2. any compound of an acid with an alkali or base. 3. a saline purgative such as Epsom salts. *S. depletion* a loss of salt from the body due to sweating, persistent diarrhoea, or vomiting. Common in hot climates where it can be prevented by the taking of salt tablets. *Smelling s's* aromatic ammonium carbonate. A restorative in fainting.

salve (salv, sahv) an ointment.

sample (ˈsahmpəl) 1. a selection of individuals made for research purposes from a larger population and intended to reflect that population in all significant aspects. 2. a small part of anything intended as representative of the whole, e.g. blood specimen. *Convenience s.* a nonprobability sampling strategy that uses the most readily accessible persons or objects as subjects in a study. *Nonprobability s.* a procedure in which elements are chosen by non-random methods. *Probability sampling* a procedure that uses some form of random selection when the sample units are chosen. *Purposive s.* a nonprobability sampling strategy in which the researcher selects subjects who are considered to be typical of the population. *Quota s.* a nonprobability sampling strategy that identifies the strata of the population and proportionately represents the strata in the sample. *Snowball effect s.* a strategy used for locating samples difficult to locate. It uses social network and the fact that friends tend to have characteristics in common; subjects who meet the eligibility criteria are asked for assistance in getting in touch with others who meet the same criteria. *Systematic s.* a probability sampling strategy that involves the selection of subjects randomly drawn from a population list at fixed intervals.

sandfly ('sand,flie) a very small fly of the genus *Phlebotomus*, common in tropical climates and the vector of most types of LEISHMANIASIS. *S. fever* a fever transmitted by the bites of sandflies and common in Mediterranean countries. Similar to DENGUE and sometimes known as 'three-day fever'.

sanguineous (sang'gwini·əs) pertaining to or containing blood.

saphena (sə'feenə) one of two superficial veins that carry blood from the foot upwards.

saphenous (sə'feenəs) relating to the saphena veins.

sapphism ('safizəm) female homosexuality; lesbianism.

sarcoid ('sahkoyd) 1. tuberculoid; characterised by non-caseating epithelioid cell tubercles. 2. pertaining to or resembling SARCOIDOSIS. 3. sarcoidosis.

sarcoidosis (,sahkoy'dohsəs) a chronic, progressive, generalised disease resembling tuberculosis which can affect any part of the body but most frequently involves the lymph nodes, liver, spleen, lungs, skin, eyes, and small bones of the hands and feet.

sarcoma (sah'kohmə) a malignant tumour developed from connective tissue cells and their stroma. *Chondro-s.* one arising in cartilage. *Fibro-s.* one containing much fibrous tissue; this can arise in the fibrous sheath of a muscle. *Kaposi's s.* one principally involving the skin, although visceral lesions can be present; it usually begins on the distal parts of the extremities, most often on the toes or feet, as reddish-blue or brownish soft nodules and tumours. It is viral in origin and is frequently seen in AIDS. *Melanotic s.* a highly malignant type pigmented with melanin. *Round-celled s.* a highly malignant growth composed of a primitive type of cell.

sarcomatosis (,sahkohmə'tohsəs) multiple sarcomatous growths in various parts of the body.

sarcomere (,sahkoy'miə) the smallest functional unit of a myofibril.

Sarcoptes (sah'kopteez) a genus of mites. *S. scabiei* the cause of scabies.

SARS (sahz) *See* SEVERE ACUTE RESPIRATORY SYNDROME

sartorius (sah'tor·ri·əs) a long muscle of the thigh which flexes both the thigh and the lower leg.

satyriasis (,satə'rieəsəs) abnormally excessive sexual appetite in men.

scab (skab) the crust on a superficial wound consisting of dried blood, pus, etc.

scabies ('skaybeez) 'the itch'; a contagious skin disease caused by the itch mite (Sarcoptes scabiei), the female of which burrows beneath the skin and deposits eggs at intervals. It is intensely irritating and the rash is aggravated by scratching. The sites affected are chiefly between the fingers and toes, the axillae, and groins.

scald ('skawld) a burn caused by hot liquid or vapour.

scale (skayl) 1. a scheme or instrument by which something can be measured. 2. a self-report inventory that provides a set of response symbols for each item. A rating or score is assigned to each response. A pair of scales is a balance for measuring weight. 3. compact layers of dead epithelial tissue shed from the skin. 4. to scrape deposits of tartar from the teeth.

scalenus (skə'leenəs) one of four muscles which move the neck to either side and raise the first and second ribs during inspiration. *S. syndrome* symptoms of pain and tenderness in the shoulder with sensory loss and wasting of the medial aspect of the arm. It can be caused by pressure on the brachial plexus, by spasm of the scalenus anterior muscle, or by a cervical rib.

scalp (skalp) the hairy skin that covers the cranium.

scalpel ('skalpəl) a small, pointed surgical knife with a convex edge to the blade.

scan (skan) an image produced using a moving detector or a sweeping beam of radiation, as in scintiscanning. B-mode ultrasonography, scanography, or computed tomography.

scanning ('skaning) 1. visual examination of an area. 2. a speech disorder that can be present in cerebellar disease. The syllables are inappropriately separated from each other and are evenly stressed with rhythmically occurring pauses between them.

scaphoid ('skayfoyd) boat-shaped. *S. bone* a boat-shaped bone of the wrist which articulates with the radius and with the trapezium and the trapezoid bones.

scapula ('skapyəla) the large flat triangular bone forming the shoulder-blade.

scar (skah) the mark left after a wound has healed with the formation of connective tissue.

scarification (ˌskarəfə'kayshən, ˌskair·ri-) the making of small cuts or punctures of the skin to allow a vaccine to enter the body.

scarlet fever ('skahlət) scarlatina; an acute, notifiable, rare, infectious disease of childhood. It is caused by group A beta-haemolytic streptococcus. There is sore throat, high fever, and a punctate rash. Now it is readily treated by antibiotics, and the complications of NEPHRITIS and middle ear infection are less common than used to be the case.

Schick test (shik) *B. Schick, Austrian paediatrician, 1877–1967.* A skin test of susceptibility to diphtheria. A small amount of diphtheria toxin is injected intradermally.

Schilling test ('shiling) *R.F. Schilling, American haematologist, b. 1919.* A test used to confirm the diagnosis of PERNICIOUS ANAEMIA by estimating the absorption of ingested radioactive vitamin B_{12}.

Schistosoma (ˌshistə'sohmə) a genus of minute blood flukes, some of which are parasitic in humans. *S. haematobium* a species which infests the urinary bladder; widely found in Africa and the Middle East, especially in Egypt. *S. japonicum* and *S. mansoni* species which infest the large intestine. They are found respectively in China, Japan, and the Philippines, and in Africa, the West Indies, and tropical America.

schistosomiasis (ˌshistəsoh'mieəsəs)

a parasitic infection of the intestinal or urinary tract by *Schistosoma.* The parasite enters the skin from contaminated water and causes diarrhoea, HAEMATURIA, and anaemia. The secondary hosts are freshwater snails. Bilharziasis.

schizoid ('skitsoyd) resembling schizophrenia. *S. personality* one that is marked by introspection, self-consciousness, solitariness, and a failure in affection towards others. Some schizophrenics have this personality, but only a few who are schizoid become schizophrenic.

schizophrenia (ˌskitsə'freeni·ə) a general term encompassing a large group of mental disorders (the schizophrenic disorders) characterised by mental deterioration from a previous level of functioning and disturbances of multiple psychological processes, including delusions, loosening of associations, poverty of the content of speech, auditory hallucinations, inappropriate affect, disturbed sense of self, and withdrawal from the external world. *Paranoid s.* predominance of delusions of a persecutory nature. *Simple s.* a progressive deterioration of the patient's efficiency with increasing social withdrawal. *See* HEBEPHRENIA and CATATONIA.

Schlemm's canal (shlemz) *F. Schlemm, German anatomist, 1795–1858.* A venous channel at the junction of the cornea and sclera for the draining of aqueous humour.

Schönlein–Henoch purpura or **syndrome** (ˌshərnlien'henok) *J.L. Schönlein, German physician, 1793–1864; E.H. Henoch, German paediatrician, 1820–1910. See* PURPURA.

Schwann cells (shwon) cells of ectodermal origin that compose the NEURILEMMA.

sciatica (sie'atikə) pain down the back of the leg in the area supplied by the sciatic nerve. It is usually caused by pressure on the nerve roots by a protrusion of an intervertebral disc.

scintigraphy (sin'tigrəfee) the recording of the distribution of radioactivity in an organ after injection of a small dose of a radioactive substance specifically taken up by that organ.

sclera ('skliə·rə) the fibrous coat of the eyball, the white of the eye, which covers the posterior part and in front becomes the cornea.

scleroderma (ˌskliə·roh'dərmə) a autoimmune disease marked by progressive hardening of the skin in patches or diffusely, with rigidity of the underlying tissues. It is often a chronic condition. *See* RAYNAUD'S PHENOMENON.

scleroma (sklə'rohmə) a patch of hardened tissue.

sclerosis (sklə'rohsəs) the hardening of any part from an overgrowth of fibrous and connective tissue, often due to chronic inflammation. *Amyotrophic lateral s.* rapid degeneration of the pyramidal (motor nerves) tract and anterior horn cells in the spinal cord. Characterised by weakness and spasm of limb muscles, with wasting of the muscle, difficulty with talking and swallowing. *Arterio-s.* the changes occurring in walls of arteries causing hardening and loss of elasticity. *Athero-s.* the deposition of fatty plaques and hardening and fibrosis of the artery lining. *Disseminated s. see* SCLEROSIS.

(multiple). *Mönckeberg's s.* extensive degeneration with atrophy and calcareous deposits in the middle muscle coat of arteries, especially of the small ones. *Multiple s.* scattered (disseminated) patches of degeneration in the nerve sheaths in the brain and spinal cord. Characterised by relapses and remissions. Symptoms include disturbances of speech, vision, micturition, and muscular weakness of a limb or limbs. *Systemic s.* (scleroderma) a generalised multisystem disease characterised by dense fibrosis of involved organs and a widespread vascular disorder. *See* RAYNAUD'S PHENOMENON.

sclerotherapy (ˌskleroh'therəpee) treatment of varicose veins and haemorrhoids by the injection of sclerosing solutions to produce fibrosis.

sclerotic (sklə'rotik) 1. hard; indurated; affected by sclerosis. 2. pertaining to the sclera of the eye. *S. coat* the tough membrane forming the outer covering of the eyeball, except in front of the iris where it becomes the clear horny cornea.

sclerotomy (sklə'rotəmee) incision of the sclerotic coat usually for the removal of a foreign body or for the relief of GLAUCOMA.

scoliosis (ˌskohli'ohsəs) lateral curvature of the spine. *See* LORDOSIS and KYPHOSIS.

scopolamine (skoh'poləˌmeen) HYOSCINE.

scorbutic (skaw'byootik) affected with or related to scurvy.

scotoma (skoh'tohmə) a blind area in the field of vision due to some lesion of the retina. It is also found in GLAUCOMA and in detachment of the retina.

screening ('skreening) 1. fluoroscopy. 2. the carrying out of a test on a large number of people to determine the proportion of them that have a particular disease.

scrotum ('skrohtəm) the pouch of skin and soft tissues containing the testicles.

scurf (skərf) dandruff.

scurvy ('skərvee) avitaminosis C. A deficiency disease caused by lack of vitamin C (which is found in raw fruits and vegetables). Clinical features of scurvy include fatigue, oozing of blood from the gums, and bruising. The condition rapidly improves with adequate diet.

seasonal affective disorder syndrome (ˌseezənəl əˌfektiv ˌdis'awdə ˌsinˌdrohm) a condition in which the person notices a change in mood or feelings according to the season of the year and hence the amount of exposure to (sun)light. SADS.

sebaceous (sə'bayshəs) fatty, or pertaining to the SEBUM. *S. cyst see* CYST. *S. glands* are found in the skin, communicating with the hair follicles and secreting sebum.

seborrhoea (ˌsebə'reeə) a disease of the sebaceous glands marked by an excessive secretion of sebum which collects on the skin in oily scales.

sebum ('seebəm) the fatty secretion of the sebaceous glands.

secondary ('sekəndree) second in order of time or importance. *S. deposits see* METASTASIS.

secretin (sə'kreetən) the hormone originating in the duodenum which, in the presence of bile salts, is absorbed into the bloodstream and stimulates the secretion of pancreatic juice.

secretion (sə'kreeshən) a substance formed or concentrated in a gland

and passed into the alimentary tract, the blood, or to the exterior. The secretions of the endocrine glands include various hormones and are important in the overall regulation of body processes.

sedation (sə'dayshən) the allaying of irritability or the relief of pain or mental distress, particularly by drugs.

sedative ('sedətiv) a drug or agent that lessens excitement and relieves tension. Sedative drugs are used to induce sleep.

sedentary ('sedəntree) pertaining to sitting; physically inactive.

sedimentation (ˌsedəmen'tayshən) the deposit of solid particles at the bottom of a liquid. *Erythrocyte s. rate* abbreviated ESR. *See* ERYTHROCYTE.

segregation (ˌsegrə'gayshən) the separation during meiosis of allelic genes as the chromosomes migrate towards opposite poles of the cell.

seizure ('seezhə) a sudden involuntary contraction of a group of muscles.

self (self) 1. a term used to denote an animal's own antigenic constituents, in contrast to 'not-self', denoting foreign antigenic constituents. 2. the complete being of an individual, comprised of physical and psychological characteristics and including conscious and unconscious components.

self-actualisation (selfˌakshooəlie'zayshən) a level of psychological development in which innate potential is realised to the full, allowing transcendence of the environment.

self-care (self'kair) the personal care carried out by the patient, e.g. bathing, personal grooming, eating, and toilet hygiene. This might require assistance or instruction from a healthcare worker. The aim of rehabilitative care is to maximise self-care and personal independence.

self-examination of breast *see* BREAST and BREAST SELF-EXAMINATION.

self-examination of testes *see* TESTICULAR SELF-EXAMINATION.

self-image (self'imij) an individual's concept of his or her own personality and abilities based on his or her own ideas and perceptions.

sella turcica (ˌselə 'tərsika) a depression in the sphenoid body which protects the pituitary gland.

semen ('seemən) the secretion of the testicles containing spermatozoa which is ejaculated from the penis during sexual intercourse. Seminal fluid.

semicircular (ˌsemee'sərkyələ) formed in a half-circle. *S. canals* part of the labyrinth of the internal ear consisting of three canals in the form of arches which contain fluid and are connected with the cerebellum by their nerve supply. Impressions of change of position of the body are registered in these canals by oscillation of the fluid, and are conveyed by the nerves to the CEREBELLUM.

semicomatose (ˌsemee'kohmatohs, -tohz) in a condition of unconsciousness from which the patient can be roused.

semilunar (ˌsemee'loonə) shaped like a half-moon. *S. cartilages* two crescent-shaped cartilages in the knee joint. *S. valve see* VALVE.

seminoma (ˌsemee'nohmə) a malignant tumour of the testis that is highly radiosensitive.

semipermeable (ˌsemee'pərmi·əbəl)

of a membrane, permitting the passage of some molecules and hindering that of others.

semiprone (ˌsemee'prohn) partly prone. Applied to a position in which the patient is lying face down but the knees are turned to one side.

senescence (sə'nesəns) the process of growing old.

Sengstaken–Blakemore tube (ˌsengztayken 'blaykmor) *R.W. Sengstaken, American neurosurgeon, b. 1923; A.H. Blakemore, American surgeon, 1879–1970.* A compression tube used in the treatment of bleeding oesophageal varices.

senile ('seeniel) related to the involutional changes associated with old age. *S. dementia* deterioration of mental activity in the elderly associated with an impaired blood supply to the brain.

senna ('senə) a laxative derived from the cassia plant. Proprietary standardised preparations are available as tablets or granules.

sensation (sen'sayshən) a feeling resulting from impulses sent to the brain by the sensory nerves.

sense (sens) the faculty by which conditions and properties of things are perceived, e.g. hunger or pain. *S. organ* one that receives a sensory stimulus, for instance, the eyes and ears. *Special s.* any one of the faculties of sight, hearing, touch, smell, taste, and muscle sense, through which the consciousness receives impressions from the environment.

sensible ('sensəbəl) 1. capable of being perceived. *S. perspiration* that obvious on the skin as moisture. 2. sensitive.

sensitisation (ˌsensətie'zayshən) 1. the process of rendering susceptible. 2. an increase in the body's response to a certain stimulus, as in the development of an allergy. *Protein s.* the condition occurring in an individual when a foreign protein is absorbed into the body, e.g. shellfish causing URTICARIA when eaten. *See* DESENSITISATION.

sensory ('sensə·ree) relating to sensation. *S. cortex* that part of the cerebral cortex to which information is relayed by the sensory nerves. *S. nerve* an afferent nerve conveying impression from the peripheral nerve endings to the brain or spinal cord.

sentiment ('sentəmənt) an emotion directed towards some object or person. Sentiments are acquired and profoundly influence a person's actions.

sepsis ('sepsəs) an infection of the body by pus-forming bacteria. *Focal s.* a local focus of infection which produces general symptoms. *Oral s.* infection of the mouth which causes general ill-health by absorption of toxins. *Puerperal s.* infection of the uterus occurring after labour.

septicaemia (ˌseptə'seemi·ə) the presence in the blood of large numbers of bacteria and their toxins. The symptoms are a rapid rise of temperature (which is later intermittent), rigors, sweating, and all the signs of severe fever.

septum ('septəm) a division or partition. *Atrial s., atrioventricular s., ventricular s.* the partitions dividing the various cavities of the heart. *Nasal s.* the structure made of bone and cartilage which separates the nasal cavities.

sequela (sə'kweelə) a morbid

condition occurring after a disease and resulting from it.

sequestrum (sə'kwestrəm) a piece of dead bone. Inflammation in bone leads to THROMBOSIS of blood vessels resulting in necrosis of the affected part, which separates from the living structure.

serological (ˌsiə·rə'lojikəl) relating to serum. *S. tests* those that are dependent on the formation of antibodies in the blood as a response to specific organisms or proteins.

serology (siə'roləjee) the scientific study of serum.

serosa (sə'rohsə) a serous membrane. It consists of two layers: the visceral (in close contact with the organ) and the parietal (lining the cavity).

serotonin (ˌsiə·roh'tohnən, ˌserə-) an amine present in blood platelets, the intestine, and the central nervous system, which acts as a vasoconstrictor. It is derived from the amino acid tryptophan and is inactivated by monoamine oxidase.

serous ('siə·rəs) related to serum. *S. effusion* an effusion of serous exudate.

serum ('siə·rəm) the clear, fluid residue of blood from which the corpuscles and fibrin have been removed. *S. hepatitis* jaundice caused by hepatitis B virus, usually after a blood transfusion or an inoculation with contaminated material. *S. sickness* an allergic reaction usually 8–10 days after a serum injection. It can be manifested as an irritating urticaria, pyrexia, and painful joints. It readily responds to adrenaline and antihistaminic drugs. *See* ANAPHYLAXIS.

sessile ('sesiel) attached by a base.

severe acute respiratory syndrome (SARS) (səˌviər əˌkyoot rə'spirətree ˌsindrohm; sahz) (SARS) a disease which had it origins in Guangdong Province, China. Caused by a newly characterised *Coronavirus*, it is marked by severe pneumonitis with cough or breathlessness, high fever (greater than 38°C), one of more positive assays for SARS *CoV*, and an appropriate travel or contact history. Transmission of SARS appears to be by close person-to-person contact with respiratory secretions or infected body fluids of a known or suspected case of SARS. Healthcare facilities should ensure effective infection-control standards to minimise risk to other patients and healthcare employees.

sex (seks) 1. either of the two divisions of organic organisms described respectively as male and female. *S. chromosome* a chromosome that determines sex. Women have two X chromosomes and men have one X chromosome and one Y chromosome. *S. hormone* a steroid hormone produced by the ovaries or the testes and controlling sexual development. *S.-limited* pertaining to a characteristic found in only one sex. *S.-linked* pertaining to a characteristic that is transmitted by genes that are located on the sex chromosomes, e.g.HAEMOPHILIA. 2. to discover the sex of an organism.

sexual ('sekshooəl) pertaining to sex. *S. development* the biological and psychosocial changes that lead to sexual maturity. *S. deviation* aberrant sexual activity; expression of the sexual instinct in practices which are socially prohibited or unacceptable, or biologically undesirable.

sexuality (ˌsekshoo'alətee) 1. the characteristic quality of the male and female reproductive elements.

2. the constitution of an individual in relation to sexual attitudes and behaviour.

sexually transmitted disease ('sekshooəlee) abbreviated STD. An infectious disease is transmitted by means of sexual intercourse (heterosexual or homosexual) or by intimate contact with the genitals, mouth, and rectum. STDs include syphilis, gonorrhoea, human immuno-deficiency virus (HIV) infection, chlamydial infection, genital herpes, non-specific urethritis, trichomoniasis, genital lice, scabies, genital warts, hepatitis B infection, and yaws.

SGOT serum glutamic-oxalacetic transaminase, an enzyme excreted by damaged heart muscle. A raised serum level occurs in MYOCARDIAL INFARCTION.

SGPT serum glutamic-pyruvic transaminase, an enzyme excreted by the parenchymal cells of the liver. There is a raised blood level in infectious hepatitis.

sheath (sheeth) 1. an enveloping tubular structure or part. 2. a condom worn on the erect penis during sexual intercourse to trap seminal fluid with a view to: (i) preventing the transmission of organisms that cause sexually transmitted diseases and/or (ii) reducing the risk of pregnancy.

shiatsu (shee'atsoo) a form of manipulation in which the practitioner uses the thumbs, fingers, and palms of the hands, knees, forearms, elbows, and feet to apply pressure to the client's body in order to promote and maintain health.

Shigella (shi'gelə) a genus of Gram-negative rod-like bacteria. Some species cause bacillary dysentery. *S. flexneri* and *S. shiga* are common in Asia, *S. dysenteriae* in the USA and *S. sonnei* in Western Europe.

shin (shin) the bony front of the leg below the knee. The tibia.

shingles ('shing·gəlz) HERPES ZOSTER.

Shirodkar's operation (shi'rodkəz) *Shirodkar, Indian obstetrician.* A 'purse-string' suture that is placed round an incompetent cervix during pregnancy to prevent abortion. It is removed at the 38th week.

shock (shok) a condition produced by severe illness or trauma in which there is a sudden fall in blood pressure. This leads to lack of oxygen in the tissues and greater permeability of the capillary walls, so increasing the degree of shock by greater loss of fluid. The patient has a cold, moist skin, a feeble pulse, and a low blood pressure, and is distressed, thirsty, and restless. *Allergic* or *anaphylactic s.* shock produced by the injection of a protein to which the patient is sensitive. *Cardiogenic s.* shock as a result of an acute heart condition such as MYOCARDIAL INFARCTION. *Hypovolaemic s.* shock resulting from a reduction in the volume of blood in the circulation after haemorrhage or severe burns. *Neurogenic s.* shock due to nervous or emotional factors. *Shell s.* a psychoneurotic condition caused by the stresses of warfare.

short-sightedness (ˌshawt'sietədnəs) MYOPIA.

shoulder ('shohldə) the junction of the clavicle and the scapula where the arm joins the body. *S. lift see* AUSTRALIAN LIFT.

show (shoh) the blood-stained discharge that occurs at the onset of labour.

shunt (shunt) a diversion, particularly of blood, due to a congenital defect, disease, or surgery.

SIADH syndrome of inappropriate antidiuretic hormone secretion.

sialography (ˌsieə'logrəfee) radiographic examination of the salivary ducts after the introduction of a radio-opaque contrast medium.

sialolith ('sieəlohˌlith) a salivary calculus.

sibilant ('sibələnt) hissing or whistling.

sibling ('sibling) one of a family of children having the same parents. Applied in psychology to one of two or more children of the same parent or substitute parent figure. *S. rivalry* jealousy, compounded of love and hate of one child for its sibling.

sickle-cell anaemia ('sikəl) an inherited blood disease. *See* ANAEMIA.

siderosis (ˌsidə'rohsəs) 1. chronic inflammation of the lung due to inhalation of particles of iron. 2. excess iron in the blood. 3. the deposit of iron in the tissues.

SIDS (sidz) sudden infant death syndrome.

sigmoid ('sigmoyd) shaped like the Greek letter Σ. *S. colon* or *flexure* that part of the colon in the left iliac fossa just above the rectum.

sigmoidoscope (sig'moydəˌskohp) an instrument by which the interior of the rectum and sigmoid colon can be seen.

sign (sien) 1. any objective evidence of disease or dysfunction. 2. an observable physical phenomenon so frequently associated with a given condition as to be considered indicative of its presence. *S. language* hand and body language used by totally deaf people to communicate with others. *Vital s's* the signs of life, namely pulse, respiration, and temperature.

silicosis (ˌsilə'kohsəs) fibrosis of the lung due to the inhalation of silica dust particles. It occurs in miners, stonemasons, and quarry workers.

Sims' position (simz) *J.M. Sims, American gynaecologist, 1813–83.* A semiprone position. *See* POSITION.

sinew ('sinyoo) a tendon or ligament.

sinoatrial (ˌsienoh'aytri·əl) situated between the SINUS venosus and the atrium of the heart. *S. node* the pacemaker of the heart. *See* NODE.

sinus ('sienəs) 1. a cavity in a bone. *Air s.* a cavity in a bone containing air. *Ethmoidal s.* air spaces in the ethmoid bone. *Frontal s.* air spaces in the frontal bone. *Sphenoidal s.* air spaces in the sphenoid bone. 2. a venous channel, especially within the cranium. *S. arrhythmia see* ARRHYTHMIA. *Cavernous s.* a venous sinus of the DURA MATER which lies along the body of the sphenoid bone. *Coronary s.* the vein that returns the blood from the heart muscle into the right atrium. *S. thrombosis* clotting of blood in a cranial venous channel. In the lateral sinus it is a complication of MASTOIDITIS 3. an unhealed passage leading from an abscess or internal lesion to the surface.

sinusitis (ˌsienə'sietəs) inflammation of the lining of a sinus, especially applied to the bony cavities of the face.

sinusoid ('sienəˌsoyd) like a sinus. Used to describe the irregular channels by which blood vessels anastomose in certain organs, such as the liver and suprarenal glands.

skeleton ('skelətən) the bony framework of the body, supporting and protecting the organs and soft tissues.

Skene's gland (skeenz) one of a pair of glands which open into the posterior urethral orifice in the female.

skin (skin) the outer protective covering of the body. It consists of an outer layer, the epidermis or cuticle, and an inner layer, the dermis or CORIUM, which is known as 'true skin'. *S. grafting* transplantation of pieces of healthy skin to an area where loss of surface tissue has occurred. *S. patch* a drug-impregnated adhesive patch which is applied to the skin. The drug is slowly absorbed, allowing its level in the blood to be maintained over a given period of time. *S. test* application of a substance to the skin, or intradermal injection of a substance, to permit observation of the body's reaction to it.

skull (skul) the bony framework of the head consisting of the cranium and facial bones.

sleep (sleep) a period of rest for the body and mind during which volition and consciousness are in partial or complete abeyance and the bodily functions partially suspended. It occurs in a 24-hour biological rhythm. Sleep occurs in cycles which have two distinct phases. Each phase lasts approximately 60–90 min: orthodox or non-rapid eye movement sleep (NREM), and paradoxical or rapid eye movement sleep (REM).

sleeping sickness ('sleeping) TRYPANOSOMIASIS. A tropical fever occurring in parts of Africa caused by a protozoal parasite (Trypanosoma) which is conveyed by the tsetse fly.

slipped disc (slipt) a prolapsed intervertebral disc which causes pressure on the spinal nerves. It can be very painful.

slit lamp ('slit ˌlamp) a special light source so arranged with a microscope that examination of the interior of the eye can be carried out at the level of each layer.

slough (sluf) dead tissue caused by injury or inflammation. It separates from the healthy tissue and is ultimately washed away by exuded serum leaving a granulating surface.

smallpox ('smawlˌpoks) variola. Eradicated from the world in 1980. Smallpox vaccination is no longer required for travellers to any part of the world.

smear (smiə) a specimen for microscopic examination that has been prepared by spreading a thin film of the material across a glass slide.

smegma ('smegmə) the secretion of sebaceous glands of the clitoris and prepuce.

Smith-Petersen nail (ˌsmith-'peetəsən) *M.N. Smith-Petersen, American surgeon, 1886–1953.* A metal nail used to fix the fragments of bone in intracapsular fracture of the head of the femur (*see* figure).

smoking ('smohking) the act of drawing into the mouth and puffing out the smoke of tobacco contained in a cigarette, cigar, or pipe. Close relationships between smoking and lung cancer, heart disease, bronchitis, and emphysema have been definitely established. Smoking is also harmful in pregnancy because the inhaled carbon monoxide reduces oxygen transportation in the body and the nicotine causes vasoconstriction of the arterioles.

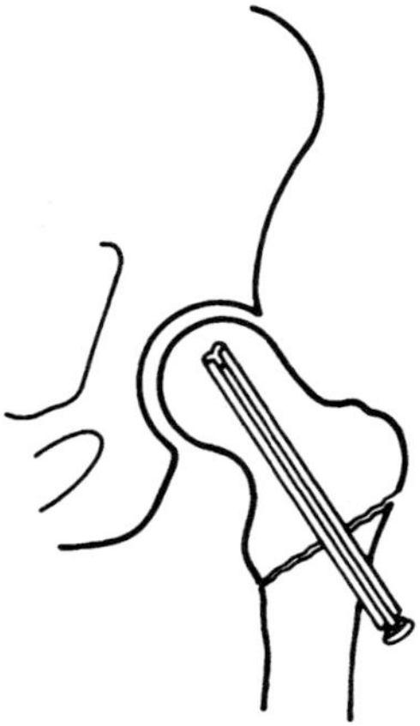

Smith-Petersen Nail

The result is a diminished supply of food and oxygen to the fetus leading to fetal growth retardation.

snake (snayk) a limbless reptile; a serpent. The bites of many snakes are poisonous to humans. *S. venom antitoxin* antivenin. A serum made from animals, usually horses, which have been immunised against the venom of a specific type of snake.

Snellen's test letters ('snelənz) *H. Snellen, Dutch ophthalmologist, 1834–1908.* Square-shaped letters on a chart used for sight testing.

snow (snoh) frozen water vapour. *S. blindness* photophobia due to the glare of snow. *Carbon dioxide s.* solid CO_2 which is used as a refrigerant; 'dry ice'.

snuffles ('snufəlz) a chronic discharge from the nose occurring in children as a result of infection of the nasal mucous membrane.

social class ('sohshəl) a category arising from the division of society into economic or occupational groupings.

social worker ('sohshəl ˌwərkə) a professional trained in the treatment of individual and social problems of patients and their families.

socialisation (ˌsohshəlie'zayshən) the process by which society integrates the individual, and the individual learns to behave in socially acceptable ways.

sociology (ˌsohsee'oləjee) the scientific study of the development of man's social relationships and organisation, i.e. interpersonal and intergroup behaviour as distinct from the behaviour of an individual.

sociopath ('sohseeohˌpath) a person with an antisocial personality; a psychopath.

sodium ('sohdi·əm) *symbol* Na. A metallic alkaline element widely distributed in nature and forming an important constituent of animal tissue. *S. aminosalicylate* an antituberculous drug used in conjunction with streptomycin and isoniazid. *S. bicarbonate* an antacid widely used to treat digestive disorders, especially flatulence. Repeated use can cause ALKALOSIS. *S. chloride* common salt. Its presence in the diet is necessary to health. *S. citrate* compound used to prevent clotting of blood during blood transfusions. *S. cromoglycate* a drug used as an inhalant in the treatment of asthma. *S. fluoride* a salt used in the fluoridation of water and also in toothpastes to prevent the formation of caries. *S. hydroxide* caustic soda. A powerful corrosive drug used to destroy warts. It can cause severe chemical burns. *S. hypochlorite* a compound with germicidal properties used in solution to disinfect utensils, and diluted as a topical antibacterial agent. *S. phosphate* a purgative. *S. salicylate* an antipyretic drug used in the treatment of rheumatic fever. *S. sulphate* a purgative; also used in 25% solution as a wound dressing. *S. valproate* a drug used in the treatment of epilepsy.

solar plexus ('sohlə) coeliac plexus. A network of sympathetic nerve ganglia in the abdomen; the nerve supply to abdominal organs below the diaphragm.

solute ('solyoot) a substance that is dissolved in a solution.

solution (sə'looshən) a liquid in which one or more substances have been dissolved.

solvent ('solvənt) a liquid that dissolves or has power to dissolve. *S. abuse see* ABUSE.

soma ('sohmə) 1. the body as distinct from the mind. 2. the body tissue as distinct from the germ cells.

somatic (sə'matik) 1. relating to the body as opposed to the mind. 2. relating to the body wall as distinct from the viscera.

somnambulism (som'nambyə-ˌlizəm) walking and carrying out other complex activities during a state of sleep.

Somogyi effect (soh'mohgee) *M. Somogyi, American biochemist, 1883–1971*. A rebound phenomenon occurring in DIABETES mellitus; overtreatment with insulin induces HYPOGLYCAEMIA resulting in rebound HYPERGLYCAEMIA and KETOSIS.

sorbitol ('sawbətˌtol) a sweetening agent which is converted into sugar in the body although it is slowly absorbed from the intestine. It is used in some diabetic foods and in intravenous feeding.

sordes ('sawdeez) brown crusts which form on the teeth and lips of unconscious patients, or those suffering from acute or prolonged fevers.

sore (sor) a general term for any ulcer or open skin lesion. *Cold s.* herpes simplex. *Hard s.* a syphilitic chancre. *Pressure s.* a sore caused by pressure from the bed (decubitus ulcer) or a splint. *Soft s.* a chancroid ulcer. *S. throat* inflammation of the larynx or pharynx including tonsillitis.

souffle ('soofəl) a blowing sound heard on auscultation. *Uterine s.* is due to the blood passing through the uterine arteries of the mother, particularly over the placental site. It is synchronous with the maternal pulse.

sound (sownd) an instrument shaped like a probe for exploring cavities, detecting the presence of foreign bodies, or dilating a stricture.

spasm ('spazəm) a sudden involuntary muscle contraction. *Carpopedal s.* spasm of the hands and feet. A sign of tetany. *Clonic s.* alternate muscle rigidity and relaxation. *Habit s.* a tic. *Nictitating s.* spasmodic twitching of the eyelid. *Tetanic s.* violent muscle spasms, including OPISTHOTONOS. *Tonic s.* a sustained muscle rigidity.

spasmolytic (ˌspazmə'litik) a drug that reduces spasm.

spastic ('spastik) 1. caused by spasm; convulsive. *S. colon* irritable bowel syndrome. *S. paralysis* paralysis associated with lesions of the upper motor neurone, as in cerebral vascular accidents, and characterised by increased muscle tone and rigidity. 2. one affected by spasticity, often applied to persons suffering from congenital paralysis due to some cerebral lesion or impairment.

spasticity (spa'stisətee) marked rigidity of muscles.

spatial ('spayshəl) pertaining to space.

spatula ('spatyələ) 1. a flexible, blunt blade used for spreading ointment. 2. a rigid blade-shaped instrument for depressing the tongue in throat examination, etc.

specific (spə'sifik) 1. relating to a species. 2. a remedy that has a distinct curative influence on a particular disease, e.g. quinine in malaria. 3. related to a unit mass of a substance. *S. gravity* the density of fluid compared with that of an equal volume of water.

specimen ('spesəmən) a sample or part taken to show the nature of the whole, e.g. for chemical testing or microscopic survey.

spectacles ('spektəkəlz) a frame containing lenses worn in front of the eyes to correct errors of vision or to protect from glare.

spectrometer (spek'tromətə) an instrument for measuring the strength and wavelengths of visible or invisible electromagnetic radiations.

spectroscope ('spektrə͵skohp) an instrument used for analysing the spectra of light and other radiations.

speech (speech) the act of communicating by sounds by means of a linguistic code. *Clipped s.* speech in which the words are cut short. *Deaf s.* the characteristic utterance of people with severe hearing loss. *Explosive s.* loud, sudden utterances; a sign of mental disorder. *Incoherent s.* disconnected utterances made when the sequence of thought is disturbed, as in delirium. *Oesophageal s.* speech produced after LARYNGECTOMY by swallowing air and using it to vibrate within the oesophagus against the closed cricopharyngeal spincter. *S. pathologist* a professional trained to identify, assess, and rehabilitate persons with speech or language disorders, learning difficulties, and feeding difficulties. *Scanning s.* speech in which the syllables are inappropriately separated from each other and are evenly stressed. Characteristic of cerebellar damage. *Staccato s.* speech in which each syllable is separately pronounced. Characteristic of multiple sclerosis.

sperm (spərm) 1. a spermatozoon. 2. the semen.

spermatocele ('spərmətoh͵seel) a cystic swelling in the EPIDIDYMIS containing semen.

spermatozoon (͵spərmətoh'zoh·ən) a mature male germ cell consisting of a flat-shaped head, a short middle part, and a long tail. There are 300–500 billion spermatozoa in a normal ejaculate.

spermicide ('spərmə͵sied) any agent that will destroy SPERMATOZOA.

sphenoid ('sfeenoyd) wedge shaped. *S. bone* the central part of the base of the skull.

spherocytosis (͵sfiə·rohsie'tohsəs) the presence in the blood of erythrocytes that are more nearly spherical than biconcave. Characteristic of ACHOLURIC jaundice, it can also be hereditary.

sphincter ('sfingktə) a ring-shaped muscle, contraction of which closes a natural orifice.

sphincterectomy (ˌsfingktə'rektəmee) 1. the excision of a sphincter. 2. in ophthalmology, an operation to free the sphincter of the iris when it has become attached to the back of the cornea.

sphygmic ('sfigmik) relating to the pulse.

sphygmocardiograph (ˌsfigmoh'kahdeeəˌgrahf, -ˌgraf) an instrument that records both the pulse waves and the heart beat.

sphygmograph ('sfigmohˌgrahf, -ˌgraf) an instrument which registers graphically the force and character of the arterial pulse.

sphygmomanometer (ˌsfigmohmə'nomətə) an instrument for measuring the arterial blood pressure.

spica ('spiekə) a bandage applied to a joint in a series of 'figures of eight'.

spigot ('spigət) a small plastic peg to close the opening of a tube.

spina ('spienə) spine; a slender, thorn-like projection that occurs on many bones. *S. bifida* a congenital defect of non-union of one or more vertebral arches, allowing protrusion of the meninges and possibly their contents. *See* MENINGOCELE and MENINGOMYELOCELE.

spinal ('spienəl) relating to the spine. *S. anaesthesia see* ANAESTHESIA. *S. canal* the hollow in the spine formed by the neural arches of the vertebrae. It contains the spinal cord, meninges, and cerebrospinal fluid. *S. caries* disease of the vertebrae, usually tuberculous. *See* POTT'S DISEASE. *S. column* the backbone; the vertebral column. *S. cord see* CORD. *S. curvature* abnormal curving of the spine. If associated with caries, it is known as Pott's disease. *See* KYPHOSIS, LORDOSIS, and SCOLIOSIS. *S. jacket* a support for the spine, made of plaster of Paris or other material, used to give rest after injury to or operation on the spine. *S. nerves* the 31 pairs of nerves which leave the spinal cord at regular intervals throughout its length. They pass out in pairs, one on either side between each of the vertebrae, and are distributed to the periphery. *S. puncture* lumbar or cisternal puncture.

spine (spien) 1. the backbone or vertebral column consisting of 33 vertebrae, separated by fibrocartilaginous discs and enclosing the spinal cord. 2. a sharp process of bone.

spinnbarkeit ('spinbahˌkiet) [Ger.] a thread of mucus secreted by the cervix uteri. Used to determine ovulation because this usually coincides with the time at which the mucus can be drawn out on a glass slide to its maximum length.

spirochaete ('spieraˌkeet) one of a group of microorganisms in the form of a spiral, some of which are found in impure fresh or salt water. The group includes the species *Treponema*, *Borrelia*, and *Leptospira*.

spirograph ('spieraˌgrahf, -ˌgraf) an instrument for registering respiratory movements.

spirometer (spie'romətə, spi'rom-) an instrument for measuring the air capacity of the lungs.

spironolactone (ˌspierənoh'laktohn) a diuretic drug used when there is excess secretion of aldosterone. It promotes the excretion of sodium and water but the retention of potassium.

Spitz–Holter valve (ˌspits 'holtə) *Spitz, American engineer; J.W. Holter, American engineer.* A device used in the treatment of HYDROCEPHALUS to drain the cerebrospinal fluid from the ventricles into the superior vena cava or the right atrium.

splanchnic ('splangknik) pertaining to the viscera. *S. nerves* sympathetic nerves to the viscera.

spleen (spleen) a large, vascular, gland-like but ductless organ, coloured a reddish purple and situated in the left HYPOCHONDRIUM under the border of the stomach. It manufactures lymphocytes and breaks down red blood cells.

splenectomy (splə'nektəmee) excision of the spleen.

splenomegaly (ˌspleenoh'megəlee) enlargement of the spleen.

splenorenal (ˌspleenoh'reenəl) relating to the spleen and the kidney. *S. anastomosis* an operation carried out to treat portal hypertension. The spleen is excised and the splenic vein is inserted into the renal vein.

splint (splint) an appliance used to support or immobilise a part while healing takes place, or to correct or prevent deformity.

spondylitis (ˌspondə'lietəs) inflammation of the vertebrae. *Ankylosing s.* a rheumatic disease, chiefly of young males, in which there is abnormal ossification with pain and rigidity of the intervertebral, hip, and sacroiliac joints.

spondylolisthesis (ˌspondəlohlis'theesəs) a sliding forwards or displacement of one vertebra over another, usually the 5th lumbar over the sacrum, causing symptoms such as low back pain as a result of pressure on the nerve roots.

spondylosis (ˌspondə'lohsəs) ANKYLOSIS of the vertebral joints usually caused by a degenerative disease of the intervertebral discs such as OSTEOARTHRITIS.

spongioblastoma (ˌspunjeeohbla'stohmə) a rapidly growing brain tumour that is highly malignant. A GLIOMA.

spontaneous (spon'tayni·əs) occurring without apparent cause. Applied to certain types of fracture and to recovery from a disease without any specific treatment.

sporadic (spə'radik) pertaining to isolated cases of a disease that occurs in various and scattered places (compare endemic and epidemic).

spore (spaw) 1. a reproductive stage of some of the lowest forms of vegetable life, e.g. moulds. 2. a protective state which some bacteria are able to assume in adverse conditions such as lack of moisture, food, or heat. In this form, the organism can remain alive but inert for years.

spotted fever ('spotəd) a febrile disease characterised by a skin eruption, such as Rocky Mountain spotted fever, boutonneuse fever, and other infections due to tick-borne RICKETTSIAE.

sprain (sprayn) wrenching of a joint, producing laceration of the capsule or stretching of the ligaments with consequent swelling which is due to effusion of fluid into the affected part.

sprue (sproo) a disease of malabsorption in the intestine which can be tropical or non-tropical in form. There is STEATORRHOEA, diarrhoea, glossitis, and anaemia.

sputum ('spyootəm) material expelled from the air passages through the mouth. It consists chiefly of mucus and saliva, but in diseased conditions of the air passages it can be purulent, blood-stained, and frothy, and can contain many bacteria. It must always be regarded as highly infectious. *Rusty s.* that in which altered blood permeates the mucus. Characteristic of acute lobar pneumonia.

squamous ('skwayməs) scale. *S. bone* the thin part of the temporal bone which articulates with the parietal and frontal bones. *S. cell carcinoma* a malignancy of the squamous cells of the skin or bronchus. *S. epithelium* epithelium composed of flat and scale-like cells.

squint (skwint) *see* STRABISMUS.

stability (stə'bilətee) an instruments ability to produce the same results with repeated testing.

staging ('stayjing) 1. the determination of distinct phases or periods in the course of a disease. 2. the classification of neoplasms according to the extent of the tumour. *TNM s.* staging of tumours according to three basic components: primary tumour (T), regional nodes (N), and metastasis (M). Subscripts are used to denote size and degree of involvement; for example, 0 indicates undetectable, and 1, 2, 3, and 4 indicate progressive increase in size or involvement.

stammering ('staməˑring) stuttering; a speech disorder in which the utterance is broken by hesitation and repetition or prolongation of words and syllables.

standard deviation (ˌstandəd ˌdeeveey'ayshən) (Σ) a measure of the dispersion of a random variable: the square root of the average squared deviation from the mean. For data that have a normal distribution, about 68% of the data points fall within 1 standard deviation from the mean and about 95% fall within 2 standard deviations.

standard error of the mean the standard deviation of a theoretical distribution of sample means. It indicates the average error in the estimation of the population mean.

standard precautions (prə'kawshənz) guidelines recommended by the National Health and Medical Research Council (NHMRC) or Centres for Disease Control and Prevention (United States of America). Standard precautions are work practices required for a basic level of infection control. They include: (a) good hygiene practices (particularly washing and drying hands before and after patient contact); (b) the use of protective barriers (which can include gloves, gowns, plastic aprons, masks, eye shields, or goggles); (c) appropriate handling and disposal of sharps and other contaminated or infectious waste; and (d) use of aseptic techniques (*See* Appendix 12).

standards ('standədz) statements of the levels of service or care related to specific topics which staff agree to provide. Often accompanied by a description of the structure (staff, equipment, etc.) and process needed to attain specified observable outcomes.

stapedectomy (ˌstaypi'dektəmee) removal of the STAPES and insertion of a vein graft or other device to re-establish conduction of sound waves in OTOSCLEROSIS.

stapediolysis (stəˌpeedee'oləsəs) an operation in which the footpiece of the stapes is mobilised to aid conduction in deafness from OTOSCLEROSIS.

stapes ('staypeez) the stirrup-shaped bone of the middle ear.

Staphylococcus (ˌstafəloh'kokəs) a genus of Gram-positive non-mobile bacteria which under the microscope appear grouped together in small masses like bunches of grapes. They are normally present on the skin and mucous membranes. *S. pyogenes* (or S. aureus) is a common cause of boils, carbuncles, and abscesses.

staphyloma (ˌstafə'lohmə) a protrusion of the cornea or the sclerotic coat of the eyeball as a result of inflammation or a wound.

stasis ('staysəs) the stagnation or stoppage of the flow of a fluid. *Intestinal s.* sluggish movement of faeces through the bowel owing to partial obstruction or to impairment of the action of the intestinal muscles. *Venous s.* congestion of blood in the veins.

statistics (ˌstə'tistiks) 1. numerical facts pertaining to a particular subject or body of objects. 2. the science dealing with the collection, tabulation, and analysis of numerical facts.

status (ˌstaytəs) condition. *S. asthmaticus* a severe and prolonged attack of asthma. *S. epilepticus* a condition in which there is rapid succession of epileptic fits. *S. lymphaticus* a condition in which all lymphatic tissues are hypertrophied, especially the thymus gland.

STD sexually transmitted disease.

steapsin (stee'apsən) the fat-splitting enzyme (lipase) of the pancreatic juice.

steatoma (stie'tohma) 1. a sebaceous cyst. 2. a LIPOMA; a fatty tumour.

steatorrhoea (ˌstiətə'reeə) the presence of an excess of fat in the stools due to malabsorption of fat by the intestines.

steatosis (stiə'tohsəs) fatty degeneration.

Steinmann pin ('stienmən) *F. Steinmann, Swiss surgeon, 1872–1932.* A fine metal rod passed through a bone by which extension is applied to overcome muscle contraction in certain fractures. *See* KIRSCHNER WIRE.

stellate ('stelayt) star shaped. *S. fracture* a radiating fracture of the patella. *S. ganglion* the inferior cervical ganglion. A star-shaped collection of nerve cells at the base of the neck.

stenosis (stə'nohsəs) abnormal narrowing or contraction of a channel or opening. *Aortic s.* narrowing of the opening of the aortic valve due to scar tissue formation as the result of inflammation. *Mitral s.* narrowing of the orifice of the mitral valve, usually following rheumatic fever. *Pulmonary s.* a congenital narrowing of the opening from the right ventricle of the heart into the pulmonary artery. *Pyloric s.* narrowing of the pyloric orifice of the stomach due to scar tissue, new growth, or congenital hypertrophy.

Stensen's duct ('stensənz) *H. Stensen, Danish physician, 1638–86.* The duct of the parotid gland opening into the mouth opposite the second upper molar.

stercobilin (ˌstərkoh'bielən) a brown-orange pigment derived from bile and present in faeces.

stereognosis (ˌstereeog'nohsəs, ˌstiə-) the ability to visualise the shape of an object by touch alone.

stereotypy ('stereeohˌtiepee, 'stiə-)

repetitive actions carried out or maintained for long periods in a monotonous fashion.

Sterets (ste'rets) a proprietary brand of swabs impregnated with 70% isopropyl alcohol. These swabs are rubbed on to a skin site before an injection.

sterile ('steriel) 1. aseptic; free from microorganisms. 2. barren; incapable of producing young.

sterility (stə'rilətee) 1. the state of being free from microorganisms. 2. the inability of a woman to become pregnant, or of a man to produce potent SPERMATOZOA.

sterilisation (ˌsterəlie'zayshən) 1. rendering dressings, instruments, etc. aseptic by destroying or removing all microbial life. 2. rendering incapable of reproduction by any means.

steriliser ('sterəˌliezə) an apparatus in which objects can be sterilised. *See* AUTOCLAVE.

Steri-Strips ('steriˌstrips) proprietary skin closure strips which are placed across a wound. A final strip is placed on either side parallel to the wound.

sternotomy (stər'notəmee) the operation in which the sternum is cut through to enable the heart to be reached.

sternum ('stərnəm) the breastbone; the flat narrow bone in the centre of the anterior wall of the thorax.

steroid ('steroyd, 'stiə-) one of a group of hormones chemically related to cholesterol. They include oestrogen, androgen, progesterone, and the corticosteroids. They can be naturally occurring or synthetic.

sterol ('sterol, 'stiə·rol) one of a group of steroid alcohols which includes cholesterol and ergosterol.

stertorous ('stərtə·rəs) snore-like; applied to a snoring sound produced in breathing during sleep or in coma.

stethoscope ('stethəˌskohp) an instrument used for listening to internal body sounds, especially from the heart and lungs. It consists of a hollow tube, one end of which is placed over the part to be examined and the other at the ear of the examiner.

Stevens–Johnson syndrome (ˌsteevənz'jonsən) *A.M. Stevens, American paediatrician, 1884–1945; F.C. Johnson, American paediatrician, 1894–1934.* A severe form of ERYTHEMA multiforme in which the lesions can involve the oral and anogenital mucosa, eyes, and viscera, associated with such constitutional symptoms as malaise, headache, fever, ARTHRALGIA, and conjunctivitis.

stigma ('stigmə) 1. a small spot or mark on the skin. 2. any mark characteristic of a condition or defect, or of a disease. It refers to visible signs rather than symptoms.

stilboestrol (stil'beestrol) a synthetic oestrogen preparation used in the treatment of cancer of the prostate and less commonly for postmenopausal breast cancer.

stillbirth ('stilˌbərth) a baby which has issued forth from its mother after the 24th week of pregnancy and has not, at any time after being completely expelled from its mother, breathed or shown any sign of life.

Still's disease (stilz) *Sir G.F. Still, British paediatrician, 1868–1941.* A form of rheumatoid arthritis in children, sometimes associated with enlargement of the lymph glands.

stimulant ('stimyələnt) an agent that

causes increased energy or functional activity of any organ.

stimulus ('stimyələs) *pl. stimuli* (L.) any agent, act or influence that produces functional or trophic reaction in a receptor or an irritable tissue. *Conditioned s.* a neutral object or event that is psychologically related to a naturally stimulating object or event and which causes a CONDITIONED RESPONSE (*see also* CONDITIONING). *Discriminative s.* a stimulus associated with reinforcement which exerts control over a particular form of behaviour; the subject discriminates between closely related stimuli and responds positively only in the presence of that stimulus. *Eliciting s.* any stimulus, conditioned or unconditioned, that elicits a response. *Structured s.* a well-organised and unambiguous stimulus, the perception of which is influenced to a greater extent by the characteristics of the stimulus than by those of the perceiver. *Threshold s.* a stimulus that is just strong enough to elicit a response. *Unconditioned s.* any stimulus that is capable of eliciting an unconditioned response (*see also* CONDITIONING). *Unstructured s.* an unclear or ambiguous stimulus, the perception of which is influenced to a greater extent by the characteristics of the perceiver than by those of the stimulus.

stitch (stich) 1. a popular term used to describe a sudden sharp pain usually due to spasm of the diaphragm or other internal abdominal organ. 2. a suture. *S. abscess* pus formation where a stitch has been inserted.

Stokes–Adams syndrome (ˌstohks-'adəmz) *Sir W. Stokes, Irish surgeon, 1804–78; R. Adams, Irish physician, 1791–1875.* Attacks of SYNCOPE or fainting due to cerebral hypoxia as a result of cardiac arrhythmia, especially complete heart block. It is treated by using an artificial pacemaker.

stoma ('stohmə) 1. a mouth or mouth-like opening. 2. an artificial opening in the skin surface leading into one of the tubes forming the alimentary canal. *See* COLOSTOMY and ILEOSTOMY.

stomach ('stumək) the dilated portion of the alimentary canal between the oesophagus and the duodenum, just below the diaphragm. *Bilocular* or *hourglass s.* one divided into two parts by a constriction. *Leather bottle s.* induration and thickening of the gastric wall, usually the result of malignant disease. *S. pH electrode* apparatus used to measure gastric contents in situ. *S. pump* one that removes the contents of the stomach by suction. *S. tube* a flexible tube used for washing out the stomach or for the administration of liquid food.

stomatitis (ˌstohmə'tietəs) inflammation of the mouth, either simple or with ulceration caused by vitamin deficiency, or by bacterial or fungal infection. *Angular s.* cracking at the corners of the mouth usually due to riboflavin deficiency. *Aphthous s.* that characterised by small, white, painful ulcers on the mucous membrane. *Ulcerative s.* painful shallow ulcers on the tongue, cheeks, and lips. A severe type that can produce serious constitutional effects.

stone (stohn) a CALCULUS.

stool (stool) a motion or discharge

from the bowels. *Fatty s.* that which contains undigested fat. *Hunger s.* stool passed by underfed infants: frequent, small, and green. *Rice-water s.* the water stool containing small white flakes seen in cholera. *Tarry s.* a black tarry stool due to the presence of blood from high in the gastrointestinal tract (such as from a peptic ulcer or oesophageal varices). MELAENA.

strabismus (strə'bizməs) squint; HETEROTROPIA. A deviation of the eye from its normal direction. It is called 'convergent' when the eye turns in towards the nose, and 'divergent' when it turns outwards. *Concomitant s.* a squint in which the angle of deviation stays constant.

strabotomy (strə'botəmee) the division of ocular muscles in the treatment of STRABISMUS.

strain (strayn) 1. overuse or stretching of a part, e.g. a muscle or tendon. 2. a group of microorganisms within a species. 3. to pass a liquid through a filter.

strangulated ('strang·gyə,laytəd) compressed or constricted so that the circulation of the blood is arrested. *S. hernia see* HERNIA.

strangulation (,strang·gyə'layshən) 1. choking caused by compression of the air passages. 2. arrested circulation to a part, which results in GANGRENE.

strangury ('strang·gyə,ree) a painful, frequent desire to micturate, but in which only a few drops of urine are passed with difficulty.

stratified ('stratə,fied) arranged in layers. *S. tissue* a covering tissue in which the cells are arranged in layers. The germinating cells are the lowest and, as surface cells are shed, there is continual replacement.

stratum ('strahtəm, 'stray-) a layer; applied to structures such as the skin and mucous membranes. *S. corneum* the outer, horny layer of the epidermis.

Streptococcus (,streptə'kokəs) a genus of Gram-positive spherical bacteria occurring in chains or pairs. Divided into various groups. The first group includes the beta-haemolytic human and animal pathogens; the second and third include alpha-haemolytic parasitic forms occurring as normal flora in the body; and the fourth is made up of saprophytic forms. *S. mutans* implicated in dental caries. *S. pneumoniae* pneumococcus, the most common cause of lobar pneumonia; also causes serious forms of meningitis, septicaemia, empyema, and peritonitis. *S. pyogenes* beta-haemolytic, toxigenic, pyogenic streptococci causing septic sore throat, scarlet fever, rheumatic fever, PUERPERAL fever, and acute GLOMERULONEPHRITIS.

streptokinase (,streptə'kienayz) an enzyme derived from a streptococcal culture and used to liquefy clotted blood and pus.

Streptomyces (,streptoh'mieseez) a genus of soil bacteria from which a large number of antibiotics are derived.

streptomycin (,streptə'miesən) an antiobiotic drug derived from *Streptomyces griseus*; used particularly in the treatment of tuberculosis when treatment is combined with other drugs to reduce drug resistance.

stress (stres) any factor, mental or physical, the pressure of which can adversely affect the functioning of the body. *S. disorders* those resulting from an individual's inability to withstand stress. *S. incontinence* incontinence, usually of urine, when the intra-abdominal pressure is raised, such as in coughing, sneezing, or laughing.

stria ('strieə) *pl.* striae. A line or stripe. *Striae gravidarum* the lines that appear on the abdomen of pregnant women. They are red in first pregnancy but white subsequently, and are due to stretching and rupture of the elastic fibres.

striated (strie'aytəd) striped. *S. muscle* voluntary muscle. *See* MUSCLE.

stricture ('strikchə) a narrowing or local contraction of a canal. It can be caused by muscle spasm, new growth, or scar tissue formation after inflammation.

stridor ('striedaw) a harsh, vibrating, shrill sound, produced during respiration when there is partial obstruction of the larynx or trachea.

stroke (strohk) a popular term to describe the sudden onset of symptoms, especially those of cerebral origin. *Apoplectic s.* cerebral haemorrhage. *Heat s.* a HYPERPYREXIA accompanied by cerebral symptoms. It can occur in someone newly arrived in a very hot climate.

stroma ('strohmə) the connective tissue forming the ground substance, framework, or matrix of an organ, as opposed to the functioning part or PARENCHYMA.

Strongyloides (stronjə'loydeez) a genus of nematode worms, one of which, *S. stercoralis*, is common in tropical countries and causes diarrhoea and intestinal ulcers.

strontium ('stronti·əm) *symbol* Sr. A metallic element. Isotopes of strontium are used in bone scanning to detect abnormalities. *S.-90* a radioactive isotope used in radiotherapy in the treatment of skin and eye malignancies.

strychnine ('strikneen) a highly poisonous alkaloid made from the seeds of *Strychnos nux-vomica.* Formerly used in small amounts in 'tonics'.

Stryker frame ('striekə) an apparatus especially designed for care of patients with injuries of the spinal cord or paralysis. It is constructed of pipe and canvas and is designed so that one nurse can turn the patient without difficulty.

stupor ('styoopə) a state of semi-unconsciousness occurring in the course of many varieties of mental illness in which the patient does not move or speak, and makes no response to stimuli.

Sturge–Weber syndrome (ˌstərj-'webə) *W.A. Sturge, British physician, 1850–1919; Sir H.D. Weber, British physician, 1824–1918.* A congenital abnormality in which there is a port wine stain on the face with an ANGIOMA of the meninges on the same side. Common symptoms are epilepsy, HEMIPLEGIA, and associated learning difficulties.

stuttering ('stutə·ring) *see* STAMMERING.

stye *see* HORDEOLUM.

stylet ('stielət) a wire or rod for keeping clear the lumen of catheters, cannulae, and hollow needles.

styloid ('stieloyd) like a pen. *S. process* a long pointed spine, particularly one projecting from the temporal bone. Also processes on the ulna and radius.

styptic ('stiptik) an astringent which,

applied locally, arrests haemorrhage, e.g. alum and tannic acid.

subacute (ˌsubəˈkyoot) moderately acute. Between ACUTE and CHRONIC.

subarachnoid (ˌsubəˈraknoyd) below the arachnoid. *S. space* between the arachnoid and pia mater of the brain and spinal cord; contains cerebrospinal fluid.

subclavian (subˈklayvi·ən) beneath the clavicle. *S. artery* the main vessel of supply to the neck and arms.

subclinical (subˈklinikəl) without clinical manifestations; said of the early stages or a very mild form of a disease.

subconscious (subˈkonshəs) 1. not conscious yet able to be recalled to consciousness. 2. in psychoanalysis, the part of the mind that retains memories which cannot, without much effort, be recalled to mind.

subcutaneous (ˌsubkyooˈtayni·əs) beneath the skin. *S. injection* one given hypodermically.

subdural (subˈdyoo·rəl) below the DURA MATER. *S. haematoma* a blood clot between the arachnoid and dura mater. It can be acute or arise slowly from a minor injury.

subinvolution (ˌsubinvəˈlooshən) incomplete or delayed return of the uterus to its pregravid size during the PUERPERIUM, usually as the result of retained products of conception and infection.

subjective (səbˈjektiv) related to the individual. *S. symptoms* those of which the patient is aware by sensory stimulation, but which cannot easily be seen by others. *See also* OBJECTIVE.

sublimate (ˈsubləˌmayt) a substance obtained by sublimation.

sublimation (ˌsubləˈmayshən) 1. the vaporisation of a solid and its condensation into a solid deposit. 2. in psychoanalysis, a redirecting of energy at an unconscious level. The transference into socially acceptable channels of tendencies that cannot be expressed. An important aspect of maturity.

subliminal (subˈlimənəl) below the threshold of perception.

sublingual (subˈling·gwəl) beneath the tongue. *S. glands* two small salivary glands in the floor of the mouth.

subluxation (ˌsublukˈsayshən) partial dislocation of a joint.

submaxillary (ˌsubmakˈsilə·ree) beneath the lower jaw. *S. glands* two salivary glands situated under the lower jaw.

submucous (subˈmyookəs) beneath mucous membrane. *S. resection* an operation to correct a deflected nasal septum.

subnormal (subˈnawməl) below normal.

subphrenic (subˈfrenik) beneath the diaphragm. *S. abscess* one that develops below the diaphragm usually after peritonitis or from postoperative infection.

substitution (ˌsubstəˈtyooshən) the act of putting one thing in place of another. In psychology, this might be the nurse or foster mother in the place of the child's own mother. In psychotherapy, the nurse or therapist might be substituted for someone in the patient's background.

substrate (ˈsubstrayt) a substance on which an enzyme acts.

succus (ˈsukəs) a juice. *S. entericus* a digestive fluid secreted by intestinal glands. *S. gastricus* gastric juice.

succussion (su'kushən) a method of determining when free fluid is present in a cavity in the body. A sound of splashing is heard when the patient moves or is deliberately moved.

sucrose ('sookrohz, -ohs) a disaccharide obtained from cane or beet sugar.

suction ('sukshən) 1. the process of sucking. 2. the removal of gas or fluid from a cavity or other container by means of reduced pressure. *Post-tussive s.* a sucking noise heard in the lungs just after a cough.

sudamen (soo'daymən) a small white vesicle formed in the sweat glands after prolonged sweating.

sudden infant death syndrome (sudən) abbreviated SIDS. The sudden and unexpected death of an apparently healthy infant, typically occurring between the ages of 3 weeks and 5 months, and not explained by careful postmortem studies. Called 'crib death' or 'cot death' because the infant is often found dead in the cot.

sudor ('syoodaw) sweat; perspiration.

sudorific (ˌsyoodə'rifik) DIAPHORETIC; an agent causing sweating.

suffocation (ˌsufə'kayshən) asphyxiation; a cessation of breathing caused by occlusion of the air passages causing unconsciousness and, ultimately, to death.

suffusion (sə'fyoozhən) a process of diffusion or overspreading, as in flushing of the skin; blushing.

sugar ('shuhgə) a group of sweet carbohydrates classified chemically as monosaccharides or disaccharides. The following are included: *beet s.* obtained from sugar beet; *cane s.* obtained from sugar cane; *fructose* fruit sugar; *grape s.* dextrose, glucose; *milk s.* lactose. *Muscle s.* INOSITOL; a sugar-like compound found in animal tissue, particularly in muscle, and also in many plant tissues.

suggestibility (səˌjestə'bilətee) inclination to act on suggestions of others.

suggestion (sə'jeschən) a tool of psychotherapy in which an idea is presented to, and accepted by, a patient. *Posthypnotic s.* one implanted in a patient under hypnosis which lasts after his or her return to normal condition.

suicide ('sooəˌsied) the taking of one's own life; also any person who voluntarily and intentionally takes his or her own life. Legally, a death suspected of being due to violence that is self-inflicted is not termed a suicide unless the victim leaves positive evidence of the intention to take his or her own life, or the method of death is such that a verdict of suicide is inevitable. Some religious faiths consider it to be a sin and can refuse a consecrated burial.

sulcus ('sulkəs) a furrow or fissure; applied especially to those of the brain.

sulphacetamide (ˌsulfə'setəˌmied) a soluble sulphonamide used as eyedrops to treat corneal and conjunctival infections.

sulphadiazine (ˌsulfə'dieəˌzeen) a slow-acting sulphonamide drug which is relatively non-toxic. Used in the treatment of MENINGOCOCCAL MENINGITIS.

sulphadimidine (ˌsulfə'diemәˌdeen) a sulphonamide with which a high blood level can be obtained with fewer side-effects. Used in the treatment of urinary tract infections.

sulphafurazole (ˌsulfə'fyoo·rəzohl) a soluble, rapidly excreted sulphonamide.

sulphaguanidine (ˌsulfə'gwahnəˌdeen) a mild sulphonamide used in the treatment of bacillary dysentery.

sulphamethizole (ˌsulfə'methəˌzohl) a sulphonamide used in urinary infection because it is rapidly excreted in an active form.

sulphasalazine (ˌsulfə'saləˌzeen) a sulphonamide used in the treatment of ulcerative colitis.

sulphonamide (sul'fonəˌmied) the generic term for all aminobenzenesulphonamide preparations, including the bactericidal sulpha drugs.

sulphone ('sulfohn) one of a group of drugs which, with prolonged use, have been successful in treating leprosy. Dapsone is the most widely used.

sulphonylurea (ˌsulfonə'lyoo·ri·ə) one of a group of oral hypoglycaemic agents used in the treatment of DIABETES mellitus.

sulthiame (sul'thieˌaym) an anticonvulsant drug used in the treatment of epilepsy.

sunburn ('sunˌbərn) a dermatitis due to exposure to the sun's rays causing burning and redness.

sunstroke ('sunˌstrohk) a profound disturbance of the body's heat-regulating mechanism caused by prolonged exposure to excessive heat from the sun. Persons over 40 and those in poor health are most susceptible to it.

superego (ˌsoopə'reegoh, -'regoh) that part of the personality that is concerned with moral standards and ideals that are derived unconsciously from parents, teachers, and the environment, and which influence a person's whole mental make-up, acting as a control on impulses of the ego.

superfecundation (ˌsoopəˌfekən-dayshən, -ˌfee-) the fertilisation of two or more ova produced during the same menstrual cycle by SPERMATOZOA from separate coital acts.

superfetation (ˌsoopəfee'tayshən) the fertilisation of a second ovum when pregnancy has already started, producing two fetuses of different maturity.

superior (soo'piə·ri·ə) above; the upper of two parts.

supine ('soopien) 1. lying on the back, with the face upwards. 2. the turning of the palm of the hand upwards. *See* PRONATION.

suppository (sə'pozətree) a medicated solid substance prepared for insertion into the rectum or vagina which will dissolve at body temperature.

suppression (sə'preshən) 1. complete cessation of a secretion. *S. of urine* no secretion of urine by the kidneys. 2. in psychology, conscious inhibition as distinct from repression, which is unconscious.

suppuration (ˌsupyə'rayshən) the formation of pus.

supracondylar (ˌsooprə'kondələ) above the condyles. *S. fracture* one above the lower end of the humerus or femur.

supraorbital (ˌsooprə'awbət'l) above the orbit of the eye.

suprapubic (ˌsooprə'pyoobik) above the pubic bones. *S. cystotomy* surgical incision of the urinary bladder just above the pubic bones.

suprarenal (ˌsooprə'reenəl) above the kidney. *S. gland* adrenal gland. One of a pair of triangular endocrine glands situated on the upper surface of the kidneys. *See* ADRENAL.

surfactant (sər'faktənt) a surface-active agent. A mixture of phospholipids that is secreted into the pulmonary alveoli and reduces the surface tension of pulmonary fluids, thus contributing to the elastic properties of pulmonary tissue. Surfactant can be instilled via a tracheal catheter as treatment for respiratory distress syndrome. *See also* RESPIRATORY distress syndrome of newborn.

surgeon ('sərjən) a medical practitioner who specialises in surgery.

surgery ('sərjə·ree) the branch of medicine that treats disease by operative measures.

surrogate ('surəgət) a real or imaginary substitute for a person or object in someone's life. *S. mother* a woman who carries a child for another (the commissioning parent) with the intention that the child be handed over after birth.

survey ('sərˌvay) the systematic collection of information, not forming part of a scientific epidemiological study.

susceptibility (səˌseptə'bilətee) lack of resistance to infection. The opposite to immunity.

suspensory (sə'spensə·ree) supporting a part. *S. bandage* one applied to support a part of the body, particularly the scrotum or the lower jaw. *S. ligament* a ligament that supports or suspends an organ, e.g. that of the lens of the eye.

suture ('soochə) 1. a stitch or series of stitches used to close a wound (*see* figure). *Atraumatic s.* a suture fused to the needle to obtain a single thickness through each puncture of the needle. *Continuous s.* a form of oversewing with one length of suture. *Everting s.* a type of mattress stitch that turns the edges outwards to give a closer approximation. *Fascial s.* a strip of fascia taken from the patient and used to form a suture. *Interrupted s.* a series of separate sutures. *Mattress s.* one in which each suture is taken twice through the wound, giving a loop one side and a knot the other. *Purse-string s.* a circular continuous suture around a small wound or appendix stump. *Subcuticular s.* a continuous suture placed just below the skin. *Tension s.* or *relaxation s.* one taking

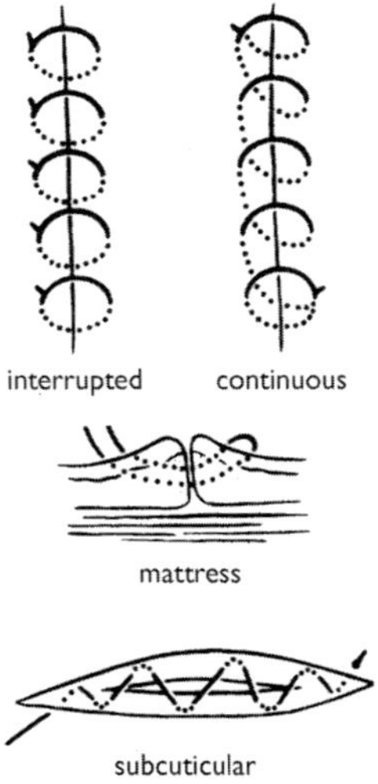

Sutures

a large bite and relieving the tension on the true stitch line. 2. the jagged line of junction of the bones of the cranium. *Coronal s.* the junction between the frontal and parietal bones. *Lambdoid s.* the junction between the parietal and occipital bones. *Saggital s.* the junction between the two occipital bones.

suxamethonium (ˌsuksəmee'thohni·əm) a short-acting muscle-relaxant drug which can be used to get good muscle relaxation during surgery performed under general anaesthesia and during electroconvulsive therapy.

swab (swob) 1. a small piece of cotton wool or gauze. 2. in pathology, a dressed stick used in taking bacteriological specimens.

swallowing ('swoloh·ing) the taking in of a substance through the mouth and pharynx and into the oesophagus. It is a combination of a voluntary act and a series of reflex actions. Once begun, the process operates automatically. Called also deglutition.

Swan-Ganz catheter (ˌswon'gants) a flow-directed, balloon-tipped catheter passed through the right side of the heart to be positioned in the pulmonary vasculature.

sweat (swet) perspiration; a clear watery fluid secreted by the sweat glands. *S. glands* coiled tubular glands situated in the dermis with long ducts to the skin surface.

sycosis (sie'kohsəs) a pustular inflammation of the hair follicles, usually of the beard and moustache.

Sydenham's chorea ('sidənəmz) *T. Sydenham, British physician, 1624–89.* A disorder of the central nervous system closely linked with rheumatic fever; also called 'Saint Vitus' dance'. The condition, usually self-limited, is characterised by purposeless, irregular movements of the voluntary muscles that cannot be controlled by the patient.

symbiosis (ˌsimbie'ohsəs) in parasitology, an intimate association between two different organisms for the mutual benefit of both.

symblepharon (sim'blefə·ron) adhesion of an eyelid to the eyeball.

symbolism ('simbəˌlizəm) in psychology, an abnormal mental condition in which events or objects are interpreted as symbols of the patient's own thoughts. In psychiatry, the re-entry into consciousness of repressed material in an acceptable form.

sympathectomy (ˌsimpə'thektəmee) division of autonomic nerve fibres which control specific involuntary muscles. An operation performed for many conditions, among them RAYNAUD'S DISEASE.

sympathetic (ˌsimpə'thetik) 1. exhibiting sympathy. *S. ophthalmia* inflammation leading to loss of sight in the opposite eye after a perforating injury in the ciliary region. 2. relating to the autonomic nervous system. *S. nervous system* one of the two divisions of the autonomic nervous system. It supplies involuntary muscle and glands; it stimulates the ductless glands and the circulatory and respiratory systems but inhibits the digestive system.

sympatholytic (ˌsimpəthə'litik) pertaining to drugs that oppose the action of the sympathetic nervous system.

sympathomimetic (ˌsimpəthəmi'metik) pertaining to drugs that produce effects similar to those caused by a stimulation of the sympathetic nervous system.

symphysis ('simfisəs) a cartilaginous joint along the line of union of two bones. *S. pubis* the cartilaginous junction of the two pubic bones.

symptom ('simptəm) any indication of disease perceived by the patient. *Cardinal s's* 1. symptoms of greatest significance to the doctor, establishing the identity of the illness. 2. the symptoms associated with temperature, pulse, and respiration. *Dissociation s.* anaesthesia to pain and to heat and cold, without impairment of tactile sensibility. *Objective s.* one perceptible to others than the patient, such as pallor, rapid pulse or respiration, restlessness, etc. *Presenting s.* the symptom or group of symptoms about which the patient complains or from which relief is sought. *Signal s.* a sensation, aura, or other subjective experience indicative of an impending epileptic or other seizure. *Subjective s.* one perceptible only to the patient, such as pain, pruritus, vertigo, etc. *Withdrawal s's* symptoms that follow sudden abstinence from a drug on which a person is dependent.

symptomatology (ˌsimptəmə'toləjee) 1. the study of the symptoms of a disease. 2. the symptoms of a particular disease taken together.

synalgia (si'nalji·ə) pain felt in one part of the body but caused by inflammation of or injury to another part. Referred pain.

synapse ('sienaps) the junction between the termination of an axon and the dendrites of another nerve cell. Chemical transmitters pass the impulse across the space.

syncope ('singkəpee) a simple faint or temporary loss of consciousness due to cerebral ischaemia, often caused by dilatation of the peripheral blood vessels and a sudden fall in blood pressure.

syndactylism (sin'daktəˌlizəm) possessing webbed fingers or toes. A condition in which two or more fingers or toes are joined together.

syndrome ('sindrohm) a group of signs or symptoms typical of a distinctive disease which frequently occur together and form a distinctive clinical picture.

synechia (si'neeki·ə) adhesion of the iris to the cornea in front (anterior s.) or the capsule of the lens behind (posterior s.).

synergist ('sinəjəst, si'nər-) 1. a muscle that works in conjunction with another muscle. 2. a drug that works in combination with another drug, the two drugs having a greater effect when taken together than when taken separately.

synovectomy (ˌsienoh'vektəmee, ˌsi-) excision of a diseased synovial membrane to restore joint movement.

synovial fluid (sie'nohvi·əl, si-) the fluid that surrounds a joint and is secreted by the synovial membrane. It is a thick, colourless, lubricating substance.

synovial membrane (sie'nohvi·əl 'membrayn, si-) a serous membrane lining the articular capsule of a movable joint and terminating at the edge of the articular cartilage.

synovitis (ˌsienə'vietəs) inflammation of a synovial membrane usually with an effusion of fluid within the joint.

synthesis ('sinthəsəs) the building up of a more complex structure from simple components. This can apply to drugs or to plant or animal tissues.

syphilis ('sifələs) an infectious venereal disease leading to many structural and cutaneous lesions; called also lues. Syphilis is caused by a spiral-shaped bacterium (spirochaete), *Treponema pallidum.* It is a SEXUALLY TRANSMITTED DISEASE, with the exception of congenital syphilis acquired by an infant from the mother in utero. There is an early infectious stage followed by a latent period of many years before the non-infectious late stage when serious disorders of the nervous and vascular systems arise. *Congenital s.* that transmitted by the mother to the fetus; it is preventable if the mother receives a full course of penicillin during her pregnancy. *Non-venereal s.* a chronic treponemal infection mainly seen in children, occurring in many areas of the world, caused by an organism indistinguishable from *Treponema pallidum* and transmitted by direct non-sexual contact. Lesions are usually oral mucous patches; subsequent lesions occur in the axillae, inguinal region, and rectum. Then, after a latent period, destructive lesions of the skin and bones develop.

syringe (si'rinj) an instrument for injecting fluids or for aspirating or irrigating body cavities. It consists of a hollow tube with a tight-fitting piston. A hollow needle or a thin tube can be fitted to the end.

syringomyelia (si,ring·gohmie'eeli·ə) the formation of cavities filled with fluid inside the spinal cord. Impairment of muscle function and sensation result at the level of and below the lesion. Painless injury can be the first symptom. It is a progressive disease.

syringomyelitis (si,ring·goh,mieə-'lietəs) inflammation of the spinal cord, as the result of which cavities are formed in it.

syringomyelocele (si,ring·goh-'mieəloh,seel) a type of SPINA BIFIDA in which the protruded sac of fluid communicates with the central canal of the spinal cord.

systemic (si'stemik) pertaining to or affecting the body as a whole. *S. circulation* circulation of the blood throughout the whole body, other than the pulmonary circulation. *See* SCLEROSIS.

systole ('sistəlee) the period of contraction of the heart. *See* DIASTOLE. *Atrial s.* the contraction of the heart by which the blood is pumped from the atria into the ventricles. *Extra-s.* a premature contraction of the atrium or ventricle, without alteration of the fundamental rhythm of the pacemaker. *Ventricular s.* the contraction of the heart by which the blood is pumped into the aorta and pulmonary artery.

systolic (si'stolik) relating to a systole. *S. murmur* an abnormal sound produced during systole in heart affections. *S. pressure* the highest pressure of the blood reached during systole.

Tt

T symbol for *thymine*.

T cell ('tee ˌsel) a lymphocyte which is derived from the thymus and is responsible for cell-mediated immunity.

t statistic ('tee stə'tistik) commonly used in nursing research; it tests whether two group means are more different than would be expected by chance. Groups can be related or independent.

TAB typhoid-paratyphoid A and B vaccine. A sterile suspension of the killed salmonellae causing these diseases. Used as a preventive, it provides an active immunity.

tabes ('taybeez) a wasting away. *T. dorsalis* LOCOMOTOR ATAXIA. A slowly progressive disease of the nervous system affecting the posterior nerve roots and spinal cord. It is a late manifestation of syphilis.

taboo (ˌtə'boo) any ritual prohibition of certain activities, e.g. incest in many societies, or the open discussion of death and dying.

taboparesis (ˌtaybohpə'reesəs) the presence of the symptoms of both tabes dorsalis and general paralysis of the insane in a patient suffering from late syphilis.

tachycardia (ˌtakee'kahdi·ə) abnormally rapid action of the heart and consequent increase in pulse rate. *See* BRADYCARDIA. *Paroxysmal t.* spasmodic increase in cardiac contractions of sudden onset lasting a variable time from a few seconds to hours.

tachyphasia (tachyphrasia) (ˌtakee'fayzi·ə; ˌtakee'frayzi·ə) extreme volubility of speech. It can be a sign of mental disorder.

tachyphrenia (ˌtakee'freeni·ə) hyperactivity of the mental processes.

tachypnoea (ˌtakip'neeə) rapid, shallow respirations; a reflex response to stimulation of the VAGUS nerve endings in the pulmonary vessels.

tactile ('taktiel) relating to the sense of touch.

Taenia ('teeniə) a genus of tapeworms. *T. saginata* the beef tapeworm. The most common type of tapeworm found in the human intestine. *T. solium* the pork tapeworm. Can also be parasitic in man, causing CYSTICERCOSIS. *See* TAPEWORM.

taeniacide ('teeni·əˌsied) an agent that is lethal to tapeworms.

taeniafuge ('teeni·əˌfyooj) a drug that expels tapeworms.

taeniasis (tee'nieəsəs) an infestation with tapeworms.

TAF toxoid-antitoxin floccules. A

vaccine used for diphtheria immunisation. *See* TOXOID.

t'ai chi (ˌtie'chee) system of movement, Chinese in origin, promoting general health and wellbeing.

talipes ('taləpeez) clubfoot. A deformity caused by a congenital or acquired contraction of the muscles or tendons of the foot. *T. calcaneous* the heel alone touches the ground on standing. *T. equinus* the toes touch the ground but not the heel. *T. valgus* the inner edge of the foot only is in contact with the ground. *T. varus* the person walks on the outer edge of the foot.

talus ('tayləs) the ASTRAGALUS or ankle bone.

tampon ('tampon) a plug of absorbent material inserted in the vagina, the nose, or other orifice to restrain haemorrhage or absorb secretion.

tamponade ('tampəˌnayd) the surgical use of tampons. *Cardiac t.* impairment of heart action by haemorrhage or effusion into the pericardium; can be due to a stab wound or can follow surgery.

tantalum ('tantələm) *symbol* Ta. Metallic element used for prostheses and wire sutures.

tantrum ('tantrəm) an outburst of ill temper. *Temper t.* a behaviour disorder of childhood. A display of bad temper in which the child performs uncontrolled actions in a state of emotional stress.

tapeworm ('taypwərm) any of a group of cestode flatworms including the *Taenia* genus which are parasitic in the intestines of humans and many animals. The adult consists of a round head with suckers or hooklets for attachment (scolex). From this, numerous segments (proglottids) arise, each of which produces ova capable of independent existence for a considerable length of time. Treatment is by ANTHELMINTIC drugs.

tapotement (ˌtapoht'monh) [Fr.] a tapping movement used in massage.

tapping ('taping) *see* PARACENTESIS.

tarsal ('tahsəl) relating to a tarsus. *T. bones* the seven small bones of the ankle and instep. *T. cyst* MEIBOMIAN cyst; CHALAZION. *T. glands* meibomian glands of the eyelids. *T. plates* small cartilages in the upper and lower eyelids.

tarsalgia (tah'salji·ə) pain in the foot, usually associated with flattening of the arch.

tarsorrhaphy (tah'so·rəfee) stitching of the eyelids together to protect the cornea or to allow healing of an abrasion.

tartar ('tahtə) a hard incrustration deposited on the teeth and on dentures. *T. emetic* antimony potassium tartrate. A salt used in the treatment of SCHISTOSOMIASIS and LEISHMANIASIS.

task allocation ('tahsk ˌaləkayˌshən) a method of organising care whereby each specific type of care is carried out by a separate nominated nurse, e.g. for the same patient, one nurse records the blood pressure and another nurse gives the prescribed medications.

taste (tayst) the sense by which it is possible to identify what is eaten and drunk. Taste receptors (buds) lie on the tongue and give the sensations of sweet, sour, salt, and bitter.

tattoo (ta'too) a permanent discolouration of the skin due to a foreign pigment.

taxis ('taksəs) manipulation by hand to restore any part to its normal position. It can be used to reduce a hernia or a dislocation.

taxonomy (tak'sonəmee) the theory and practice of the classification of animals and plants.

Tay–Sachs disease (ˌtay'saks) *W. Tay, British physician, 1843–1927; B. Sachs, American neurologist, 1858–1944. See* AMAUROTIC (familial idiocy).

team nursing ('teem ˌnərsing) a method of organising care based on the allocation of each nurse to a team that cares for a group of patients, usually for a number of shifts.

tears (tiəz) the watery, slightly alkaline and saline secretion of the lacrimal glands that moistens the conjunctiva.

teat (teet) 1. a nipple of the breast. 2. a manmade nipple used on infants' feeding bottles.

technetium (tek'neeshi·əm) *symbol* Tc. A metallic element. *Radioactive t.* isotope (^{99m}Tc) used in a number of diagnostic tracer tests. Because it has a short half-life (6 hours), a large dose can be given for scanning organs, but the patient receives only a low radiation dose.

teeth (teeth) *see* DENTITION.

tegument ('tegyəmənt) the skin.

tela ('teelə) a web-like tissue. *T. choroidea* the fold of PIA MATER containing a network of blood vessels found in the ventricles of the brain from which the cerebrospinal fluid originates.

telangiectasis (təˌlanjee'ektəsəs) a group of dilated capillary blood vessels, weblike or radiating in form.

telangioma (təˌlanjee'ohmə) a tumour of the blood capillaries.

telepathy (tə'lepəthee) the transmission of thought without any normal means of communication between two persons.

telereceptor (ˌteleerə'septə) a sensory nerve ending which can respond to distant stimuli. Those of the eyes, ears, and nose are examples. Teleceptor.

telophase ('telohˌfayz) the last stage in the division of cells when the chromosomes have been reconstituted in the nuclei at either end of the cell and the cell cytosplasm divides to form two new cells.

temperature ('temprəchə) the degree of heat of a substance or body as measured by a thermometer. *Normal t.* of the human body is 37°C, with a slight decrease in the early morning and a slight increase at night. It indicates the balance between heat production and heat loss.

template ('templayt) a mould or pattern. In radiotherapy, a map of the area of the patient requiring treatment and of those areas to be protected from radiation.

temple ('tempəl) the region on either side of the head above the zygomatic arch.

temporal ('tempə·rəl) pertaining to the side of the head. *T. arteritis* giant cell arteritis. A chronic inflammatory condition of the carotid arterial system, occurring usually in elderly people. There is persistent headache and partial or total blindness can result. *T. bone* one of a pair of bones on either side of the skull and containing the organ of hearing. *T. lobe* the part of the cerebrum below the lateral SULCUS.

temporomandibular (ˌtempə·rohman'dibyələ) relating to the temporal bone and the mandible.

T. joint the hinge of the lower jaw. *T. j. syndrome* painful dysfunction of the temporomandibular joint, marked by a clicking or grinding sensation in the joint; commonly associated with malocclusion of the teeth.

tenacious (tə'nayshəs) thick and viscid, as applied to sputum or other body fluids.

tendinitis (ˌtendə'nietəs) inflammation of a tendon and its attachments.

tendon ('tendən) a band of fibrous tissue forming the termination of a muscle and attaching it to a bone. *Achilles t.* that inserted into the CALCANEUM. *T. grafting* an operation which repairs a defect in one tendon by a graft from another. *T. insertion* the point of attachment of a muscle to a bone which it moves. *T. reflex* the muscular contraction produced on percussing a tendon.

tenesmus (tə'nezməs) a persistent, painful, ineffectual straining to empty the bowel or bladder.

tennis elbow ('tenəs) a painful disorder which affects the extensor muscles of the forearm at their attachment to the lateral EPICONDYLE.

Tenon's capsule (tə'nonhz) *J.R. Tenon, French surgeon, 1724–1816.* The fibrous tissue in which the eyeball is situated.

tenonitis (ˌtenə'nietəs) inflammation of Tenon's capsule. PROPTOSIS of the eyeball occurs, often accompanied by pain and PYREXIA.

tenorrhaphy (te'no·rəfee) the suturing together of the ends of a divided tendon.

tenosynovitis (ˌtenohˌsienə'vietəs) inflammation of a tendon sheath.

TENS abbreviation for transcutaneous electrical nerve stimulation. A method of treating persistent pain by passing small electrical currents into the spinal cord or sensory nerves by means of electrodes applied to the skin. TENS is non-invasive and non-addictive, with no known side-effects.

tension ('tenshən) the act of stretching or the state of being stretched. *Arterial t.* the pressure of blood on the vessel wall during cardiac contraction. *Intraocular t.* the pressure of the contents of the eye on its walls, measured by a tonometer. *Intravenous t.* the pressure of blood within the veins. *Premenstrual t.* symptoms of abdominal distension, headache, emotional lability, and depression, occurring a few days before the onset of menstruation. *See* PREMENSTRUAL. *Surface t.* tension or resistance which acts to preserve the integrity of a surface, particularly the surface of a liquid.

tensor ('tensə, -saw) a muscle that stretches a part.

teratogen ('terətəjən) an agent or influence that causes physical defects in the developing embryo.

teratoma (ˌterə'tohmə) a solid tumour containing tissues similar to those of a dermoid cyst. Found most often in the ovaries and testes; many of these tumours are malignant.

tertian ('tərshən) recurring every 48 hours. *See* MALARIA.

tertiary ('tərshə·ree) third. *T. prevention* prevention of ill health, mitigating the effects of illness and disease that have already occurred. *T. syphilis* the non-infectious stage of neurosyphilis.

test (test) 1. an examination or trial. 2. analysis of the composition of a substance by the use of chemical reagents. *Agglutination t.* one whose results depend on agglutination of bacteria or other cells: used in diagnosing certain infectious diseases and rheumatoid arthritis; the cross-matching of blood; and in pregnancy tests, in which no agglutination indicates a positive pregnancy test, whereas agglutination indicates a negative result. *Complement-fixation t's* tests that utilise antigen–antibody reaction and result in haemolysis, to determine the presence of various organisms in the blood. *Concentration t.* a test of renal function based on the patient's ability to concentrate urine. *Creatinine clearance t.* a test for renal function based on the rate at which ingested creatinine is filtered through the renal GLOMERULI. *Early pregnancy t.* a do-it-yourself immunological test for pregnancy, performed as early as 9 days after menstruation was expected. *Glucose tolerance t.* a metabolic test of carbohydrate tolerance used to diagnose diabetes mellitus. *Glycosylated haemoglobin t.* measurement of the percentage of haemoglobin A_1 (HbA_1) molecules which helps to assess diabetic control. HbA_1 is a type of adult haemoglobin where one part of the beta chain has been combined with glucose and increases in diabetes, especially when the blood glucose control is poor. *Histamine t.* after a rapid intravenous injection of histamine phosphate, the blood pressure normally falls, but in patients with PHAECHROMOCYTOMA, after the fall, there is a marked rise in blood pressure. *Pregnancy t's* laboratory procedures for early determination of pregnancy. *Sickling t.* a method to demonstrate haemoglobin S and the sickling phenomenon in erythrocytes, performed by reducing the oxygen concentration to which the red cells are exposed. *Treponema pallidum haemagglutination* (TPHA) *t., Treponema pallidum immobilisation* (TPI) *t.* serological tests related directly to the causative organism, used in the diagnosis of syphilis. *vdrl t.* a slide flocculation test for syphilis designed by the Venereal Disease Research Laboratory, USA. *T. weighing* a method of determining the amount of breast milk taken, by weighing the baby before and after the feed without changing any of its clothes, so that the difference equals the feed. Sometimes called test feeding. With successful demand feeding there should be no need for this regimen.

testicle ('testikəl) a testis; one of the two glands in the scrotum which produce SPERMATOZOA. *Undescended t.* condition in which the organ remains in the pelvis or inguinal canal.

testicular self-examination (tes'tikyələ ˌselfˌegzamə'nayshən) should be performed regularly once a month for the detection of early tumours of the testis which are curable if detected at an early stage. Self-examination should take place after a warm bath or shower, which relaxes the scrotal skin. (a) Standing in front of a mirror, look for any swelling. One testis might appear larger than the other or hang lower; this is normal. (b) Examine each testis with both hands and gently roll each testis between the fingers and thumb. A small lump is felt for and, if found, almost always occurs in only one testis and is usually painless. (c) A cord-like structure found on the top and back of each testis should be found and examined.

testis ('testəs) a testicle.

testosterone (tes'tostə,rohn) the hormone produced by the testes which stimulates the development of sex characteristics. Now made synthetically. It is used medicinally in cases of failure of sex function and as a palliative treatment in some cases of advanced metastatic breast cancer in females.

tetanus ('tetənəs) an acute disease of the nervous system caused by the contamination of wounds by the spores of a soil bacterium, *Clostridium tetani*. Muscle stiffness around the site of the wound occurs followed by rigidity of face and neck muscles; hence 'lockjaw'. All muscles are then affected and OPISTHOTONOS can occur. *T. vaccine* or *toxoid* provides active immunity. *T. antitoxin* a serum that gives short-term passive immunity and can be used with penicillin for immediate treatment of a case of tetanus.

tetany ('tetənee) an increased excitability of the nerves due to a lack of available calcium, accompanied by painful muscle spasm of the hands and feet (carpopedal spasm). The cause can be HYPOPARATHYROIDISM or ALKALOSIS as a result of excessive vomiting or hyperventilation.

tetrachloroethylene (,tetrə,klor-·roh'ethə,leen) an anthelmintic drug widely used to treat hookworm disease.

tetracycline (,tetrə'siekleen) an antibiotic drug belonging to the group known as the tetracyclines which are effective against many different microorganisms, including RICKETTSIAE, Gram-negative and Gram-positive organisms, and mycoplasma.

tetralogy (te'traləjee) a series of four. *T. of Fallot see* FALLOT'S TETRALOGY.

tetraplegia (,tetrə'pleeji·ə) quadriplegia. Paralysis of all four limbs.

thalamus ('thaləməs) a mass of nerve cells at the base of the cerebrum. Most sensory impulses from the body pass to this area and are transmitted to the cortex.

thalassaemia (,thalə'seemi·ə) a group of haemolytic anaemias mostly found in the Mediterranean region and the Far East caused by the inheritance of abnormal haemoglobin. *T. major* Cooley's anaemia; the severest form of THALASSAEMIA with death usually occurring before adolescence. *T. minor* a mild form of the disease with few symptoms. Those suffering from it can pass the disease on to their children.

thalassotherapy (thə,lasoh'therəpee) treatment involving sea bathing or a sea voyage.

thalidomide (thə'lidə,mied) a drug used as a sedative in the early 1960s; associated with severe malformities in early uterine life.

thanatology (,thanə'toləjee) 1. the study of death and dying. 2. the forensic study of the causes of death.

theca ('theekə) a sheath, such as the covering of a tendon. *T. folliculi* the covering of a Graafian follicle. *T. vertebralis* the membranes enclosing the spinal cord; the DURA MATER.

thenar ('theenə) 1. the palm of the hand. 2. the fleshy part at the base of the thumb.

theobromine (ˌtheeoh'brohmeen) an alkaloid derived from the cocoa bean. Used as a heart stimulant and as a mild diuretic.

theophylline (thee'ofəˌleen) an alkaloid derived from tea-leaves and with action similar to that of theobromine. Used mainly in the treatment of bronchospasm.

theory (ˌthiəree) set of interrelated concepts, definitions, and propositions that present a systematic view of phenomena for the purpose of explaining and making predictions about those phenomena.

therapeutic (ˌtherə'pyootik) pertaining to therapeutics or treatment of disease; curative. *T. abortion see* ABORTION. *T. community* any treatment setting (usually psychiatric) which provides a living–learning situation through group processes emphasising social, environmental and personal interactions and which encourages the individual to learn socially from these processes. *T. use of self* the ability of a psychiatric nurse to use therapy, experimental knowledge, self-awareness, and the ability to explore and use personal impact on others.

therapeutics (ˌtherə'pyootiks) the science and art of healing and the treatment of disease.

therapy ('therəpee) the treatment of disease.

thermal ('thərməl) relating to heat.

thermistor ('thərmistə) a type of thermometer used to measure minute changes in temperature.

thermocautery (ˌthərmoh'kawtə·ree) the deliberate destruction of tissue by means of heat. *See* CAUTERY.

thermogenesis (ˌthərmoh'jenəsəs) the production of heat.

thermography (ˌthər'mogrəfee) a method of measuring the amount of heat produced by different areas of the body using infra-red photography. Used as a diagnostic aid in the detection of breast tumours and the assessment of rheumatic joints; also used in the study of pain.

thermolysis (thər'moləsəs) the loss of body heat by radiation, by excretion and by the evaporation of sweat.

thermometer (thə'momətə) an instrument for measuring temperature. *Clinical t.* one used to measure the body temperature. *Electronic t.* a clinical thermometer which works electrically. It contains electronic devices whose characteristics change with temperature. The reading is recorded within seconds and displayed visually.

thermoreceptor (ˌthərmohrə'septə) a nerve ending that responds to heat and cold.

thermostat ('thərməˌstat) an apparatus which automatically regulates the temperature and maintains it at a specified level.

thermotaxis (ˌthərmoh'taksəs) the normal regulation of body temperature by the maintenance of the balance between heat production and heat loss.

thermotherapy (ˌthərmoh'therəpee) the treatment of disease by application of heat.

thiamine ('thieəˌmeen) vitamin B_1, or aneurine. An essential vitamin involved in carbohydrate metabolism. A deficiency causes beriberi. The source is liver and unrefined cereals.

thiazides ('thieəˌziedz) any of a group of diuretics that act by inhibiting the reabsorption of sodium in the proximal renal tubule and stimulating chloride excretion, with resultant increase in excretion of water.

thioguanine (ˌthieoh'gwahneen) an antimetabolite used in the treatment of acute leukaemia.

thiopentone (ˌthieoh'pentohn) a basal narcotic of the barbiturate group given intravenously as a short-acting anaesthetic and in preoperative preparation.

thiopropazate (ˌthieoh'prohpəˌzayt) a tranquilliser used in the treatment of SCHIZOPHRENIA and psychoneuroses.

thiotepa (ˌthieoh'teepə) an intravenous cytotoxic drug used in the treatment of cancer, particularly of the bladder or ovary.

thiouracil (ˌthieoh'yoo·rəsil) a drug used in the treatment of thyrotoxicosis. A derivative, propylthiouracil, which is more active and less toxic, is now more often used.

thirst (thərst) an uncomfortable sensation of dryness of the mouth and throat with a desire for oral fluids. *Abnormal t.* POLYDIPSIA.

Thomas splint ('tomas) *H.O. Thomas, British orthopaedic surgeon, 1834–91*. A splint consisting of an oval iron ring that fits over the lower limb. Attached to the ring are two round iron rods which are bent into a W-shape at the lower end. It is used to support the limb and move the weight from the knee joint to the pelvis. (*See* figure.)

thoracic (thaw'rasik) relating to the thorax. *T. duct* the large lymphatic vessel situated in the thorax along the spine. It opens into the left subclavian vein.

thoracocentesis (ˌthaw·rəkohsen'teesəs) puncture of the wall of the thorax to allow aspiration of pleural fluid.

thoracoscopy (ˌthaw·rə'koskəpee) examination of the pleural cavity by means of an endoscopic instrument.

thoracotomy (ˌthaw·rə'kotəmee) a surgical incision into the thorax.

thorax ('thaw·raks) the chest; a cavity containing the heart, lungs, bronchi, and oesophagus. It is bounded by the diaphragm, the sternum, the thoracic vertebrae, and the ribs. *Barrel-shaped t.* a development in EMPHYSEMA when the chest is malformed like a barrel.

threadworm ('thredˌwərm) a species of roundworm, *Enterobius vermicularis*, parasitic in the large intestine, particularly of children.

threonine ('threeəˌneen) one of the essential amino acids.

thrill ('thril) a tremor discerned by palpation.

throat (throht) 1. the anterior surface of the neck. 2. the pharynx. *Clergyman's sore t.* laryngitis. *Sore t.* PHARYNGITIS.

thrombectomy (throm'bektəmee) surgical excision of a clot from a vein or an artery.

thrombin ('thrombən) an enzyme that converts fibrinogen to fibrin during the later stages of blood clotting.

thromboangiitis (ˌthrombohˌanjee'ietəs) inflammation of blood vessels with clot formation. *T. obliterans* inflammation of the arteries, usually of the legs of young males, causing intermittent claudication and gangrene. Buerger's disease.

thrombocyte ('thrombohˌsiet) a

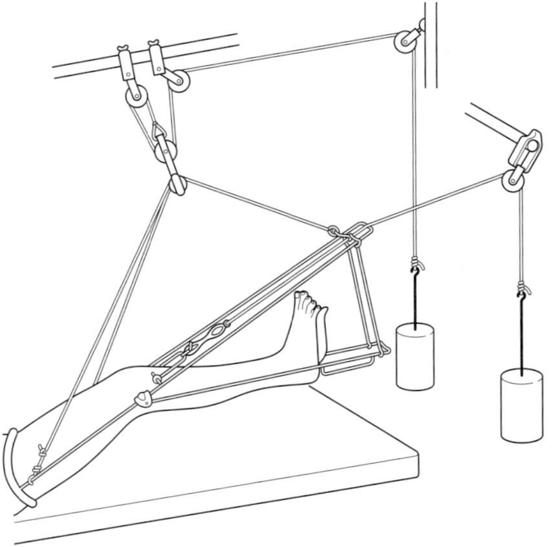

Thomas splint in use with skeletal traction.
A Pearson knee flexion piece is attached.

Thomas splint

blood platelet. Disc-shaped; essential for the clotting of shed blood.

thrombocytopaenia (ˌthrombohˌsietoh'peeni·ə) a reduction in the number of platelets in the blood; bleeding can occur. Destruction of platelets can be caused by infections, certain drugs, transfusion-related purpuras, idiopathic thrombocytopaenic PURPURA and disseminated intravascular coagulopathy.

thrombocytosis (ˌthrombohsie'tohsəs) an increase in the number of platelets in the blood.

thromboendarterectomy (ˌthrombohˌendahtə'rektəmee) surgical removal of a clot from an artery together with a portion of the lining of the artery.

thromboendarteritis (ˌthrombohˌendahtə'rhietəs) inflammation of the lining of an artery with clot formation as a result.

thrombokinase (ˌthromboh'kienayz) THROMBOPLASTIN. A lipid-containing protein activated by blood platelets and injured tissues which is capable of activating prothrombin to form thrombin, which, combined with fibrinogen, forms a clot.

thrombolysis (throm'boləsəs) the disintegration or dissolving of a clot.

thrombophlebitis (ˌthrombohflə'bietəs) the formation of a clot, associated with inflammation of the lining of a vein.

thromboplastin (ˌthromboh'plastən) *see* THROMBOKINASE.

thrombosis (throm'bohsəs) the formation of a thrombus. *Cavernous sinus t.* thrombosis of the cavernous sinus, usually the result of infection of the face, when the veins in the sinus are affected via ophthalmic vessels. *Cerebral t.* the occlusion of a cerebral artery, the most common cause of cerebral infarction (a 'stroke'). *Coronary t.* the occlusion of a coronary vessel, by which the heart muscle is deprived of blood causing myocardial ischaemia and often causing MYOCARDIAL INFARCTION (a 'heart attack'). *Lateral sinus t.* a complication of mastoiditis when infection of the lateral sinus of the DURA MATER occurs and there is clot formation.

thrombus ('thrombəs) a stationary blood clot caused by coagulation of the blood in the heart or in an artery or a vein.

thrush (thrush) an infection of the mucous membranes, most commonly of the mouth and vagina, by a fungus, *Candida albicans. See* CANDIDIASIS.

thymectomy (thie'mektəmee) surgical removal of the thymus.

thymine ('thiemeen) one of the pyrimidine bases found in DNA.

thymokesis (ˌthiemoh'keesəs) persistence of the thymus gland in an adult.

thymol ('thiemol) an aromatic antiseptic used in solution as a mouthwash.

thymoma (thie'mohmə) a tumour that originates in thymus tissue.

thymus ('thieməs) a gland-like structure situated in the upper thorax and neck. Present in early life, it reaches its maximum development during puberty and continues to play an immunological role throughout life, although its function declines with age.

thyrocricotomy (ˌthierohkrie'kotəmee) incision of the cricothyroid membrane to achieve TRACHEOSTOMY.

thyroglossal (ˌthieroh'glosəl) relating to the thyroid and the tongue. *T. cyst see* CYST.

thyroid ('thieroyd) 1. shaped like a shield. 2 pertaining to the thyroid gland. *T. cartilage* the largest cartilage of the larynx. It forms the 'Adam's apple' in the front of the throat. *T. gland* a ductless gland consisting of two lobes situated in front and on either side of the trachea. It secretes the hormones thyroxine and triiodothyronine which are concerned with regulating the metabolic rate. *Intrathoracic* or *retrosternal t.* position of the gland low in the neck and wholly or in part behind the sternum. *T.-stimulating hormone* abbreviated TSH. Thyrotrophin; a hormone produced by the anterior pituitary gland which controls the activity of the thyroid gland.

thyroidectomy (ˌthieroy'dektəmee)

partial or complete removal of the thyroid gland.

thyroiditis (ˌthieroy'dietəs) inflammation of the thyroid. Acute thyroiditis, usually due to a viral infection, is characterised by sore throat, fever, and painful enlargement of the gland. *Hashimoto's t.* a progressive autoimmune disease of the thyroid gland with degeneration of its epithelial elements and replacement by lymphoid and fibrous tissue.

thyroparathyroidectomy (ˌthierohˌparəˌthieroy'dektəmee) surgical removal of the thyroid and parathyroid glands.

thyrotoxicosis (ˌthierohˌtoksə'kohsəs) hyperthyroidism. The symptoms arising when there is overactivity of the thyroid gland. The metabolism is speeded up and there is enlargement of the gland and EXOPHTHALMOS.

thyrotrophin (ˌthieroh'trohfən) *see* THYROID-STIMULATING HORMONE.

thyroxine (thie'rokseen) one of the two hormones secreted by the thyroid gland. It is used in the treatment of HYPOTHYROIDISM.

TIA transient ischaemic attack.

tibia ('tibi·ə) the shin bone; the larger of the two bones of the leg, extending from knee to ankle.

tic (tik) a spasmodic twitching of certain muscles, usually of the face, neck, or shoulder. *T. douloureux* paroxysmal trigeminal neuralgia.

tick (tik) a blood-sucking parasite which can transmit the organisms of various diseases.

tidal volume ('tied'l) the amount of gas passing into and out of the lungs in each respiratory cycle.

tine test (tien) a tuberculin skin test employing a multiple-puncture, disposable device. It is especially useful in mass screening of children, but is less accurate than the Mantoux test.

tinea ('tini·ə) a group of skin infections caused by a variety of fungi and named after the area of the body affected, thus: *T. barbae*, the beard; *T. capitis*, the head; *T. circinata* or *T. corporis*, the body; *T. cruris*, the groin; and *T. pedis*, the feet. *See* RINGWORM.

tinnitus (ti'nietəs) a ringing, buzzing, or roaring sound in the ears.

tissue ('tisyoo, 'tishoo) a group or layer of similarly specialised cells that together perform certain special functions.

titration (tie'trayshən) determination of a given component in solution by addition of a liquid reagent of known strength until a given end-point, e.g. change in colour, is reached, indicating that the component has been consumed by reaction with the reagent.

tobacco (tə'bakoh) the dried leaves of the plant *Nicotiana tabacum*, containing the drug nicotine, which can be smoked, chewed, or inhaled. All these activities are potentially dangerous to health.

tobramycin (ˌtohbrə'miesən) an antibiotic drug used chiefly in the treatment of *Pseudomonas* infection.

tocography (to'kogrəfee) the measurement of alterations in the intrauterine pressure during labour.

tocopherol (to'kofə·rol) vitamin E, present in wheat germ, green leaves, and milk.

token economy program (ˌtohkən ə'konəmee) a behavioural approach to modifying troublesome behaviours and restoring lost self-help behaviours by the systematic rewarding of desired behaviour by giving tokens which can be exchanged for goods or privileges.

tolazamide (to'lazə,mied) an oral hypoglycaemic drug used in the treatment of DIABETES mellitus.

tolazoline (to'lazoh,leen) a vasodilator drug of the peripheral blood vessels, used in the treatment of peripheral vascular disease.

tolbutamide (tol'byootə,mied) an oral drug that stimulates the release of insulin from the pancreas. Used in the treatment of DIABETES mellitus.

tolerance ('tolə·rəns) the ability to endure without effect of injury. *Drug t.* decrease of susceptibility to the effects of a drug due to its continued administration. *Immunological t.* specific non-reactivity of lymphoid tissues to a particular antigen capable, under other conditions, of inducing immunity.

tomography (tə'mogrəfee) body section radiography in which X-rays or ultrasound waves are used to produce an image of a layer of tissue at any depth.

tone (tohn) 1. the normal degree of tension, e.g. in a muscle. 2. a particular quality of sound.

tongue (tung) a muscular organ attached to the floor of the mouth and concerned in taste, mastication, swallowing, and speech. It is covered by a mucous membrane from which project numerous PAPILLAE.

tonic ('tonik) 1. a term popularly applied to any drug supposed to brace or tone up the body or any particular part or organ. 2. possessing tone in a state of contraction, e.g. muscles. *T. spasm* a prolonged contraction of one or several muscles, as seen in epilepsy, for example. *See* CLONIC.

tonography (to'nogrəfee) the measurement made by a tonometer recording the intraocular pressure and so, indirectly, the drainage of aqueous humour from the eye.

tonsil ('tonsəl) a mass of lymphoid tissue, particularly one of two small, almond-shaped bodies, situated one on each side between the pillars of the FAUCES. It is covered by mucous membrane and its surface is pitted with follicles (*see* figure). *Pharyngeal t.* the lymphadenoid tissue of the pharynx between the pharyngotympanic tubes. Adenoids.

tonsillectomy (,tonsə'lektəmee) excision of one or both tonsils.

tonus ('tohnəs) the normal state of partial contraction of the muscles.

tooth (tooth) a structure in the mouth designed for the mastication

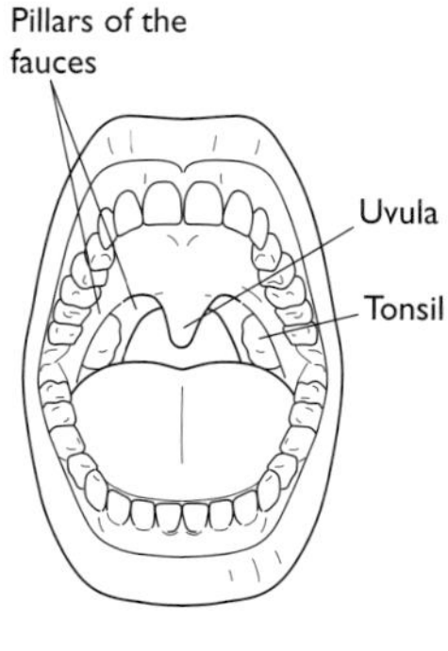

Tonsil

of food. Each is composed of a crown, neck, and root with one or more fangs. The main bulk is of dentine enclosing a central pulp; the crown is covered with a hard white substance called 'enamel'. *See* DENTITION.

tophus ('tohfəs) a small, hard, chalky deposit of sodium urate in the skin and cartilage, occurring in gout and sometimes appearing on the auricle of the ear.

topical ('topikəl) relating to a particular spot; local. *T. lotion* one for local or external application.

topography (tə'pografee, toh-) the study of the surface of the body in relation to the underlying structures.

torpor ('tawpə) a sluggish condition in which response to stimuli is absent or very slow.

torsion ('tawshən) twisting: (a) of an artery to arrest haemorrhage; (b) of the pedicle of a cyst which produces venous congestion in the cyst and consequent gangrene (a possible complication of ovarian cyst).

torso ('tawsoh) the body, excluding the head and the limbs; the trunk.

torticollis (ˌtawtə'koləs) wryneck, a contracted state of the cervical muscles producing torsion of the neck. The deformity can be congenital or hysterical, or secondary to pressure on the accessory nerve, to inflammation of glands in the neck, or to muscle spasm.

tourniquet ('tooənəˌkay, 'tawnə-) a constrictive band applied to a limb to arrest arterial haemorrhage. No longer used in first aid because its use can cause permanent damage to muscles or nerve supply.

toxaemia (tok'seemi·ə) poisoning of the blood by the absorption of bacterial toxins. *T. of pregnancy* a condition affecting pregnant women and characterised by ALBUMINURIA, hypertension, and oedema, with the possibility of pre-eclampsia and ECLAMPSIA developing.

toxic ('toksik) 1. poisonous, relating to a poison. 2. caused by a toxin. *T. shock syndrome* a severe illness characterised by high fever of sudden onset, vomiting, diarrhoea and, in severe cases, death. A sunburn-like rash with peeling of the skin occurs. The syndrome affects almost exclusively menstruating women using tampons, although a few women who do not use tampons and a few males have been affected. It is thought to be caused by infection with *Staphylococcus aureus*.

toxicity (tok'sisətee) the degree of virulence of a poison.

toxicology (ˌtoksə'koləjee) the science dealing with poisons.

toxin ('toksən) any poisonous compound, usually referring to that produced by bacteria.

Toxocara (ˌtoksoh'kair·rə) a genus of nematode worms, parasitic in the intestines of dogs and cats, which can also infest humans, especially children. The spleen, liver, and lungs are most often affected but the parasite can also infest the retina, causing inflammation and granulation.

toxoid ('toksoyd) a toxin which has been deprived of some of its harmful properties but is still capable of producing immunity and can be used in a vaccine. *Diphtheria* **t.** toxin which has been treated with formaldehyde. Used for immunisation against diphtheria. *See* TAF and ALUM PRECIPITATED TOXOID.

Toxoplasma (ˌtoksoh'plazmə) a genus of protozoa which infests birds and animals and can be transmitted from them to humans.

toxoplasmosis (ˌtoksohplaz'mohsəs) a disease due to *Toxoplasma gondii*. The congenital form is marked by central nervous system lesions which can lead to blindness, brain defects, and death. The acquired infection is often asymptomatic but can result in pneumonia, skin rashes, and NEPHRITIS.

TPN total parenteral nutrition. The adminstration of a nutritionally adequate solution through a central venous catheter.

trabecula (trə'bekyələ) a dividing band or septum extending from the capsule of an organ into its interior and holding the functioning cells in position.

trabeculectomy (trəˌbekyə'lektəmee) an operation to lower the intraocular pressure in glaucoma that cannot be controlled by medication.

tracer ('traysə) a means by which something may be followed, as (1) a mechanical device by which the outline or movements of an object can be graphically recorded, or (2) a material by which the progress of a compound through the body can be observed, e.g. a radioactive isotope tracer.

trachea (trə'keeə, 'traki·ə) the windpipe: a cartilaginous tube lined with ciliated mucous membrane extending from the lower part of the larynx to the commencement of the bronchi.

tracheitis (ˌtrakee'ietəs) inflammation of the trachea causing pain in the chest, with coughing.

tracheobronchitis (ˌtrakeeohbrong'kietəs) acute infection of the trachea and bronchi due to viruses or bacteria.

tracheostomy (ˌtrakee'ostəmee) a surgical opening into the 3rd and 4th cartilage rings of the trachea. *T. tubes* those used to maintain an airway after tracheotomy, either permanently or until the normal use of the air passages is regained.

tracheotomy (ˌtrakee'otəmee) surgical incision of the trachea. *Inferior* or *low t.* that in which the opening is made below the thyroid isthmus. *Superior* or *high t.* that in which the opening is made above the thyroid isthmus.

trachoma (trə'kohmə) a chronic infectious disease of the conjunctiva and cornea, producing photophobia, pain, and lacrimation, caused by an organism once thought to be a virus but now classified as a strain of the bacteria *Chlamydia trachomatis*. Trachoma is more prevalent in Africa and Asia than in other parts of the world.

traction ('trakshən) the exertion of a pulling force, as that applied to a fractured bone, dislocated joint or to relieve muscle spasm to maintain proper position and facilitate healing. In obstetrics, that along the axis of the pelvis to assist in delivery of a fetal part, or the placenta and membranes. *Hamilton–Russell t.* a form of traction of the leg (*see* figure) in which there is an upward pull over a beam (A) and the cord is continuous with a series of pulleys (B) attached to the limb by skin traction horizontally (C). *Head t.* traction exerted on the head in the treatment of cervical injury. *Skeletal t.* a method of keeping the fractured ends of bone in position

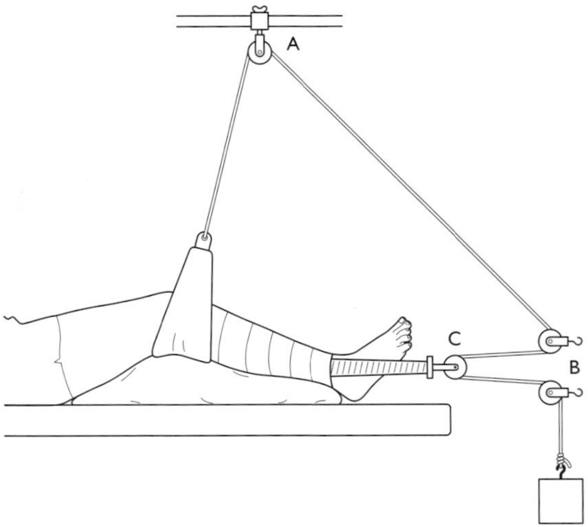

Hamilton-Russell Traction

by traction on the bone. A metal pin or wire is passed through the distal fragment or adjacent bone to overcome muscle contraction.

trait (trayt) an inherited or developed physical or mental characteristic.

trance (trans) a condition of semi-consciousness of hysterical, cataleptic, or hypnotic origin. It is not due to organic disease.

tranquilliser ('trangkwəˌliezə) a drug which allays anxiety, relieves tension, and has a calming effect on the patient.

transabdominal (ˌtranzab'domənəl, ˌtrahnz-) across the abdominal wall or through the abdominal cavity.

transactional analysis (tran'zakshənəl, trahn-) a theory of personality structure and a psychotherapeutic method. The human personality is viewed as consisting of three ego states: the parent, the adult, and the child. The aim is to allow the adult ego to take control over the child and parent egos.

transaminase (tran'zaməˌnayz) one of a group of enzymes which catalyses the transfer of an amine group from one amino acid into another. Transaminases include *glutamic-oxalacetic t.* (GOT) and *glutamic-pyruvic t.* (GPT).

transcendental meditation (ˌtran-sənˌdent'l ˌmedə'tayshən, ˌtrahn-) a technique for attaining a state of physical relaxation and psychological calm by the regular practice of a relaxation procedure which entails the repetition of a mantra. Has been successfully used by some patients to reduce hypertension.

transcutaneous blood gas monitors (tranzˌkyooˌtaynee·əs ˌblud 'gas ˌmonitəz) the application of a probe to a baby's skin which is heated to a temperature of 44°C and enables measurements of PO_2 and PCO_2 to be made. Accuracy depends on the quality of the peripheral circulation; transcutaneous blood gas monitoring is therefore usually used in conjunction with intermittent arterial sampling.

transcutaneous electrical nerve stimulation (transˌkyooˌtaynee·əs əˌlektrikəl 'nərv ˌstimyəlayshən) *see* TENS.

transference ('transfə·rəns, trans-'fər·rəns, 'trahns-) in psychiatry, the unconscious transfer by the patient on to the psychiatrist of feelings that are appropriate to other people significant to the patient.

transfusion (trans'fyoozhən) the introduction of whole blood or a blood component into a vein, performed in cases of severe loss of blood, shock, septicaemia, etc. It is used to supply actual volume of blood or to introduce constituents, such as clotting factors or antibodies, that are deficient in the patient. *Direct t.* the transfer of blood directly from a donor to a recipient. *Exchange* or *replacement t.* the removal of most or all of the recipient's blood and its replacement with fresh blood. Used with infants suffering from ERYTHROBLASTOSIS. *See* RHESUS FACTOR. *Intra-arterial t.* the passing of blood into an artery under positive pressure in cases in which large quantities are required rapidly, as in cardiovascular surgery.

transient ischaemic attack ('tran-zeeənt) abbreviated TIA. A sudden episode of temporary or passing symptoms caused by diminished blood flow through the carotid or VERTEBROBASILAR blood vessels.

transillumination (ˌtranzəˌloomə-'nayshən, ˌtrahnz-) the illumination of a translucent body structure by a strong light as an aid to diagnosis, particularly of tumours of the retina and of abnormalities in the ethmoidal and frontal sinuses.

translocation (ˌtranzloh'kayshən, ˌtrahnz-) in morphology, the transfer of a segment of a chromosome to a different site on the same chromosome or to a different chromosome. It can be a cause of congenital abnormality.

translucent (tranz'loosnət, trahnz-) allowing light rays to pass through indistinctly.

transmigration (ˌtranzmie'grayshən, ˌtrahnz-) a movement from one place to another, as in the passage of blood cells through the walls of the capillaries. DIAPEDESIS. *External t.* the passage of an ovum from an ovary to the uterine tube on the opposite side. *Internal t.* the movement of an ovum from one uterine tube to the other through the uterus.

transplacental (ˌtransplə'sent'l, ˌtrahns-) across the placenta. Movement can be from mother to fetus, or vice versa. *T. infection* can affect an unborn child.

transplant ('transplant, 'trahnsplahnt) 1. an organ or tissue taken from the body and grafted into another area of the same individual or another individual. 2. to transfer tissue from one part to another or from one individual to another.

transplantation (ˌtransplan'tayshən, ˌtrahnsplahn-) the transfer of living organs from one part of the body to another (autotransplant) or from one individual to another (allograft). Transplantation is often called grafting, although the term 'grafting' is more commonly used to refer to the transfer of skin.

transposition (ˌtranzpə'zishən, ˌtrahnz-) 1. displacement of any of the viscera to the opposite side of the body. 2. the operation which partially removes a piece of tissue from one part of the body to another, the complete severance being delayed until it has become established in its new position. *T. of the great vessels* a congenital abnormality of the heart in which the positions of the pulmonary artery and aorta are reversed.

transsexualism (tranz'sekshooəˌlizəm, trahnz-) a disturbance of gender identity in which there is a prolonged and persistent desire to discard one's biological sex characteristics and live as a member of the opposite sex.

transudate ('transyəˌdayt, 'trahn-) any fluid that passes through a membrane.

transverse (trans'vərz, trahnz-) cross-wise. *T. presentation* position of the fetus whereby it lies across the pelvis, which position must be corrected before normal birth can take place.

transvestite (tranz'vestiet) a person who experiences a habitual and strongly persistent desire to dress as a member of the opposite sex ('cross-dressing'), often for reasons of sexual gratification. The majority are male and have no desire to change sex physically (by surgery).

tranylcypromine (ˌtranəl'sieprohmeen) a monoamine oxidase inhibitor used in psychiatry for the treatment of depression.

trapezius (trə'peezi·əs) the large triangular muscle of the upper back and shoulder.

trauma ('trawmə) injury. *Birth t.* an injury to the infant sustained during the process of being born. In some psychiatric theories, the psychological shock produced in an infant by the experience of being born. *Psychological t.* an emotional shock that makes a lasting impression.

treatment ('treetmənt) the mode of dealing with a patient or disease. *Active t.* that in which specific medical or surgical treatment is undertaken. *Conservative t.* that which aims at preserving and restoring injured parts by natural means, e.g. rest, fluid replacement, etc., as opposed to radical or surgical methods. *Empirical t.* treatment based on observation of symptoms and not on theory. *Palliative t.* that which relieves distressing symptoms but does not cure the disease. *Prophylactic t.* that which aims at the prevention of disease.

Trematoda (ˌtremə'tohdə, ˌtree-) a class of fluke worms, some of which are parasitic in man. Many of them have freshwater snails as secondary hosts.

tremor ('tremə) an involuntary, muscular quivering which can be due to fatigue, emotion, or disease. Tremor, first of one hand and later affecting the other limbs, is the first symptom of PARKINSONISM. *Intention t.* one that occurs on attempting a movement, as in disseminated SCLEROSIS.

Trendelenburg's position (tren-'delən,bərgz) *F. Trendelenburg, German surgeon, 1844–1924. See* POSITION.

Trendelenburg's sign a test of the stability of the hip. The patient stands on the affected leg and flexes the other knee and hip. If there is dislocation, the pelvis is lower on the side of the flexed leg, which is the reverse of normal.

trephine (trə'fien, -'feen) an instrument for cutting out a circular piece of bone, usually from the skull. *Corneal t.* one used to cut out a piece of cornea in KERATOPLASTY.

Treponema (,trepə'neemə) a genus of spirochaetes. Anaerobic bacteria, they are motile, spiral, and parasitic in humans and animals. *T. careatum* the causative agent of PINTA. *T. pallidum* the causative agent of syphilis. *T.p. immobilisation test* a serological test for syphilis. *T. pertenue* the causative agent of YAWS (framboesia).

triage (tree'ahzh) [Fr.] 1. 'to choose, classify, or sort'. 2. 'a process by which a patient is assessed upon arrival to determine the urgency of the problem, and to designate appropriate healthcare resources to care for the identified problem'. *T. nurse* a registered nurse with specialist skills and knowledge who carries out the assessment and classification of casualties according to the type and severity of their injuries in order to assign them for treatment in the accident and emergency department.

triamcinolone (,trieam'sinə,lohn) a glucocorticoid steroid which does not cause salt and water retention; used to treat inflammatory disorders.

triamterine (trie'amtə,reen) a diuretic that acts by antagonising aldosterone and does not cause potassium loss. Used in the treatment of OEDEMA.

triangulation (trie,ang·gyə'layshən) the expansion of research methods in a single study or multiple studies to enhance diversity, enrich understanding, and accomplish specific goals.

triceps ('trieseps) having three heads. *T. muscle* that situated on the back of the upper arm, which extends the forearm.

trichiasis (tri'kieəsis) 1. a condition of ingrowing hairs about an orifice, or ingrowing eyelashes. 2. the appearance of hair-like filaments in the urine.

trichinosis (,trikə'nohsəs) a disease caused by eating underdone pork containing a parasite, *Trichinella spiralis*. This becomes deposited in muscle and causes stiffness and painful swelling. There can also be nausea, diarrhoea, and fever. Trichiniasis.

trichloroethylene (trie,klaw·roh-'ethə,leen) a weak inhalation anaesthetic. Used in midwifery for painful dressings and in general anaesthesia in combination with other anaesthetics.

trichology (tri'koləjee) the study of hair.

trichomonas (,trikoh'mohnas) a

genus of flagellate protozoa that is parasitic to humans. *T. hominis* infests the bowel and can cause dysentery. *T. tenax* infests the mouth and can be present in cases of PYORRHOEA. *T. vaginalis* is commonly present in the vagina and can cause LEUCORRHOEA and VAGINITIS.

trichomoniasis (ˌtrikohmə'nieəsəs) infestation with a parasite of the genus *Trichomonas*.

Trichophyton (ˌtrikoh'fieton) a genus of fungi that affect the skin, nails, and hair.

trichophytosis (ˌtrikohfie'tohsəs) infection of the skin, nails or hair with one of the genus *Trichophyton*. *See* TINEA.

trichosis (tri'kohsəs) any abnormal growth of hair.

trichuriasis (ˌtrikyə'rieəsəs) infestation by the whipworm.

Trichuris (tri'kyoo·rəs) a genus of nematode worms which can infest the colon and cause diarrhoea. A whipworm.

tricuspid (trie'kuspəd) having three flaps or cusps. *T. valve* that at the opening between the right atrium and the right ventricle of the heart.

trifluoperazine (ˌtriefloo·oh'perəˌzeen) a potent tranquillising drug that is used in the treatment of SCHIZOPHRENIA and psychoneuroses.

trifocal (trie'fohkəl) pertaining to a spectacle lens that has three foci, one for distant vision, one for intermediate vision, and one for near vision.

trigeminal (trie'jeminəl) divided into three. *T. nerves* the 5th pair of cranial nerves, each of which is divided into three main branches and supplies one side of the face. *T. neuralgia* pain in the face which is confined to branches of the trigeminal nerve. Tic douloureux.

trigeminy (trie'jemənee) the type of pulse in which there are three beats and then a missed beat. A regular irregularity. Pulsus trigeminus.

trigger finger ('trigə ˌfing·gə) a stenosing of the tendon sheath at the metacarpophalangeal joint, allowing flexion of the finger but not extension without assistance when it 'clicks' into position.

triglyceride (trie'glisəˌried) 'human fat', an ester of glycerol and three fatty acids.

trigone ('triegohn) a triangular area. *T. of the bladder* the triangular space on the floor of the bladder, between the ureteric openings and the urethral orifice.

tri-iodothyronine (trieˌieədoh'thierəˌneen) a hormone produced by the thyroid gland together with thyroxine.

trimeprazine (trie'meprəˌzeen) a sedative drug used for preoperative medication in the treatment of PRURITUS and to sedate children.

trimester (trie'mestə) a period of three months. *First t. of pregnancy* the first three months during which rapid development is taking place.

trimipramine (trie'miprəˌmeen) an antidepressant drug used particularly when anxiety and insomnia accompany depression.

triplopia (tri'plohpi·ə) a condition in which thre images of an object are seen at the same time.

trismus ('trizməs) lockjaw; a tonic spasm of the muscles of the jaw.

trisomy ('triesəmee) the presence of an extra chromosome in each cell in addition to the normal paired set of 46. The cause of several chromosome disorders including DOWN'S SYNDROME and KLINEFELTER'S SYNDROME.

trocar ('trohkah) a pointed instrument used with a cannula for performing PARACENTESIS.

trochanter (troh'kantə) either of two bony prominences below the neck of the femur. *Greater t.* that on the outer side forming the bony prominence of the hip. *Lesser t.* that on the inner side at the neck of the femur.

trochlea ('trokli·ə) any pulley-shaped structure, but particularly the fibrocartilage near the inner angular process of the frontal bone through which passes the tendon of the superior oblique muscle of the eye.

trochlear ('trokli·ə) relating to nutrition. *T. nerves* those that control the nutrition of a part. *T. ulcer* one arising from a failure in the nutrition of a part.

trophoblast ('trofəˌblast) the layer of cells surrounding the blastocyst at the time of, and responsible for, implantation.

tropia ('trohpi·ə) a manifest squint, one that is present when both eyes are open.

tropical ('tropikəl) relating to the areas north and south of the equator, termed the tropics. *T. medicine* that concerned with diseases that are more prevalent in hot climates.

Trousseau's sign ('troosohz) *A. Trousseau, French physician, 1801–67.* 1. spontaneous peripheral venous thrombosis. 2. a sign of tetany in which carpal spasm can be elicited by compressing the upper arm and causing ischaemia to the nerves distally.

truancy ('trooənsee) absence of a child from school without leave. A disorder of conduct which can result from emotional insecurity or a feeling of unfairness.

truncus ('trungkəs) a trunk; the main part of the body, or a part of it, from which other parts spring. *T. arteriosus* the arterial trunk connected to the fetal heart which develops into the aortic and pulmonary arteries.

truss (trus) an apparatus in the form of a belt with a pressure pad for retaining a hernia in place after reduction.

Trypanosoma (ˌtripənoh'sohmə) a genus of protozoan parasites which pass some of their life cycle in the blood of vertebrates, including humans. *T. gambiense* and *T. rhodensiense* are transmitted by the bite of the tsetse fly and are the cause of sleeping sickness.

trypanosomiasis (ˌtripənohsə'mieəsəs) a disease caused by infestation with *Trypanosoma*. Sleeping sickness.

trypsin ('tripsən) a digestive enzyme that converts protein into amino acids.

trypsinogen (trip'sinəjən) the precursor of trypsin. It is secreted in the pancreatic juice and activated by the enterokinase of the intestinal juices into trypsin.

tryptophan ('triptəˌfan) one of the essential amino acids.

tsetse fly ('tetsee, 'tse-) a fly of the genus *Glossina* which transmits the parasite *Trypanosoma* to humans, causing TRYPANOSOMIASIS.

tsutsugamushi disease (ˌtsootsoogə'mooshee) scrub typhus which occurs in Japan and is transmitted by the bite of a mite.

tubal ('tyoobəl) relating to a tube. *T.*

ligation tying of the fallopian tubes as method of female sterilisation. *T. pregnancy* extrauterine pregnancy where the embryo develops in the uterine tube. Ectopic pregnancy.

tube feeding (tyoob) administration of liquid and semisolid foods through a nasogastric tube, gastrostomy tube, or enterostomy tube. Tube feeds are administered to patients who are unable to take foods by mouth.

Tubegauz ('tyoob,gawz) a proprietary brand of woven circular bandage applied with a special applicator.

tubercle ('tyoobəkəl) 1. a small nodule or a rounded prominence on a bone. 2. the specific lesion (a small nodule) produced by the tubercle bacillus.

tubercular (tyə'bərkyələ) pertaining to tubercles.

tuberculin (tyə'bərkyələn) the filtrate from a fluid medium in which *Mycobacterium tuberculosis* has been grown and which contains its toxins. *Old t.* is prepared from the human bacillus. It is used in skin tests in diagnosing tuberculosis. *See* MANTOUX TEST.

tuberculosis (tyə,bərkyə'lohsəs) an infectious, inflammatory, notifiable disease produced by the tubercle bacillus, *Mycobacterium tuberculosis*, that is chronic in nature. *Bovine t.* a form found in cattle and spread by infected milk. *Military t.* a severe form with small tuberculous lesions spread throughout the body and severe toxaemia. *Open t.* any type of tuberculosis in which the organisms are being excreted from the body. *Pulmonary t.* that affecting the lungs; also termed phthisis. *T. of the spine* Pott's disease.

tuberosity (,tyoobə'rosətee) an elevation or protuberance on a bone to which tendons are attached.

tuberous ('tyoobə·rəs) covered with tubers. *T. sclerosis* a familial disease with tumours on the surfaces of the lateral ventricles of the brain and sclerotic patches on its surface, and marked by mental deterioration and epileptic attacks.

tubocurarine (,tyoobohkyoo'rahreen) a preparation of curare used to secure skeletal muscle relaxation.

tubule ('tyoobyool) a small tube. *Renal* or *uriniferous t.* the essential secreting tube of the kidney.

tularaemia (,toolə'reemi·ə) a plague-like disease of rodents, caused by *Francisella* (Pasteurella) *tularensis*, which is transmissible to humans. The illness can be contracted by handling diseased animals or their hides, eating infected wild game, or being bitten by insects that have fed on infected animals. It causes fever and headache; the lymph glands enlarge and can suppurate.

tumefaction (,tyoomə'fakshən) a swelling or the process of becoming swollen. Tumescence.

tumescence (,tyoo'mesəns) 1. a swelling or enlarging of a part. 2. a swollen condition. 3. a penile erection.

tumour ('tyoomə) an abnormal swelling. The term is usually applied to a morbid growth of tissue which can be benign or malignant. A neoplasm. *Benign* or *innocent t.* one that does not infiltrate or cause metastases, and is unlikely to recur if removed. *Malignant t.* one that invades and destroys tissue and can spread to neighbouring tissues, and to more distant sites via the blood and the lymphatic systems.

tunica ('tyoonikə) a coat, a covering, or the lining of a vessel. *T. adventitia*, *t. media*, *t. intima* the outer, middle, and inner coats of an artery, respectively. *T. vaginalis* the membrane covering the front and sides of the testis.

tuning fork ('tyooning) a metal instrument used for testing hearing by means of the sounds produced by its vibration. *See* RINNE'S TEST and WEBER TEST.

tunnel ('tunəl) in anatomy, a canal through a structure. *Carpal t.* the osteofibrous channel in the wrist between the carpal bones and tissue covering the flexor tendons. *C.t. syndrome* pain and tingling in the hand and fingers caused by compression of the median nerve in the carpal tunnel. *T. vision* vision that is restricted to the central field. Occurs in chronic GLAUCOMA and in RETINITIS PIGMENTOSA.

turbinate ('tərbənət, -ˌnayt) scroll shaped. *T. bone* one of the three thin long plates that form the walls of the nasal cavity.

turbinectomy (ˌtərbə'nektəmee) excision of a turbinate bone.

turgid ('tərjid) swollen and congested.

Turner's syndrome ('tərnəz) *H.H. Turner, American physician, 1892–1970.* A chromosomal defect in females causing short stature. Classically, an absence of one X chromosome. Affects 1 in 3000 live female births. The majority have streak ovaries leading to an absence of puberty and infertility. Other features can include webbing of the neck, CUBITUS VALGUS, nail abnormalities, and coarctation of the aorta. Intelligence is usually normal.

twin (twin) one of a pair of individuals who have developed in the uterus together. *Binovular* (dizygotic) *t.* each twin has developed from a separate ovum; fraternal twins. *Uniovular* (monozygotic) *t.* both twins have developed from the same cell; identical twins.

tympanectomy (ˌtimpə'nektəmee) excision of the tympanic membrane.

tympanites (ˌtimpə'nieteez) distension of the abdomen by accumulation of gas in the intestine or the peritoneal cavity.

tympanitis (ˌtimpə'nietəs) inflammation of the middle ear; otitis media.

tympanoplasty ('timpənəˌplastee) an operation to reconstruct the eardrum and restore conductivity to the middle ear. MYRINGOPLASTY.

tympanosclerosis (ˌtimpənoh-sklə'rohsəs) fibrosis and the formation of calcified deposits in the middle ear which leads to deafness.

tympanum ('timpənəm) 1. the middle ear. 2. the eardrum or tympanic membrane.

type (tiep) the general or prevailing character of any particular case of disease, person, substance, etc. *Asthenic t.* a type of physical constitution, with long limbs, small trunk, flat chest, and weak muscles. *Athletic t.* a type of physical constitution with broad shoulders, deep chest, flat abdomen, thick neck, and good muscular development. *Blood t's see* BLOOD GROUP. *Phage t.* a sub-group of a bacterial species susceptible to a particular bacteriophage and demonstrated by PHAGE TYPING. Called also lysotype and phagotype. *Pyknic t.* a type of physical constitution marked by rounded body, large chest, thick shoulders, broad head, and short neck.

type I diabetes *See* DIABETES

type 2 diabetes *See* DIABETES

type I error the rejection of a null hypothesis that is actually true.

type II error the acceptance of a null hypothesis that is actually false.

type A behaviour (ˌtiep 'ay) a behaviour pattern associated with the development of coronary heart disease, characterised by excessive competitiveness and aggression, and a fast-paced lifestyle. Research has shown that this type of behaviour is associated with coronary artery disease and MYOCARDIAL INFARCTION. The opposite type of behaviour, exhibited by individuals who are relaxed, unhurried, and less aggressive, is called type B and is associated with a lower risk of heart disease.

typhoid fever ('tiefoyd) enteric fever. A notifiable infectious disease caused by *Salmonella typhi* which is transmitted by water, milk, or other foods, especially shellfish, that have been contaminated. There is high fever, a red rash, delirium and, sometimes, intestinal haemorrhage. Recovery usually begins during the 4th week of the disease. A person who has had typhoid fever gains immunity from it but can become a carrier. Although perfectly well, he or she harbours the bacteria and passes them out in the faeces or urine. The typhoid bacillus often lodges in the gallbladder of carriers.

typhus ('tiefəs) an acute, notifiable, infectious disease caused by species of the parasitic microorganism *Rickettsia*. There is high fever, a widespread red rash, and severe headache. Typhus is likely to occur where there is overcrowding, lack of personal cleanliness, and bad hygienic conditions, because the infection is spread by bites of infected lice or by rat fleas. *Scrub t.* a form spread by mites and widespread in the Far East. TSUTSUGAMUSHI DISEASE.

tyramine ('tierəˌmeen, 'ti-) an enzyme present in cheese, game, broad-bean pods, yeast extracts, wine, and strong beer, which has a similar effect in the body to that of adrenaline. Foodstuffs containing tyramine should be avoided by patients taking monoamine oxidase inhibitors.

tyrosine ('tierəˌseen, 'ti-) an essential amino acid which is the product of phenylalanine metabolism. In some diseases, especially of the liver, it is present as a deposit in the urine. It is a precursor of catecholamines, melanin, and thyroid hormones.

tyrosinosis (ˌtierohsə'nohsəs, ˌti-) a congenital condition in which there is an error of metabolism and phenylalanine cannot be reduced to tyrosine. Hepatic failure can occur.

Uu

ulcer ('ulsə) an erosion or loss of continuity of the skin or of a mucous membrane, often accompanied by suppuration. *Decubitus u.* a pressure sore caused by lying immobile for long periods of time on a bony area. *Duodenal u.* a peptic ulcer in the duodenum. *Gastric u.* a peptic ulcer in the lining of the stomach. *Gravitational u.* a varicose ulcer of the leg which is difficult to heal because of its dependent position and the poor venous return. *Gummatous u.* one arising in late non-infective syphilis; it is slow to heal. *Indolent u.* one that is painless and heals slowly. *Peptic u.* one that occurs on the mucous membrane of either the stomach or duodenum. *Perforating u.* one that erodes through the thickness of the wall of an organ. *Rodent u.* a slow-growing EPITHELIOMA of the face which can cause local destruction and ulceration but does not give rise to metastases. BASAL CELL CARCINOMA. *Trophic u.* one due to a failure of nutrition of a part. *Varicose u.* gravitational ulcer.

ulcerative ('ulsə͵raytiv) characterised by ulceration (the formation of ulcers). *U. colitis* inflammation and ulceration of the colon and rectum of unknown cause.

ulna ('ulnə) the medial and larger bone of the forearm.

ultrasonic (͵ultrə'sonik) relating to sound waves having a frequency range beyond the upper limit perceived by the human ear. These waves are widely used instead of X-rays, particularly in the examination of structures not opaque to X-rays.

ultrasound ('ultra͵sownd) ultrasonic waves used to examine the interior organs of the body. These waves can also be used in the treatment of soft-tissue pain, and to break up renal calculi or the crystalline lens when cataract is present. *U. screening* a method of body imaging based on the reflectivity of sound. Ultrasound scanning is non-invasive and is widely used in obstetrics to detect the site of the placenta, the presence of fetal abnormalities, and the sex of the fetus; it will reveal a multiple pregnancy at an early stage. Is also used by other medical disciplines.

ultraviolet rays (͵ultrə'vielət) short wavelength electromagnetic rays. They are present in sunlight, and cause tanning and sunburn. *U. light* is used to promote vitamin D formation and for treatment of certain skin conditions.

umbilical cord (um'bələkəl ˌkawd) arises from the placenta and enters the fetus at the site of the future navel; it has two arteries and one vein which provide the nutritional, hormonal, and immunological link between mother and fetus during pregnancy.

umbilicus (um'biləkəs, ˌumbi'liekəs) the navel; the circular depressed scar in the centre of the abdomen where the umbilical cord of the fetus was attached.

unconscious (un'konshəs) 1. insensible; incapable of responding to sensory stimuli and of having subjective experiences. 2. that part of mental activity which includes primitive or repressed wishes, concealed from consciousness by the psychological censor. *Collective u.* in Jungian psychology, the portion of the unconscious which is theoretically common to human beings.

unconsciousness (un'konshəsnəs) the state of being unconscious. This can vary in depth from *deep u.*, when no response can be obtained, through to lesser degrees of unconsciousness, when the patient can be roused by painful simuli, to a level when the patient can be roused by speech or non-painful stimuli. Deep prolonged unconsciousness is known as coma. *See* COMA.

undine ('undeen) a glass flask with a spout used for irrigation of the eye.

undulant ('undyələnt) rising and falling like a wave. *U. fever see* BRUCELLOSIS.

Unguent *pl* **unguentum** (ung-'gwentəm) an ointment or salve.

uni a prefix meaning one.

unilateral (ˌyoonee'latə·rəl) on one side only.

union ('yooni·ən) 1. a joining together. 2. the repair of tissue after separation by incision or fracture. *See* CALLUS and HEALING. *Immediate u* healing by first intention.

uniovular (ˌyoonee'ohvyələ, -'ov-) from one ovum. *U. twins* identical twins, developed from one ovum.

unipara (ˌyoonee'parə) a woman who has had only one pregnancy that has resulted in a live infant.

unit ('yoonət) 1. a single thing. *Intensive care u.* a hospital department reserved for those with severe medical or surgical disorders. 2. a standard of measurement. *International insulin u.* a measurement of the pure crystalline insulin arrived at by biological assay. *SI u.* one of the various units of measurement making up the Système International d'Unités (International System of Units).

urachal (ˌyoo'raykəl) referring to the urachus. *U. cyst* a congenital abnormality in which a small cyst persists along the course of the urachus. *U. fistula* one that forms when the urachus fails to close. Urine can leak from the umbilicus.

urachus (ˌyoo'raykəs) a tubular canal existing in the fetus, connecting the bladder with the umbilicus. In the adult, it persists in the form of a solid fibrous cord.

uraemia (yə'reemi·ə) 1. an excess in the blood of urea, creatinine, and other nitrogenous end-products of protein and amino acid metabolism; sometimes referred to as azotaemia. 2. in current usage, the entire complex of signs and symptoms of chronic renal failure. Depending upon the cause it might or might not be reversible. Uraemia leads to vomiting and nausea, headache, weakness, metabolic disturbances, convulsions, and coma (*see* RENAL FAILURE).

urate ('yoo·rayt) a salt of uric acid. *Sodium u.* a compound found in concentration around joints in cases of gout.

urea (yə'reeə, 'yoo·ri·ə) carbamide. A white crystalline substance which is an end-product of protein metabolism and the chief nitrogenous constituent of urine. It is a diuretic. The normal daily output is about 33 g. *Blood u.* that which is present in the blood. Normal value is 3–8 mmol/L.

ureter (yə'reetə, 'yoo·rətə) one of the two long narrow tubes that convey the urine from the kidneys to the bladder.

ureterectomy (yə,reetə'rektəmee) the surgical removal of a ureter.

ureteric (yə'reetərik) relating to the ureter. *U. catheter* a fine catheter for insertion via the ureter into the pelvis of the kidney, either for drainage or for retrograde urography. *U. transplantation* operation in which the ureters are divided from the bladder and implanted in the colon or loop of ileum. Congenital defects or malignant growth can make this necessary.

ureterocele (yə'reetə·rə,seel) a cystic enlargement of the wall of the ureter at its entry into the bladder.

ureterocolostomy (yə,reetə-·rohkə'lostəmee) anastomosis of a ureter to the colon.

ureteroenterostomy (yə,reetə·roh-,entə'rostəmee) surgical implantation of a ureter into the intestine.

ureterolith (yə'reetə·rə,lith) a calculus in a ureter.

ureterolithotomy (yə,reetə·rohli-'thotəmee) removal of a calculus from the ureter.

ureteronephrectomy (yə,reetə-·rohnə'frektəmee) surgical removal of a kidney and its ureter.

ureterosigmoidostomy (yə,reetə-·roh,sigmoy'dostəmee) surgical implantation of the ureters into the sigmoid colon.

ureterostomy (yə,reetə'rostəmee) the surgical creation of a permanent opening through which the ureter discharges urine.

ureterovaginal (yə,reetə·rohvə-'jienəl, -'vajinəl) relating to the ureter and vagina. *U. fistula* an opening into the ureter by which urine escapes via the vagina.

urethra (yə'reethrə) the canal through which the urine is discharged from the bladder. The male urethra also discharges reproductive secretions and is about 18 cm long whereas the female urethra is about 3.5 cm in length.

urethritis (,yoo·ree'thrietəs) inflammation of the urethra with resulting frequency, urgency, and scalding when passing urine. The condition is frequently a symptom of gonorrhoea but can be caused by other infectious organisms. *Non-specific u.* abbreviated NSU. A sexually transmitted inflammation of the urethra caused by a variety of organisms other than gonococci. *See* NON-SPECIFIC urethritis.

urethrocele (yə'reethroh,seel) a prolapse of the female urethral wall through the urinary meatus which can result from damage to the pelvic floor during childbirth.

urethrography (,yoo·ree'throgrəfee)

radiographic examination of the urethra. A radio-opaque contrast medium is inserted by catheter.

urethroplasty (yə'reethroh,plastee) a surgical repair of the urethra.

urethroscope (yə'reethrə,skohp) an instrument for examining the interior of the urethra.

urethrostenosis (yə,reethroh-stə'nohsəs) stricture of the urethra.

urethrostomy (yə'reeth,rostəmee) surgical formation of a permanent opening of the urethra at the perineal surface.

urethrotomy (,yoo·ree'throtəmee) incision of the urethra to remedy stricture.

-uria (-yooreeə) a word termination (suffix) denoting a characteristic or constituent of the urine indicated by the stem to which it is affixed, as in oliguria and proteinuria.

uric acid ('yoo·rik) lithic acid, the end-product of nucleic acid metabolism, a normal constituent of urine. Its accumulation in the blood produces uricacidaemia. Renal calculi are frequently formed of it.

uricosuric (,yoo·rikoh'syoo·rik) any drug that promotes the excretion of uric acid in the urine.

urinalysis (,yoo·rə'naləsəs) the bacteriological or chemical examination of the urine.

urinary ('yoorənree) relating to urine. *U. tract* the system that conducts urine from the kidneys to the exterior, including the ureters, the bladder, and the urethra.

urination (,yoo·rə'nayshən) micturition. The act of passing urine.

urine ('yoo·rən) the clear fluid of a varying straw colour secreted by the kidneys and excreted through the bladder and urethra. It is composed of 96% fluid and 4% solid constituents, including cells and casts. Important chemicals excreted in urine include urea and uric acid. Specific gravity = 1.010–1.025; slightly acidic. *Residual u.* that which remains in the bladder after micturition. *u. retention* the inability to urinate voluntarily or to empty a full bladder.

urobilin (,yoo·roh'bielən) the main pigment of urine, also found in faeces, derived from urobilinogen.

urobilinogen (,yoo·rhobie'linəjən) a pigment derived from BILIRUBIN which, on oxidation, forms urobilin.

urochrome ('yoo·roh,krohm) the yellow pigment which colours urine derived from the breakdown of haemoglobin.

urodynamics (,yoo·rohdie'namiks) the dynamics of the propulsion and flow of urine in the urinary tract.

urogenital (,yoo·roh'jenət'l) relating to the urinary and genital organs. Urinogenital.

urography (yə'rografee) radiographic examination of the urinary tract after the injection of a radio-opaque, water-soluble, iodine-containing medium.

urogram ('yoo·roh,gram) a radiographic image obtained by urography.

urokinase (,yoo·roh'kienayz) an enzyme in urine which is secreted by the kidneys and causes FIBRINOLYSIS. In certain diseases it can cause bleeding from the kidneys.

urolith ('yoo·roh,lith) a calculus in the urinary tract.

urology (yə'roləjee) the study of diseases of the urinary tract.

uropathy (yə'ropəthee) any disease condition affecting the urinary tract.

urostomy (yə'rostəmee) an artificial

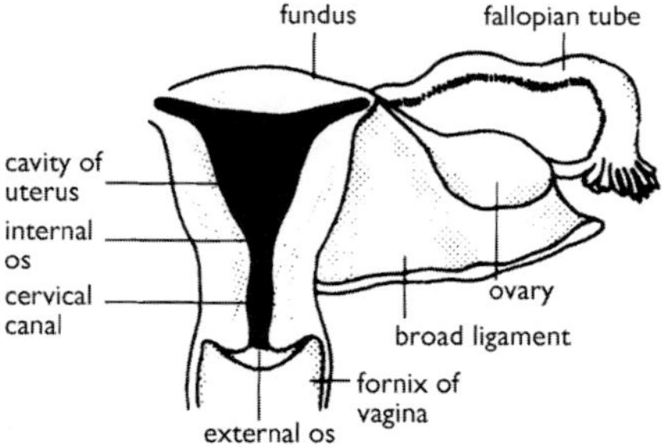

The Uterus and Adnexa

urinary conduit for deflecting urine from the ureters to the abdominal wall.

urticaria (ˌərtəˈkair·ri·ə) nettle rash or hives. An acute or chronic skin condition characterised by the recurrent appearance of an eruption of weals, causing great irritation. The cause can be certain foods, infection, drugs, or emotional stress. *See* ALLERGY.

uterine (ˈyootəˌrien) relating to the uterus.

uterocele (ˈyootə·rəˌseel) a hernia of the uterus; a hysterocele.

uterosalpingography (ˌyootə·roh-ˌsalpingˈgogrəfee) radiographic examination of the uterus and the uterine tubes.

uterovesical (ˌyootə·rohˈvesikəl) referring to the uterus and bladder. *U. pouch* the fold of peritoneum between the two organs.

uterus (ˈyootə·rəs) the womb: a triangular, hollow, muscular organ situated in the pelvic cavity between the bladder and the rectum (*see* figure). Its function is the nourishment and protection of the fetus during pregnancy, and its expulsion at term. *Bicornuate u.* one having two horns. A congenital malformation. *Gravid u.* the pregnant uterus. *U. didelphys* a double uterus caused by the failure of union of the two müllerian ducts from which it is formed.

utricle (ˈyootrikəl) any small sac. The delicate membranous sac in the bony vestibule of the ear.

uvea (ˈyoovi·ə) uveal tract. The pigmented layer of the eye consisting of the iris, ciliary body, and choroid.

uveitis (ˌyooveeˈietis) inflammation of the uveal tract.

uvula (ˈyoovyələ) the small fleshy appendage which is the free edge of the soft palate, hanging from the roof of the mouth.

uvulectomy (ˌyoovyəˈlektəmee) the surgical excision of the uvula.

uvulitis (ˌyoovyəˈlietəs) inflammation of the uvula.

Vv

vaccination (ˌvaksəˈnayshən) the introduction of vaccine into the body to produce immunity to a specific disease.

vaccine (ˈvakseen) a suspension of killed or attenuated organisms (viruses, bacteria, or rickettsiae) administered for prevention, amelioration, or treatment of infectious diseases. *Attenuated v.* one prepared from living organisms which, through long cultivation, have lost their virulence. *Bacille Calmette–Gurin v.* an attenuated bovine bacillus vaccine giving immunity from tuberculosis. *Sabin v.* an attenuated poliovirus vaccine that can be administered by mouth, in a syrup, or on sugar. *Salk v.* one prepared from an inactivated strain of poliomyelitis virus. *tab v.* a sterile solution of the organisms that cause typhoid and paratyphoid A and B. Paratyphoid C can now be included. *Triple v.* one that protects against diphtheria, tetanus, and whooping cough.

vaccinia (vakˈsini·ə) cowpox; a virus infection of cows, which can be transmitted to humans by contact with the lesions. A local pustular eruption is produced.

vacuum (ˈvakyoom) a space from which air or gas has been extracted. *V. extractor* an instrument used to assist delivery of the fetus. A suction cup is attached to the head and a vacuum created slowly. Gentle traction is applied which is synchronised with the uterine contractions.

vagal (ˈvaygəl) relating to the VAGUS nerve.

vagina (vəˈjienə) the canal, lined with mucous membrane, that leads from the uterus to the external genetalia.

vaginismus (ˌvajəˈnizməs) a painful spasm of the muscles of the vagina occurring usually when the vulva or vagina is touched resulting in painful sexual intercourse or dyspareunia.

vaginitis (ˌvajəˈnietəs) inflammation of the vagina. *Atrophic* or *postmenopausal v.* inflammation caused by degenerative changes in the mucous lining of the vagina and insufficient oestrogen secretion. Adhesions can occur, partially closing the vagina. *Trichomonas v.* infection caused by *T. vaginalis*, a protozoon that causes a thin, yellowish discharge, giving rise to local tenderness and PRURITUS.

vaginocele (ˈvajənohˌseel) vaginal hernia

vaginoplasty (ˈvajənohˌplastee) surgical repair of the vagina; called also colpoplasty.

vaginovesical (ˌvajənoh'veesikəl) pertaining to the vagina and bladder.

vagotomy (vay'gotəmee) surgical incision of the vagus nerve or any of its branches. A treatment for gastric or duodenal ulcer. *Highly selective v.* division of only those vagal fibres supplying the acid-secreting glands of the stomach. *Medical v.* interruption of impulses carried by the vagus nerve by administration of suitable drugs.

vagus ('vaygəs) the 10th cranial nerve arising in the medulla. It provides sensory fibres to the ear, tongue, pharynx, and larynx, and provides the parasympathetic and visceral afferent fibres to the organs in the thorax and abdomen. *V. resection see* VAGOTOMY.

valgus ('valgəs) a displacement outwards, particularly of the feet. *Genu valgum* knock-knee, with the ankles set apart. *Hallux v.* twisting of the big toe towards the other toes. *Talipes v.* clubfoot with the inner edge only in contact with the ground, and the foot turned outwards.

validity (və'lidəˌtee) the extent to which a measure, indicator, or method of data collection possesses the quality of being sound or true, as far as can be judged. *Construct v.* the extent to which an instrument is said to measure a theoretical construct or trait. *Content v.* the degree to which the content of the measure represents the universe of content, or the domain of a given behaviour. *External v.* the degree to which findings of a study can be generalised to other populations or environments. *Face v.* a type of content validity that uses an expert's opinion to judge the accuracy of an instrument. *Internal v.* the degree to which it can be inferred that the experimental treatment, rather than an uncontrolled condition, resulted in the observed effects.

valine ('valəən) an essential amino acid required for nitrogen equilibrium which is formed by the digestion of dietary protein.

Valium ('vali·əm) trade name for a preparation of diazepam, an anxiolytic and skeletal muscle relaxant.

Valsalva's manoeuvre (val'salvəz) *A.M. Valsalva, Italian anatomist, 1666–1723.* Technique for increasing the intrathoracic pressure by closing the mouth and nostrils and blowing out the cheeks, thereby forcing air back into the nasopharynx. When the breath is released, the intrathoracic pressure drops and the blood is quickly propelled through the heart, producing an increase in the heart rate (tachycardia) and the blood pressure. Immediately after this event a reflex BRADYCARDIA ensues. Valsalva's manoeuvre occurs when a person strains to defaecate or urinate, uses the arm and upper trunk muscles to move up in bed, or strains during coughing, gagging, or vomiting. The increased pressure, immediate tachycardia, and reflex bradycardia can bring about cardiac arrest in vulnerable heart patients.

valve (valv) 1. a means of regulating the flow of liquid or gas through a pipe. 2. a fold of membrane in a passage or tube, so placed as to permit passage of fluid in one direction only. They are important structures in the heart, in veins, and in lymph vessels. *Semilunar v.* either of two valves at the junction of the pulmonary artery and aorta, respectively, with the heart.

valvotomy (val'votəmee) valvulotomy. A surgical operation to open up a fibrosed valve, e.g. mitral valvotomy to relieve MITRAL STENOSIS.

valvulitis (ˌvalvyə'lietəs) inflammation of a valve, particularly of the heart.

vancomycin (ˌvankoh'miesən) an antibiotic highly effective against Gram-positive bacteria, especially staphylococci. The toxic effects are quite severe and can include damage to the 8th cranial (vestibulocochlear) nerve and renal disorders.

vanillylmandelic acid (vəˌniləlman-'delik) abbreviated VMA. A metabolite of catecholamines which is excreted in small amounts in the urine. Excessive amounts of VMA in the urine can indicate that the patient has an adrenal medullary tumour.

vaporisation (ˌvaypərie'zayshən) the alteration of a liquid or solid to a gaseous form.

vaporiser ('vaypəˌriezə) an apparatus for producing a very fine spray of a liquid.

variable ('vairee·əbəl) in social research, a characteristic which can be measured and which can vary along a continuum (e.g. recording of foot size in a population being studied), be more discrete (e.g. in family size) or be bipolar (e.g. sex). *Dependent v.* in experimental studies, the presumed effect of the independent or experimental variable on the outcome. *Independent v.* the antecedent or the variable that has the presumed effect on the dependent variable.

varicella (ˌvaree'selə) chickenpox. An infectious disease of childhood with an incubation period of 12–20 days. On the first day of disease, there is slight fever and an eruption of transparent vesicles on the chest, which appear in successive crops all over the body. The vesicles soon dry up, sometimes leaving shallow pits in the skin. The disease is usually mild, but can be severe in neonates, adults, and those who are immunocompromised.

varicocele ('varikəˌseel) a dilatation of the veins of the spermatic cord.

varicocelectomy (ˌvarikohsə-'lektəmee) surgical removal of dilated veins *see* VARICOCELE from the scrotum.

varicose ('varəˌkohs) swollen or dilated . *V. ulcer* gravitational ulcer. *See* ULCER. *V. veins* a dilated and twisted condition of the veins (usually those of the leg) caused by structural changes in the walls or valves of the vessels.

variola (və'rieələ) smallpox.

varix *pl* **varices**('vair·riks) an enlarged tortuous vein, artery, or lymphatic vessel.

varus ('vair·rəs) a displacement inwards. *Genu varum* bowleg, with the ankles close together. *Hallux v.* twisting of the big toe away from the other toes. *Talipes v.* clubfoot with the outer edge only in contact with the ground and foot turned inwards.

vas (vas) *pl.* vasa. A vessel or duct. *V. deferens* one of a pair of excretory ducts conveying the semen from the epididymis to the urethra. *V. efferens* one of the many small tubes that convey semen from the testis to the epididymis. *Vasa vasorum* the minute nutrient vessels that supply the walls of the arteries and veins.

vascular ('vaskyələ) relating to or consisting largely of blood vessels. *V. system* the cardiovascular system.

vascularisation (ˌvaskyələ·rie-'zayshən) the development of new blood vessels within a tissue.

vasculitis (ˌvaskyə'lietəs) angiitis; inflammation of a blood vessel. *Allergic v.* a severe allergic response to drugs or to cold. Arising in small arteries or veins, with fibrosis and thrombi formation.

vasectomy (və'sektəmee) excision of a part of the vas deferens. If performed bilaterally, sterility results. Employed as a method of contraception.

vasoconstriction (ˌvayzohkən-'strikshən) decrease in the diameter of a blood vessel

vasoconstrictor (ˌvayzohkən'striktə) any agent that causes contraction of a blood vessel wall which results in a decrease in the blood flow and an increase in the blood pressure.

vasodilator (ˌvayzohdie'laytə) any agent that causes an increase in the lumen of blood vessels and therefore an increase in the blood flow and a fall in the blood pressure.

vasomotor (ˌvayzoh'mohtə) controlling the muscles of blood vessels, both dilator and constrictor. *V. centre* nerve cells in the MEDULLA OBLONGATA controlling the vasomotor nerves. *V. nerves* sympathetic nerves regulating the tension of the blood vessels.

vasopressin (ˌvayzoh'presən) antidiuretic hormone (ADH). A hormone from the posterior lobe of the pituitary gland which causes constriction of plain muscle fibres and reabsorption of water in the renal tubules. Used in the treatment of DIABETES insipidus and bleeding from oesophageal varices.

vasospasm ('vayzohˌspazəm) constriction of a blood vessel.

vasovagal (ˌvayzoh'vaygəl) vascular and vagal. *V. attack* fainting or syncope stress, often evoked by emotional stress associated with fear and pain. There is postural hypotension.

vasovesiculitis (ˌvasohvəˌsikyə-'lietəs) inflammation of the vas deferens and seminal vesicles.

VDRL test Venereal Disease Research Laboratory test for syphilis.

vector ('vektə) 1. an animal that carries organisms or parasites from one host to another, either of the same species or to one of another species; for example, dogs which carry rabies, and mosquitoes, which carry malaria. 2. a quantity with magnitude and direction. *Electrocardiograph v.* the method of recording the direction and magnitude of the electrical activity of the heart.

vegan ('veegən) a vegetarian who excludes all animal protein from the diet.

vegetarian (vejə'tair·reeyən) a person who eats only food of vegetable origin. *V. diet* one in which no meat is eaten. A *lacto-vegetarian* diet prohibits the intake of meat, poultry, fish, and eggs. An *ovo-lacto-vegetarian* diet allows all foods from plants plus eggs, milk, and other dairy products. An *ovo-vegetarian* diet allows eggs and foods of plant origin, but prohibits all animal and dairy products.

vegetation (ˌvejə'tayshən) in pathology, a plant-like outgrowth. *Adenoid v.* overgrowth of lymphoid tissue in the nasopharynx.

vehicle (ˈveeəkəl) in pharmacy, a substance or medium in which a drug is administered.

vein (vayn) a vessel carrying blood from the capillaries back to the heart. It has thin walls and a lining endothelium from which the venous valves are formed.

vena cava (ˈveenə ˈkayvə) large veins returning blood to the right atrium of the heart.

venepuncture (ˈvenəˌpungkchə) the insertion of a needle into a vein for the introduction of a drug or fluid or for the withdrawal of blood.

venereal (vəˈniə·ri·əl) pertaining to, or caused by, sexual intercourse. *V. disease* a disease transmitted by sexual intercourse or other genital contact. GONORRHOEA, SYPHILIS, and CHANCROID are defined in law as venereal diseases. The term venereal disease (VD) is being replaced by the term SEXUALLY TRANSMITTED DISEASE (STD).

venereology (vəˌniə·reeˈoləjee) the study and treatment of venereal diseases.

venesection (ˈvenəˌsekshən) PHLEBOTOMY. Surgical blood-letting by opening a vein or introducing a wide-bore needle. Performed on blood donors and occasionally to relieve venous congestion.

venogram (ˈveenəˌgram) 1. a graphic recording of the pulse in a vein. 2. a radiograph taken during venography.

venography (veeˈnogrəfee) radiographic examination of a vein after the instillation of a contrast medium to trace its pathway.

venom (ˈvenəm) a poison secreted by an insect, snake, or other animal. *Russell's viper v.* the venom of the Russell viper (Vipera russelli) which acts in vitro as an intrinsic THROMBOPLASTIN and is useful in defining deficiencies of clotting factor X.

venous (ˈveenəs) pertaining to the veins. *V. sinus* one of 14 channels, similar to veins, by which blood leaves the cerebral circulation.

ventilation (ˌventəˈlayshən) 1. the process or act of supplying a house or room continuously with fresh air. 2. in respiratory physiology, the process of exchange of air between the lungs and the ambient air. *Pulmonary v.* (usually measured in litres per minute) refers to the total exchange, whereas *alveolar v.* refers to the effective ventilation of the alveoli, where gas exchange with the blood takes place. 3. in psychiatry, the free discussion of one's problems or grievances.

ventilator (ˈventəˌlaytə) an apparatus designed to qualify the air that is breathed through it or to control pulmonary ventilation either intermittently or continuously. Ventilators provide an intermittent flow of air and/or oxygen under pressure and are connected to the patient by a tube inserted through the mouth, the nose, or an opening in the trachea.

ventimask (ˈventiˌmahsk) an oxygen mask that provides oxygen enrichment of the inspired air while eliminating the need to rebreathe the expired carbon dioxide.

Ventolin (ˈventələn) trade name for a salbutamol metered-dose inhaler; a bronchodilator.

ventouse (ˈvenˌtooz) *see* VACUUM (extractor).

ventral (ˈventrəl) pertaining to a hollow structure or belly.

ventricle (ˈventrikəl) a small pouch

or cavity; applied especially to the lower chambers of the heart and to the four cavities of the brain.

ventricular (ven'trikyələ) pertaining to a ventricle. *V. folds* the outer folds of mucous membrane forming the false vocal cords. *V. septal defect* abbreviated VSD. Congenital abnormality in which there is communication between the two ventricles of the heart as a result of maldevelopment of the intraventricular septum.

ventriculography (ven,trikyə'lografee) 1. radiographic examination of the ventricles of the heart using a radio-opaque contrast medium. 2. radiographic examination of the ventricles of the brain after the injection of air or a contrast medium through a burr hole.

ventriculoscope (ven'trikyələ-,skohp) an instrument for viewing the inside of the ventricles of the brain.

ventrofixation (,ventrohfik'sayshən) stitching a retroverted uterus or other abdominal organ to the abdominal wall.

ventrosuspension (,ventrohsə-'spenshən) an abdominal operation performed to remedy a displacement of the uterus.

Venturi mask (ven'tyoo·ree) *G.B. Venturi, Italian physicist, 1746–1822.* A type of disposable mask used to deliver a controlled oxygen concentration to a patient. The flow of 100% oxygen through the mask draws in a controlled amount of room air (21% oxygen). Commonly available masks deliver 24%, 28%, 35%, or 40% oxygen. At concentrations above 24%, humidification might be required.

Venturi nebuliser ('nebyəliezə) a type of nebuliser used in AEROSOL therapy. The pressure drop of gas flowing through the nebuliser draws liquid from a capillary tube. As the liquid enters the gas stream, it breaks up into a spray of small droplets.

venule ('venyool) a minute vein which collects blood from the capillaries.

verapamil (ve'rapə,mil) a coronary dilator used in the treatment of supraventricular TACHYCARDIA and of ANGINA PECTORIS.

verbigeration (,vərbijə'rayshən) the monotonous repetition of phrases or meaningless words.

vermicide ('vərmə,sied) an agent that destroys intestinal worms; an anthelmintic.

vermiform ('vərmə,fawm) worm shaped. *V. appendix* the worm-shaped structure attached to the CAECUM.

vermifuge ('vərmə,fyooj) an agent that expels intestinal worms; an anthelmintic.

verminous ('vərmənəs) infested with worms or other animal parasites, such as lice.

vernix ('vərniks) [L.] *varnish. V. caseosa* the fatty covering on the skin of the fetus during the last months of pregnancy. It consists of cells and sebaceous material.

verruca (və'rookə) a wart. Hypertrophy of the prickle cell layer of the epidermis and thickening of the horny layer. A virus is the causative organism. *V. acuminata* a venereal wart that appears on the external genitalia. *V. plana* a small, smooth, usually skin-coloured or light-brown, slightly raised wart, sometimes occurring in great numbers; seen most often in children. *V. plantaris* a viral epidermal tumour on the sole of the foot.

version ('vərshən, -zhən) the turning of a part; applied particularly to the turning of a fetus in order to facilitate delivery. *External v.* manipulation of the uterus through the abdominal wall in order to change the position of the fetus. *Internal v.* rotation of the fetus by means of manipulation with the finger of one hand in the vagina. *Podalic v.* turning of the fetus so that the head is uppermost and the feet presenting. *Spontaneous v.* one that occurs naturally without the application of force.

vertebra ('vərtəbrə) one of the 33 irregular bones forming the spinal column: 7 cervical, 12 thoracic, 5 lumbar, 5 sacral (sacrum), and 4 coccygeal (coccyx) vertebrae.

vertebral ('vərtəbrəl) pertaining to a vertebra. *V. column* the spine or backbone.

vertebrobasilar (ˌvərtəbroh'basələ) pertaining to the vertebral and the basilar arteries. *V. disease* a condition affecting the flow of blood through the vertebral and basilar arteries which can cause recurrent attacks of blindness, DIPLOPIA, vertigo, DYSARTHRIA, and HEMIPARESIS.

vertex ('vərteks) the crown of the head. *V. presentation* position of the fetus such that the crown of the head appears in the vagina first.

vertigo ('vərtəˌgoh) a feeling of rotation or of going round, in either oneself or one's surroundings, particularly associated with disease of the CEREBELLUM and the vestibular nerve of the ear. It can occur in DIPLOPIA or MENIÈRE'S SYNDROME.

vesica ('vesikə) a bladder; usually referring to the urinary bladder.

vesicle ('vesikəl) 1. in anatomy, a small bladder or blister, usually containing fluid. *Seminal v.* one of a pair of sacs which arise from the VAS DEFERENS near the bladder and contain semen. 2. a very small blister, usually containing serum.

vesicoureteric (ˌvesikoh·yoorə'terik) relating to the urinary bladder and the ureters. *V. reflex* the passing of urine backwards up the ureter during micturition. A cause of PYELONEPHRITIS in children.

vesicovaginal (ˌvesikohvə'jienəl) relating to the bladder and vagina. *See* FISTULA.

vesicular (ve'sikyələ) relating to or containing vesicles. *V. breathing* the soft murmur of normal respiration, as heard on auscultation. *V. mole* hydatidiform mole.

vesiculitis (veˌsikyə'lietəs) inflammation of a vesicle, particularly the seminal vesicles.

vessel ('vesəl) a tube, duct or canal for conveying fluid, usually blood or lymph.

vestibular (ve'stibyələ) relating to a vestibule. *V. glands* those in the vestibule of the vagina, including BARTHOLIN'S GLANDS. *V. nerve* a branch of the auditory nerve supplying the semicircular canals and concerned with balance and equilibrium.

vestibule ('vestəˌbyool) a space or cavity at the entrance to another structure. *V. of the ear* the cavity at the entrance to the cochlea. *V. of the vagina* the space between the LABIA MINORA at the entrance to the vagina.

vestibulocochlear (veˌstibyəloh-'kokli·ə) pertaining to the vestibule of the ear and the cochlea. *V. nerve* the 8th cranial nerve. Also known as the auditory nerve.

vestigial (və'stijəl) rudimentary. Referring to the remains of an anatomical structure which, being of no further use, has atrophied.

viable ('vieəbəl) capable of independent life.

Vibrio ('vibreeoh) a genus of Gram-negative bacteria, curved and motile by means of flagellae. *V. cholerae* or *comma* that which causes cholera.

vicarious (və'kairi·əs) 1. obtained or undergone at second-hand through sympathetic participation in another's experiences. 2. substituted for another; used when one organ functions instead of another.

villus ('viləs) a small finger-like process projecting from a surface. *Chorionic v. see* CHORIONIC. *Intestinal v.* those of the mucous membrane of the small intestine, each of which contains a blood capillary and a LACTEAL.

vinblastine (vin'blasteen) a vinca alkaloid used as an antineoplastic in the treatment of Hodgkin's disease and testicular germinal cell cancer, usually in combination with other antineoplastic agents.

Vincent's angina ('vinsənts) *J.H. Vincent, French physician, 1862–1950. See* ANGINA.

Vincent's stomatitis an infection of the mouth characterised by bleeding, pain, fever, and swelling of the nodes in the neck.

vincristine (vin'kristeen) a vinca alkaloid used as an antineoplastic in the treatment of acute leukaemias, Hodgkin's disease, non-Hodgkin's lymphomas, and some solid tumours, usually in combination with other antineoplastic agents.

vinyl ('vienəl) a plastic material now used extensively for medical equipment. *V. ether* a short-acting inhalation anaesthetic drug used mainly for inducing anaesthesia and for minor surgery.

viraemia (vie'reemi·ə) the presence of viruses in the blood.

virilism ('virə,lizəm) masculine traits exhibited by a female owing to the production of excessive amounts of androgenic hormone either in the adrenal cortex or from an ovarian tumour. *See* ARRHENOBLASTOMA.

virology (vie'roləjee) the scientific study of viruses, their growth, and the diseases caused by them.

virulence ('virələns) the power of a microorganism to produce toxins or poisons. This depends on: (a) the number and power of the invading organisms; and (b) the power of the microorganism to overcome host resistance.

virulent ('virələnt) dangerously poisonous.

virus ('vierəs) any member of a class of infectious agents which were originally distinguished by their smallness and their inability to replicate outside a living host cell; because these properties are shared by certain other microorganisms (rickettsiae, chlamydiae), viruses are now characterised by their simple organisation and their unique mode of replication. A virus consists of genetic material, which can be either DNA or RNA, and is surrounded by a protein coat and, in some viruses, by a membranous envelope. They cause many diseases, including chicken pox (varicella), herpes zoster (shingles), herpes infections, measles (rubeola), German measles (rubella), mumps, infectious mononucleosis, hepatitis A and B, yellow fever, the common cold, acquired immune deficiency syndrome (AIDS), influenza, certain types of pneumonia and croup and other respiratory infections, poliomyelitis, and several types of encephalitis. There is evidence that certain viruses might be capable of causing cancer.

viscera ('visə·rə) plural of viscus.

visceroptosis (ˌvisə·rop'tohsəs) a general tendency of the abdominal organs to prolapse.

viscid ('visəd) sticky and glutinous.

viscosity (vi'skosətee) resistance to flowing. A sticky and glutinous quality.

viscus ('viskəs) any of the organs contained in the body cavities, especially in the abdomen.

vision ('vizhən) the faculty of seeing. Sight.

visual ('vizhyooəl) relating to sight. *V. acuity* sharpness of vision. It is assessed by reading test types. *V. cells* the rods and cones of the retina. *V. field* the area within which objects can be seen when looking straight ahead. *V. purple* the pigment in the outer layers of the retina. RHODOPSIN.

vital ('viet'l) relating to life. *V. capacity* the amount of air that can be expelled from the lungs after a full inspiration. *V. signs* the signs of life, namely pulse, respiration, and temperature. *V. statistics* the records kept of births and deaths among the population, including the causes of death and the factors that seem to influence their rise and fall.

vitallium (vie'tali·əm) a metal alloy used in dentistry and for prostheses in bone surgery.

vitamin ('vitəmən) any of a group of accessory food factors which are contained in foodstuffs and are essential to life, growth and reproduction. *See* Appendix 7.

vitiligo (ˌvitə'liegoh) a skin disease marked by an absence of pigment, producing white patches on the face and body. LEUKODERMA.

vitrectomy (vi'trektəmee) surgical extraction of the vitreous humour and its replacement by a physiological solution in the treatment of vitreous haemorrhage in diabetic RETINOPATHY.

vitreous ('vitri·əs) glassy. *V. humour* the transparent jelly-like substance filling the posterior of the eye from lens to retina.

vocal ('vohkəl) pertaining to the voice or the organs that produce the voice. *V. cords* the two folds of tissue in the larynx, formed of fibrous tissue covered with squamous epithelium. *V. resonance* the normal sounds of speech heard through the chest wall by means of a stethoscope.

voice (voys) the acoustic sounds of speech produced by the vibrations of the vocal cords of the larynx.

void (voyd) empty or expel waste products from the body, such as urine from the bladder.

volar ('vohlə) pertains to the palms of the hand or soles of the feet.

volatile ('voləˌtiel) having a tendency to evaporate readily.

volition (və'lishən) the conscious adoption by the individual of a line of action.

Volkmann's contracture ('vohlkmənz) *R. von Volkmann, German surgeon, 1830–89.* Contraction of the fingers and sometimes of the wrist or of analogous parts of the foot, with loss of power, after severe injury or improper use of a tourniquet or cast.

volume ('volyoom) the space occupied by a substance. *Minute v.* the total volume of air breathed in or out in 1 min. *Packed cell v.* that occupied by the blood cells after centrifuging (about 45% of the blood sample). *Residual v.* the amount of air left in the lungs after breathing out fully.

voluntary ('voləntree) under the control of the will. *See* INVOLUNTARY.

volvulus ('volvyələs) twisting of a loop of bowel causing obstruction. Most common in the sigmoid colon.

vomer ('vohmə) a thin plate of bone forming the posterior septum of the nose.

vomit ('vomət) 1. matter ejected from the stomach through the mouth (vomitus). 2. to eject material in this way. *Bilious v.* vomit mixed with bile. The vomit is stained yellow or green. *Coffee-ground v.* ejected matter that contains small quantities of altered blood, which has this appearance. *Faecal* or *stercoraceous v.* vomit mixed with faeces. Occurs in intestinal obstruction when the contents of the upper intestine regurgitate back into the stomach. It is dark brown with an unpleasant odour.

vomiting ('voməting) a reflex act of expulsion of the stomach contents via the oesophagus and mouth. It can be preceded by nausea and excess salivation if the cause is local irritation in the stomach. *Cyclical v.* recurrent attacks of vomiting often occurring in children and associated with acidosis. *V. of pregnancy* vomiting occurring more frequently in the first trimester of pregnancy. MORNING SICKNESS. *Projectile v.* the forcible ejection of the gastric contents, usually without warning. Present in hypertrophic PYLORIC STENOSIS and in cerebral diseases.

von Recklinghausen's disease (von 'rekling,howzənz) *see* RECKLINGHAUSEN'S DISEASE.

von Willebrand's disease (von 'vili,brants) *E.A. von Willebrand, Finnish physician, 1870–1949.* A bleeding disorder inherited as an autosomal dominant trait (rarely recessive), characterised by a prolonged bleeding time, deficiency of coagulation factor VIII, and associated with EPISTAXIS and increased bleeding after trauma or surgery, MENORRHAGIA, and postpartum bleeding.

vulnerability (,vulnə·rə'bilətee) weakness. Susceptibility to injury or infection.

vulva ('vulvə) the external female genital organs.

vulvectomy (vul'vektəmee) excision of the vulva.

vulvitis (vul'vietəs) inflammation of the vulva.

vulvovaginitis (,vulvoh,vajə'nietəs) inflammation of the vulva and vagina.

Ww

Waldeyer's ring ('valdieəz) *H.W.G. von Waldeyer-Hartz, German anatomist, 1836–1921.* The circle of lymphoid tissue in the pharynx formed by the lingual, faucial, and pharyngeal tonsils.

Wangensteen tube ('wangen,steen) *O.H. Wangensteen, American surgeon, 1898–1981.* A gastrointestinal aspiration tube with a tip that is opaque to X-rays.

warfarin ('wawfə·rən) an oral anticoagulant drug that depresses the PROTHROMBIN level. Used mainly in the treatment of coronary and venous thrombosis.

wart (wawt) an elevation of the skin often of a brownish colour caused by hypertrophy of papillae in the dermis due to a virus infection. *See* VERRUCA and CONDYLOMA.

Wassermann test (reaction) ('vasəmən) *A.P. von Wassermann, German bacteriologist, 1866–1925.* A complement-fixation test used in the diagnosis of syphilis.

water ('wawtə) a clear, colourless, tasteless liquid composed of hydrogen and oxygen (H_2O). *W. balance* fluid balance. That between the fluid taken in by all routes and the fluid lost by all routes. *W.-borne* descriptive of certain diseases that are spread by contaminated water. *W.-brash* the eructation of dilute acid from the stomach to the pharynx, giving a burning sensation. PYROSIS. Heartburn. *W.-seal drainage* a closed method of drainage from the pleural space allowing the escape of fluid and air but preventing air entering because the drainage tube discharges under water.

Waterhouse–Friderichsen syndrome (,wawtəhows'freedriksən) A rare disorder. The malignant or fulminating form of meningococcal MENINGITIS, which is marked by sudden onset and short course, fever, coma, CYANOSIS, haemorrhages from the skin and mucous membranes, and haemorrhage into the adrenal glands.

Watson–Crick helix (,wotsən 'krik) Double helix; a representation of the structure of DEOXYRIBONUCLEIC ACID (DNA), consisting of two coiled chains, each of which contains information completely specifying the other chain.

wave (wayv) a uniform disturbance in which energy moves through a medium without altering the constituents of the medium.

waxy flexibility (,waksee ,fleksə'bilətee) a cataleptic state in which a patient's limbs are held indefinitely in any position in which they have been placed. *See* CATATONIA.

wean (ween) 1. to discontinue breast-feeding or bottle-feeding, and to substitute other foods. This should be effected gradually at about the 4th to 6th month. 2. in respiratory therapy, to decrease gradually dependence on assisted ventilation until the patient is able to breathe spontaneously.

webbing ('webing) the state of being connected by a membrane or a fold of skin. *W. of the hands* or *feet* congenital abnormality in which the digits are not separated from each other. SYNDACTYLY. *W. of the neck* folds of skin in the neck giving it a webbed appearance. Occurs in certain congenital conditions, e.g. TURNER'S SYNDROME.

Weber test ('vaybə) *F.E. Weber-Liel, German otologist, 1832–91.* A test for hearing. A vibrating tuning fork is held in the centre of the forehead. Sound is normally heard equally in both ears. If the sound is heard louder in one ear, it can be indicative of conductive deafness in that ear.

Weil's disease ('vielz) *A. Weil, German physician, 1848–1916.* Spirochaetal jaundice. The causative organism, *Leptospira icterohaemorrhagiae*, is harboured and excreted by rats and enters through a bite, a skin abrasion, or via infected food or water.

Weil–Felix reaction (ˌviel'feeliks) *E. Weil, Austrian physician, 1880–1922; A. Felix, Czech bacteriologist, 1887–1956.* An agglutination test of blood serum used in the diagnosis of typhus.

well-baby clinic (ˌwel'baybee) mothers are encouraged to bring their infants to these clinics for assessment and monitoring of the child's health. Immunisation is available and there are opportunities for 'family' health promotion.

wellness ('welnəs) the development of a personal lifestyle that promotes feelings of wellbeing, achieves the highest level of health within one's capability, and minimises chances of becoming ill. It is guided by a developing sense of self-awareness and self-responsibility encompassing emotional, mental, physical, social, spiritual, and environmental health.

wen (wen) a small sebaceous cyst; a STEATOMA.

Werdnig–Hoffmann disease (ˌvərdnig'hofmən) *G. Werdnig, Austrian neurologist, 1844–1919; J.E. Hoffmann, German neurologist, 1857–1919.* Disease characterised by progressive spinal muscular atrophy affecting the shoulder, neck, pelvis and, eventually, the respiratory muscles of infants.

Werner's syndrome ('vərnəz) *C.W.O. Werner, German physician, 1879–1936.* An hereditary condition characterised by cataracts, OSTEOPOROSIS, stunted growth, and premature greying of the hair.

Wernicke–Korsakoff syndrome (ˌvərnikə'kawsəkof) *K. Wernicke, German neurologist, 1848–1905; S.S. Korsakoff, Russian neurologist, 1854–1900.* A disorder of the central nervous system usually associated with chronic alcoholism, nutritional deficiency, and severe deficiency of vitamin B_1. It is characterised by a combination of motor and sensory disturbances and disordered memory function. One form is Wernicke's ENCEPHALOPATHY, a

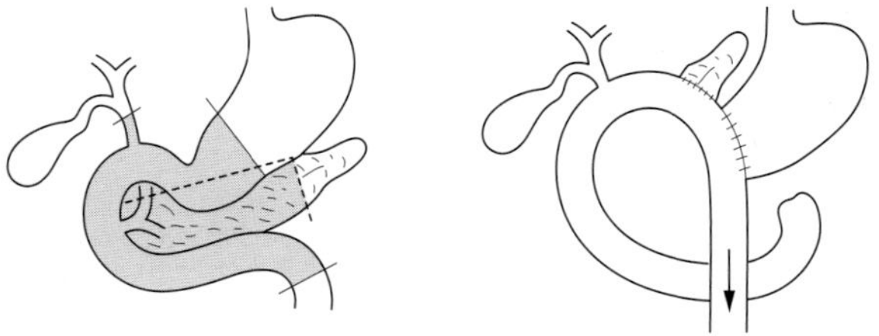

Whipple's Operation

neurological condition due to vitamin B_1 deficiency. Untreated, it progresses from mental confusion and double vision to lethargy and coma.

Wertheim's operation ('vərt·hiemz) *E. Wertheim, Austrian gynaecologist, 1864–1920. See* HYSTERECTOMY.

Wharton's jelly ('wawtənz) *T. Wharton, British physician, 1614–73.* The connective tissue of the umbilical cord.

wheal (weel) a raised stripe on the skin as is caused by the lash of a whip. Typical of URTICARIA.

wheezing ('weezing) breathing with a rasp or whistling sound. It results from constriction or obstruction of the throat, pharynx, trachea, or bronchi.

whiplash injury ('wip,lash) injury to the spinal cord, nerve roots, ligaments, or vertebrae in the cervical region due to a sudden jerking back of the head and neck. Common in road traffic accidents in which there is sudden acceleration or deceleration of the vehicle.

whiplash shake syndrome ('wip,lash 'shayk) a constellation of injuries to the brain and eye that can occur when a child under three years of age is shaken vigorously with the head unsupported. This causes stretching and tearing of the cerebral vessels and brain substance, commonly leading to subdural haematomata and retinal haemorrhages. It can result in paralysis, blindness and other visual disturbances, convulsions, and death. Also known as 'shaken baby syndrome'.

Whipple's operation ('wipəlz) *A.O. Whipple, American surgeon, 1881–1963.* Radical pancreatoduodenectomy performed for carcinoma of the head of the pancreas. (*See* figure on page 454.)

whipworm ('wip,wərm) *see* TRICHURIS.

white blood cell *see* LEUKOCYTE

white leg (wiet) milk leg. *See* PHLEGMASIA.

whitlow ('witloh) a felon; a suppurating inflammation of a finger near the nail. *Melanotic w.* a malignant tumour of the nail bed characterised by formation of melanotic tissue. *Subperiosteal w.* one in which the infection involves the bone covering. *Superficial w.* a pustule between the true skin and cuticle. *See* PARONYCHIA.

WHO World Health Organization.

whooping cough ('hooping ˌkof) a notifiable infectious disease characterised by catarrh of the respiratory tract and paroxysms of coughing, ending in a prolonged whooping respiration; also called pertussis. The causative organism is *Bordetella pertussis.* Whooping cough is a serious disease; most cases occur in children. All babies should be immunised against whooping cough unless there is a sound medical objection.

Widal reaction (vee'dahl) *G.F.I. Widal, French physician, 1862–1929.* A blood agglutination test for typhoid fever.

Willebrand's disease (ˌvilə'brants) *E. A. von Willebrand, Finnish physician 1879–1940.* A common genetic disorder linked to a missing blood factor, von Willebrands' Factor (vWF), which assists with the clotting of blood. The disorder is not sex linked, meaning that both males and females can have the disorder. Generally, the disease is divided into three types: Type I (mild), Type II (medium) and Type III (severe). The lower the type, the fewer the signs and symptoms that occur.

Wilms' tumour (vilmz) *M. Wilms, German surgeon, 1867–1918.* A highly malignant tumour of the kidney occurring in young children. A NEPHROBLASTOMA.

Wilson's disease ('wilsənz) *S.A.K. Wilson, British neurologist, 1878–1937.* Hepatolenticular degeneration. A congenital abnormality in the metabolism of copper leading to neurological degeneration.

window (ˌwindoh) an opening 1. specific time period during which an event can be observed, a reaction monitored or a procedure commenced. 2. a surgical opening in the surface of a structure or between the chambers of a structure.

wiring ('wieəring) the fixing together of a broken or split bone by the use of a wire. Commonly used for the jaw, the patella, and the sternum.

wisdom teeth ('wizdəm) the back molar teeth, the eruption of which is often delayed until maturity.

wish fulfilment ('wishˌfuhlˌfilmənt) a desire, not always acknowledged consciously by the person, which is fulfilled through dreams or by day-dreaming.

withdrawal (widh'drawrəl) 1. a pathological retreat from reality. 2. abstention from drugs to which one is habituated or addicted; also denoting the symptoms occasioned by such withdrawal. *W. symptoms* symptoms brought about by abrupt withdrawal of a narcotic or other drug to which a person has become addicted; also called 'abstinence syndrome'. The usual reactions to withdrawal include anxiety, weakness, gastrointestinal symptoms, nausea and vomiting, tremor, fever, rapid heartbeat, convulsions, and delirium.

Wolff–Parkinson–White syndrome (ˌwuhlfˌpahkinsən'wiet) *L. Wolff, American cardiologist, 1898–1972; Sir J. Parkinson, British physician, 1885–1976; P.D. White, American cardiologist, 1886–1973.* Abnormal heart rhythm caused by an accessory bundle between the atria and ventricles. A congenital disorder.

womb (woom) the uterus.

Wood's light (wuhdz) *R.W. Wood, American physicist, 1868–1953.* Ultraviolet light transmitted through a glass filter containing nickel oxide. It produces fluorescence of infected hairs when placed over a scalp affected with ringworm.

woolsorter's disease ('wuhl,sawtəz) pulmonary anthrax.

word blindness ('wərd) *see* DYSLEXIA.

word salad ('wərd,saləd) speech in which the words are strung together without meaning.

World Health Organization (wərld) abbreviated WHO. The specialised agency of the United Nations that is concerned with health on an international level.

worm (wərm) any one of a number of groups of long soft-bodied invertebrates, some of which are parasitic to humans.

wound (woond) a cut or break in continuity of any tissue caused by injury or operation. It is classified according to its nature. *Abrased w.* the skin is scraped off but there is no deeper injury. *Contused w.* with bruising of the surrounding tissue. *W. healing* the restoration of integrity to injured tissues by replacement of dead tissue with viable tissue. The process starts immediately after an injury and can continue for months or years. *See* HEALING. *Incised w.* usually the result of operation and produced by a knife or similar instrument. The edges of the wound can remain in apposition, and it should heal by first intention. *Lacerated w.* one with torn edges and tissues, usually the result of accident or injury. It is often septic and heals by second intention. *Open w.* a gaping wound on the body surface. *Penetrating w.* often made by gunshot, shrapnel, etc. There can be an inlet and outlet hole, and vital organs are often penetrated by the missile. *Punctured w.* made by a pointed or spiked instrument. *Septic w.* any type into which infection has been introduced, causing suppurative inflammation. It heals by secondary intention.

wrist (rist) the point of the carpus and bones of the forearm. *W. drop* loss of power in the muscles of the hand. It can be due to nerve or tendon injury, but can result from lack of sufficient support by splint or sling.

writer's cramp (,rietəz 'kramp) a colloquial term for painful spasm of the hand and forearm, caused by excessive writing and poor posture. *See* REPETITIVE STRAIN INJURY

wryneck ('rie,nek) *see* TORTICOLLIS.

Wuchereria (,vookə'riə·ri·ə) a genus of nematode worms which is the principal vector of FILARIASIS. *W. bancrofti* the most common species in tropical and subtropical areas.

Xx

X chromosome ('eks,krohmə,sohm) the female sex chromosome, being present in all female gametes and only half the male gametes. When union takes place, two X chromosomes result in a female child (XX) but one of each results in a male child (XY). *See* Y CHROMOSOME.

X-rays ('eks,rayz) electromagnetic waves of short length which are capable of penetrating many substances and of producing chemical changes and reactions in living matter. They are used both to aid diagnosis and to treat disease. Called also Roentgen rays.

xanthelasma (,zanthə'lazmə) a disease marked by the formation of flat or slightly raised yellow cholesterol deposits on the eyelids.

xanthine ('zantheen) a compound found in plant and animal tissues; the forerunner of uric acid in nucleoprotein metabolism.

xanthochromia (,zanthoh'krohmi·ə) 1. the presence of yellow patches on the skin. 2. the yellow colouring of cerebrospinal fluid seen in patients who have had a subarachnoid haemorrhage.

xanthoma (zan'thohmə) the presence in the skin of flat areas of yellowish pigmentation due to deposits of lipids. There are several varieties. *X. palpebrarum* XANTHELASMA.

xanthopsia (zan'thopsi·ə) a disturbance of vision in which all objects appear yellow.

xanthosis (zan'thohsəs) a yellow skin pigmentation, seen in some cases of DIABETES and POLIOMYELITIS.

xenophobia (,zeenə'fohbi·a) a fear of strangers.

Xenopsylla (,zenop'silə) a genus of fleas, some of which are vectors of plague. *X. cheopis* the rat flea which transmits bubonic plague.

xero- combining form meaning drynesss.

xeroderma (,ziə·roh'dərmə) an hereditary condition in which there is excessive dryness of the skin. A mild form of ICHTHYOSIS. *X. pigmentosum* a rare hereditary and often fatal disease in which there is extreme sensitivity of the skin and eyes to light. It begins in childhood and rapidly progresses. The formation of malignant neoplasms is common.

xerophthalmia (,ziə·rof'thalmi·ə) a condition in which the cornea and conjunctiva become horny and necrosed owing to a deficiency of vitamin A. Xeroma.

xerosis (zə'rohsəs) a condition of

dryness, especially of the eyes, mouth, vagina, or skin.

xerostomia (ˌziə·roh'stohmi·ə) dryness of the mouth due to a failure of salivary gland secretion.

xiphoid process ('zifoyd) the smallest of the three parts of the sternum.

X linked ('eksˌlinkt) pertaining to the genes, or the effect of these genes, situated on the X chromosome. X-linked disorders are those caused by the genes on the X chromosome.

xylene ('zieleen) xylol; dimethylbenzene. A clear inflammable liquid resembling benzene. Used as a solvent for rubber and in microscopy.

Xylocaine ('zieləˌkayn) a proprietary preparation of lignocaine used for local anaesthesia.

xylose ('zielohz) a pentose sugar found in connective tissue and sometimes in urine which is not metabolised in the body.

XYY syndrome (ˌeksˌwie'wie) an extremely rare condition in males in which there is an extra Y chromosome, making a total of 47 chromosomes in each body cell. *See* KLINEFELTER'S SYNDROME.

Yy

Y chromosome ('wie,krohmə, sohm) the male sex chromosome, being present in half the male gametes and none of the female. It carries few major genes. *See* X CHROMOSOME.

yawning ('yawning) an involuntary act in which the mouth is opened wide and air is drawn in and exhaled. It can accompany tiredness or boredom.

yaws (yorz) framboesia. A skin infection common in tropical countries. Caused by *Treponema pertenue*, it is common among people (especially children) who live in primitive conditions in equatorial Africa, South America, and the East and West Indies.

yeast (yeest) any of the fungi of the genus *Saccharomyces*. They produce fermentation in malt and in sweetened fruit juices, resulting in the formation of alcoholic solutions such as beer and wines.

yellow fever ('yeloh) an acute, notifiable, infectious disease of the tropics caused by a virus and transmitted by a mosquito (Aëdes aegypti). The virus attacks the liver and kidneys and the symptoms include rigor, headache, pain in the back and limbs, high fever, and black vomit. Haemorrhage from the intestinal mucous membrane can occur. There is a high mortality rate.

yin and yang ('yin,ənd'yang) the two complementary principles of Chinese philosophy incorporated into traditional Chinese medicine. Yin is feminine, dark, and negative; yang is masculine, bright, and positive. Together, the yin–yang interaction and balance is believed to maintain the harmony of the body and, in a healthy person, to maintain a state of dynamic balance.

yoga ('yohgə) one of the six systems of Indian philosophy which emphasises personal physical preparation using isometric exercises, relaxation, breathing techniques, and the attainment of defined body positions to achieve relaxation, with physical and emotional harmony and wellbeing.

yogurt ('yohgət) a semisolid curdled milk preparation made from whole or skimmed milk solid by fermentation with from the genus *Lactobacillus*.

yoke (yohk) a structure that connects small cylinders of medical gases, such as portable oxygen or respiratory equipment.

yolk (yohk) the stored nutrients of an egg or ovum that also supplies nourishment to the developing embryo.

Zz

Z-plasty ('zed,plastee) a plastic operation for removing and repairing deformity resulting from a contraction scar.

Z-track ('zed ,trak) the injection of irritating substances without tracking through sensitive tissues.

zidovudine (,ziedoh'vədeen) an antiviral drug used to retard the progress of AIDS. Also known as azidothymidine or AZT.

Ziehl–Neelsen method (,ziel'neelsən) *F. Ziehl, German bacteriologist, 1857–1926; F.K.A. Neelsen, German pathologist, 1854–94.* A method of staining tubercle baccili for microscopic study.

zimmer ('zimə) the trade name of a metal, lightweight walking aid, and commonly applied to other products of similar design and weight. Predominantly used by the elderly to assist in rehabilitation.

zinc (zingk) *symbol* Zn. A trace element which is essential in the body for cell growth and multiplication. The recommended daily intake of zinc is 15 mg for an adult. A severe deficiency of zinc can retard growth in children, cause a low sperm count in adult males, and retard wound healing.

Zollinger–Ellison syndrome (,zolinjə'elisən) A rare condition in which a pancreatic tumour causes excessive outpouring of gastric juice. Peptic ulcers can occur.

zona ('zohnə) 1. a zone. *Z. pellucida* the membrane surrounding the ovum. 2. herpes zoster; shingles. *Z. facialis* herpes of the face.

zone therapy ('zohn ,therəpee) in reflex zone therapy the feet are palpated in order to alleviate pain and/or treat symptoms by stimulating the self-healing capacity of the body.

zonula ('zonyələ) a zonule. In anatomy, a small, usually circular, area. *Ciliary z.* the area surrounded by the suspensory ligaments of the eye.

zonulolysis (,zonyə'loləsəs) dissolving of the zonular fibres by zonulysin to aid cataract extraction.

zonulysin (,zonyə'liesən) a proteolytic enzyme that can be used in eye surgery to dissolve the suspensory ligament.

zoonosis (,zoh·ə'nohsəs, ,zooə-'nohsəs) a disease of animals that is transmissible to humans, e.g. anthrax, cat-scratch fever, etc.

zoster ('zostə) *see* HERPES.

zygoma (zie'gohmə, zi-) the arch formed by the union of the temporal bone with the malar bone in front of the ear.

zygote ('ziegoht, 'zi-) a single fertilised cell formed from the union of a male and a female gamete.

zymase (ˌziemayz) an enzyme.

zymosis (zie'mohsəs) 1. fermentation. 2. the development of an infectious disease.

Appendices

Appendix 1

Commonly Used Combining Forms

a- without, not
ab- away from
abdomin/o- pertaining to the abdomen
acanth/o- thorny
acou- pertaining to hearing
acr/o- pertaining to the extremities
ad- to, towards
aden/o- pertaining to the glands
adip/o- pertaining to fat
aer/o- pertaining to air
-aemia, -emia pertaining to blood
-aesthesia, -esthesia pertaining to feeling or sensation
-agog, -agogue an agent that promotes the expulsion of a substance
alg-, algesi- pertaining to pain
-algia painful
allo- reversed or differing from normal
ambi- pertaining to both sides
andr/o- pertaining to the male
angi/o- pertaining to a vessel, especially a blood vessel
ant-, -anti- against
ante- before, in front of
arthr/o- pertaining to a joint
-asthenia depleted vitality
audi/o- hearing
aur/i, aur/o- ear
aut/o- pertaining to the self
bar/o- pertaining to pressure
-basia ability to walk
bi- two or twice, double
bili- pertaining to bile
blephar/o- pertaining to the eyelids or eyelash
brachy- short
brady- slow

bronch/o-	pertaining to the bronchus
bucc/o-	pertaining to the cheek
carcin-	pertaining to cancer
cardi/o-	heart
cata-	against
-cele	swelling or tumour
-centesis	to puncture or cut
cephal/o-	pertaining to the head
cerebr/o-	pertaining to the cerebrum
cervic-	pertaining to the neck
cheir/o-, chir/o-	pertaining to the hand
-chesia	pertaining to the discharge of substances
chol/e-, chol/o-	pertaining to bile
circum-	around
-clasia	crushing or breaking up
col/o-	colon
colp/o-	vagina
contra-	opposed, against
copr/o-	pertaining to faeces
cortic-	pertaining to the cortex
crani/o-	pertaining to the cranium or skull
cry/o-	cold
crypt/o-	concealed or hidden
cut-	pertaining to the skin
cyan-	blue
cyst/o-	pertaining to the bladder
cyt/o-	cell or cytoplasm
-dactyl	digit
de-	away from
derm/a-, derm/o-	pertaining to the skin
di-	twice or two
dipl/o-	double
-dipsia	thirst
dors/i-, dors/o-	pertaining to the dorsum or back
duoden/o-	duodenum of intestine
dys-	painful or disordered
ecto-	outside
-ectomy	the surgical removal of, excision
-ectopia	the displacement of a part or organ
end-, endo-, ent-, ento-	within, inner
enter/o-	pertaining to the intestines
epi-	upon, on, over
eu-	good or well
erythr/o-	red
faci/o-	face
-faction	the process of making

-fibroma	benign tumour consisting of fibrous tissue
fiss-	split, cleft
flex-	bend
galact/o-	pertaining to milk
gastr/o-	stomach
-genesis	beginning process, origin
gen/o-	producing
glio-	pertaining to the neurolgia, or a gluey substance
gloss/o-	pertaining to the tongue
gluc/o-, glyc/o-	pertaining to glucose, or sweetness
gnath-	pertaining to the jaw
-gram, -gramme	drawing
gynec/o-, gyn/o-	pertaining to woman
haem-, hem-	pertaining to blood
hemi-	half
hepat-	pertaining to the liver
heter/o-	pertaining to another
hist/o-	pertaining to the tissues
holo-	pertaining to the whole
home/o-, hom/o-	the same
hydr/o-	meaning water or hydrogen
hyper-	excess or above
hypo-	beneath or deficient
hyster/o-	pertaining to the uterus
-iasis	disease produced or producing
ile/o-	ileum of intestine
ili/o-	ilium (upper part of hip bone)
inter-	situated between
intra-	situated within
ischi/o-	pertaining to the hip, or ischium
iso-	equal
jejun/o-	jejunum of intestine
kin/e-, kin/o-, kinesi/o-	movement , motion
-lalia	a disorder of speech
lamin-	layer
laryng/o-	pertaining to the larynx
later/o-	pertaining to the side
leuco-, leuko-	white, pertaining to the white corpuscles
lip/o-	pertaining to fat, fatty acids
-lipoma	tumour consisting of fatty tissue
lith/o-	stone or calculus
lymph/o-	lymph

-lysis detachment or breaking down, dissolving
macr/o- large or abnormal size
mal- bad or abnormal
-malacia softening of tissue
man- pertaining to the hand
mast/o- pertaining to the breast
mega- large or great
melan- black
mening/o- meninges
meta- change, beyond
micro- small
mon/o- one
morph/o- form, structure, shape
multi- many
myc/o- pertaining to fungus
myel/o- pertaining to bone marrow or spinal cord
my/o- pertaining to muscle
myring/o- eardrum
narc/o- pertaining to stupor
nas/o- pertaining to the nose
necr/o- pertaining to death
neo- new, recent
nephr/o- pertaining to the kidneys
neur/o- pertaining to the nerves
nutri- pertaining to nourishment
ocul/o- pertaining to the eye
-odynia a state of pain
olig/o- few or little
-oma a tumour
onc/o- pertaining to a swelling or tumour
oo- pertaining to an egg or ovum
ophthalm/o- pertaining to the eye(s)
orch/i-, orchi/do-, orch/o- testis or testes
-orexia pertaining to the appetite
or/o- mouth
orth/o- straight or normal
-osis a pathological condition
oste/o- pertaining to bone
-ostomy a surgical procedure where an opening is made to allow the contents of the intestines or the bladder to drain through the abdominal wall

oto-	pertaining to the ear
paedia-, pedia-	pertaining to a child
pan-	all
para-	beside, beyond, after
path/o-	related to disease
ped-, pod-	foot
pell-	pertaining to the skin
-paenia, -penia	deficiency of, lack of
-pepsia	pertaining to digestion
peri-	around
-pexy	surgical fixation
phag/o-	eating
pharyng/o-	pharynx
-phasic	speech disorder
-phily	fondness or affinity for something
phleb/o-	pertaining to a vein
-phobe	one who fears
-phyma	a swelling or tumour
pil/o-	resembling hair
-plasty	surgical shaping or forming
-plegic	pertaining to paralysis
plex-	a stroke
-pnea, -pnoea	breathing or breath
pneum/o-	of or related to the lungs, air or breathing
-poiesis, -poesis	production of
poli/o-	pertaining to the grey matter in the central nervous system
poly-	many
post-	after or behind
-praxia	pertaining to the performance of movements
pre-	before
proct/o-	pertaining to the rectum
psor-	pertaining to itching
pseud/o-	false
psych-	pertaining to the mind
-ptosis	a prolapse
pulm/o-	pertaining to the lungs
pyel/o-	pertaining to the pelvis or the kidney
py/o-	pertaining to pus
quadr/i-	four
rachi/o-	pertaining to the spine
re-	back or again
ren-	pertaining to the kidneys
retin/o-	retina
retro-	located behind
rhin/o-	pertaining to the nose
-rrhagia	to pour or burst forth
-rrhoea, -rrhea	flow or discharge

ruber-, rubor- red, redness
sacr/o- pertaining to the sacrum
salping/o- fallopian tube or Eustachian tube
sangui- pertaining to blood
sarc/o- flesh or muscular substance
scler/o- hard
scoli/o- twisted, crooked
-scope instrument for examining
semi- meaning half
somat/o- body
sphygm/o- pulse
spondyl/o- vertebra or spinal column
-stasis a stoppage or inhibition
sten/o- narrow
steth/o- pertaining to the chest
-stomy a surgical opening
-strophy twisting
sub- under, beneath
super-, supra- above, superior, excess
sym-, syn- together, with
tachy- fast or rapid
tend/o-, ten/o-, tenont/o, tendin/o- tendon
-thelioma a tumour in cellular tissue
therm/o- pertaining to heat
thorac/o- pertaining to chest or thorax
thromb/o- pertaining to a clot, or thrombus
-tomy a surgical incision
-tony pertaining to motor control
trache/o- pertaining to trachea
trans- across or though
-tresia a perforation
tri- three
-trophy a condition of growth
uni- one
ure- pertaining to urine or the urinary tract
-uria the presence of a substance in the urine
vas/o- pertaining to a vessel
ven/e-, ven/i, ven/o- pertaining to vein(s)
ventr/i-, ventr/o- front of body or belly
vesic/o- pertaining to the bladder or a blister
xen/o- strange
xer/o- dry

Appendix 2
Commonly Used Abbreviations

Abbreviations in use can vary widely from place to place. Each institution's list of acceptable abbreviations is the best authority for its records.

Abbreviation	*Meaning*
ABG	arterial blood gases
ABO	three basic blood groups
ACE	angiotensin-converting enzyme
ACTH	adrenocorticotropic hormone
ADHD	attention deficit-hyperactivity disorder
ADH	antidiuretic hormone
ADL	activities of daily living
AF	atrial fibrillation
AFB	acid-fast bacillus
AIDS	acquired immunodeficiency syndrome
AK	above the knee
ALS	advanced life support; amyotrophic lateral sclerosis
AMI	acute myocardial infarction
BK	below the knee
BMI	body mass index
BMR	basal metabolic rate

Abbreviation	*Meaning*
BP	blood pressure
BPH	benign prostatic hypertrophy
bpm	beats per minute
BSE	breast self-examination
Bx	biopsy
·/c	with
CABG	coronary artery bypass graft
CAT	computed (axial) tomography
CCU	coronary care unit; critical care unit
CF	cystic fibrosis
CHF	congestive heart failure
CHO	carbohydrate
CI	cardiac index; cardiac insufficiency; cerebral infarction
CMV	cytomegalovirus
CNC	clinical nurse consultant
CNS	central nervous system; clinical nurse specialist
c/o	complains of/complaints of
COAD	chronic obstructive airways disease
COLD	chronic obstructive lung disease
COPD	chronic obstructive pulmonary disease
CPAP	continuous positive airway pressure
CPR	cardiopulmonary resuscitation
CSF	cerebrospinal fluid
CT	computed tomography
CVA	cerebrovascular accident

Abbreviation	*Meaning*
CVP	central venous pressure
CVS	chorionic villi sampling
CXR	chest X-ray
D&C	dilation (dilatation) and curettage
DIC	desseminated intravascular coagulopathy/coagulation
DKA	diabetic ketoacidosis
DNA	deoxyribonucleic acid
DOA	dead on arrival
DOB	date of birth
DOE	dyspnoea on exertion
DRG	diagnostic-related groups
DT	delirium tremens
EBP	evidence-based practice
ECG	electrocardiogram; electrocardiograph
ECHO	echocardiography
ED	emergency department
EEG	electroencephalogram; electroencephalograph
ENT	ears, nose and throat
ESR	erythrocyte sedimentation rate
ESRD	end-stage renal disease
F	fahrenheit
FEV	forced expiratory volume
FH, Fhx	family history
FSH	follicle-stimulating hormone
GI	gastrointestinal; glycaemic index

Abbreviation	*Meaning*
GP	general practitioner
GTT	glucose tolerance test
GU	genitourinary
Hb; Hgb	haemoglobin
HCT	haematocrit
HDL	high-density lipoprotein
HIV	human immunodeficiency (AIDS) virus
Hx; hx	history
ICP	intracranial pressure
ICU	intensive care unit
IDC	indwelling catheter
IDDM	insulin dependent diabetes mellitus (type I diabetes)
Ig	immunoglobulin
IM	intramuscular
IOP	intraocular pressure
IPPB	intermittent positive pressure breathing
IQ	intelligence quotient
IV	intravenous
IVP	intravenous pyelogram
KVO	keep vein open
lab	laboratory
LMP	last menstrual period
LOC	level of consciousness; loss of consciousness
LP	lumbar puncture
MI	myocardial infarction

Abbreviation	*Meaning*
MRI	magnetic resonance imaging
MS	multiple sclerosis
MVA	motor vehicle accident
N/A	not applicable; not available
NAD	no abnormalities detected; non-adherent dressing
NBM	nil by mouth
NG, ng	nasogastric
NICU	neonatal intensive care unit
NIDDM	non-insulin dependent diabetes mellitus (type 2 diabetes)
NS	normal saline
NSAID	non-steroidal anti-inflammatory drug
OTC	over-the-counter
Pap test	Papanicolaou smear
PCA	patient-controlled analgesia
pH	hydrogen ion concentration (alkalinity and acidity in urine and blood analysis)
PID	pelvic inflammatory disease
PKU	phenylketonuria
PM	evening
PMT	premenstrual tension
PUO	pyrexia of unknown origin
PVC	premature ventricular contraction
RBC	red blood cell; red blood count
Rh	rhesus factor
ROM	range of motion

Abbreviation	*Meanings*
rpm	revolutions per minute
SGOT	serum glutamic oxaloacetic transaminase
SIDS	sudden infant death syndrome
SLE	systemic lupus erythematosus
SOB	shortness of breath
SG; sp.gr.	specific gravity
SR	sedimentation rate
s/s	signs and symptoms
Staph	Staphylococcus
stat	immediately (*statim*)
STD	sexually transmitted disease
Strep	Streptococcus
TB	tuberculosis; tubercle bacillus
TENS	transcutaneous electrical nerve stimulation
TIA	transient ischaemic attack
TPN	total parenteral nutrition
TPR	temperature, pulse, and respiration
Tx; Rx	treatment
UA	urinalysis
URI	upper respiratory infection
UTI	urinary tract infection
VSD	ventricular septal defect
WBC; wbc	white blood cell; white blood count
wt	weight
X-ray	Roentgen ray

Appendix 3
Units of Measurement

SI Units (Systeme Internationale d'Unites)

Base units

Physical quantity	***Name of unit***	***Symbol***
Mass	kilogram	kg
Length	metre	m
Time	second	s
Electric current	ampere	A
Temperature	kelvin	K
Luminous intensity	candela	cd
Amount of substance	mole	mol

Derived units

Derived units to measure other quantities are obtained by multiplying or dividing any two or more of the seven base units. Some of these have their own names and symbols. For example:

Physical quantity	***Name of unit***	***Symbol***	***Base or derived units***
Force	newton	N	$kg{\cdot}m{\cdot}s^{-2}$
Pressure	pascal	Pa	$N{\cdot}m^{-2}$
Energy, work, heat	joule	J	$N{\cdot}m$
Power	watt	W	$J{\cdot}s^{-1}$

Prefixes used for multiples

Factor	**Prefix**	**Symbol**
10^{-12}	pico	p
10^{-9}	nano	n
10^{-6}	micro	μ
10^{-3}	milli	m
10^{-2}	centi	c
10^{-1}	eci	d
10	deca	da
10^{2}	hecto	h
10^{3}	kilo	k
10^{6}	mega	M
10^{9}	giga	G
10^{12}	tera	T

Capacity

The SI unit of volume is the cubic metre (m^3), but the litre (L) is more commonly used and accepted.

1000 microlitres (μL)	= 1 millilitre (mL)
1000 millilitres	= 1 litre (L)
1 cubic centimetre (cm^3)	= 1 millilitre
1 teaspoon	= 5 mL
1 dessertspoon	= 10 mL
1 tablespoon	= 15 mL
1 cup	= 250 mL
1 tumbler	= 285 mL

Weight

1000 micrograms (μg)	= 1 milligram (mg)
1000 milligrams	= 1 gram (g)

1000 grams	= 1 kilogram (kg)
1000 kilograms	= 1 metric tonne

Energy

A dietetic Calorie is the amount of heat required to raise the temperature of 1 litre of water by 1°C and is equal to 4.184 kilojoules.

1 g fat will produce 38 kilojoules or 9 Calories.
1 g protein will produce 17 kilojoules or 4 Calories.
1 g carbohydrate will produce 17 kilojoules or 4 Calories.

Comparative temperatures

Celsius (°C)	*Fahrenheit (°F)*	*Celsius (°C)*	*Fahrenheit (°F)*
100.0 (boiling point)	212	38.5	101.3
95	203	38	100.4
90	194	37.5	99.5
85	185	37	98.6
80	176	36.5	97.7
75	167	36	96.8
70	158	35.5	96
65	149	35	95
60	140	34	93.2
55	131	33	91.4
50	122	32	89.6
45	113	31	87.8
44	112.2	30	86
43	109.4	25	77
42	107.6	20	68
41	105.8	15	59

Celsius (°C)	Fahrenheit (°F)	Celsius (°C)	Fahrenheit (°F)
40	104	10	50
39.5	103.1	5	41
39	102.2	0 (freezing point)	32

To convert readings on the Fahrenheit scale into Celsius, subtract 32, multiply by 5, and divide by 9. For example:

$98 - 32 = 66 \times 5 = 330 \div 9 = 36.6$.
Therefore 98°F = 36.6°C.

To convert readings on the Celsius scale into Fahrenheit, multiply by 9, divide by 5, and add 32. For example:

$36.6 \times 9 = 330 \div 5 = 66 + 32 = 98$
Therefore 36.6°C = 98°F.

The term 'Celsius' (after the Swedish astronomer who invented the scale in 1742) is now being internationally used instead of 'centigrade', which term is employed in some countries to denote fractions of an angle.

Appendix 4

Table of Normal Values

Normal values for adults based on those obtained from major teaching hospitals. These reference ranges can vary, depending on the assay used in particular laboratories

Haematology	
Basophil granulocytes	0.01–0.1 × 10^9/L
Eosinophil granulocytes	0.04–0.4 × 10^9/L
Erythrocyte sedimentation rate (ESR)	0–10 mm/h
Haemoglobin (male)	13–18 g/dL
Haemoglobin (female)	11.5–16.5 g/dL
Leukocytes	4.3–10.8 × 10^9/L
Mean corpuscular haemoglobin (MCH)	1.7–2.0 fmol
Mean corpuscular haemoglobin concentration (MCHC)	32–36 g/dL
Mean corpuscular volume (MCV)	76–96 fL
Monocytes	0.2–0.8 × 10^9/L
Neutrophil granulocytes	3.5–7.5 × 10^9/L
Packed cell volume (PCV) (male)	42–63mL/dL
Packed cell volume (PCV) (female)	36–45 mL/dL
Plasma volume	45 ± 5mL/kg

Haematology	
Platelet count	150–400 × 10^9/L
Red cell folate	> 160 μg/L
Reticulocyte count	0.5–2.5% of red cells
Serum B_{12}	160–925 ng/L
Serum folate	5–63 nmol/L (3–20μg/L)
Total blood volume (male)	75 ± 10mL/kg
Total blood volume (female)	70 ± 10 mL/kg

Coagulation	
Bleeding time (Ivy method)	2.5–9 min
Partial thromboplastin time (PTTK)	30–40 seconds
Prothrombin time	12–15 seconds

Biochemistry	
Acid phosphatase (phostatic)	<0.8 U/L
Alanine aminotransferase (ALT)	<30 U/L
Albumin	36–47 g/L
Alkaline phosphatase	30–100 U/L
Alpha-1-Antitrypsin	2–4 g/L
Alpha-fetoprotein	<10kU/L
Amylase	<220 U/L
Angiotensin-converting enzyme	5.5–28 IU/L
Aspartate aminotransferase (AST)	5–40 U/L
Bicarbonate	23–31 mmol/L
Bilirubin	<18 μmol/L

Biochemistry	
Calcium	2.2–2.67 mmol/L (8.5–10.5 mg/dL)
Chloride	100–106 mmol/L (100–106 mEq/L)
Cholinesterase	7–9 U/mL
Copper	12–25 μmol/L (100–200 μg/dL)
Complement (total haemolytic)	150–250 U/mL
Creatinine	0.06–0.12 mmol/L (0.6–1.5 mg/dL)
Creatinine kinase (CPK)	<195 U/L
Ferritin	5.8–120 nmol/L (15–250 mmol/L μg/L)
Gamma glutamyl transferase (γGT)	10–40 U/L
Glucose	3–5.8 mmol/L
Glycosylated haemoglobin (Hb_1Ac)	3.8–6.4%
Hydroxybutyric dehydrogenase (HBD)	40–125 U/L
Iron	10–30 μmol/L
Iron binding capacity (total)	42–80 μmol/L (250–410 μg/dL)
Lactate dehydrogenase	<150 U/L
Lead	1.8 μmol/L
Magnesium	0.7–1.1 mmol/L
Osmolality	275–295 mosmol/kg
Phosphate	0.8–1.4 mmol/L
Potassium	3.5–5.0 mmol/L
Protein (total)	61–84 g/L

Biochemistry	
Sodium	135–146 mmol/L
Urate	0.2–0.5 mmol/L
Urea	3–8 mmol/L
Vitamin A	0.5–2.1 μmol/L (0.15–0.6 μg/mL)
Vitamin D (25–hydroxy)	19.4–137 nmol/L (8–55 ng/mL)
Vitamin D (1,25–dihydroxy)	62–155 pmol/L (26–65 pg/mL)
Zinc	10–18 μmol/L

Blood gases	
Arterial PCO_2	4.8–6.1 kPA (36–46 mm Hg)
Arterial PO_2	10–13.3 kPa (75–100 mm Hg); for every year over 60, add 0.13 kPa
Arterial $[H^+]$	35–45 nmol/L
Arterial pH	7.35–7.45

Cerebrospinal fluid	
Pressure (adult)	50–200 mm water
Cells	0–5 lymphocytes/mm^3
Glucose	2.5–5.6 mmol/L
Protein	100–400 mg/L

Faeces (normal fat content)	
daily output on normal diet	<7g
fat (as stearic acid)	11–18 mmol/24 h

Lipids and lipoproteins

Cholesterol	<5.5 mmol/L
Triglyceride	<2.0 mmol/L
Lipoproteins HDL (male)	0.90–1.80 mmol/L
Lipoproteins HDL (female)	0.90–2.10 mmol/L
Lipids (total)	4.0–10g/L (400–1000 mg/dL)

Urine

Total quantity in 24 h	1000–1500 mL
Specific gravity	1.010–1.025
pH	4–8

Urine: average solids excreted in 24 h

Calcium	<7.5 mmol
Copper	<1.1 μmol
Creatinine	8–16 mmol
5-Hydroxyindole acetic acid	<40 μmol
4-Hydroxy-3-methoxymandelic acid	<40 μmol
Hydroxyproline	0.08–0.25 mmol
Lead	0.14–0.40 μmol
Magnesium	3.3–5.0 mmol
Oestriol	varies widely during pregnancy (μmol)
Phosphate	15–50 mmol
Protein (quantitative)	<0.15 g
Urea	300–600 mmol

Appendix 5
Drug Control

Terry Maunsell, Director of Pharmacy,
Royal Prince Alfred Hospital, Sydney

The manufacture, supply, and use of drugs are subject to regulation and control. Federal and state legislation both apply, and restrictions can therefore differ somewhat from state to state. In addition, there can be state health department guidelines and institutional policies that apply to the use of drugs in public hospitals and institutions. Nurses must be aware of the laws and regulations that relate to drug use in the state in which they are working, and must observe these carefully.

Medicines are classified into groupings (or schedules) known as 'Poisons Schedules'. The Poisons Schedules list all poisons, hazardous substances, restricted substances, drugs of addiction, and prohibited substances. They specify packaging, storage, and labelling requirements, as well as the restrictions that apply to the supply and use of substances in each schedule. All states have substantially adopted uniform scheduling practices. From time to time, amendments are made to the various Poisons Schedules.

In all states, restricted drugs and drugs of addiction must be ordered by a medical practitioner on a prescription or a medication order. In hospitals and other institutions, this usually applies to all drugs. A prescription or medication order must be legible and written in ink or biro and must include, in the prescriber's own handwriting, the patient's name and address (or unique identifying number), the name and strength of the drug, the route of administration, the dose and frequency, and the prescriber's signature. All orders for drugs of addiction must include the quantity required in words and numbers. An order written by another person is not a legal order even if signed by a medical practitioner. In certain circumstances, provision exists for medical officers to generate prescriptions via computer. However, strict protocols apply to the use of such computerised systems and, in all cases, the prescription must be generated only by the medical practitioner.

Legislation requires that the dispensing, storage, and administration of drugs of addiction be recorded in a drug register reserved for this purpose. Drugs of addiction include opioids (such as morphine, pethidine, methadone, papaveretum, and oxycodone), cocaine and other stimulants (such as dexamphetamine), and other substances (such as pentazocine).

In hospitals, institutional policy might also require that the administration of other substances such as sedatives and some analgesics be similarly recorded. For security and safety reasons, the storage and supply of accountable drugs in hospital is subject to tight control.

In hospitals and other health institutions, the prescribing and administration of all drugs should be clearly noted in the medication record or in another appropriate place in the patient's medical record.

Abbreviations used in prescriptions

English is the preferred language for the writing of prescriptions, rather than the traditional Latin. *The use of abbreviations in prescriptions in either English or Latin is potentially dangerous and should be discouraged..* However, nurses might still encounter the following Latin abbreviations.

Abbreviation	*Latin*	*English*
a.c.	ante cibum	before food
ad lib.	ad libitum	to the desired amount
b.d. or b.i.d.	bis in die	twice a day
c.	cum	with
o.m. or m.	omni mane	every morning
o.n. or n.	omni nocte	every night
o.d	omni die	every day
p.c.	post cibum	after food
p.r.n.	pro re nate	whenever necessary
q.d.s.	quaque die sumendum	four times daily

Abbreviation	*Latin*	*English*
q.i.d.	quater in die	four times a day
q.q.h.	quater quaque hora	every four hours
R	recipe	take
s.o.s.	si opus sit	if necessary
stat.	statim	at once
t.d.s.	ter die sumendum	three times daily
t.i.d.	ter in die	three times a day

Administration of drugs

Administration of drugs accurately, safely, and appropriately is an extremely important aspect of nursing. Nurses must exercise professional judgment and satisfy themselves that they are competent to administer the prescribed medication and are prepared to be accountable for that action. The exercise of professional judgment involves the application of knowledge and experience to the situation faced. This must be based on a sound knowledge of the diagnosis, the condition of the patient, and the environment in which care is given.

Throughout the administration process, the underlying principle must be the safety and wellbeing of the patient. The appropriate application of this principle results in a sequence of events that ensures the '5 rights' of drug administration. These are that the *right* patient receives the *right* drug in the *right* dose by the *right* route, at the *right* time.

Nurses administer medications that have been prescribed (ordered) by a medical practitioner. If there is any doubt in either reading or interpreting the order, the prescriber must be contacted and clear instructions obtained.

Before the medication is given, the patient's identity should be confirmed. This can be done by verbal confirmation and by checking the patient's identity band, or by other appropriate documentation. This is particularly important for infants and for patients who are unconscious or mentally incompetent.

Drugs have both generic names and trade names. Generic names should be used rather than trade names. Any unfamiliar generic or trade names should be checked to ensure that the intended medication is, in fact, being administered. If there is any doubt, the pharmacist should be contacted.

Labelling information on the container should be thoroughly checked three times before the medication is administered. If the label is illegible, the contents of the container should not be used. Expiry dating on the container label should be checked. If the expiry date has been passed, a new supply of medication should be obtained. Before use, medication should be inspected and any unusual effects such as colour changes, cloudiness of solution, or moisture absorption by tablets should be noted. Such changes can indicate loss or change of activity due to incorrect storage. In such situations, a new supply of medication should be obtained. If the contents of the container are non-uniform in any way, the contents should not be used and the container should be returned to the pharmacy. Medications must be kept in their original packaging.

The prescribed dose should be carefully considered before medication is given. If there is any doubt, the nurse should consult the pharmacist or the prescriber before proceeding. If, after checking, the nurse still has doubts about the dose, he or she should withhold the medication, inform the nursing supervisor and the prescriber of his or her actions, indicate the reasons, and document in the patient's medical records that the medication has not been given.

The dosage form should also be considered. The dosage form provided by the manufacturer should not be divided, crushed, or in any other way altered unless it has been ascertained that it is appropriate to do so. The nurse should check that the dosage form provided is appropriate to the route of administration available. Although the medical practitioner prescribes the drug and the route of administration, the nurse should question such an order when it seems inappropriate—for example, if an oral medication has been prescribed for a patient who is vomiting.

Throughout the process of drug administration, the effects and side-effects of treatment should be noted. Both positive effects and adverse reactions relating to medication should be recorded and reported to the appropriate medical officer. Assessment of the situation is especially important when administering drugs which are to be taken 'when necessary' (p.r.n.).

It is important, especially with drugs whose efficacy depends on reaching or maintaining adequate blood levels, that drugs be given at the correct time. The effects of drugs can be substantially affected when administered with or after food. The nurse should ensure that the patient receives the drug and swallows the medication.

Thorough and accurate records of drug administration must be maintained. The administration record should be made after the medication has been given and the dose, route, time, and signature or initials of the administering nurse recorded. If the patient refuses the drug or if the medication is not administered, the reason for non-administration should be noted and reported.

The responsibility of the nurse can vary in the setting of a patient's home. Patients have greater freedom in their own setting. The implications of self-medication, possession of over-the-counter medications, and alternative therapies (such as herbal remedies or Chinese medicines) must also be considered. If nurses working in the community become involved in obtaining prescribed medicines for patients, they must recognise responsibility for their safe transit and correct delivery.

These guidelines apply to the administration of drugs in all healthcare settings, but do not replace the need for the nurse to be conversant with the laws and policies that apply in the particular setting in which he or she is working.

Appendix 6
Resuscitation

Andrea Marshall (with assistance of Ella Tyler, chairman, Basic Life Support Committee, Australian Resuscitation Council)

The central focus of resuscitation is the protection of the brain and heart from ischaemia, and the steps involved in resucitation are systematic and implemented in order of priority. The principles of basic life support (BLS) include: (i) establishing and maintaining an airway; (ii) breathing; and (iii) circulation—the objective being to provide the brain and heart with an oxygenated blood supply. Effective BLS techniques rely on rapid assessment of the situation and initiating procedures that facilitate and maintain an adequate supply of oxygenated blood to the brain before irreversible damage occurs.

Advanced life support (ALS) techniques include a range of therapeutic and technological interventions carried out by trained health personnel. These are not discussed here.

Basic life support

If a person collapses, the rescuer must assess the situation quickly, ensure the safety of the rescuer, victim, and bystanders, call for help, and commence basic life support (BLS).

When calling for help the 'phone first' approach is recommended because the vast majority of cardiac arrests are due to ventricular fibrillation, which is treatable by defibrillation.

The level of consciousness is determined by the use of verbal and tactile stimuli. These stimuli should never reach a level that causes or aggravates injury, and infants and small children should never be shaken. The shoulders should be firmly grasped and squeezed to elicit a response. Verbal stimuli should also be used. If conscious, the person will respond. Allow the person to adopt a comfortable position, and observe him or her closely for any changes in condition.

If there is no response to the stimuli, the person is unconscious and should be turned on his or her side. Help should be summoned. Anyone who fails to respond to touch or the spoken word is considered to be unconscious and more vigorous efforts to obtain a response (such as painful stimuli) are not warranted.

The priorities of BLS are:

- airway;
- breathing; and
- circulation.

Airway

The key to successful resuscitation is a clear airway. When an unconscious person is lying on his or her back, the lower jaw tends to drop which causes the tongue to fall to the back of the pharynx and occlude the airway. The problem is compounded by relaxation of soft palate tissues and the epiglottis. In addition, an unconscious person is unable to swallow or cough, and any foreign material in the mouth or pharynx can contribute to obstruction of the airway. Simply turning the person on his or her side, and supporting the jaw, can often prevent death. This often relieves the obstruction, and gravity assists any foreign material to drain from the mouth. Visible material or debris that could be blocking the airway can be actively removed by sweeping a gloved pointer finger around the mouth.

Airway management

Airway assessment and management can take place with the person lying on his or her side or back. In many instances, lying on the side is preferable for the reasons stated above. However, because many cardiac arrests result from ventricular defibrillation, it might be appropriate to manage a person on his her back to facilitate early defibrillation.

The steps involved in airway management include:

- *Clear the airway:* Remove loose-fitting dentures and any visible foreign material from the mouth. Allow fluids or vomitus to drain by turning the face slightly downwards.
- *Open the airway:* Tilt the head backwards and support the jaw. The head is tilted backwards by placing one hand on the forehead and

supporting the jaw at the point of the chin in such a way that there is no pressure on the soft tissues of the neck. This brings the jaw and tongue forwards, thus opening the airway. If it is suspected that the person has injured his or her neck or back, the head should not be moved; the jaw thrust method to open the airway should be used (see next).

- *Jaw thrust:* pressure is applied behind the angle of the jaw to thrust it forwards.

Recognition of airway obstruction

If the airway is partially or completely occluded, attempts to breathe result in:

- flaring of the nostrils;
- use of accessory muscles, evidenced by sucking in of the soft tissues of the neck and upper chest, indrawing of the chest, and outpushing of the abdomen;
- noisy and laboured respiratory efforts if the airway is partially obstructed, and no movement of air if completely obstructed; and
- increasing peripheral and central cyanosis, particularly if obstruction is complete.

Note: There might be no attempt to breathe at all.

Breathing

Once the airway is open, the unconscious person's breathing should be checked. With an ear placed over the person's nose and mouth:

- *look* for movement of the chest and abdomen;
- *listen* for the passage of air into and out of the mouth and nose; and
- *feel* for the escape of exhaled air on your face.

If breathing is *present*, leave the person on his or her side, ensuring that the airway remains open, and observe closely for any changes in condition.

If breathing is *absent*, turn the person on his or her back and begin expired air resuscitation (EAR) by giving five full breaths within 10 seconds and observing for the rise and fall of the chest.

If the chest does not rise and/or EAR is not effective:

- check the head tilt and jaw support technique in order to prevent an air leak; and
- ensure that the breaths delivered are full inflations.

Note: Distension of the stomach with air occurs if the breaths delivered

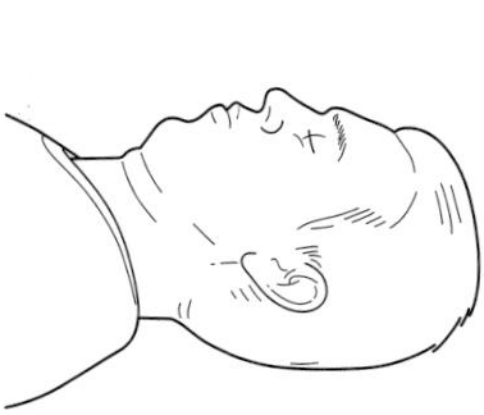

Blocked airway

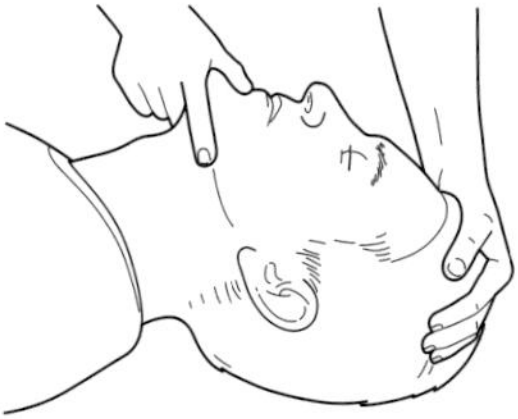

Backward head tilt
jaw support

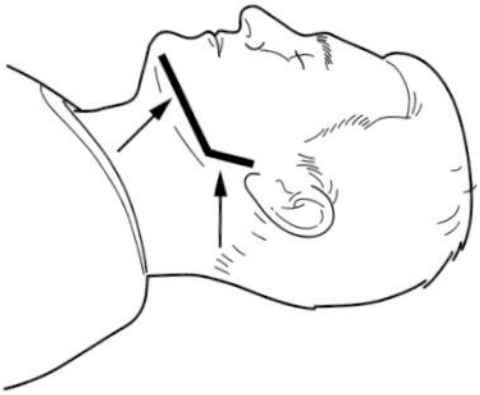

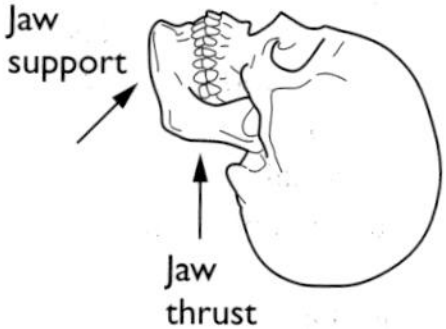

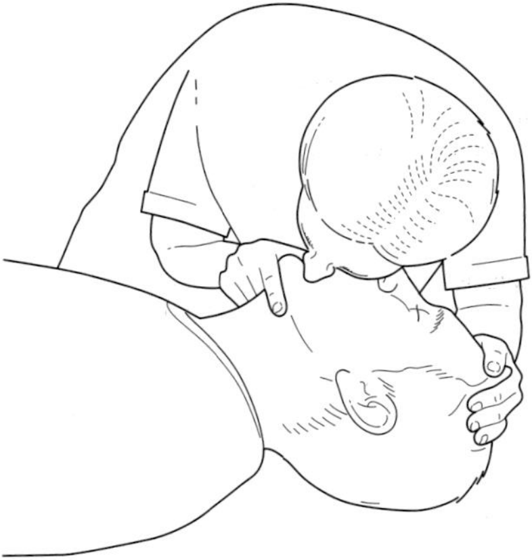

are too hard or are delivered when the airway is partially obstructed. This can precipitate regurgitation and vomiting, and can further compromise the airway.

Methods of EAR include mouth-to-mouth respiration, mouth-to-nose respiration, mouth-to-stoma respiration, and mouth-to-mask respiration.

Circulation

After delivering five full breaths, feel for the carotid pulse while maintaining maximum head tilt. If the pulse is *present*, continue EAR at a rate of 12–15 breaths per minute until breathing returns. Check for the continued presence of the carotid pulse every two minutes. If breathing is re-established, turn the person on his or her side and observe closely for airway, breathing, and circulation.

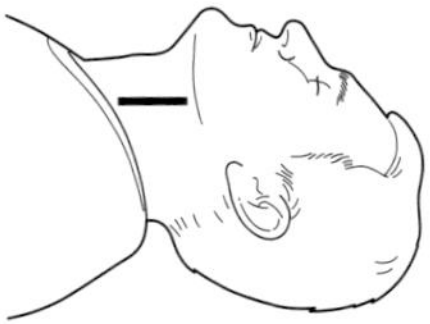

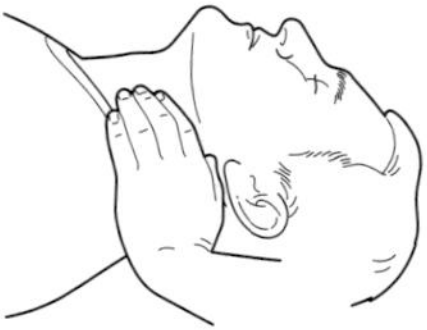

If the pulse is *absent*, a cardiac arrest has occurred, and cardiopulmonary resuscitation (CPR) should be initiated immediately, as follows.

- Ensure the person is on a firm flat surface.
- Begin external cardiac compression (ECC) by locating the middle of the lower half of the sternum:

The *caliper method* involves placing a finger at the upper and lower ends of the sternum. Locate the mid-sternum by extending the thumbs of each hand an equal distance to meet in the middle. Leaving the thumb of the upper hand in position, place the heel of the other hand against it and along the lower half of the sternum.

The *xiphisternal method* involves identifying the lower margin of the ribcage and moving the fingers up to the notch where the ribs meet at the lower end of the sternum. Place an index finger at the lower end of the sternum (just above the notch) and the heel of the other hand alongside the finger.

With either method, the end result is that the heel of one hand is lying on the long axis of the lower half of the sternum. The other hand is used to provide additional force, so that all pressure is exerted through the heel of the bottom hand. Fingers do not touch the chest. Shoulders should be vertically over the sternum, with the compressing arm straight.

Depth and rate of compression

The sternum should be compressed 4–5 cm (1Ω–2 inches) with each compression. The rate of compression is at least 60 times per minute. During ECC, the heel of the hand remains on the sternum.

Rate of compressions to inflations

With one operator, the ratio is 2 breaths to 15 compressions. For two operators the ratio is 1 breath to 5 compressions. Feel for the carotid pulse every 2 minutes.

CPR is continued until the person recovers, or until appropriate assistance arrives.

Correctly performed, CPR can re-establish cardiac function, or at least maintain an artificial circulation sufficient to preserve neurological function until personnel trained in ALS arrive at the scene.

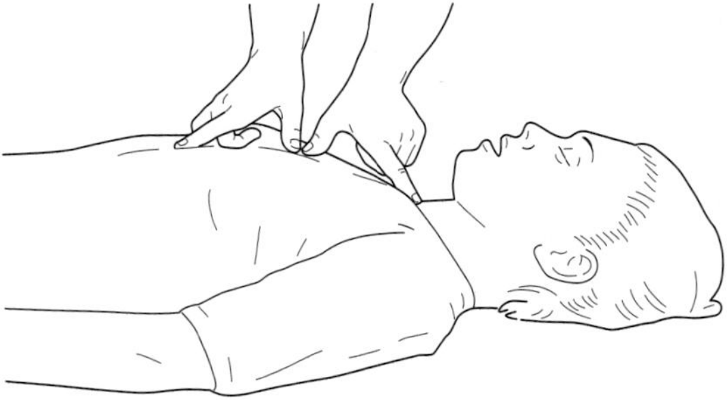

(a)

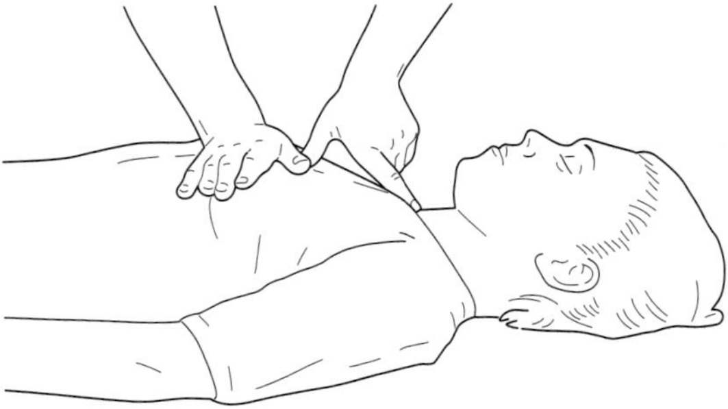

(b)

Flow chart of basic life support

COLLAPSE
Check response to verbal and tactile stimuli

CONSCIOUS
Make comfortable
Observe: Airway
Breathing
Circulation

UNCONSCIOUS
Turn victim on side
Turn face slightly downwards
Clear airway
Apply head tilt and jaw support/jaw thrust
Check for breathing

BREATHING
Leave on side in stable position
Observe: Airway
Breathing
Circulation

NOT BREATHING
Turn victim on back
Give 5 full inflations within 10 seconds
Check for carotid pulse

PULSE PRESENT
Continue EAR
Check carotid pulse and breathing after one minute and then at least every two minutes

PULSE ABSENT
Begin CPR (EAR & ECC)
Check carotid pulse and breathing after one minute and then at least every two minutes

EAR = Expired Air Resuscitation
ECC = External Cardiac Compression
CPR = Cardiopulmonary Resuscitation

(Australian Resuscitation Council, 2002).

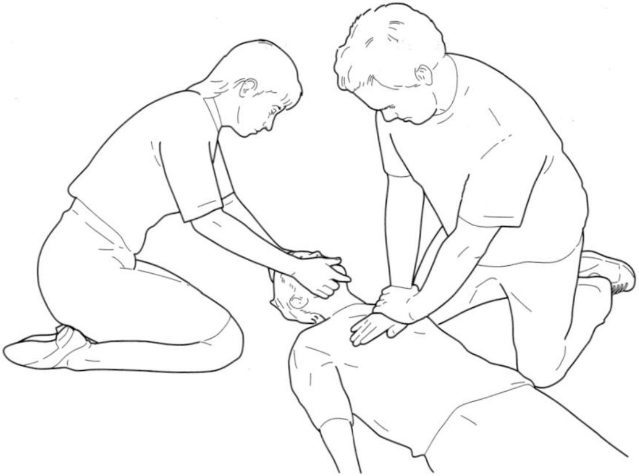

(c)

BLS for infants and children

BLS for infants (less than 1 year) and children (1–8 years) is essentially the same as for adults, with the following exceptions.

Airway

- Keep the head horizontal.
- Avoid over-extension of the head and neck when opening the airway, especially with infants.

Breathing

- *Infants*: Obtain a firm seal over the mouth and nose and deliver a volume that is less than for a child but enough to ensure that the chest rises. The ventilation rate is 20 puffs per minute.
- *Children*: As for adults, but the ventilation rate is 15–20/minute.

Circulation

- *Infants*: Using two fingers, compress the sternum below the mid-point. Depth of compression is approximately one-third of the depth of the chest at a rate of 100/minute.

- *Children*: For children between the ages of 1 and 8 years, use the heel of one hand to compress the sternum below the mid-point. For children older than 8 years perform compressions as for adults. For children 1 year and older the depth of compression is approximately one-third the depth of the chest at a rate of 100/minute.

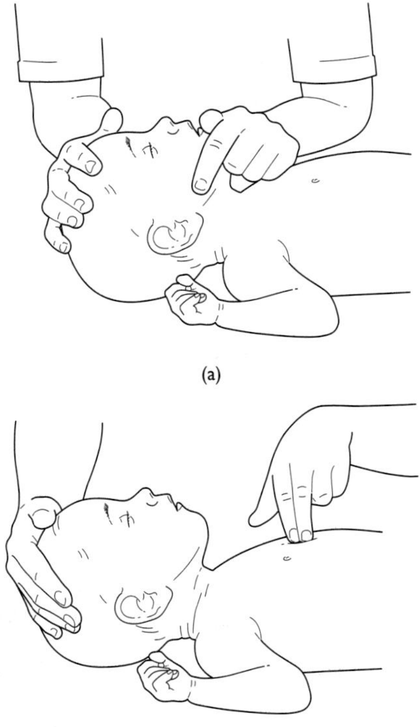

(a)

(b)

Circulation, assistance for infants

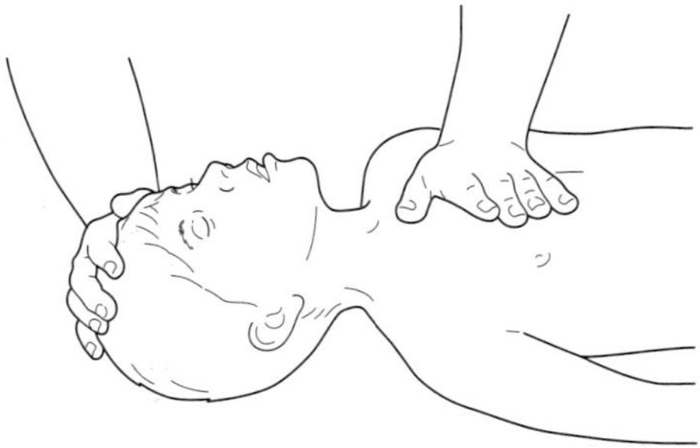

Circulation, assistance for children

Cardiopulmonary resuscitation management steps

Condition	*Breathing*	*Pulse*	*Management steps*
Conscious	Present	Present	Place patient in most comfortable position. Observe airway, breathing, and circulation (ABC).
Unconscious	Present	Present	Leave patient on side. Maintain a clear airway. Observe breathing and circulation.
Unconscious	Absent	Present	Turn victim on back. Commence expired air resuscitation (EAR) with 5 full inflations. Continue at about 15 breaths per minute. Check pulse after one minute, then at least every two minutes.
Unconscious	Absent	Absent	With victim on back give cardiopulmonary resuscitation (CPR). One rescuer: 2 inflations to 15 compressions. Two rescuers: 1 inflation to 5 compressions is also acceptable if the rescuers are highly skilled. Check pulse after 1 minute and then at least every 2 minutes.

Infants less than 1 year

Airway	*Breathing*	*Circulation*
Do not extend the neck; provide jaw support	Cover mouth and nose. Inflate enough to observe chest rise 20/minute.	2–3 fingers, just below mid-sternum. Compress one-third chest depth. Rate 100/minute

Children 1–8 years

Airway	*Breathing*	*Circulation*
Tilt head (more than infants, less than adults); provide jaw support.	Rate 15–20/minute	Heel of one hand just below mid-sternum.Compress one-third chest depth. Rate 100/minute

SOURCE: AUSTRALIAN RESUSCITATION COUNCIL, *POLICY STATEMENTS ON CARDIOPULMONARY RESUSCITATION*. ARC, MELBOURNE, 2002.

Appendix 7
Nutrition

Wendy Gray, Lecturer, Department of Family and Community Health, University of Sydney

The Australian dietary guidelines

1. Enjoy a wide variety of nutritious foods.
2. Eat plenty of breads and cereals (preferably wholegrain), vegetables (including legumes), and fruits.
3. Eat a diet low in fat and, in particular, low in saturated fat.
4. Maintain a healthy body weight by balancing physical activity and food intake.
5. If you drink alcohol, limit your intake.
6. Eat only moderate amounts of sugars and foods containing added sugars.
7. Choose low-salt foods and use salt sparingly.
8. Encourage and support breastfeeding.

The Healthy Diet Pyramid

The 12345+ Food and Nutrition Plan

Indulgences or extras: *No more than 2*

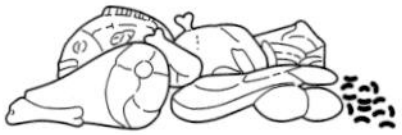

Meats & alternatives: *1 serve*

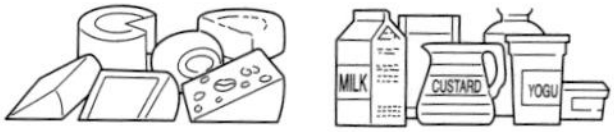

Milk & milk products: *2 serves*

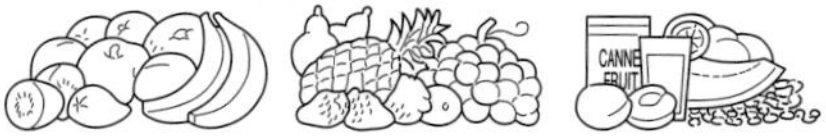

Fruits: *3 serves*

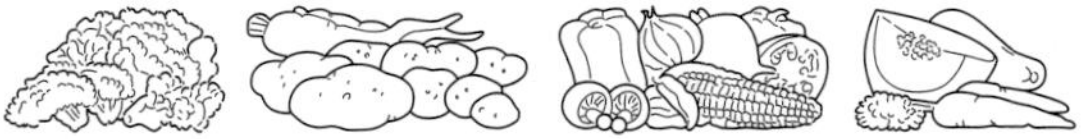

Vegetables: *4 serves*

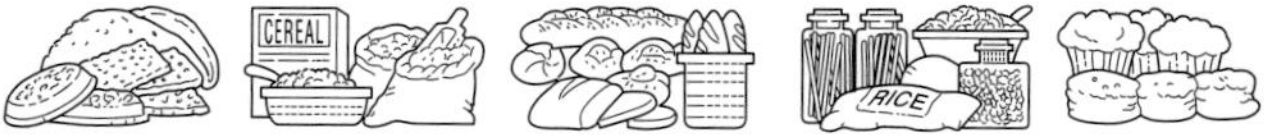

Breads & cereals: 5 serves

A Simple Guide to Healthy Eating and Weight Control

Reproduced from 12345+ Food and Nutrition Plan (Baghurst et. al., 1990) by permission of CSIRO and the Anti-Cancer Foundation of South Australia.

An average daily intake should include:
1 serve from the meats and alternatives group;
2 serves from the milk and milk products group;
3 serves from the fruit group;
4 serves from the vegetable group; and
5 *or more* serves from the wholegrain breads and cereals group.

Note: Each day, pregnant women and teenagers need one extra serve of both (i) milk and milk products; and (ii) meats and alternatives.

Energy balance

The body needs energy for growth, metabolism and activity. Individual energy needs depend on age, sex, size, body composition, activity level, nutritional status, and health.

Energy is provided by carbohydrates, fat, proteins, and alcohol. It is measured in either kilocalories (usually called 'Calories' with a capital 'C') or kilojoules.

- 1 Calorie (1 kilocalorie) = 4.184 kilojoules.
- 1 g of carbohydrate (sugar and starches) yields 4 Calories = 17 kilojoules.
- 1 g of fat yields 9 Calories = 38 kilojoules.
- 1 g of protein yields 4 Calories = 17 kilojoules.
- 1 g of alcohol yields 7 Calories = 29 kilojoules.

Dietary fats/oils have more than twice the energy of carbohydrates and protein. Dietary fat is more readily converted to, and stored as body fat, than are dietary carbohydrates and protein. It is recommended that no more than 30% of total kilojoules consumed should come from fat (and that saturated fat should constitute no more than 8–10 % of this).

Healthy weight range

The following table sets out desirable weights for men and women 18 years of age and older.

Height (cm)	*Healthy body weight range (kg)*
142	40–50
145	42–52
147	44–55

Height (cm)	*Healthy body weight range (kg)*
150	45–56
152	46–58
155	48–60
157	50–62
160	51–64
163	53–66
165	55–68
168	56–71
170	58–72
173	60–75
175	62–77
178	63–79
180	65–81
183	68–85

Notes:
(i) Height is without shoes
(ii) Weight is in light clothing without shoes

SOURCE: REPRODUCED WITH PERMISSION OF THE AUSTRALIAN NUTRITION FOUNDATION

Appendix 8

Immunisation

The Australian Standard Vaccination Schedule

The Australian Standard Vaccination Schedule (ASVS) shown below is the technical schedule recommended by the NHMRC. Over recent years a considerable variety of vaccines, which combine together various antigens, have become available in Australia. The ASVS is therefore based on antigens rather than on specific vaccines. The new immunization schedule (Table 1.) incorporates all vaccines recommended as 'best practice'. It should be noted that vaccines listed on the ASVS are not necessarily included for funding under the National Immunisation Program.

Table 1: Australian Standard Vaccination Schedule, 2003

AGE	*VACCINE*								
Birth	Hepatitis B[1]								
2 months	Hepatitis B[2,3]	DTP_a	Hib[1,2]	IPV			7vPCV[1]		
4 months	Hepatitis B[2,3]	DTP_a	Hib[1,2]	IPV			7vPCV[1]		
6 months	Hepatitis B[2]	DTP_a	Hib[1]	IPV			7vPCV[1]		
12 months	Hepatitis B[3]		Hib[1,2]		MMR			MenC	
18 months						VZV	23vPPV[1]		
2 years									
4 years		DTP_a		IPV	MMR				
10 - 13 years	Hepatitis B[4]					VZV[1]			
15 - 17 years		dTp_a						MenC[1]	
50 years and over		dT					23vPPV[2]		
65 years and over							23vPPV		Influenza (annual)

Note: Vaccines currently funded under the National Immunisation Program are shaded in Table 1. above.

Schedule key

Hepatitis B[1]	Monovalent hepatitis B vaccine
Hepatitis B[2]	Hepatitis B vaccine combinations with DTPa, 3 doses at 2, 4 and 6 months, in addition to the birth dose for a total of 4 doses.
Hepatitis B[3]	Hepatitis B vaccine in combination with Hib (PRP-OMP), 3 doses at 2, 4 and 12 months, in addition to the birth dose for a total of 4 doses.
Hepatitis B[4]	Hepatitis B vaccine for 10 to 13 year olds who have not received a primary course.
Hib[1]	PRP-T, HbOC (low risk populations).
Hib[2]	PRP-OMP (low risk or high risk populations).
7vPCV[1]	Access to free conjugate pneumococcal vaccine is provided to the following groups; all Aboriginal and Torres Strait Islanders children aged up to 2 years, Aboriginal children in central Australia aged up to 5 years, non-Indigenous children in central Australia aged up to 2 years, and all children under 5 years with medical risk factors that predispose them to high rates or high severity of pneumococcal infection.
23vPPV[1]	Pneumococcal polysaccharide vaccine (Aboriginal and Torres Strait Islander children only); this dose can be given between 18 months and 2 years of age (refer to State/Territory Public Health Units for recommended age for administration).
23vPPV[2]	National Indigenous Pneumococcal Program.
MenC[1]	Routine meningococcal C conjugate vaccine at 15 years of age for children who have not received vaccine at 12 months of age. Note that the Federal Government has announced that this program will be funded and will commence in early 2003.
VZV[1]	Vaccination only for children with a negative history of varicella disease or vaccination.

Notes:

- Aboriginal and Torres Strait Islander children receive 3 doses of PRP-OMP Hib vaccine.

- Non-Indigenous can receive 3 doses of PRP-OMP Hib vaccine or 4 doses of either PRP-T or HbOC Hib vaccine. (Mixing Hib schedules is not recommended. Infants starting with PRP-OMP should continue with PRP-OMP).
- Adolescent hepatitis B, meningococcal C conjugate and varicella vaccination is not required if a primary vaccination course has been given in early childhood.
- OPV is currently funded for the ASVS at 2, 4 and 6 months and 4 years of age. IPV is not currently funded.

Vaccine Key

Hepatitis B	Hepatitis B vaccine
DTPa	Diphtheria-tetanus-pertussis (acellular) infant/child formulation
dTpa	Adult formulation diphtheria-tetanus-pertussis (acellular) vaccine
Hib	*Haemophilus influenzae* type b (Hib) vaccine PRP-OMP, PRP-T, HbOC (as monovalent or in combination)
IPV	Inactivated Poliovirus Vaccine (in combination)
MMR	Measles, Mumps, Rubella vaccine
VZV	Varcella-zoster vaccine
7vPCV	Pneumococcal conjugate vaccine (7 valent)
23vPPV	Pneumococcal polysaccharide vaccine (23 valent)
MenC	Meningococcal C conjugate vaccine
Influenza	Influenza vaccine
dT	Adult diphtheria-tetanus vaccine

Copied with permission from Part I 8th Edition Australian Immunisation Schedule pp22-24. Full document available at http://immunise.health.gov.au/handbook.htm.

Appendix 9

Code of Ethics and Code of Professional Conduct for Nurses in Australia

In 1993 the Australian Nursing Council developed a Code of Ethics for Nurses in Australia and, in 1995, a Code of Professional Conduct. The Code of Ethics relates to the ideals of the profession and the moral values that nurses voluntarily accept, whereas the Code of Professional Conduct identifies the minimum requirements for practice in the profession. These two codes and the published practice standards for nursing in Australia provide a working framework for nursing practice.

Code of ethics for nurses in Australia

Nurses support and enable individuals, families, and groups to maintain, restore, or improve their health status, or to be cared for and comforted when deterioration of health has become irreversible. A traditional idea of nursing is concern for the care and nurture of human beings regardless of race, religion, status, age, gender, diagnosis, or any other criterion.

Nursing is based on the development of a helping relationship and the implementation and evaluation of therapeutic processes. Therapeutic processes include health promotion and education, counselling, nursing interventions, and the empowerment of individuals, families, or groups to exercise maximum choice in relation to their health care. Nurses provide care and support before and during birth and throughout life, and alleviate pain and suffering during the dying process.

The Code of Ethics has been developed for nursing in the Australian context and is relevant to all nurses working in Australia. The Code of Ethics outlines nursing's intentions in practice and is supported by policies and position statements from organisations representing nurses and nursing.

The Code of Ethics complements the International Council of Nurses (ICN) Code for Nurses (1973).

Thus, the purposes of this Code of Ethics are to:

- identify the fundamental moral commitments of the profession;
- provide nurses with a basis for professional and self-reflection and a guide to ethical practice; and
- indicate to the community the values that nurses hold.

Value statements

- Nurses respect the individual needs, values, and culture of persons in the provision of nursing care.
- Nurses respect the rights of persons to make informed choices in relation to their care.
- Nurses promote and uphold the provision of quality nursing care for all people.
- Nurses hold in confidence any information obtained in a professional capacity, and use professional judgment in sharing such information.
- Nurses respect the accountability and responsibility inherent in their roles.
- Nurses value the promotion of an ecological, social, and economic environment that supports and sustains health and wellbeing.

Code of professional conduct for nurses in Australia

Upon entering the practice of nursing each nurse accepts the responsibility and trust vested in the nursing profession and the corresponding obligation to adhere to the profession's standards of professional conduct. Nurses have a responsibility to the individual, society, and the profession to provide safe, competent nursing care which is responsive to individual, group, and community needs. The Code of Professional Conduct for Nurses in Australia is a set of national minimum standards for accountable professional nursing conduct.

Nursing is carried out in a variety of settings including clinical practice, education, administration, and research. All nurses are personally accountable for their practice in whatever setting the practice occurs. There are many factors outside the control of a nurse which can affect the practice setting and the care provided. These factors can and will be taken into consideration by professional bodies and/or courts when the nurse is called to account for the quality of nursing care given to patients/clients. This principle also applies in relation to access to appropriate educational programs for maintaining competence.

The purposes of the Code of Professional Conduct are to:

- inform the profession of the minimum standards for professional conduct;
- inform the public of the minimum standards for professional conduct; and,
- provide appropriate bodies with a basis for decisions regarding standards of professional conduct.

The Code of Professional Conduct states that each nurse will:

- provide safe and competent nursing care;
- uphold the agreed standards of the profession;
- practise in accordance with laws relevant to the nurse's area of practice;
- respect the dignity, culture, values, and beliefs of patients/clients and significant others in the provision of nursing care;
- promote and support the health, wellbeing, and informed decision-making of patients/clients in the provision of nursing care;
- promote and preserve the trust that is inherent in the privileged relationship between nurses and their patients/clients with respect to both their person and their property;
- treat as confidential personal information obtained in a professional capacity; and
- refrain from engaging in exploitation, misinformation, and misrepresentation with respect to healthcare products and nursing services.

Source: Australian Nursing Council 1993,1995, and 2000

Appendix 10
Aspects of Nursing and the Law

Rosemary Brooker

All areas of the law affect practising nurses. Two aspects of common law—negligence and assault—are briefly discussed below.

Professional negligence

'Negligence' is a tort, or civil wrong, that regulates the rights and responsibilities of one individual towards another. The concept has developed around the idea of a duty of care, or responsibility, and the harm that can result if an appropriate standard of care is not maintained.

Health professionals and healthcare institutions can become involved in legal actions if a patient, or client, suffers injury while in their care. However, not every injury that occurs to a patient is a result of negligence, and not all acts or omissions that result in injury are negligent. The law recognises that some injuries are a result of unforeseen circumstances that do not involve fault on behalf of healthcare professionals or institutions.

In an action for negligence, a plaintiff must establish, on the balance of probabilities, the following four elements, on a step-by-step basis:

1. The defendant (for example, a healthcare professional) must have owed the plaintiff (for example, a patient) a duty of care. In the nursing context, it is well established that such a duty of care is owed to patients and fellow employees. Inherent in the concept of a duty of care is the existence of an appropriate standard of care.
2. The defendant's conduct must have fallen below, or breached, the standard of care.
3. As a consequence of the breach of the standard of care, the plaintiff must have suffered some damage or harm. No compensation will be awarded if no harm was suffered, or if the harm did not arise as a direct consequence of the negligent act.

4. The damage or harm sustained must have been a reasonably foreseeable consequence of the negligent act.

In establishing a successful action for negligence all the above elements must be proved by the plaintiff. The action fails completely if one or more elements cannot be proven.

If a healthcare professional negligently injures a patient in the course and scope of his or her employment, the professional's employer might be held liable at law for the torts or wrongs of its employee. This is the doctrine of vicarious liability.

Consent

It is a well-established principle of law that every person has a right to determine what is done to his or her body. No one has the right to touch another intentionally without that person's consent, and to do so creates the possibility of a claim for assault or battery. The physical force does not have to be great and nor does damage have to result. However, an intention to carry out the non-consensual contact must be established.

The defence against an accusation of assault or battery is consent. Thus the agreement of the patient must be obtained before any physical treatment is given by a nurse. This agreement can be implied, given verbally, or given in writing. For such consent to be valid it must:

- be given freely and voluntarily;
- include information, in broad terms, regarding the nature of the procedure to be performed; and
- be given by a person with the legal capacity to do so.

The major exception to the above is in emergency situations, in which consent can be implied for life-saving treatments. However, evidence of a previously expressed refusal by the patient for such treatments might override the implied consent.

The law relating to consent for children and in emergency situations can vary in different state jurisdictions.

In addition to the above, various legislation has been enacted that affects nurses. Examples include the law relating to registration, working conditions, mental health, the administration of drugs, and refusal of treatment.

For more information regarding all the areas of law relating to nursing practice the reader is directed to a more detailed source. One such is: Forrester, K. & Griffiths, D. (2001), *Essentials of Law for Health Professionals*. Mosby, Sydney.

Appendix 11

Drug Calculations

1. Oral medications (tablets, capsules)

number required = dose required/stock strength

Example 1

Mr Smith has been ordered ranitidine 300 mg. The stock strength of the drug is 150 mg per tablet. How many tablets would you administer?

number required = dose required/stock strength
therefore, number required = 300 mg/150 mg/tab
that is, number required = 2 tablets

Example 2

A patient is ordered 0.25 mg of digoxin orally. The digoxin is available in tablets containing 125 mcg. How many tablets would you administer?

First, change both strengths to the same units: 0.25 mg = 250 mcg. Then apply the above formula:

number required = dose required/stock strength
therefore, number required = 250 mcg/125 mcg/tab
that is, number required = 2 tablets

2. Oral medications (liquids)

volume required = dose required/stock strength x volume

Example

A patient is ordered 750 mg of erythromycin orally. The stock suspension contains 250 mg/5 mL. Calculate the volume to be administered.

volume required = dose required/stock strength x volume
therefore, volume required = 750/250 x 5 mL
that is, volume required = 15 mL

3. Parenteral administration

volume required = dose required/stock strength x volume

Example 1

A patient is ordered 75 mg of pethidine for pain. The ampoule contains 100 mg in 2 mL. What volume would you administer?

volume required = dose required/stock strength x volume
therefore, volume required = 75/100 x 2 mL
that is, volume required = 1.5 mL

4. Calculation of infusion rates

Infusion rates

To determine intravenous infusion rates (mL/hr)

rate (mL/hr) = volume (mL)/time (hrs)

Example

A patient is to receive 1000 mL of normal saline over 8 hours. How many millilitres per hour should the pump be set at?

rate (mL/hr) = volume (mL)/time (hrs)
therefore, rate (mL/hr) = 1000 mL/8 hrs
that is, rate = 125 mL/hr

Drops per minute

To calculate the drops per minute:

drops per minute = volume (mL)/time (minutes) x drip factor (drops/mL)

Example 1

A patient is to receive 500 mL of normal saline over 6 hours (360 minutes). An IV set that delivers 20 drops per mL (that is, a drip factor of 20 drops/mL) will be used. Calculate the required drops per minute.

drops per minute = volume (mL)/time (minutes) x drip factor (drops/mL)
therefore, drops per minute = 500 mL/360 minutes x 20 drops/mL
that is, drops per minute = 27.7 drops/min

Example 2

An infant is ordered 150 mL of normal saline to run over 10 hours (600 minutes). The microdrip delivers 60 drops per mL (that is, a drip factor of 60 drops/mL). Calculate the required drip factor in drops per minute

drops per minute = volume (mL)/time (minutes) x drip factor (drops/mL)
therefore, drops per minute = 150 mL/600 minutes x 60 drops/mL
that is, drops per minute = 15 drops/min.

Appendix 12

Infection Control Guidelines

One of the main strategies for effective prevention of the transmission of infection from person to person within the healthcare setting is the development and implementation of infection control guidelines and policies. In 1996, the National Health and Medical Research Council (NH&MRC) and the Australian Council on AIDS Infection Control Working Party recommended that the terms 'standard precautions' and 'additional precautions' be adopted to define appropriate risk-minimisation work practices.

- *Standard precautions* are work practices required to achieve a basic level of infection control in healthcare setings; they are recommended for the management and care of all patients.
- *Additional precautions* are recommended for patients in healthcare settings known or suspected to be infected or colonised with disease agents that cause infections that might not be contained by standard precautions alone.

Standard precautions

Standard precautions are intended to prevent infection by the safe handling of:

- blood (including dried blood);
- other body fluids (excluding sweat);
- non-intact skin; and
- mucous membranes.

Examples of standard precautions are:

- aseptic technique;
- hand-washing before and after patient contact;
- use of protective equipment (such as gloves, impermeable gowns, plastic aprons, face masks, eye shields etc.);
- correct handling and disposal of sharps;

- appropriate cleaning and sterilising of equipment; and
- support services (such as cleaning services, laundry services, and food-hygiene services).

Special precautions should be applied to all people being treated with invasive procedures such as injections, catheterisation, cannulation, and intubation.

Special precautions must also be applied in the care of *all* people, regardless of their perceived or confirmed infection status, to protect healthcare workers from any possibility of contact with bloodborne pathogens.

Additional precautions

Additional precautions should be applied in a healthcare setting for patients known to be infected or colonised (or suspected of being infected or colonised) with infectious agents that might not be contained with standard precautions alone.

In these cases, infection could be transmitted by:

- airborne transmission of respiratory secretions (e.g., pulmonary tuberculosis, chickenpox, measles);
- droplet transmission of respiratory secretions (e.g., rubella, pertussis, influenza);
- contact with patients who might be disseminators of infectious agents of special concern (e.g. faecal contamination from carriers of vancomycin-resistant enterococci); or
- inherent resistance to standard sterilisation procedures or other disease-specific means of transmission in which standard precautions are not sufficient (e.g., patients with known or suspected Creutzfeldt-Jakob disease).

Additional precautions should be tailored to the particular infectious agent involved and to the mode of transmission. These might include one or more of the following:

- allocation of a single room with ensuite facilities;
- dedicated toilet (to prevent transmission of infections that are transmitted primarily by contact with faecal material, such as for patients with infectious diarrhoea or gastroenteritis caused by enteric bacteria or viruses);
- cohorting (room-sharing by people with the same infection);
- special ventilation requirements (e.g., monitored negative air pressure in relation to surrounding areas);

- additional use of personal protective equipment (e.g., well-fitting masks worn by staff members);
- rostering of immune staff members to care for certain classes of infectious patients (e.g., chickenpox);
- dedicated patient equipment; and
- restricted movement of both patients and staff memebrs.

An outline of the application of additional precautions for infections with respiratory (airborne or droplet) transmission or contact transmission is shown in the table (page 520).

Outline of requirements for specified categories of additional precautions

Requirement	*Airborne transmission*	*Droplet transmission*	*Contact transmission*
Gloves	Nil	Nil	For all manual contact with patient, associated devices and immediate environmental surfaces
Impermeable apron or gown	Nil	Nil	When staff clothing is in substantial contact with the patient, items in contact with the patient, and their immediate environment
Respirator or mask	P2 particulate respirator for tuberculosis only. All others, surgical mask.	Surgical mask (fluid repellent, paper filter mask used in surgical procedures)	Protect face if splash likely
Goggles/face-shields	Protect face if splash likely	Protect face if splash likely	Protect face if splash likely
Special handling of equipment	As per standard precautions	As per standard precautions	Single use or reprocess before reuse on next patient (includes all equipment in contact with patient)

Outline of requirements for specified categories of additional precautions (cont'd)

Requirement	*Airborne transmission*	*Droplet transmission*	*Contact transmission*
Single room	Single room or cohort patients with same. infection; door closed	Single room or cohort patients with same infection; door closed.	If possible, or cohort with patient with the same infection (e.g., methicillin-resistant Staphylococcus aureus)
Negative pressure	Essential for pulmonary TB	No	No
Transport of patients	Surgical mask for patient; notify area receiving patient	Surgical mask for patient; notify area receiving patient	Notify area receiving patient
Other	Encourage patients to cover nose and mouth when coughing or sneezing and to wash hands after blowing nose. Provide one metre of separation between patients in ward accommodation	Provide one metre of separation between patients in ward accommodation	Remove gloves and gown, and wash hands before leaving patient's room

Source: NH&MRC Guidelines for Infection Control <www.health.gov.au/pubhlth/strateg/communic/review>

Appendix 13

Useful Addresses

Australian Nursing Council

First Floor
20 Challis Street
Dickson ACT 2602
Postal address:
PO Box 873
Dickson ACT 2602
Ph: +61 2 6257 7960
Fax: +61 2 6257 7955
Email: anc@anc.org.au;
overseas@anc.org.au
Web: http://www.anci.org.au

Australian Nursing Federation

Head Office

Unit 3, 28 Eyre Street,
Kingston ACT 2604
Ph: (02) 6232 6533
Fax. (02) 6232 6610
Email: enquiries@anf.org.au
Web: www.anf.org.au

New South Wales

New South Wales Nurses Association
43 Australia St
Camperdown NSW 2050
Postal Address:
PO Box 40
Camperdown NSW 1450
Ph: 1300 367 962 (freecall)
Email: gensec@nswnurses.asn.au
Web: www.nswnurses.asn.au

Northern Territory

Unit 6/5 Tiwi Gardens Rd,
Tiwi NT 0810
Postal Address:
PO Box 42533
Casuarina NT 0811
Ph: (08) 8945 7589
Fax: (08) 8945 4171
Email: ntanf@octa4.net.au

Queensland

Queensland Nurses Union
Main Office
56 Boundary Street
West End, QLD 4101
Postal Address:
GPO Box 1289
Brisbane, QLD 4001
Ph: (07) 3840 1444
Toll Free 1800 177 273
Fax: (07) 3844 9387
Email: qnu@qnu.org.au
Web: www.qnu.org.au

South Australia

18 Dequetteville Tce,
Kent Town, SA 5067
Postal address (free postage):
Reply Paid 861
ANF (SA Branch)
PO Box 861
Kent town, SA 5071
Ph: (08) 8363 1948
Toll Free 1800 809 642
Fax: (08) 8363 1672
Web: www.sa.anf.org.au

Tasmania

Hobart Office:
182 Macquarie Street,
Hobart, TAS 7000
Tel: (03) 6223 6777
Freecall: 1800 001 241
Fax: 61 3 6224 0229
Launceston Office:
76 York Street,
Launceston, TAS 7250
Tel: (03) 6334 1411
Email: enquiries@anftas.org
Web: www.anftas.org

Victoria

Head Office:
540 Elizabeth Street,
Melbourne, VIC 3000
Postal Address:
Box 12600,
A'Beckett Street PO,
Melbourne VIC 8006
Ph: (03) 9275 9333
Fax. (03) 9275 9344
Email: records@vic.anf.org.au
Web: www.anfvic.asn.au

Western Australia

260 Pier Street,
Perth WA 6000
Postal Address:
PO Box 8240
Perth Business Centre 6849
Ph: (08) 9218 9444
Fax: (08) 9218 9455
Toll free: 1800 199 145
Email: anf@anfwa.asn.au
Web: www.anfwa.asn.au

International Council of Nurses

International Council of Nurses
3, Place Jean Marteau
1201 - Geneva
Switzerland
Ph: 41-22-908-01-00
Fax: 41-22-908-01-01
Email: icn@icn.ch
Web: www.icn.ch

Nurse Registration Authorities

Australian Capital Territory

Nurses Board of the Australian Capital Territory
PO Box 976
Civic Square ACT 2608
Ph: (02) 6205 1599
Fax: (02) 6205 1602
Web: www.nursesboard.act.gov.au

New South Wales

Nurses Registration Board of New South Wales
Postal address:
PO Box K599
Haymarket, Sydney
NSW 1238
Office address : Level 2
28–36 Foveaux Street
Surrey Hills, NSW 2010
Ph: (02) 9219 0222 or 1800 241 220
Fax: (02) 9281 2030
Email: nursesreg@doh.health.nsw.gov.au
Web: www.nursesreg.nsw.gov.au

New Zealand

The Nursing Council of New Zealand
Postal address:
PO Box 9644
Wellington
New Zealand
Ph: +64 4 385 9589
Fax: +64 4 801 8502
Email: nzreg@nursingcouncil.org.nz; oseas@nursingcouncil.org.nz
Web: <www.nursingcouncil.org.nz>

Northern Territory

Nurses Board of the Northern Territory
GPO Box 4221
Darwin NT 0801
Ph: (08) 8999 4157
Fax: (08) 8999 4196

Queensland
Queensland Nursing Council
GPO Box 2928
Brisbane QLD 4001
Office address:
Level 14, 201 Charlotte Street,
Brisbane QLD 4000
Ph: (07) 3223 5111 or 1300 139993
Fax: (07) 3223 5115
Email: general@qnc.qld.gov.au
Web: www.qnc.qld.gov.au

South Australia
Nurses Board of South Australia
PO Box 7176
Adelaide SA 5000
Ph: (08) 8223 9700
Fax: (08) 8223 9717
Email:
ceo-registrar@nursesboard.sa.gov.au

Tasmania
Nursing Board of Tasmania
PO Box 847
Sandy Bay TAS 7006
Ph: (03) 6224 3991
Fax: (03) 6224 3995
Email:
NBT@nursingboardtas.com.au

Victoria
Nurses Board of Victoria
GPO Box 4932
Melbourne VIC 3001
Ph: (03) 8635 1200
Fax: (03) 8635 1248

Western Australia
Nurses Board of Western Australia
Locked Bag 6
East Perth WA 6892
Ph: (08) 9421 1100
Fax: (08) 9421 1022
Email: info@nbwa.org.au

National Nursing Organisations (NNOs)
Web: <www.anf.org.au/nno>
The NNOs are various organisations that represent the nursing profession. The website contains a directory and links to member NNOs.

New South Wales
New South Wales College of Nursing
Locked Bag 3030
Burwood NSW 1805
Ph: (02) 9745 7500
Freecall: 1800 2655343
Fax: (02) 9745 7502
Web: www.nursing.aust.edu.au

New Zealand
New Zealand Nurses Organisation
National Office
6th Floor Westbrook House
181-183 Willis Street
PO Box 2128
Wellington
Tel: 04 931 6700
Fax: 04 382 9993
Email: nurses@nzno.org.nz
Web: www.nzno.org.nz

Royal College of Nursing, Australia (RCNA)
1 Napier Close
Deakin ACT 2600
PO Box 219
Deakin West ACT 2600
Ph: + 61 2 6282 5633
Freecall: 1800 061 660
Fax: + 61 2 6282 3565
Email: canberra@rcna.org.au
Web: www.rcna.org.au

Congress of Aboriginal & Torres Strait Island Nurses (CATSIN)
Web: www.indiginet.com.au/catsin

Physiotherapy

Australian Physiotherapy Association

National

Level 3, 201 Fitzroy Street
St. Kilda, Melbourne, VIC 3182
Ph: (03) 9534 9400
Fax: (03) 9534 9199
Email:
national.office@physiotherapy.asn.au
Web: www.physiotherapy.asn.au

Australian Capital Territory

Suite 10/1st Floor,
16 National Circuit,
Barton ACT 2600
Ph: 1300 306 622
Fax: (02) 6273 4728
Email:
act.branch@physiotherapy.asn.au

New South Wales

Unit 5, 77 Parramatta Rd,
Silverwater NSW 2141
Ph: (02) 8748 1555
Fax: (02) 9647 2244
Email:
nsw.branch@physiotherapy.asn.au

Northern Territory

PO Box 4602
Darwin NT 0801
Ph: 1300 306 622
Fax: (07) 3391 7283
Email:
nt.branch@physiotherapy.asn.au

Queensland

24 Logan Road
Woolloongabba QLD 4102
Ph: (07) 3391 7100
Fax: (07) 3391 7283
Email:
qld.branch@physiotherapy.asn.au

South Australia

8/15 Fullarton Road
Kent Town SA 5067
Ph: 1300 306 622
Fax: (08) 8362 2223
Email:
sa.branch@physiotherapy.asn.au

Tasmania

286 Macquarie Street
South Hobart TAS 7004
Ph: 1300 306 622
Fax: (03) 6224 9500
Email:
tas.branch@physiotherapy.asn.au

Victoria

6/651 Victoria Street
Abbotsford VIC 3067
Ph: (03) 9429 1799
Fax: (03) 9429 1844
Email:
vic.branch@physiotherapy.asn.au

Western Australia

Hampden House
174 Hampden Road,
Nedlands WA 6009
Ph: (08) 9389 9211
Fax: (08) 9389 9221
Email:
wa.branch@physiotherapy.asn.au

Chiropractic

National

Chiropractors Association of Australia
Web: www.chiropractors.asn.au

Australian Capital Territory

PO Box 100
Curtin ACT 2605
Phone: (02) 6281 6177

New South Wales
PO Box 4118, Penrith Plaza NSW 2750
5/148 Station Road, Penrith NSW 2750
Ph: (02) 4722 6811
Fax: (02) 4722 6810
Email: caanswAzip.com.au

Northern Territory
91 Dickward Drive
Nightcliff NT 0810
Phone: (08) 8985 3144
Fax: (08) 8948 2269
Email: flowersphil@hotmail.com

Queensland
Comsec Centre
433 Logan Road
Stones Corner QLD 4120
91 Dickward Drive
Phone: (07) 3394 8334
Fax: (07) 3847 5495
Email: caa@powerup.com.au

South Australia
GPO Box 2407
Adelaide SA 5001
Phone: (08) 8377 3279
Fax: (08) 8377 0215
Email: butters@senet.com.au

Tasmania
63 Main Road
Huonville TAS 7109
Phone: (03) 6264 1037
Fax: (03) 6264 1012
Email: jlemon@netspace.net.au

Victoria
319 Victoria Street (PO Box 336)
Brunswick VIC 3056
Phone: 03 9387 9377
Fax: 03 9380 2675
Email: caavic@clari.net.au

Western Australia
Suite 1, 1 Charles Street
South Perth WA 6151
Phone: (08) 9367 3177
Fax: (08) 9367 3577
Email: caawa@tower.net.au

Pharmacists

National
Society of Hospital Pharmacists of Australia
Web: www.shpa.org.au

Australian Capital Territory
Pharmacy Department
The Canberra Hospital
PO Box 11
Woden ACT 2606

New South Wales
PO Box M48
Missenden Road Post Office
Camperdown NSW 2050

Queensland
PO Box 761,
Fortitude Valley QLD 4006

South Australia and Northern Territory
Pharmacy Department
Repatriation General Hospital
Daw Park SA 5041

Tasmania
GPO Box 106,
Hobart TAS 7001

Victoria
GPO Box 1233L,
Melbourne VIC 3001

Western Australia
GPO Box K814
Perth WA 6847

Occupational Therapy

National

Australian Association of Occupational Therapists
OT Australia National Office
6 Spring St
Fitzroy VIC 3065
Ph: +61 3 9416 1021
Fax: +61 3 9416 1421
Email: info@ausot.com.au
Web: www.ausot.com.au

Australian Capital Territory

PO Box 803
Mawson ACT 2607
Ph: 0419 429 889
Email: jlwot@bigpond.com

New South Wales

PO Box 142
Ryde NSW 2112
Ph: +61 2 9808 1822
Fax: +61 2 9807 1609
Email: info@otausnsw.org.au
Web: www.otausnsw.org.au

Northern Territory

PO Box 41479
Casuarina NT 0811
Ph: +61 8 8945 0044
Fax: +61 8 8945 6756
Email: darwinot@octa4.net.au

Queensland

388 Cavendish Road
Coorparoo QLD 4151
Ph: +61 7 3397 6744
Fax: +61 7 3397 6599
Email: info@otqld.org.au
Web: www.otqld.org.au

South Australia

17 Bagot Street
North Adelaide SA 5006
Ph: +61 8 8239 1422
Fax: +61 8 8239 0244
Email: otsa@picknowl.com.au
Web: http://homepages.picknowl.com.au/otsa

Tasmania

PO Box 3047
Launceston TAS 7250
Ph & fax: +61 3 6331 9791
Email: carol@ilctas.asn.au

Victoria

PO Box 1286
North Fitzroy VIC 3068
Ph: +61 3 9481 6866
Fax: +61 3 9481 6844
Email: info@otausvic.com.au
Web: www.otausvic.com.au

Western Australia

4A 266 Hay Street
Subiaco WA 6008
Ph: +61 8 9388 1490
Fax: +61 8 9388 1492
Email: info@otauswa.com.au
Web: www.otauswa.com.au

Speech Pathology

National

Speech Pathology Australia
2nd Floor, 11–19 Bank Place
Melbourne VIC 3000
Ph: 03 9642 4899
Fax: 03 9642 4922
Email: office@speechpathologyaustralia.org.au
Web: www.speechpathologyaustralia.org.au

Australian Capital Territory

GPO Box 1793
Civic ACT 2601

New South Wales

PO Box 150
Concord NSW 2137
Ph: 02 9743 0013
Fax: 02 9743 0014
Email: sppathnsw@email.cs.nsw.gov.au

Northern Territory

PO Box 41328
Casuarina NT 0811

Queensland
c/o The Glenleighden School
Cubberla Street
Fig Tree Pocket QLD 4069
Ph: 07 3378 1166
Fax: 07 3378 1166
Email: sppathqld@bigpond.com

South Australia
42 Lorraine Avenue
Lockleys SA 5032
Ph: 08 8354 4738
Fax: 08 8354 3077

Tasmania
PO Box 355
Moonah TAS 7009

Victoria
c/o National Office
2nd Floor, 11–19 Bank Place
Melbourne VIC 3000
Ph: 03 9642 4899
Fax: 03 9642 4922
Email:
office@speechpathologyaustralia.org.au

Western Australia
1/37 Baldwin Street
Como WA 6152
Ph: 08 9450 8281
Fax: 08 9450 8281
Email:
sppathwa@optusnet.com.au